AF682112

Diagnostic Neuropathology

DIAGNOSTIC PATHOLOGY

1. *Diagnostic Neuropathology*, Harry V. Vinters, Michael A. Farrell, Paul S. Mischel, and Karl H. Anders

ADDITIONAL VOLUMES IN PREPARATION

Diagnostic Pulmonary Pathology, edited by Phillip Cagle

Diagnostic Neuropathology

HARRY V. VINTERS
UCLA School of Medicine
Los Angeles, California

MICHAEL A. FARRELL
Beaumont Hospital
Dublin, Ireland

PAUL S. MISCHEL
UCLA School of Medicine
Los Angeles, California

KARL H. ANDERS
Kaiser-Permanente Medical Center
Woodland Hills, California

MARCEL DEKKER, INC. NEW YORK • BASEL • HONG KONG

Drawings by Ms. Toni B. King.

ISBN: 0-8247-9888-0

The publisher offers discounts on this book when ordered in bulk quantities. For more information, write to Special Sales/Professional Marketing at the address below.

This book is printed on acid-free paper.

Copyright © 1998 by Marcel Dekker, Inc. All Rights Reserved.

Neither this book nor any part may be reproduced or transmitted in any form or by any means, electronic or mechanical, including photocopying, microfilming, and recording, or by any information storage and retrieval system, without permission in writing from the publisher.

Marcel Dekker, Inc.
270 Madison Avenue, New York, New York 10016
http://www.dekker.com

Current printing (last digit):
10 9 8 7 6 5 4 3 2 1

Printed in the United States of America

To John C. E. Kaufmann,
Henry J. M. Barnett, and
Charles G. Drake,
"masters of the nervous system"

Preface

This book is intended to be used as a "primer," rather than as an encyclopedic reference work, on the subject of neuropathology. In no way does it try to substitute for the standard (and widely used) textbooks of neuropathology that authors themselves frequently consult to come to grips with difficult cases, or the numerous outstanding atlases of neuropathology available to interested students of the discipline. It reflects the unavoidable biases, choice of emphasis, and experience of the authors—among whom two have been engaged in the practice of neuropathology in Canada, the United States, and Ireland for several years, one has had an ongoing interest in neuropathology in the context of a busy general pathology experience, and one has recently completed training with a special interest in the molecular and cellular biology of developmental disorders. We hope this results in a healthy variety of perspectives on the diseases described and on the nervous system's unique response to "insults." The entities discussed do not constitute an exhaustive list of neuropathological conditions, although we have tried to give a flavor of *all* major disease entities likely to be encountered in routine neuropathological practice. The bibliography is highly selective and reflects recent literature and key review or opinion/viewpoint/consensus articles, many of which inevitably have their *own* biases.

Throughout, we have emphasized concepts of neuropathogenesis that encompass many entities. The diagrams by Ms. King are derived from our desire to place disease mechanisms in an easily understandable conceptual framework that will "demystify" neuropathology for those exploring it for the first time. Research in many of the areas discussed (neurodegenerative diseases, developmental neuropathology, metabolic abnormalities) moves forward so rapidly that a book such as this is virtually outdated even as the manuscript is submitted to the publisher. With all these caveats in mind, we hope that the text and illustrations combine to provide selective, practical insights into a field that all of us view as a dynamic and exciting one—indeed, a discipline that is perhaps uniquely poised to apply the tools of modern molecular and cellular neurobiology to understanding how and why diseases afflict the central and/or peripheral nervous system.

ACKNOWLEDGMENTS

The individuals who have either contributed directly to the preparation of this book or facilitated its completion are legion. Among the most important are the technologists, who daily prepare materials (routine, special, and immunohistochemical stains and electron microscopy specimens), without which our work would be impossible; many of their samples have become the substrate for illustrative materials in this volume. Key among these technologists are Alex Brooks, Yan Cheng, Laurel Reed, Mari-Anne Akers, Diana Lenard Secor, Olivia Droogan, and Maureen Burke. Carol Appleton provided invaluable expertise in the preparation of illustrations. Annetta Pierro assisted with many editorial tasks. We are grateful to our colleagues in neuropathology, who have often provided helpful illustrative material or assistance with clinical tasks when chapter deadlines have loomed—particularly to Drs. M. Anthony Verity, Jeffery Twiss, Cynthia Welsh, and Francesca Brett. We appreciate the intellectual inquisitiveness and dedication of our trainees and the encouragement and scholarship of our clinical colleagues in neurology, neurosurgery, and neuroradiology. The authors' research endeavors throughout manuscript preparation were generously supported by the National Institutes of Health and a Pfizer New Faculty Scholar Award.

Parts of the book were finalized during the tenure by one of us of a Visiting/Rotary Professorship in Neurology at the Leiden University Medical Center in the Netherlands, a productive, six-month visit made extraordinarily pleasant and rewarding by many, especially Drs. Marion Maat, Remco Natté, Sjoerd van Duinen, Joost Haan, and Raymund Roos.

Family members and friends all showed remarkable patience when work on this book kept us from other activities. Special thanks to Sandra, Katie, and

Edward for their forbearance during time spent working on the book, and to Sylvia, Bryan, and Evan for their patience and loving support.

All of the authors have enjoyed tremendously many years of friendship, which has taken the form of both collegial stimulation and social interaction. We are delighted to have completed this project with those bonds intact—and perhaps even stronger than they have ever been!

Harry V. Vinters
Michael A. Farrell
Paul S. Mischel
Karl H. Anders

Contents

Preface *v*

1. Basic Neurobiology and Cellular Responses in Nervous System Diseases **1**
2. Anoxic-Ischemic Change and Cerebrovascular Disease **51**
3. Craniocerebral and Spinal Trauma **147**
4. Infections **173**
5. Diseases of White Matter **261**
6. Neoplasms **295**
7. Developmental and Pediatric Neuropathology **391**
8. Neurodegenerative Diseases **453**
9. Metabolic Abnormalities **509**
10. Muscle and Nerve Disease **569**

Index *647*

Diagnostic Neuropathology

1

Basic Neurobiology and Cellular Responses in Nervous System Diseases

I. INTRODUCTION

To the student of neuropathology, the complexity of the nervous system and its pathological responses may seem overwhelming. It has a highly specialized anatomy, and many of its basic cellular responses are unique. It is our hope that by presenting a systematic approach to the cellular components of the nervous system and their basic responses to injury, the inherent order, elegance, and clarity of neuropathology can be appreciated. Following a brief overview of nervous system embryology, we will describe the basic cellular components of the central and peripheral nervous systems (CNS and PNS) and discuss their characteristic responses to injury.

II. EMBRYOLOGY

The CNS and PNS both derive from inductive events occurring early in embryogenesis. Early in the third week of intrauterine gestation, a localized thickening referred to as the neural plate arises in the ectoderm near the developing notochord. A longitudinal groove develops within this plate (neural grove), with paired folds (neural folds) along each side of the groove. These folds fuse, giving rise to the neural tube (Fig. 1). The lumen of the neural tube develops into the ventricular system, while its cellular lining, a layer of primitive pseudostratified neuroepithelium, gives rise to the component cells of the CNS: neurons, astrocytes, oligodendrocytes, and ependymal cells (Fig. 2).

Neurons, astrocytes, and oligodendrocytes migrate to appropriate positions within the developing CNS to form the specific structures of the brain and spinal cord. (The topic of cell migration within the developing nervous system is complex; this discussed further in Chap. 7). After the migrating cells have left the germinal zone, the remaining progenitor cells differentiate into ependymal cells, which continue to line the ventricular cavities throughout adult life. The leptomeninges, which cover the external surface of the CNS, arise primarily from overlying ectoderm, although their exact developmental origin is still in question.

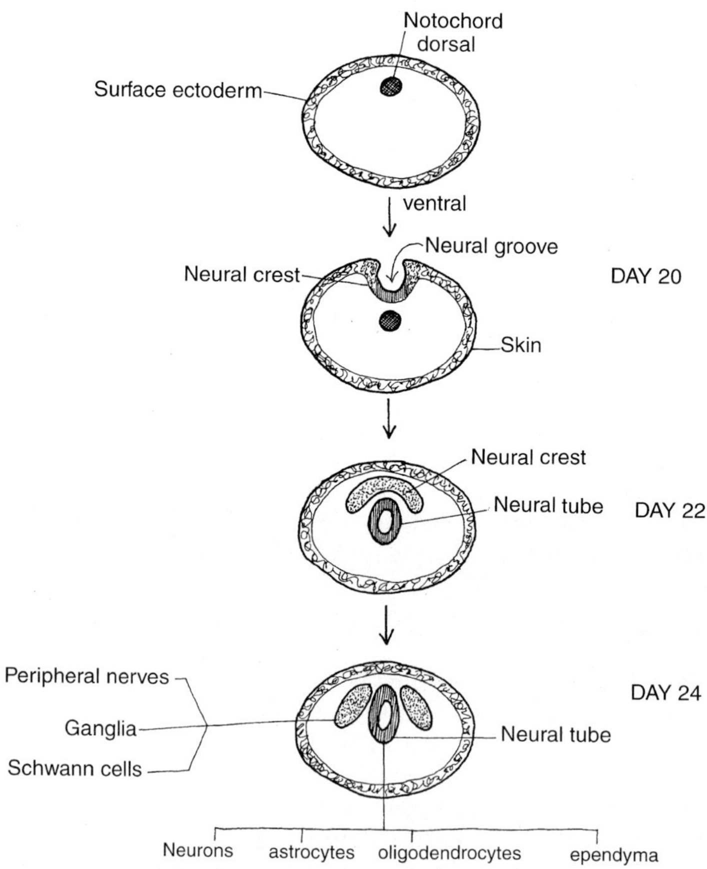

Figure 1 Schematic representation of formation of the neural tube.

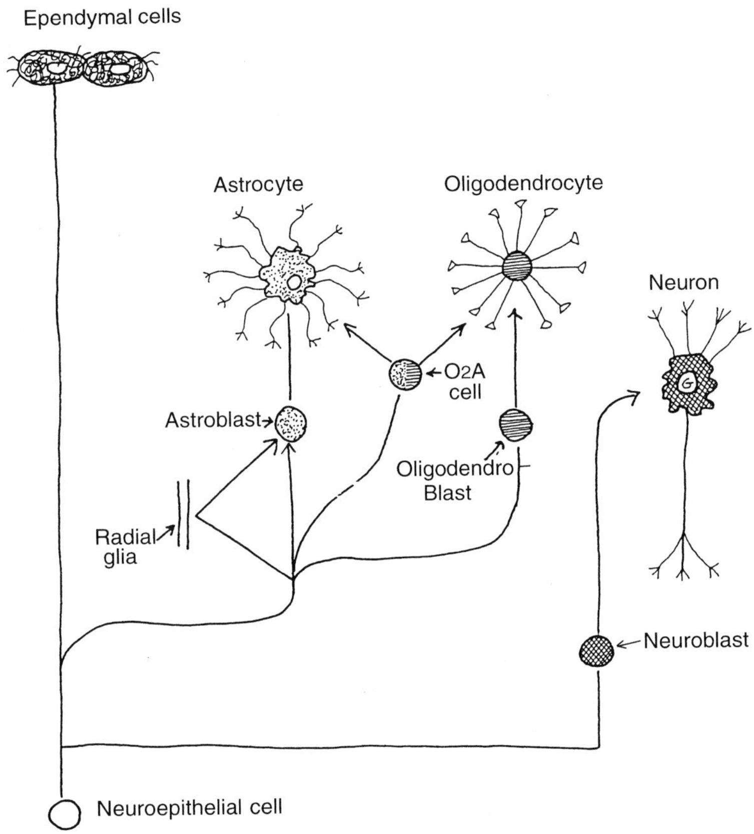

Figure 2 Schematic diagram illustrating cell lineage within the CNS.

The PNS develops from an aggregation of cells originating in the neural fold, which form the neural crest (Fig. 1). This aggregate of primitive cells, which lies between the neural tube and the surface ectoderm, gives rise to the neurons of cranial, spinal, and autonomic nerves and their ganglia, as well as the secretory cells of the adrenal medulla. Schwann cells, also neural crest-derived, eventually become associated with these peripheral nerves, and subsequently come to myelinate them. A host of other cells such as melanocytes are also derived from neural crest precursors.

III. CELLULAR ANATOMY OF THE CNS-NEURONS

Histologically, the CNS (brain and spinal cord) consists of neurons, glia (astrocytes, oligodendrocytes, ependymal cells, microglia), choroid plexus and parenchymal blood vessels. The CNS is covered by the leptomeninges and dura.

A. Neurons: Microscopic Anatomy

Neurons are the primary distinctive cells of the nervous system and are responsible for the propagation of electrical impulses. Their complex interrelationships account for the unique functional abilities of the nervous system. A neuron is composed of three main parts: 1. a cell body; 2. an axon; and 3. a dendrite. The cell bodies of neurons vary considerably in size and shape depending on their type and function. This is clearly illustrated within the cerebellum, where neurons range in shape and size from large Purkinje cells to small round neurons of the internal granule cell layer (Fig. 3). Typically, neuronal cell bodies have a polygonal shape with abundant cytoplasm and a central nucleus with a prominent single nucleolus, though these characteristic features are *not* seen in the small round neurons of the internal granule cell layer of the cerebellum or the dentate gyrus of the hippocampal formation. The cytoplasm, particularly in larger neurons, contains abundant basophilic material known as Nissl substance, which merely reflects the presence of plentiful rough endoplasmic reticulum (RER).

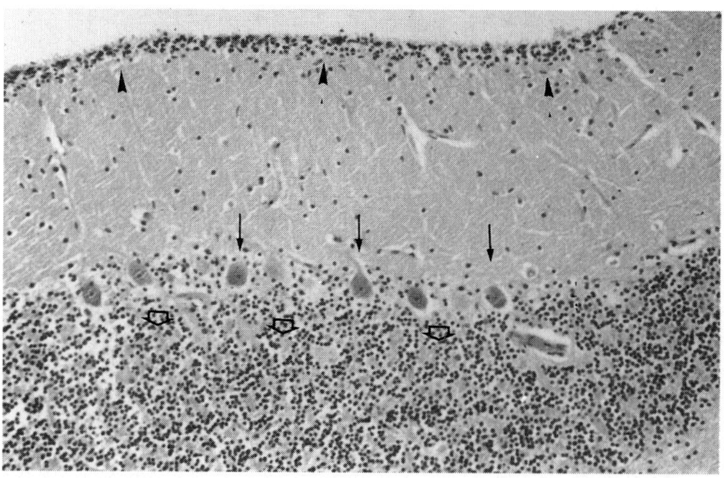

Figure 3 Neurons of the cerebellar cortex. Histologic section of the cerebellar cortex showing the range of neuron cell bodies present. Large Purkinje neurons (arrows) are seen, as are abundant small round neurons of the internal granule cell layer (open arrows). The presence of small round granule neurons on the surface (external granule cell layer) (arrowheads) indicates that this section was from a child $<$ 18 months old.

Axons and dendrites vary considerably from region to region and from neuron to neuron. Motor neurons and sensory neurons tend to have long axons while those of interneurons are quite short. The caliber of the axon and its degree of myelination vary considerably depending on the type and function of the neuron. Some authors classify neurons roughly based on their axon type and cell body size, which are usually correlated. Golgi type I neurons are large neurons with myelinated axons which extend to distant targets (e.g., motor neurons of the anterior horn of the spinal cord); Golgi type II neurons have small cell bodies and short unmyelinated axons, and serve as local interneurons (e.g., internal granule neurons of the cerebellum).

Dendrites form a highly branched tree (usually on the opposite pole of the cell body from the axon) which provides abundant surface area for synaptic contact with other neurons. These dendritic branches are not well visualized in routine (hematoxylin and eosin [H&E]-stained) histologic stains and require special techniques (e.g., Golgi-Cox) for optimal examination. Axons are also not well visualized on H&E stain and require silver impregnation techniques (e.g., Bielschowsky or other silver stains) or immunohistochemical analysis (i.e., using primary antibodies to phosphorylated neurofilaments) for optimal visualization. Immunohistochemically, neurons can be identified using antibodies against neurofilament proteins and the synaptic protein synaptophysin.

B. Neurons: Cellular Responses

1. *Changes in the Cell Body in Response to Injury*

Neuron cell bodies show five characteristic changes in response to injury: 1. chromatolytic change (in response to axonal damage); 2. acute necrosis, including anoxic/ischemic (eosinophilic) change; 3. atrophy; 4. ballooning, and 5. neuron loss. Neuronal inclusions (both normal and pathologic) are discussed separately below.

a. Chromatolytic Change. Central chromatolysis refers to an enlargement of the neuron cell body with a concomitant loss or peripheral displacement of central cytoplasmic basophilia (the characteristic bluish-purple color imparted by the ribosome-rich rough endoplasmic reticulum or RER with the H&E stain). The nucleus is displaced to the periphery, while the cytoplasm swells and the Nissl substance is pushed to the borders of the cell and ultimately reduced (Fig. 4). Central chromatolysis is a *nonspecific* response to injury, reflecting primary disruption of the basic metabolic and cellular function of the cell body. It can be seen after any disruption of the axon (as the injury progresses from distal to proximal) or with a variety of metabolic and degenerative diseases (e.g., Pick's disease) and nutritional deficiency states (e.g., pellagra). Rarely, the chromatolytic reaction is characterized by a marked central displacement of Nissl substance. This process, known as *peripheral* chromatolysis is of

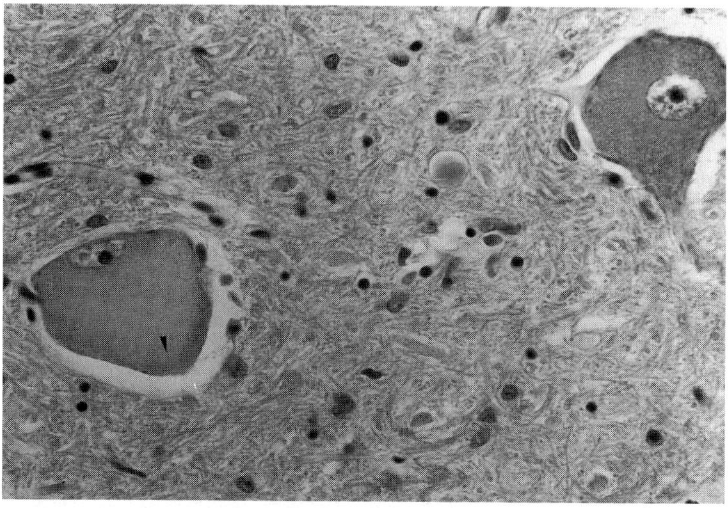

Figure 4 Central chromatolysis in anterior horn cells of spinal cord. A histologic section illustrating the characteristic changes of central chromatolysis (neuron at lower left) in contrast to a relatively normal anterior horn cell (upper right). Note the cytoplasmic swelling, with displacement of the nucleus to the periphery of the cell body. The Nissl substance (arrowhead) is also displaced to the periphery of the cell body.

unknown significance, although it may represent a possible late stage of recovery from central chromatolysis (which is not necessarily irreversible).

b. Acute Necrosis, Including Anoxic/Ischemic Change. Acute necrosis of neurons can occur in response to a number of severe injuries, the most frequent and characteristic of which constitute anoxic/ischemic change (see also Chap. 2). Acute neuronal necrosis may also be seen in patients with neurodegenerative diseases, and inflammatory and infectious conditions. After an ischemic episode, vulnerable neuron cell bodies become brightly eosinophilic and pyknotic within 6 to 8 hours after the insult (see Chap. 2). These eosinophilic neurons should not be mistaken for the darker, shrunken neurons (*lacking* eosinophilia) which occur as "contraction artifact" during tissue fixation and tissue handling. The eosinophilic neurons, if they progress to the point of irreversible cell injury, become necrotic and disappear by phagocytosis. Acute neuronal injury associated with CNS infections, inflammatory lesions, or degenerative diseases lacks the eosinophilia, and irreversible injury in those instances progress directly to shrunken necrotic neurons which are probably removed by phagocytosis. Apoptosis (programmed cell death) may play a role in neuron loss that occurs in some of these entities, especially neurodegenerative diseases. Apoptotic cell death of neurons differs from necrotic cell death. The former is characterized by single cell dropout, without the other findings seen in necrotic cell death, such as swelling and membrane rupture. Although apoptotic cell death can be detected using molecular and ultrastructural techniques, recent advances such as the TUNEL stain have made it easier to detect apoptosis in tissue sections.

Not all cells of the nervous system display the same vulnerability to an anoxic/ischemic insult. These differences form the basis for the concept of *selective vulnerability.* Anoxic/ischemic injury is the classic paradigm for understanding selective vulnerability. In response to severe and prolonged anoxia or ischemia, neurons are the most vulnerable cells, followed by vascular endothelial cells and then glia, which are relatively resistant. Mature differentiated neurons are more susceptible to anoxia than immature developing neurons; vulnerability is seemingly the price paid for the cell's high degree of specialization. Further, particular subtypes of neurons (i.e., Purkinje cells of the cerebellum and pyramidal cells of layers CA1, CA3, and CA4 of the hippocampus) are especially vulnerable to anoxic/ischemic injury (see also Chap. 2).

Reason(s) for the selective vulnerability of highly specialized neurons remain unclear, especially since the pyramidal neurons of the CA2 region of hippocampus (which are morphologically identical to other hippocampal pyramidal neurons, and sit between layers CA1 and CA3) are relatively resistant to anoxic/ischemic injury. The regional pattern of blood supply also probably contributes to the selective vulnerability of neurons to anoxic/ischemic insults. Neurons in regions near the central supply territory of a major cerebral artery are subject to less deprivation during an anoxic/ischemic insult than neurons located in an arterial borderzone. Similarly, neurons at the crest of a gyrus in the cerebral or cerebellar cortex are less likely to suffer the effects of an anoxic/ischemic episode than are neurons within the depths of a sulcus.

Lesions other than anoxic/ischemic insults also show selective vulnerability, although the basis for this is less well understood. The selective vulnerability of neurons in the anterior two-thirds of the superior temporal gyrus (with sparing of the posterior one third) in patients with Pick's disease (see Chap. 8) provides another example of selective vulnerability, presumably *unrelated* to anoxic ischemic factors.

c. Atrophy. Atrophy refers to a decrease in size of the neuronal body. Although it is not always irreversible, atrophy is often a "step along the way" to neuronal loss. Atrophy occurs in a number of contexts—degenerative diseases, retrograde degeneration, and transsynaptic degeneration—although it can be seen in any lesion which slowly but inexorably progresses toward neuronal loss. It can also be seen, to a minimal and variable degree, in normal aging.

The atrophy and loss of neurons in neurodegenerative diseases will be discussed fully in Chapter 8. Retrograde degeneration is a distal-to-proximal degeneration starting in the axon and progressing to the cell body. When there is injury to CNS axons, there is a progressive disruption from the distal to proximal axon and eventually to the cell body. One example is that of an infarct in the occipital/visual cortex, which causes retrograde degeneration extending to axons and cell bodies of the ipsilateral lateral geniculate nucleus (LGN). This process, which can also result in central chromatolysis, may furthermore lead to shrunken pyknotic neurons (in this case in the LGN), which will eventually disappear as they are removed by phagocytosis.

Transsynaptic degeneration (TSD) occurs when injury to a neuron cell body and its axon result in atrophy or loss of the next neuron in the synaptic pathway, which constitutes the main target of the injured axon. Selective atrophy and ultimate loss of neurons of the LGN (which arise in the retinal ganglion cells and synapse in the lateral geniculate nuclei) in response to injury of retinal ganglion cells is a classic example of TSD (Fig. 5).

d. Ballooning Change. Neuron cell bodies may become ballooned in response to any metabolic derangement that results in the accumulation of an undigestible product with resultant engorgement of the cell body. The classic example is Tay-Sachs disease, in which a deficiency of the enzyme hexosaminidase A results in the buildup of the cytoplasmic storage product which cannot be eliminated from the cell, with severe resultant ballooning of neuronal cell bodies (Fig. 6) and ultimately cell death. Many other metabolic storage diseases can result in ballooning of the cell body, as will be discussed in Chapter 9.

e. Neuron Loss. This represents the final common pathway for any form of severe (irreversible) neuronal injury, regardless of etiology or whether neuron death is necrotic or apoptotic. When the neuronal insult is acute (i.e., infections or anoxic/ischemic episodes), the time course of loss of neurons is relatively rapid as they pass through a stage of acute necrosis. In many other insults such as degenerative diseases or metabolic derangements, the time course of neuron loss is much slower, as they variously pass through phases of chromatolysis, ballooning, or atrophy. In some conditions, neuron loss may be due to apoptotic cell death, and these intermediate steps will not occur. In some instances of

---

Figure 5 Transsynaptic degeneration. Diagram illustrates this phenomenon in both lateral geniculate nuclei (LGN) in response to longstanding injury to the right eye. Note that right temporal retina projects to the right (ipsilateral) LGN, synapsing in layers 2, 3 and 5, while the right nasal retina projects to left (contralateral) LGN, synapsing in layers 1, 4, and 6. Injury to right eye results in loss of retinal ganglia cells with atrophy of right optic nerve, and resultant transsynaptic degeneration in the ipsilateral LGN (layers 2, 3, 5) and the contralateral LGN (layers 1, 4, 6).

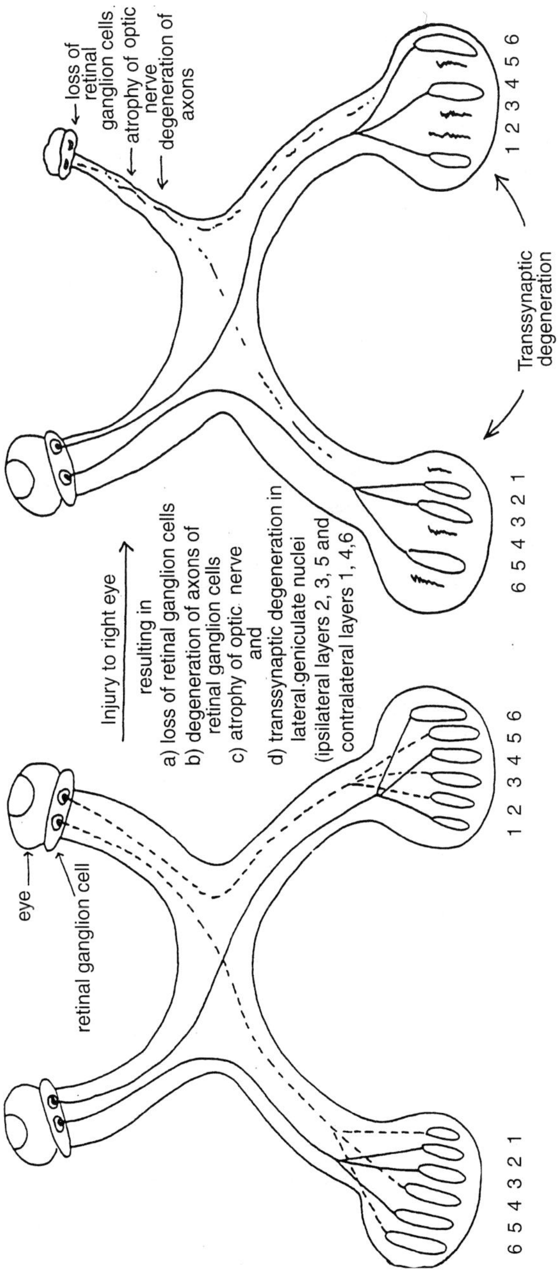
eye
retinal ganglion cell
6 5 4 3 2 1
1 2 3 4 5 6
Injury to right eye
resulting in
a) loss of retinal ganglion cells
b) degeneration of axons of retinal ganglion cells
c) atrophy of optic nerve and
d) transsynaptic degeneration in lateral.geniculate nuclei (ipsilateral layers 2, 3, 5 and contralateral layers 1, 4,6
loss of retinal ganglion cells
atrophy of optic nerve
degeneration of axons
6 5 4 3 2 1
1 2 3 4 5 6
Transsynaptic degeneration

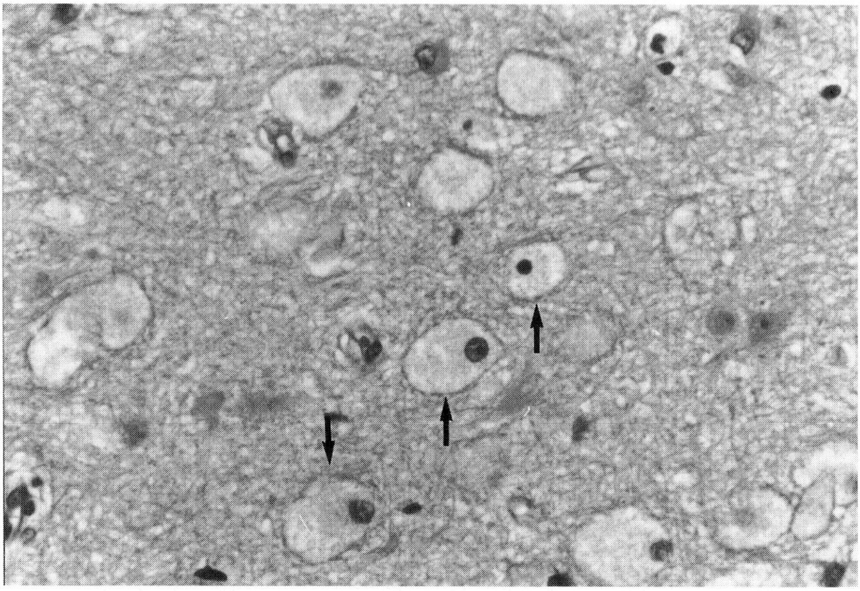

Figure 6 Tay-Sachs disease. Histologic section showing ballooned neuronal cell bodies in the brain of a child who died of Tay-Sachs disease. Note the enlarged neuronal cell bodies filled with granular and foamy storage material (arrows).

severe neuronal injury, especially old infarcts, iron and calcium salts may be precipitated at the site and in the configuration of granular deposits or the shape of the dead neuron, sometimes resulting in a mineralized deposit assuming the shape of the dead neuron and/or its axon (Fig. 7), a process referred to as "ferrugination" (see also Chap. 2).

2. Changes in the Axon in Response to Injury

In response to neuronal injury, three patterns of pathologic change are seen within axons, depending on the nature of the injury: *Wallerian degeneration* (or proximal-to-distal degeneration); *retrograde degeneration* ("dying back" or distal to proximal degeneration); and *focal axonal swelling.* Primary degenerations of the myelin sheath, which may have secondary effects on axons, are discussed in Chapter 5.

a. Wallerian Degeneration. This describes a classic response of axons to injury, characterized by degeneration proximal to the site of injury. It describes a proximal to distal degeneration of the axon. In the classic sense, Wallerian degeneration is used to describe the response of an axon to transection or some other form of severe disruption. At the site of transection, degeneration of the

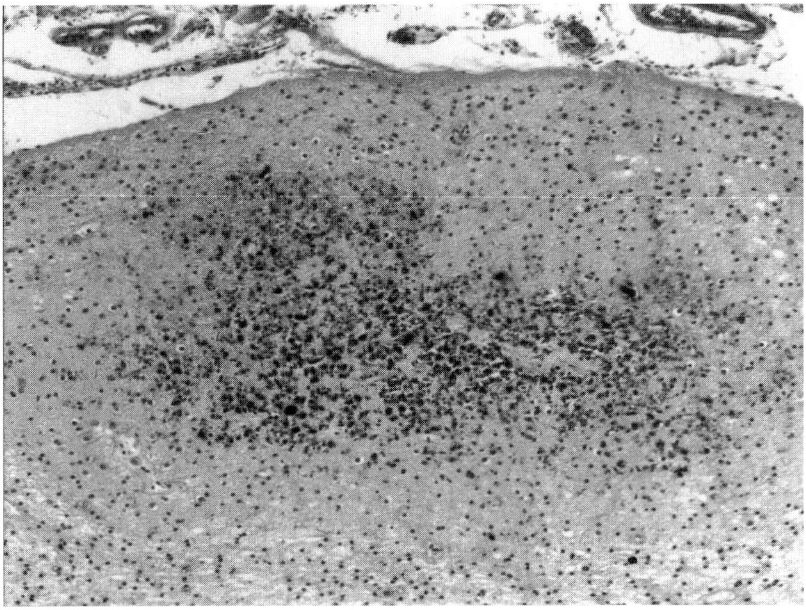

Figure 7 Mineralization of the cerebral cortex. This low-magnification view illustrates punctate calcification which can be seen after destructive injury. The mineral deposits may assume the shape of the dead neuron or its axon in a process known as ferruginization (see Chap. 2, Fig. 43).

axon progresses toward the distal tip, resulting in fragmentation and disintegration of the axon with degeneration of the surrounding myelin sheath. This imparts a characteristic beaded appearance to the axon. Wallerian degeneration of the axon also follows disruption and death of the cell body. Since many disease processes can disrupt either the axon or the cell body (in which case the degeneration begins *at* the cell body), Wallerian degeneration is a common nonspecific response to neuronal injury from insults as diverse as peripheral nerve transection, metabolic injuries and ischemia. While Wallerian degeneration progresses from proximal to distal, there may be a small amount of degeneration, progressing proximally for a short distance along the axon. Other proximal degenerative changes, such as central chromatolysis, may occur simultaneously in the injured neuron. In the PNS, partial or complete reinnervation may occur after Wallerian degeneration: an axon sprouting from the proximal stump can follow intact Schwann cell tubes as a guide. This reinnervation is inconsistent and slow, but is characteristic of the PNS, in which intact Schwann cells proliferate and form columns surrounded by intact basement membrane, providing a surface for regenerating axons. In the CNS, this kind of reinnervation does not occur. Whether this is due to a basic inability of oligodendrocytes (the glia that ensheathe and myelinate CNS axons) to guide the process, or a result of inhibitory substances secreted by glia within the CNS, remains a topic of debate and research. The spinal cord may show some partial regeneration within the PNS elements which interface with it (i.e., spinal nerves sheathed by Schwann cells).

b. Retrograde Degeneration (dying back). Retrograde degeneration reflects a metabolic derangement of the entire neuron. It is referred to by some authors as "dying-back neuropathy," and consists of a distal to proximal degeneration of the axon. Since the distal axon is the portion farthest from the cell body, it is most vulnerable to metabolic derangement. Consequently, the axon degenerates in a distal-to-proximal fashion, usually with a slowly progressive clinical course. The "stocking/glove" neuropathy often associated with diabetes mellitus is a characteristic example of this type of injury.

c. Focal Axonal Swelling. Focal axonal swelling is characterized by an enlargement of the axon as it becomes engorged with accumulated filaments and organelles. It is a nonspecific response of axons within the central or peripheral nervous system, reflecting a secondary disturbance in metabolism. In the brain, focal axonal swellings (*neuroaxonal spheroids*) are commonly seen in patients with severe axonal injury, whether ischemic, traumatic, or related to another etiology (Fig. 8). Focal axonal swellings may also be seen in some rare, inherited disorders such as infantile neuroaxonal dystrophy.

Figure 9 schematically demonstrates some common neuronal responses to injury; Table 1 lists some common neuronal responses to injury and specific insults which may cause them.

C. Neurons—Age-Related and Normal Inclusions

1. Neuromelanin

Neuromelanin is normally seen within the cell bodies of neurons in the substantia nigra (a dopaminergic nucleus in the midbrain) (Fig. 10), the locus ceruleus (a noradrenergic nucleus in the upper pons), and other, less conspicuous brainstem nuclei. It is a byproduct of the breakdown of *tyrosine*—an intermediate in the catecholamine synthesis pathway—so it accumulates within neurons that produce large amounts of the neurotransmitters dopamine and norepinephrine. Catecholamine-producing neurons are present in smaller numbers in the dorsal motor nucleus of the vagus nerve (medulla) and other brainstem nuclei.

2. Lipofuscin

Lipofuscin accumulates within neurons as the brain ages. Known as "aging pigment," it is a yellowish-brownish granular material frequently seen within the cytoplasm of larger neurons in older people. It is generally of no pathologi-

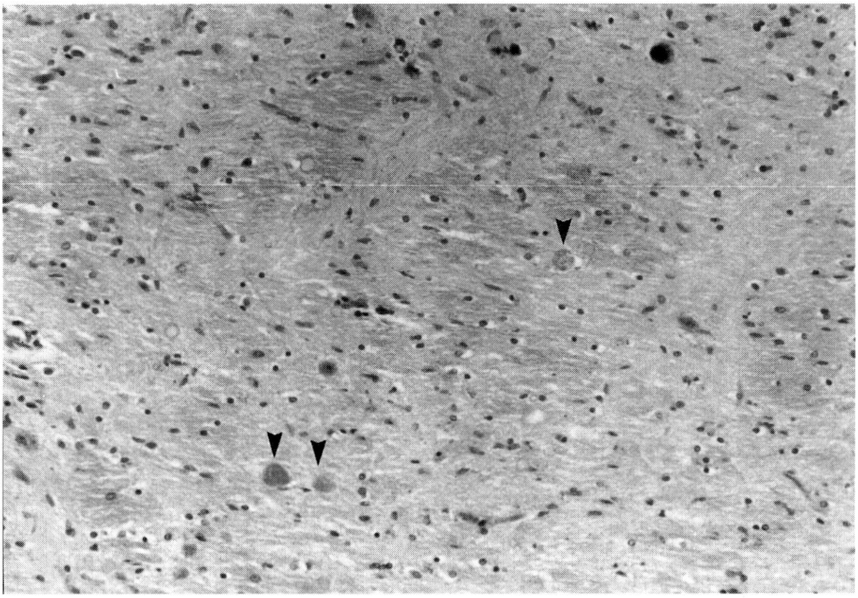

Figure 8 Focal axonal swelling. Photomicrograph from a section of brainstem illustrates focal axonal swellings or neuroaxonal spheroids. The round (eosinophilic) structures (arrows) represent enlargements or swellings of the axon which become distended by axonal filaments and organelles.

cal significance (except in the rare metabolic disease ceroid lipofuscinosis, discussed in Chap. 9.)

3. Marinesco Bodies

These are small, round, eosinophilic, glassy intranuclear inclusions seen within the neurons of the substantia nigra and locus ceruleus. Their function and pathologic significance are unknown, although they are found more frequently in the brains of older people.

D. Neurons—Pathologic Inclusions

1. Inclusions Associated with Infections

Infectious inclusions within the neuron cell body (as well as nonneuronal cells) can either be *intranuclear*, as seen with the Cowdry type A intranuclear inclusions of herpesvirus infections such as cytomegalovirus (CMV) and herpes simplex virus (HSV), or *intracytoplasmic*, as is seen with Negri bodies in cerebellar Purkinje cells or hippocampal pyramidal neurons in patients with rabies (see Chap. 4).

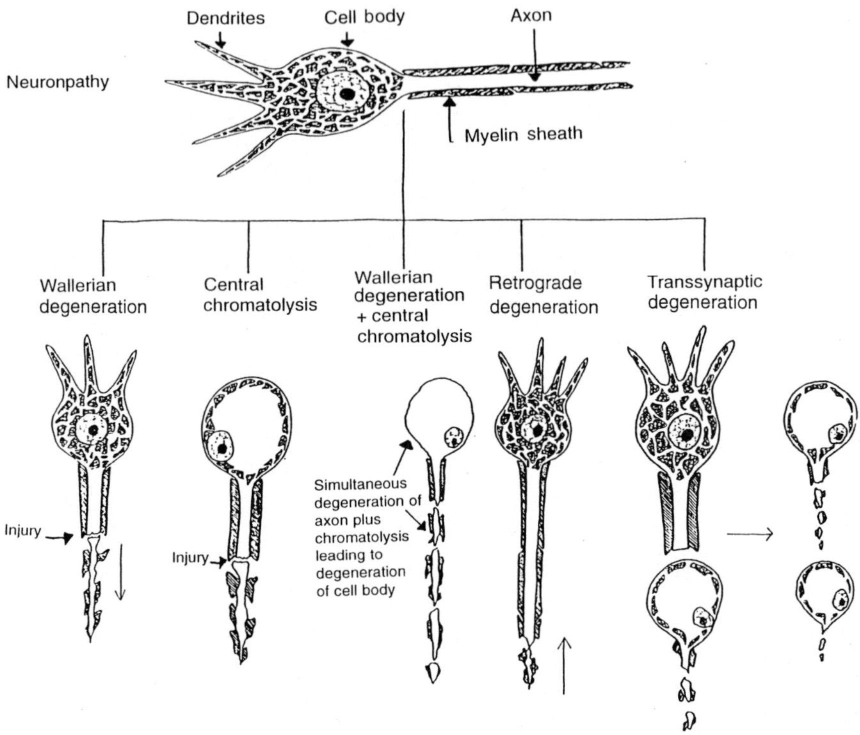

Figure 9 Schematic diagram illustrating characteristic axonal and neuronal cell body responses to injury and transsynaptic degeneration.

2. *Inclusions Associated with Degenerative Diseases*

a. Neurofibrillary Tangles (NFTs). NFTs, which are seen in large numbers in the hippocampus and neocortex of patients with Alzheimer's disease (AD) and a number of other degenerative conditions, may be seen in small numbers in the brains (usually hippocampi) of nondemented older patients. On H&E stain, NFTs appear as a faintly basophilic wisp of fibrillar material, usually best seen within pyramidal neurons (see Chap. 8). These inclusions are better visualized with the aid of a silver stain (e.g., modified Bielschowsky technique) or immunocytochemistry using antibodies to τ or other cytoskeletal epitopes.

b. Granulovacuolar Degeneration of Simchowicz (GVD). GVD refers to the presence of basophilic granules surrounded by clear vacuoles within neuronal cytoplasm (see Chap. 8). This phenomenon is seen within pyramidal neurons of the hippocampus in older patients, and more extensively in patients with AD.

Table 1 Common Neuronal Responses to Injury and Specific Clinical Examples

Response to injury	Specific clinical examples
Central chromatolysis	1. Motor neuron disease/ALS 2. Pellagra 3. Lower motor neuron transection (anterior horn cells)
Acute necrosis	1. Anoxic/ischemic insults 2. Herpes simplex encephalitis
Atrophy	1. Transsynaptic degeneration of neurons in lateral geniculate nucleus after injury to retinal ganglion cells 2. Alzheimer Disease
Ballooning	1. Tay-Sachs disease
Wallerian degeneration	1. Axon transection 2. Infarcts (causing Wallerian degeneration in descending fiber tracts)
Retrograde degeneration	1. "Stocking/glove" peripheral neuropathy of diabetes mellitus
Focal axonal swelling	1. Cerebral trauma 2. Neuroaxonal dystrophy

c. Lewy Bodies. Lewy bodies are cytoplasmic, glassy, spherical, eosinophilic or magenta-colored bodies (often surrounded by a clear halo) seen primarily within the substantia nigra and locus ceruleus of patients with idiopathic Parkinson's disease (see Chap. 8). They may also be seen within cortical neurons in patients with diffuse Lewy body disease or the Lewy body variant of AD. Although Lewy bodies are visualized on H&E stain, immunohistochemistry using primary antibodies to ubiquitin is most helpful in identifying these structures, particularly within the cerebral cortex.

d. Pick Bodies. These are cytoplasmic spherical, faintly eosinophilic, non-membrane-bound inclusions which may be seen within pyramidal and granular neurons of the hippocampal formation in patients with Pick disease (a rare, rapidly progressive dementing illness). Pick bodies are visible on H&E stain, although silver stains are more useful for their visualization (see Chap. 8).

IV. CELLULAR ANATOMY OF THE CNS—GLIA

A. Astrocytes—Microscopic Anatomy

Astrocytes are the most abundant cellular element of the brain, comprising one-third of the volume of the cerebral cortex. They are integral to CNS function and

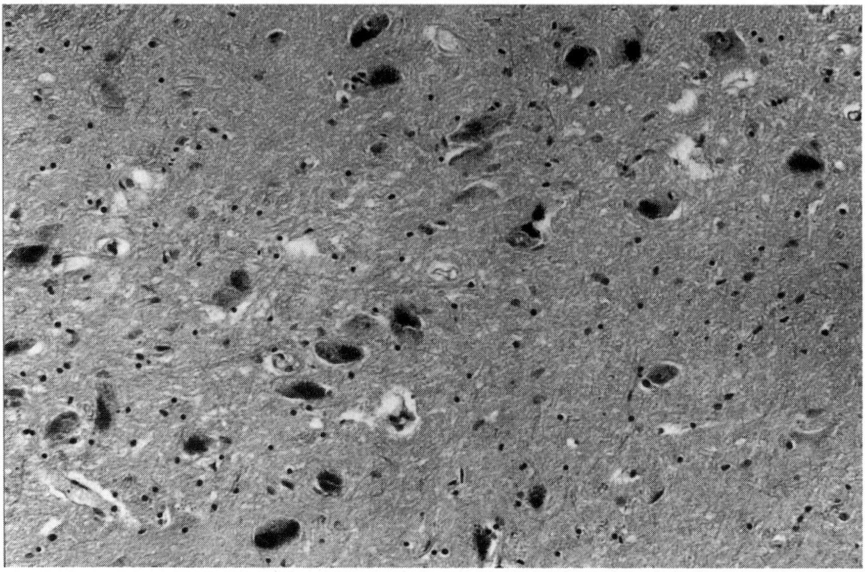

Figure 10 Neuromelanin. Histologic section of the substantia nigra showing neurons with abundant cytoplasmic pigment (neuromelanin), which is brown/black with routine stains.

participate in a number of crucial activities: neuronal migration during development; neurite outgrowth; synaptogenesis; maintenance of blood brain barrier (BBB) properties of cerebral capillaries; regulation of extracellular water, ions, neurotransmitters, and amino acids; and antigen presentation within the CNS.

Astrocytes are also the primary building blocks for the formation of a "scar" in response to neuronal injury within the CNS. They are star-shaped and tend to have long and abundant cell processes. Astrocytes have traditionally been divided into two main types: *fibrillary*—which constitute the majority of astrocytes and are most prominent in the white matter, and *protoplasmic*—which predominate in gray matter. Protoplasmic astrocytes tend to have a more delicate morphology relative to fibrillary astrocytes, which have straighter processes and more glial fibrils. Subtypes of astrocytes include pilocytic astrocytes of the periventricular cerebellar and spinal cord white matter, and Bergmann astrocytes of the cerebellar cortex. The processes of astrocytes are not well visualized on H&E stain unless particularly prominent; this requires immunohistochemistry using antibodies to glial fibrillary acidic protein (GFAP), or complex impregnation techniques. Since astrocytic processes are not well seen, astrocytes normally appear on H&E stain as oval-shaped nuclei floating within

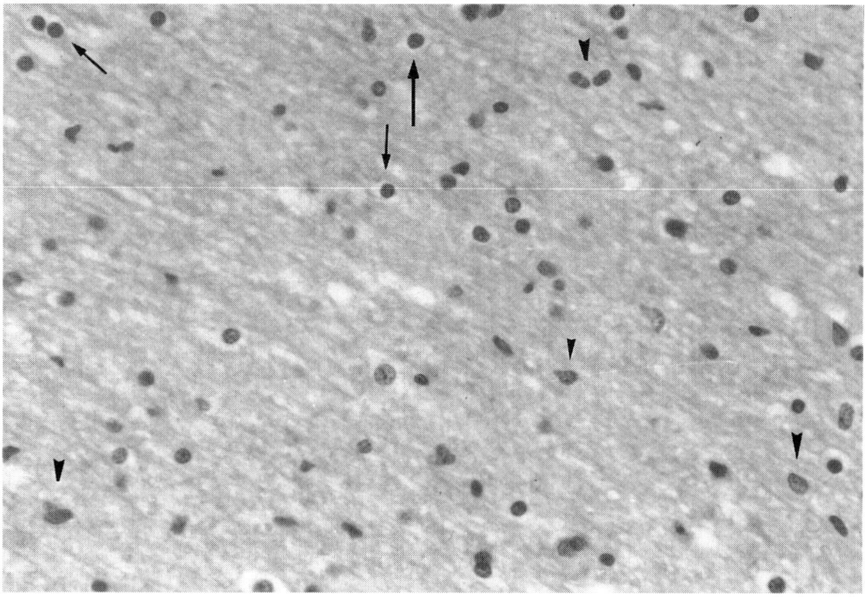

Figure 11 Astrocytes and oligodendrocytes. Section from subcortical white matter showing astrocytes and oligodendrocytes. Since astrocytic processes are not well visualized with routine stains, astrocytes appear as oval nuclei floating in a fibrillary matrix (arrowheads). Oligodendrocytes are characterized by a clear perinuclear halo, and a rounder, denser appearance (arrows), with compact nuclear chromatin.

a fibrillar matrix (Fig. 11). The oval nuclei have a delicate chromatin pattern, and a small nucleolus can often be seen.

B. Astrocytes—Cellular Responses

The primary response of astrocytes to injury in the CNS is "gliosis," or "astrocytic gliosis." Other responses include astrocyte swelling, type II astrocytosis, and, occasionally, astrocytic inclusions. Pathologic inclusions of astrocytes are far less common than those seen in neurons, although viral inclusions such as Cowdry type A intranuclear inclusions may be found.

1. Astrocytic Gliosis and Related Findings

Astrocytic gliosis (also commonly called "gliosis") has two components, which vary with the nature of the injury: *proliferation* of astrocytes, and *hypertrophy* of preexisting astrocytes. (Some authors prefer to reserve the term "astrocytosis" for proliferation and "astrogliosis" for hypertrophy, but since the response is usually mixed, this distinction is not necessary.) Hypertrophy of preexisting astrocytes tends to dominate in most cases of reactive gliosis. During reactive gliosis, the cytoplasm of some hypertrophic astrocytes becomes clearly visible (unlike the cytoplasm of astrocytes in the normal state). The resultant hypertrophic astrocytes, known as gemistocytic astrocytes, or simply "gemistocytes" (Fig. 12), can be encountered in reactive gliosis. As well, gemistocytes may predominate as the major cell component of an astrocytoma (see Chap. 6).

During reactive gliosis (or neoplasia), intermediate filaments proliferate within the cytoplasm of astrocytes. These 10-nm filaments are associated with GFAP so that during active gliosis (or neoplasia), GFAP immunostaining of the cytoplasm becomes prominent (Fig. 13). This increase in GFAP immunoreactivity is reflective of fibrillary gliosis (i.e., in reference to the increased number of glial fibers). Although GFAP immunopositivity is the hallmark of fibrillary gliosis, there are circumstances in which GFAP-positive gliosis is not seen. During development, astrocytes initially express vimentin (another intermediate cytoskeletal filament) and develop GFAP immunopositivity as they mature. GFAP is not normally expressed in developing astrocytes before the 24th week of gestation, except in radial glia (discussed in Chapter 7). Therefore, intrauterine

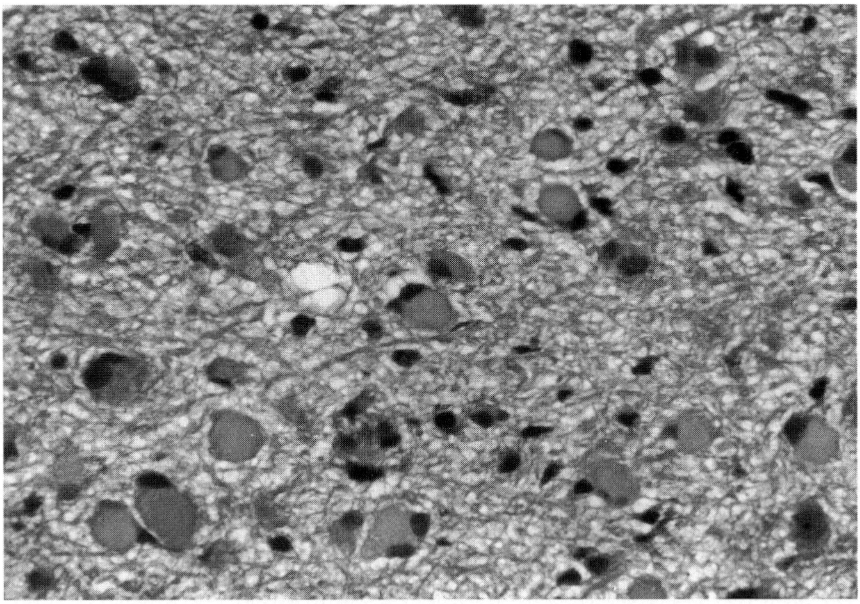

Figure 12 Hypertrophic astrocytes (gemistocytes). Reactive astrocytes which become plump and have clearly visible cytoplasmic borders. Gemistocytic astrocytes can be seen in both reactive and neoplastic conditions. Cytoplasm is glassy and eosinophilic.

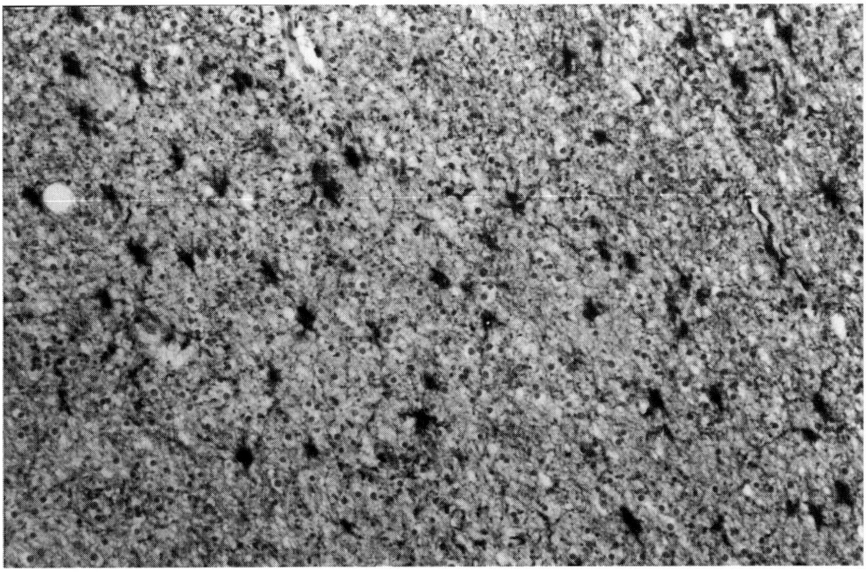

Figure 13 GFAP immunopositive astrocytes. Histologic section stained by immunohistochemistry using primary antibodies to GFAP. Antibody labels the cell bodies and their processes.

injuries prior to this time may not be associated with GFAP-positive reactive gliosis. Reactive and neoplastic astrocytes may sometimes express vimentin in addition to, or in place of, GFAP. In fibrillary gliosis, the proliferation of intermediate filaments can result in either an orderly arrangement of glial fibers (and cell bodies) parallel to the axis of nerve fiber bundles in a piloid ("hairlike") fashion known as *isomorphic gliosis*, or in a haphazard irregular fashion referred to as *anisomorphic gliosis*; the latter is the more common pattern.

Within gliotic tissue, Rosenthal fibers and cytoid bodies may be seen. Rosenthal fibers are brightly eosinophilic, corkscrew-shaped hyaline bodies (on H&E stain) which are often present in the neuropil in regions of long-standing reactive gliosis (Fig. 14). They are frequently seen around the rim of mass lesions such as craniopharyngiomas or arteriovenous malformations, but can also be present in pilocytic astrocytomas and certain metabolic diseases. Rosenthal fibers are found (ultrastructurally) to reside within astrocytic processes. They contain a major protein component of α-β crystallin. Granular cytoid bodies are rounded granular eosinophilic structures (see Chap. 2), closely related to Rosenthal fibers, and are found under similar pathological circumstances, but especially around regions of "old" brain hemorrhage.

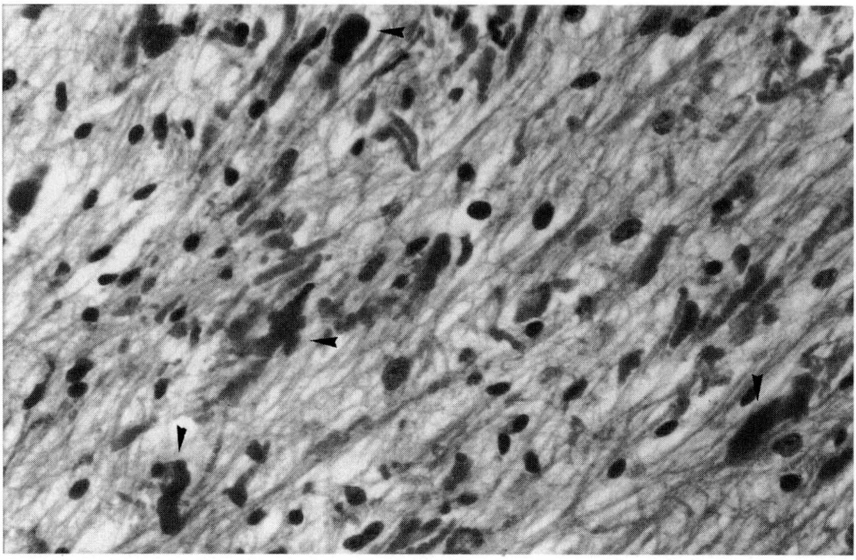

Figure 14 Rosenthal fibers. The eosinophilic corkscrew-shaped hyaline bodies of Rosenthal fibers (arrowheads) appear prominent in this histologic section, illustrating marked reactive gliosis.

2. *Astrocyte Swelling*

This is an early nonspecific response to CNS injury. Since astrocytes constitute a significant percentage of the cells of the CNS, this swelling may be significant and result in clinically hazardous cerebral edema (discussed below).

3. *Alzheimer's Type II Astrocytosis*

Unrelated to Alzheimer's disease is an uncommon form of gliosis seen in patients with metabolic abnormalities. It is seen primarily in the gray matter (especially the deep central gray matter and cerebral cortex) in patients with hepatic failure and hyperammonemic states, including especially hepatic encephalopathy. It is characterized by enlarged, pale, watery-appearing nuclei, often with prominent nucleoli (Fig. 15), but inconspicuous cytoplasm. Alzheimer type I astrocytosis, which is much less common, refers to the enlarged astrocytes bearing copper granules in patients with Wilson's disease.

C. Astrocytes—Age-Related Changes and Normal Inclusions

1. *Astrocytic Gliosis*

Gliosis is a normal part of aging and is seen most prominently in the subpial and periventricular regions. It is also frequently encountered in the inferior olivary nu-

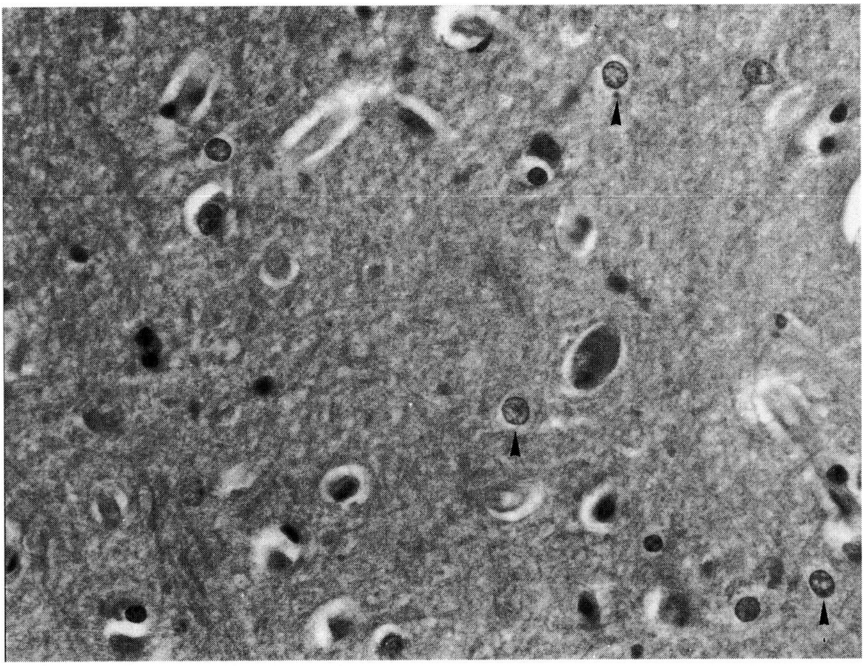

Figure 15 Alzheimer's type II astrocytosis. Magnified view illustrating the large, pale, watery-appearing nuclei (surrounded by negligible cytoplasm) of Alzheimer's type II astrocytes (arrowheads).

clei of the medulla. Whether it is pathological or a response to aging depends largely on its extent, precise location, and other evidence of CNS injury.

2. *Corpora Amylacea*

These are the most common astrocytic inclusions seen within normal brain. Corpora amylacea are present, frequently in large numbers, in the brains and spinal cords of older patients. They are round, basophilic, PAS-positive bodies, measuring 5 to 20 μm in diameter (Fig. 16). They are composed primarily of glycosaminoglycans, and have been shown to be present within astrocytic processes (although in H&E-stained sections they appear to be "floating freely" in the neuropil). Rarely, an overabundance of corpora amylacea may be associated with pathologic abnormalities.

3. *Pigment Accumulation*

Astrocytes often accumulate lipofuscin (usually in older brains) and even hemosiderin (when found adjacent to a hemorrhage). They may also accumulate intracytoplasmic material, either during the course of phagocytosis or in patients with metabolic disorders.

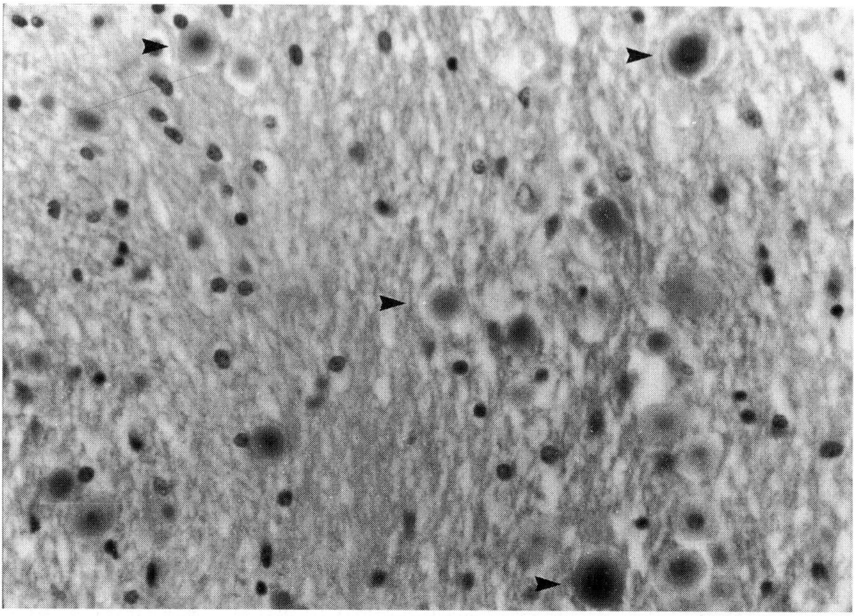

Figure 16 Corpora amylacea. These round, basophilic, PAS-positive bodies (arrowheads), which are composed of glycosaminoglycans, are present within astrocytic processes and are frequently noted on histologic sections from any area of brain, especially in subpial and perivascular locations.

D. Oligodendrocytes—Microscopic Anatomy

Oligodendrocytes are small glial cells with fewer branches than astrocytes, which are responsible for the active production of myelin in the CNS. One oligodendrocyte can be associated with, and produce myelin for, many axons (unlike the 1:1 correspondence between axon segments and Schwann cells in the PNS). In white matter, oligodendrocytes are abundant (Fig. 11) and are often oriented along fiber pathways. In gray matter, oligodendrocytes tend to surround neuronal cell bodies in a process known as satellitosis. The cells have small, round, dark nuclei, which are often surrounded by a clear halo of cytoplasm (Fig. 11). This "fried-egg" appearance is an artifact of fixation and processing, but is very useful in the identification of oligodendrocytes (and neoplasms composed of them) in formalin-fixed, paraffin-embedded material. Oligodendrocytes do not display immunoreactivity for GFAP, although immunopositivity may be seen using primary antibodies against leu-7 and galactocerebroside.

E. Oligodendrocytes—Cellular Responses

Oligodendrocytes display a limited repertoire in response to injury, namely: swelling, loss with proliferation at the rim of a lesion (usually of demyelination), and development of pathologic inclusions.

1. Oligodendrocyte Swelling

Oligodendrocyte swelling is a common nonspecific response to brain injury, and it results in an accentuation of the clear halo seen in paraffin-embedded, formalin-fixed sections.

2. Oligodendrocyte Loss

In demyelinating diseases such as multiple sclerosis, oligodendrocytes disappear, possibly in response to an autoimmune- or viral-mediated mechanism. Frequently, a rim of proliferating oligodendrocytes is seen at the edge of an actively demyelinating plaque, presumably an abortive attempt at remyelination.

3. Oligodendrocyte Inclusions

Oligodendrocytes can also develop viral inclusions. Progressive multifocal leukoencephalopathy (PML) is a brain infection caused by the JC virus (a papova virus) seen in immunosuppressed patients, especially those with AIDS (see Chap. 4). PML results in demyelination and white-matter destruction, but is also characterized by inclusions within oligodendrocytes. Oligodendrocytes are the primary target of the JC virus, and the affected oligodendrocytes display a characteristic enlarged, glassy-appearing amphophilic nucleus (Fig. 17).

F. Ependymal Cells—Microscopic Anatomy

The ependyma is a layer of cuboidal or columnar, ciliated neuroepithelium lining the ventricular system (Fig. 18). Ependymal cells arise from precursor cells surrounding the developing neural tube, which did not migrate away from this initial site, but rather differentiated into specialized neuroepithelial cells. Typically, the ependymal lining is one cell thick, is ciliated, and rests on the underlying neuropil (with no intervening basement membrane). The cilia arise from basal bodies located in the apical cytoplasm. These basal bodies can occasionally be observed using light microscopy (at high magnification often with the aid of a PTAH stain) as spherical to rod-shaped bodies referred to as *blepharoplasts*. *Tanycytes* are a specialized form of ependyma that have elongated periventricular processes that stretch into the periventricular white matter to contact subependymal blood vessels. Ependyma lines the entire ventricular system and extends along the central canal of the spinal cord, which becomes essentially obliterated (as a cavity) at around the time of puberty.

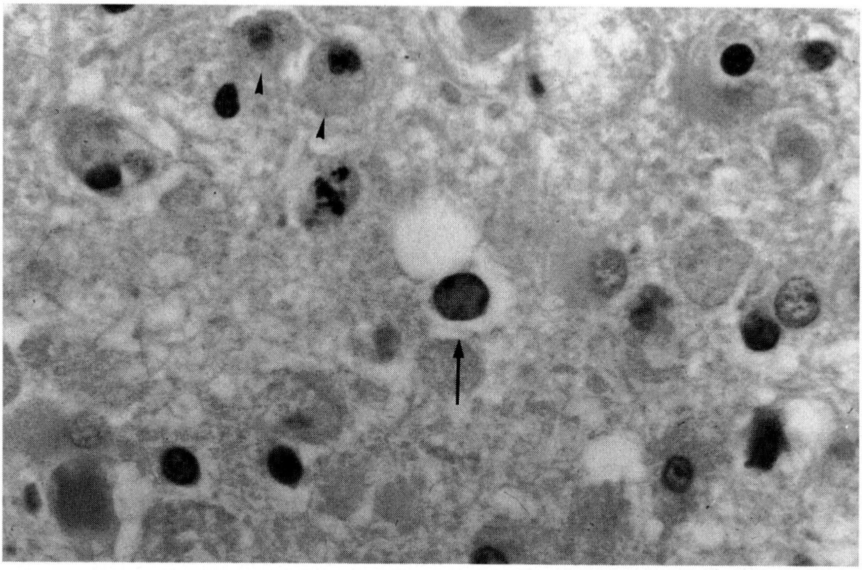

Figure 17 Oligodendrocyte inclusions in PML. A section from a patient who had AIDS and PML. Note the enlarged, glassy-appearing oligodendrocyte nucleus (arrow) which is the characteristic inclusion of PML. Note also the abundant macrophages (arrowheads) demonstrating that this is a highly destructive lesion (see also Chap. 4).

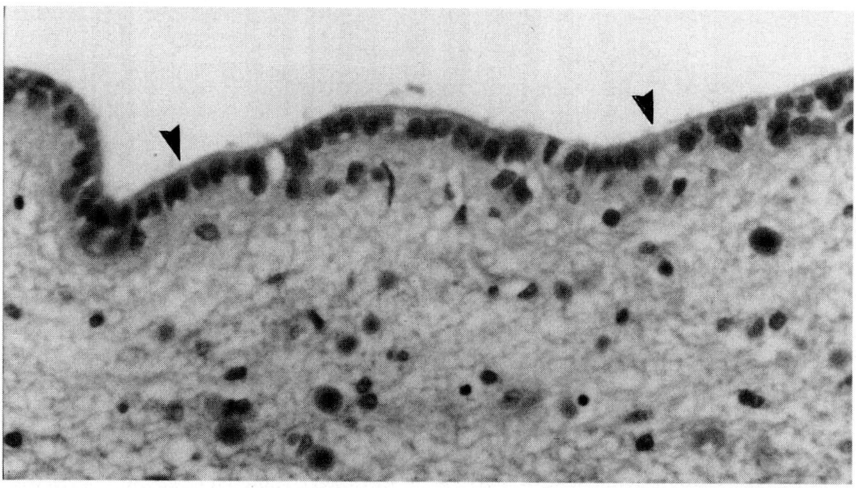

Figure 18 Ependyma. Photomicrograph showing ependymal lining of brain that interfaces with the ventricular surface (arrowheads).

G. Ependymal Cells—Cellular Responses

Ependymal cells show a limited repertoire of responses to injury. Focal loss of the ependyma with proliferation of underlying subependymal astrocytes (Fig. 19) is the most prominent ependymal response to injury. This process is referred to as "granular ependymitis," and the resultant structures "ependymal granulations." It represents a nonspecific and relatively common finding in the CNS. It may be associated with a wide range of etiologies including infection and hydrocephalus. Ependymal cells may also become atrophic (flattened shape and decreased number of cilia), usually in response to chronic hydrocephalus. CNS infections can involve the ependyma, especially CMV and other herpesviruses, in which case the classic inclusion bodies are seen.

H. Microglia—Microscopic Anatomy

Microglia are the main immune responsive cells of the CNS. Their developmental origin remains very much in debate. Most authors believe that microglia are derived primarily from bone marrow precursor cells (monocytes)

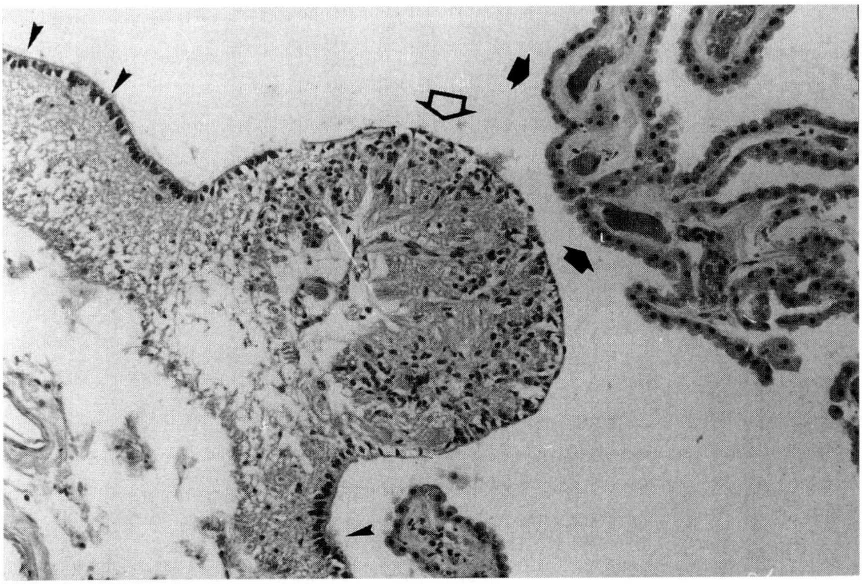

Figure 19 Granular ependymitis (and choroid plexus). Histologic section showing the "heaped-up" subependymal proliferation with focal loss of the ependymal lining (open arrow). Note the adjacent ependymal lining (arrowheads) and the choroid plexus (thick black arrows) consisting of specialized epithelial cells surrounding a fibrovascular core.

which enter the CNS after it has been vascularized; some propose that microglia arise from a neuroectodermal precursor like other glia. Microglia are involved primarily in the immune response of the CNS, since they are capable of antigen presentation, phagocytosis, and cytokine secretion. They may also serve other functions, and have been noted to be a source of trophic and other neuroregulatory factors. Although they are ubiquitous, they are not usually noticed during routine microscopic examination.

Microglia can be divided into three main types based upon their histologic appearance: ramified, perivascular, and ameboid. Ramified microglia are highly branched cells that are uniformly distributed throughout gray and white matter. They correspond to "resting" microglia. Since their processes are not seen on H&E stain, they appear as slightly elongated plump nuclei within a fibrillary background. Perivascular microglia are located around blood vessels and are not highly ramified. They appear identical to macrophages seen in the rest of the body. Ameboid microglia are ramified microglia that have become activated. They assume an elongated bipolar morphology with a plump, rod-shaped nucleus. On H&E stain, only the elongated rod shaped nucleus is visible (Fig. 20). Immunohistochemistry is useful for identifying microglia, although

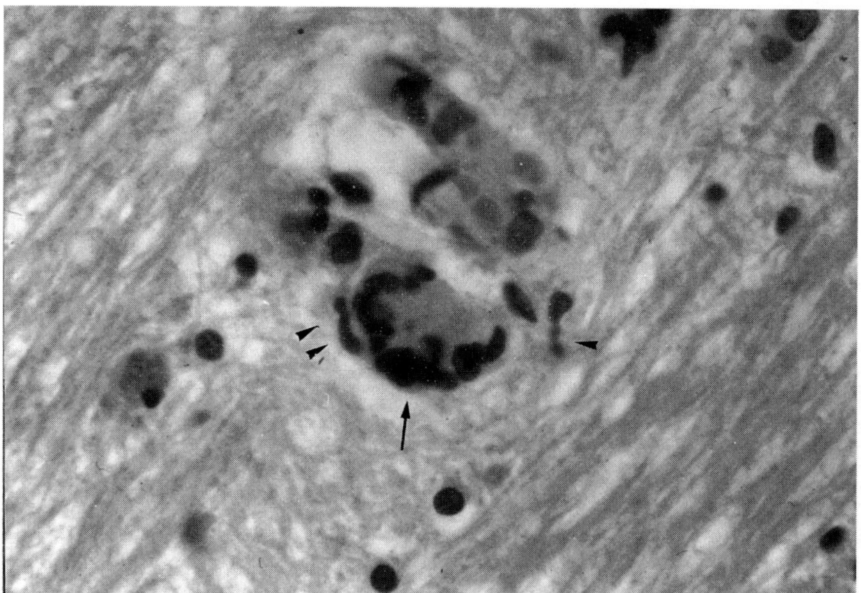

Figure 20 Activated microglia with HIV-type multinucleated giant cell (arrow), magnified view. Note the activated rod-shaped microglia surrounding the giant cell (arrowheads). (See also Chap. 4.)

no unique microglial markers are known. Immunohistochemical markers for macrophages and B-lymphocyte markers, as well as MHC class II antigens and a variety of lectins, are used to detect them.

I. Microglia—Cellular Responses

In response to injury, microglia become activated and assume a rodlike shape. In destructive lesions, macrophages are also seen, although it remains unclear whether these arise from the perivascular microglia or from bloodborne macrophages. Microgliosis consisting of proliferation of rod-shaped cells can either be diffuse (as is often seen in intraparenchymal neurosyphilis) or multifocal, with the formation of microglial nodules (Fig. 21). Microglial nodules are circumscribed, roughly circular aggregates of rod-shaped microglia, which occur most often in response to an infection (i.e., viral or rickettsial). They are, however, nonspecific, can be seen in a range of inflammatory conditions (including some of unknown etiology, e.g., Rasmussen's encephalitis), and contain some *non*microglial inflammatory cells. In poliomyelitis, microglial nodules form around infected anterior horn cells (neurons) of the spinal cord, which undergo

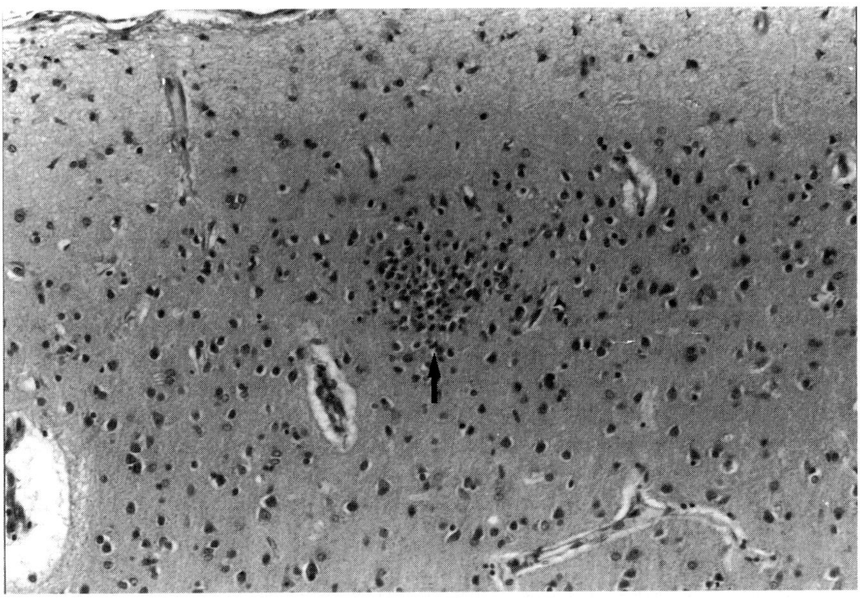

Figure 21 Microglial nodule. Section of the cerebral cortex showing a microglial nodule (arrow) consisting of a roughly circular aggregate of microglia and scattered lymphocytes. This histologic change, while relatively nonspecific, is highly characteristic of viral infections of the CNS.

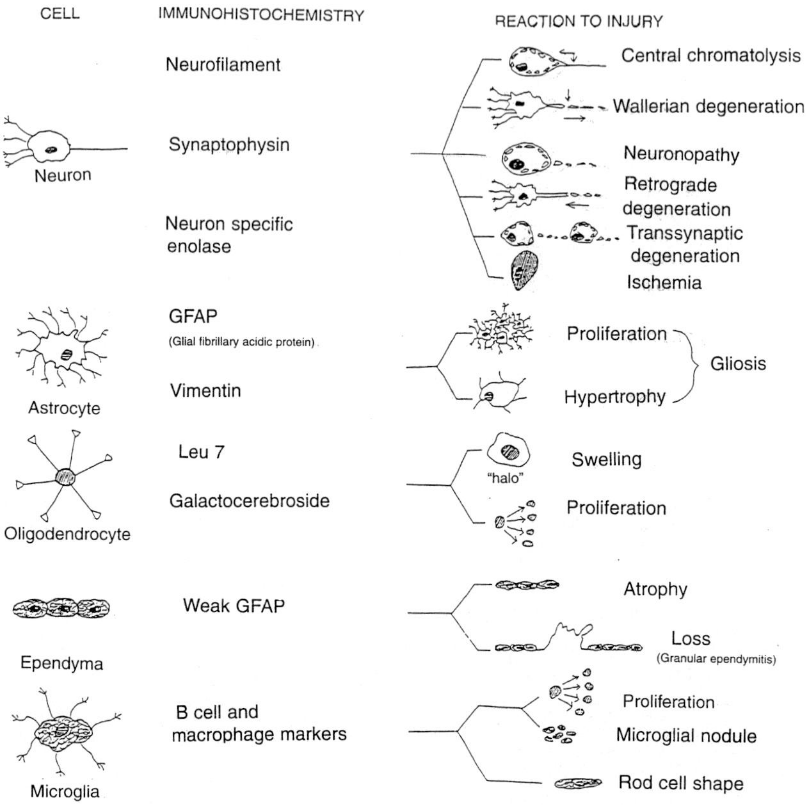

Figure 22 Schematic overview of neuron and glial responses to injury.

necrosis and phagocytosis by activated microglia in a process known as neuronophagia. Figure 22 presents an overview of glial responses to injury, and their immunohistochemical detection.

V. CELLULAR ANATOMY OF THE CNS—CHOROID PLEXUS

The choroid plexus is a frondlike intraventricular structure (located within lateral, third, and fourth ventricles) which is specialized to secrete cerebrospinal fluid (CSF). The choroid plexus projects into the subarachnoid space in the region of the cerebellopontine angle laterally (through the foramen of Luschka) and in the dorsal midline into the cisterna magna (through the foramen of Magendie). Choroid plexus develops during intrauterine gestation as a specialization of ependymal cells. The primitive mesenchymal tissue from the leptomeninges invaginates to form its fibrovascular cores, while ependymal cells line its surface and develop into choroid plexus epithelium.

The choroid plexus consists of a single layer of cuboidal or columnar epithelial cells surrounding a fibrovascular core (Fig. 19). The connective tissue core contains prominent blood vessels, collagen, macrophages, and fibroblasts, and may even contain small nests of meningothelial cells (and occasional psammoma bodies).

The choroid plexus is subject to a number of age-related changes. Xanthomatous change, consisting of a hyalinized and sclerotic stromal region surrounded by foam cells within the fibrovascular core, is common in older patients (although it can occasionally be seen in children and even fetuses). Proliferation of the stromal connective tissue with thickening of the subepithelial basement membrane, calcification, and psammoma body formation are frequently encountered in the choroid plexus of older patients.

CSF is produced primarily by epithelial cells of the choroid plexus at the rate of approximately 500 ml/day, and is secreted into the ventricles. The CSF volume "turns over" several times a day. It circulates through the ventricular system, exits through the fourth ventricular exit foramina (Luschka and Magendie), and moves around the brain and spinal cord in the subarachnoid space between the outer layer of the arachnoid and the pia. It is then reabsorbed into the blood via the arachnoidal villi, which pierce the dura and contact the dural sinuses over the cerebral convexities.

Under normal circumstances, a well-controlled balance exists between the formation and absorption of CSF; an imbalance between its formation and absorption leads to hydrocephalus (Fig. 23), defined as an excess of CSF, usually with enlargement of the ventricles. This can be symmetrical or asymmetrical, depending on the level and nature of the disruption to CSF flow. It can result from one of three mechanisms: *obstruction* to the flow of CSF; *increase* in the resistance to CSF absorption; or *primary overproduction* of CSF. Hydrocephalus secondary to an obstruction of CSF flow is commonly seen in patients with tumors and congenital malformations, and frequently results in asymmetrically enlarged ventricles, especially if obstruction is at the foramen of Monro. Increased resistance to CSF absorption may also cause hydrocephalus. Mechanical obstruction of the arachnoidal villi by inflammatory cells and eventual fibrosis (as seen in patients with meningitis) impedes CSF resorption and can lead to symmetrical hydrocephalus. Primary increases in CSF production are very rare, seen only with some choroid plexus papillomas (see Chap. 6).

True hydrocephalus must be distinguished from hydrocephalus *ex vacuo*, defined as enlargement of the ventricles secondary to a loss of brain parenchymal tissue (brain atrophy). It does not represent an imbalance in CSF circula-

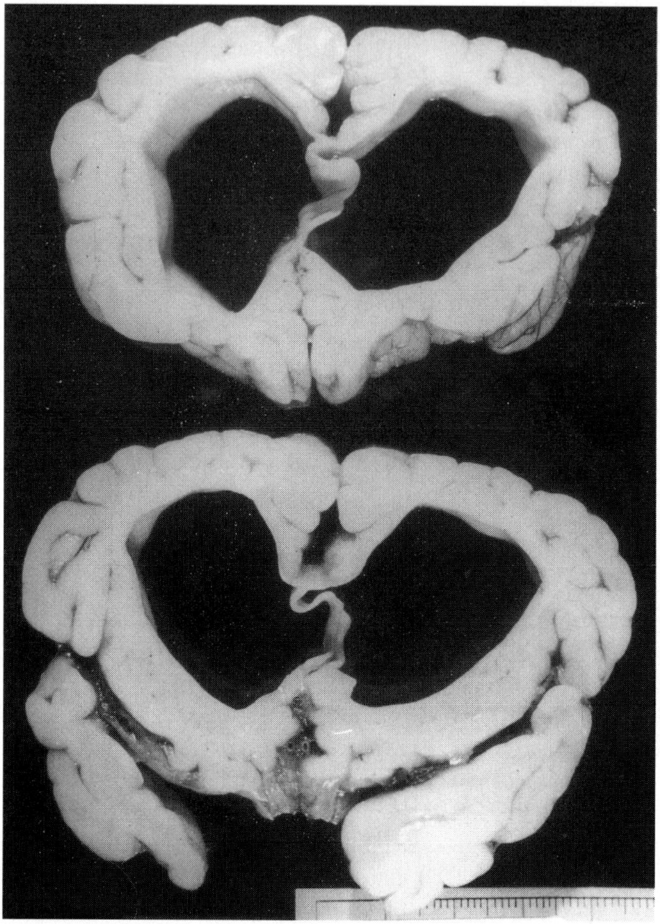

Figure 23 Hydrocephalus. Coronal sections through the cerebral hemispheres, illustrating marked dilatation of the lateral ventricles characteristic of hydrocephalus.

tion, and is associated primarily with degenerative diseases (i.e., dementia) and, in a milder form, normal aging.

VI. CELLULAR ANATOMY OF THE CNS—MENINGES

A. Microscopic Anatomy

The meninges consist of the dura (pachymeninges) and the leptomeninges (pia and arachnoid). The dura consists of two layers: an *outer* layer, which is adherent to the skull and serves as the inner periosteum, and an *inner* layer, which follows the contour of the arachnoid membrane. The inner layer of dura also gives rise to the four major dural folds: the falx cerebri, falx cerebelli, tentorium cerebelli, and diaphragma sellae. The dural arteries and venous sinuses run within these folds. The inner layer of the dura is pierced by arachnoidal granulations and draining veins. The dura is composed of highly organized, densely packed, laminated collagen with scattered elastic fibers and fibroblasts.

The pia and arachnoid (leptomeninges) form a delicate covering for the brain and spinal cord. The arachnoid consists of an outer layer of spindle-shaped cells beneath the dura, and an inner layer of loosely arranged meningothelial cells, collagen, fibroblasts, and blood vessels. The meningothelial cells are concentrated in the region of the arachnoid villi, where they may form whorls and psammoma bodies. The arachnoid is connected to the pia via delicate strands (*arachnoid trabeculae*). The pia, which is immediately adjacent to the CNS parenchyma, consists of an outer connective tissue layer (epipia) and an inner mesothelial layer (intima pia). However, on H&E, the pia appears as a thin, delicate membrane on the surface of the CNS parenchyma (Fig. 24).

B. Age-Related Changes and Normal Variants

In children, the leptomeninges are grossly thin and translucent. With increasing age, they become thicker and more fibrotic, especially over the parasagittal areas. This is appreciated microscopically, as the collagen is deposited within the subarachnoid space, especially within the region of the arachnoid villi. Small proliferations of meningothelial cells may be present, occasionally with whorls and psammoma bodies ("minimeningioma"). In the leptomeninges surrounding the spinal cord in older patients, thin, white hyaline plaques are often grossly apparent (Fig. 25). These plaques represent a normal aging change, and consist of laminated hyalinized fibrous tissue. *Arachnoiditis ossificans*, consisting of true bone formation (ossification) within a plaque, is rare and usually occurs in response to a spinal cord lesion. Abundant, heavily pigmented melanocytes can occasionally be seen within the leptomeninges, especially within darker-skinned people. These pigmented cells should not be misinterpreted as an abnormality (e.g., evidence of a previous subarachnoid hemorrhage). They are most prominent over the upper cervical spinal cord and medulla.

VII. CELLULAR ANATOMY OF THE CNS—BLOOD BRAIN BARRIER (BBB)

The BBB is a protective filter which tightly regulates the microenvironment of the CNS. (A similar *blood-nerve barrier* exists for the PNS.) This barrier occurs at the capillary level and consists of tight intercellular junctions between capil-

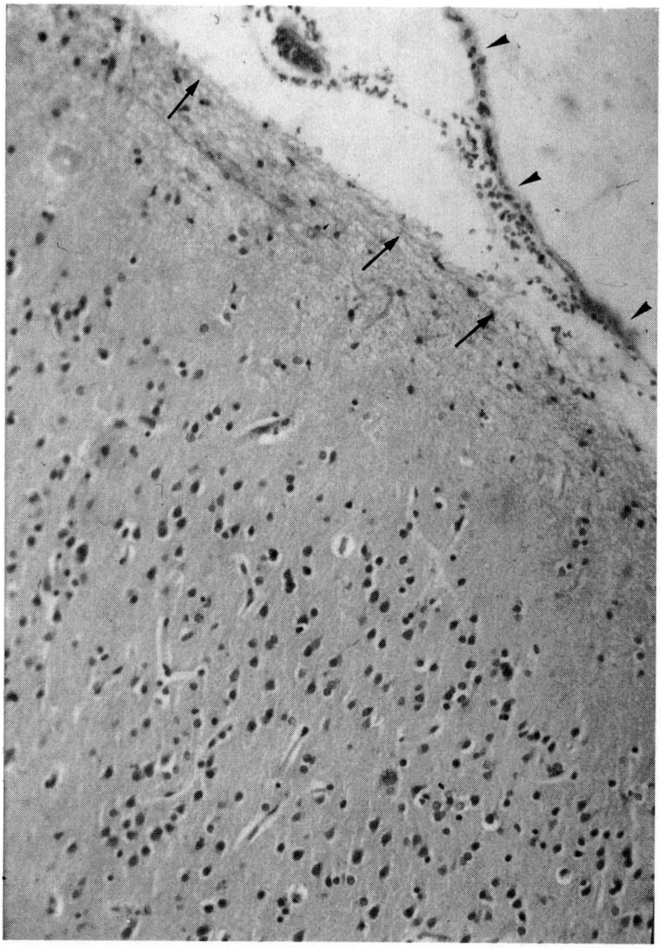

Figure 24 Leptomeninges. Section of surface of the cerebral cortex illustrating the pial surface (arrows) and the arachnoid (arrowheads). Note also the delicate blood vessels within the subarachnoid space. The pia and arachnoid are joined by delicate strands.

lary endothelial cells, surrounded by astrocytic foot processes which exert "inductive" influences on cerebral capillary endothelium. The endothelial cells themselves differ from endothelium in visceral capillaries in that they have a relatively high mitochondrial content, very few pinocytotic vesicles, and no fenestrations. These endothelial cells also contain elevated levels of enzymes

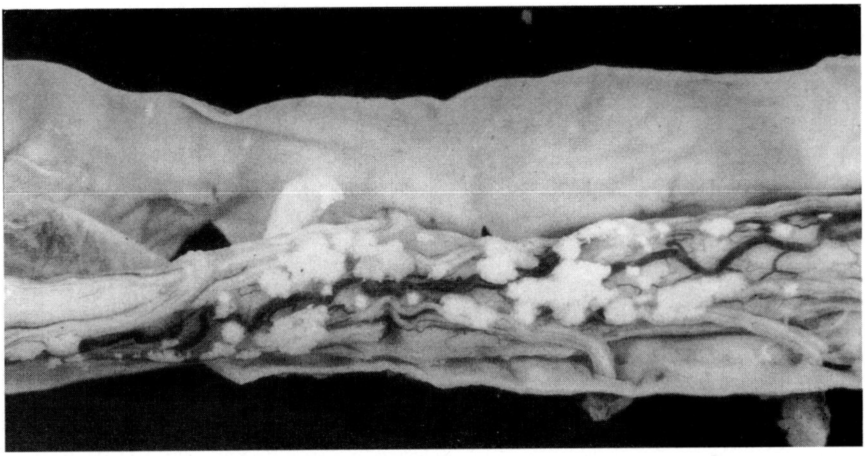

Figure 25 Arachnoid plaques. These thin, white, hyaline "eggshell" plaques surrounding the spinal cord are a common finding at autopsy, especially in older individuals.

(e.g., γ-glutamyl transpeptidase and aromatic amino acid decarboxylase) which modify peptides so that they cannot enter the extracellular fluid surrounding neurons. All of these anatomic and metabolic properties fit with the primary function of the BBB—fine regulation of the content of the extracellular fluid surrounding neurons. Comparable specializations occur within microvessels of the choroid plexus, in the arachnoid, and around peripheral nerves, forming (respectively) the *blood CSF* and *blood-nerve barriers.*

VIII. CEREBRAL EDEMA AND ITS CONSEQUENCES

Cerebral edema is defined as an abnormal accumulation of fluid associated with an increase in size of the brain. Since the brain is enclosed by (and largely fills) a nonflexible, bony casing, the skull, there is little room for its expansion. For this reason, cerebral edema is a common pathway for serious morbidity and mortality resulting from diverse "insults" to the brain. On a cellular level, cerebral edema can be classified into two main types: vasogenic, and cytotoxic (cellular). A third form, interstitial edema, is described by some authors and is associated with hydrocephalus. Cerebral edema may be focal, multifocal, or global, depending on the nature of the primary disease process. Grossly, edematous brains appear enlarged, softened, and heavy. The convexities appear flattened and the sulci may be partially effaced (Fig. 26). Microscopically, cerebral

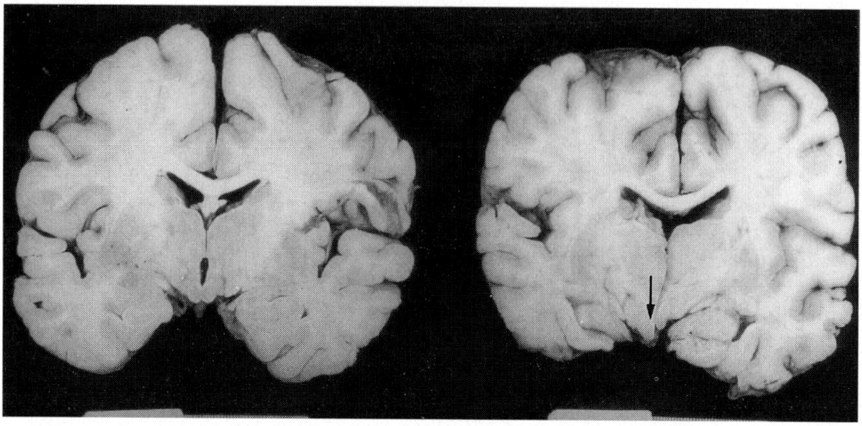

Figure 26 Cerebral edema. Comparison photograph showing similar coronal sections through two brains. Brain on the left is normal, while brain on the right shows marked cerebral edema. Note the full, flattened appearance of gyri in brain on the right, with effacement of the sulci. Note also the presence of central diencephalic herniation (arrow).

edema imparts a vacuolated appearance to the neuropil. Hypertrophic gliosis may also be seen in patients with chronic cerebral edema.

Vasogenic edema is caused by injury to the walls of cerebral capillaries resulting in breakdown of the BBB and a leakage of fluid into the brain parenchyma. This can be considered as an increase in *inter*cellular fluid volume. Vasogenic edema is associated with insults that result in disruptions of the capillary endothelium/BBB, which tend to be localized and result in focal edema. It has many etiologies including tumors, abscesses, infarcts, hemorrhages, trauma, and ischemia.

Cytotoxic (cellular) edema is caused by direct injury to the cells of the brain parenchyma (neurons, astrocytes, oligodendrocytes, etc.). The accumulation of fluid is primarily *intra*cellular and does not involve an increase in capillary permeability. It is associated with hypoxia/ischemia, infections, and a variety of metabolic disturbances. Cytotoxic edema can be either focal or global, depending on the primary disease. Clearly, many factors that cause vasogenic edema also result in cytotoxic edema—e.g., a cerebral infarct.

The third type of cerebral edema, *interstitial*, is specifically associated with hydrocephalus. In patients with hydrocephalus, ventricular expansion with stretching of their walls results in small tears in the ependymal lining, resulting in escape of CSF into the surrounding periventricular brain parenchyma.

Cerebral edema exerts its most serious and life-threatening effects by causing brain herniations, of which there are three main types: *transtentorial* (also referred to as mesial temporal/uncal) and often associated with central diencephalic herniation); *cerebellar tonsillar*; and *subfalcine*. Some authors consider a fourth type, "fungus cerebri," which occurs when brain tissue herniates through a cranial defect, whether as a result of trauma or neurosurgical intervention. These herniations have secondary consequences, which are usually responsible for most of the morbidity and mortality of any brain lesion. These can be grouped into three categories: focal tissue compression and necrosis; vascular compression/infarction; and vascular tearing/hemorrhage. The main types of cerebral herniation and their secondary consequences are summarized in Table 2.

Transtentorial herniation occurs when the medial temporal lobes are compressed over the edge of the rigid and fixed tentorium cerebelli (Figs. 27, 28). This usually results from ipsilateral hemispheric cerebral edema, although bilateral transtentorial herniations may also occur. This process can cause compression of the third cranial (oculomotor) nerve, resulting in a fixed dilated pupil.

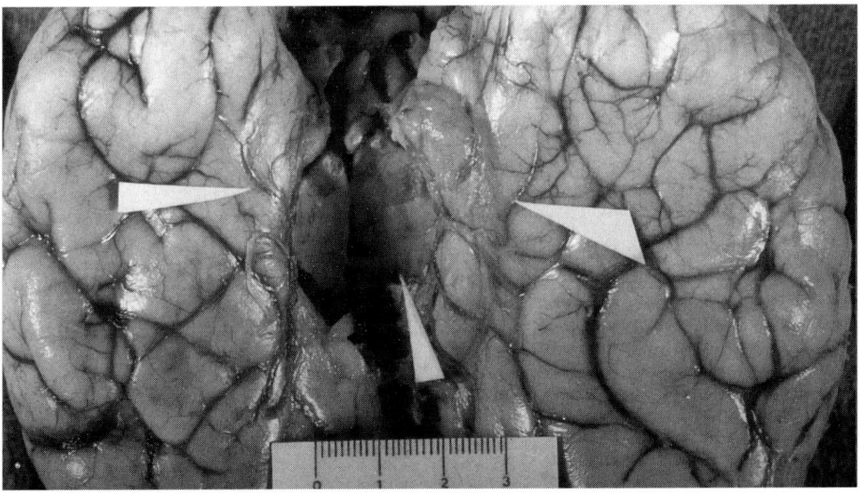

Figure 27 Transtentorial herniation. View from the inferior surface of the brain with the brainstem removed, illustrating the effect of transtentorial herniation of the left temporal lobe (right side of photograph) caused by an underlying tumor. The compression of the uncal (mesial temporal) region of the lobe against the rigid tentorium cerebelli results in this grooved appearance (white arrow at right). Arrow at bottom illustrates severe side-to-side compression of the midbrain, while arrow at left (patient's right temporal lobe) shows *absence* of uncal herniation.

Table 2 Cerebral Herniations and Their Potential Consequences

Herniation	Focal tissue compression	Vascular compression/ infarction	Vascular tearing/ hemorrhage
Transtentorial	1. 3rd and 6th cranial nerves 2. Cerebral aqueduct obstruction with hydrocephalus 3. Ipsilateral medial temporal (uncal grooving) 4. Contralateral cerebral peduncle compression necrosis (Kernohan's notch)	1. PCA compression with infarct in PCA territory 2. Proximal MCA and perforating artery compression with infarct in deep central gray matter	1. Duret hemorrhages (secondary brainstem hemorrhages)
Cerebellar tonsillar	1. Medulla (including respiratory center) 2. Cerebellar tonsils (sometimes with necrosis and fragmentation into subarachnoid space)	None	None
Subfalcine	1. Cingulate gyrus	1. Distal ACA compression with infarct in ACA territory	None

Key: PCA = posterior cerebral artery; MCA = middle cerebral artery; ACA = anterior cerebral artery.

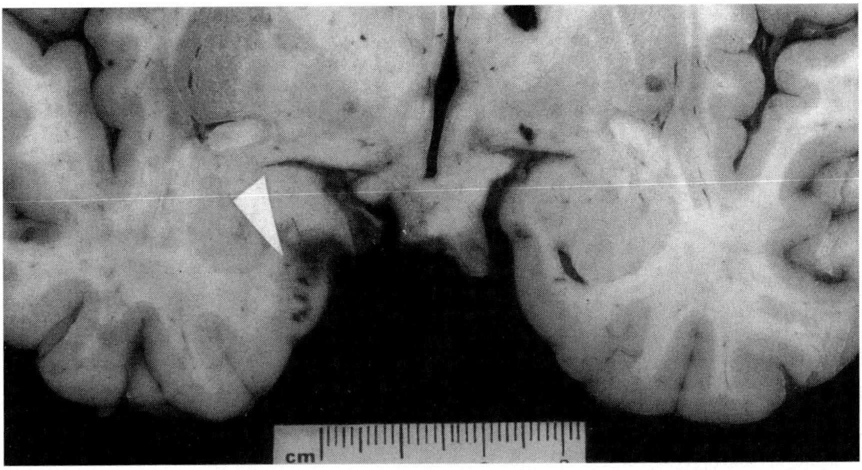

Figure 28 Transtentorial herniation. Coronal section of a brain showing transtentorial herniation with hemorrhagic necrosis of the left mesial temporal lobe (arrow).

The sixth cranial nerve can also be involved. The brainstem is frequently deformed by this compression and assumes an elongated shape (compressed from the sides and elongated in the anterior-posterior axis). As a consequence, the aqueduct of Sylvius may become narrowed or obstructed, and the perforating arteries to the midbrain and pons may become sheared, leading to midline hemorrhages in the upper pons and midbrain—so-called Duret hemorrhages (Fig. 29). The proximal posterior cerebral artery (PCA) and occasionally the proximal middle cerebral artery (MCA) and its perforating branches may be intermittently compressed, causing infarcts in the medial occipital lobe and deep central gray matter, respectively. Injury to the contralateral cerebral peduncle against the rigid tentorium (Kernohan's notch) can occur as the midbrain is shifted to the contralateral side (Fig. 30). This complication can produce false localizing signs on neurologic examination, suggesting an additional primary lesion referable to the *same* side as that on which the Kernohan's notch phenomenon is occurring.

Herniation of the cerebellar tonsils through the foramen magnum is frequently seen with mass lesions in the posterior fossa, or with massive focal or global cerebral edema (Fig. 31). It can also be seen in a more benign form in certain congenital malformations, as will be discussed in Chapter 7. The cerebellar tonsils undergo compression necrosis, and the floor of the medulla is displaced. This can be fatal, since the critical cardiorespiratory centers are located in this region. Rarely, fragments of the herniated cerebellar tonsils may even be seen within the subarachnoid space around the spinal cord.

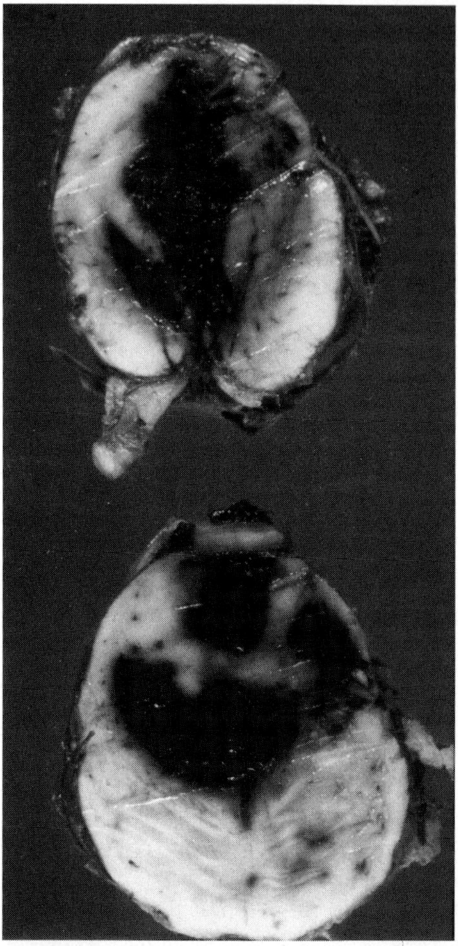

Figure 29 Duret hemorrhages. Midline hemorrhages in the upper pons and midbrain resulting from shearing of the perforating arteries or veins during side-to-side compression of the midbrain (with downward displacement) which may occur with transtentorial herniation.

Subfalcine herniation occurs when there is a midline shift, as the cingulate gyrus passes under the rigid falx cerebri (Fig. 32). It is observed frequently in the setting of a unihemispherical mass lesion. The cingulate gyrus may undergo compression necrosis, and the distal anterior cerebral artery (ACA) may be intermittently occluded, resulting in an ACA territory infarct.

The student of neuropathology must keep in mind that cerebral edema

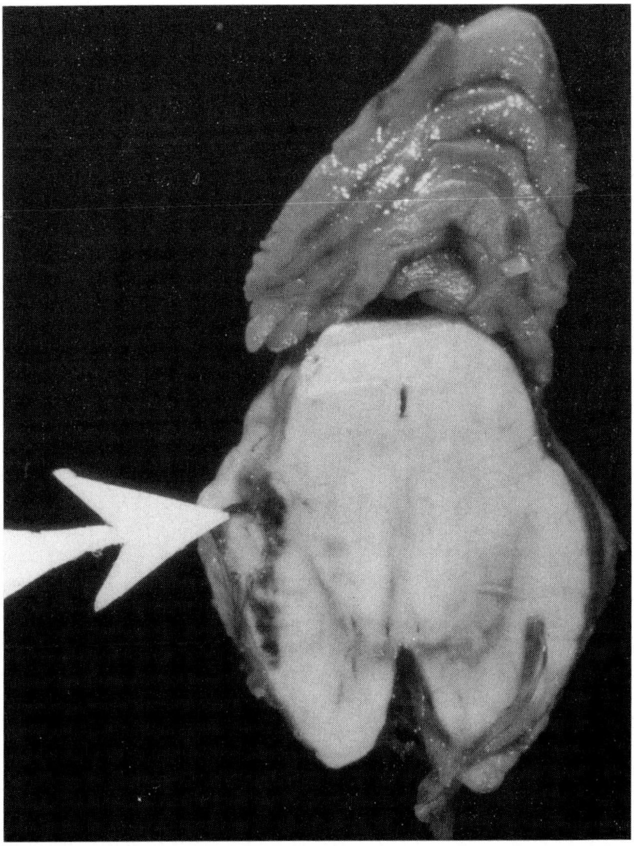

Figure 30 Kernohan's notch. Patient had a large ***right*** cerebral hemispheric mass. Injury to the contralateral (***left***) cerebral peduncle (arrow, opposite side from the space-occupying lesion) as the brainstem is compressed against the rigid tentorial notch may produce false clinical localizing signs.

and its secondary consequences account for the bulk of morbidity and mortality from a wide variety of brain injuries (especially mass lesions), and must therefore be assessed carefully in brains examined at autopsy.

IX. PERIPHERAL NERVOUS SYSTEM

A. Microscopic Anatomy of Peripheral Nerves

The anatomy of the PNS, like that of the CNS, is highly complex. It differs significantly from the CNS, both in its structural anatomy and in its capacity

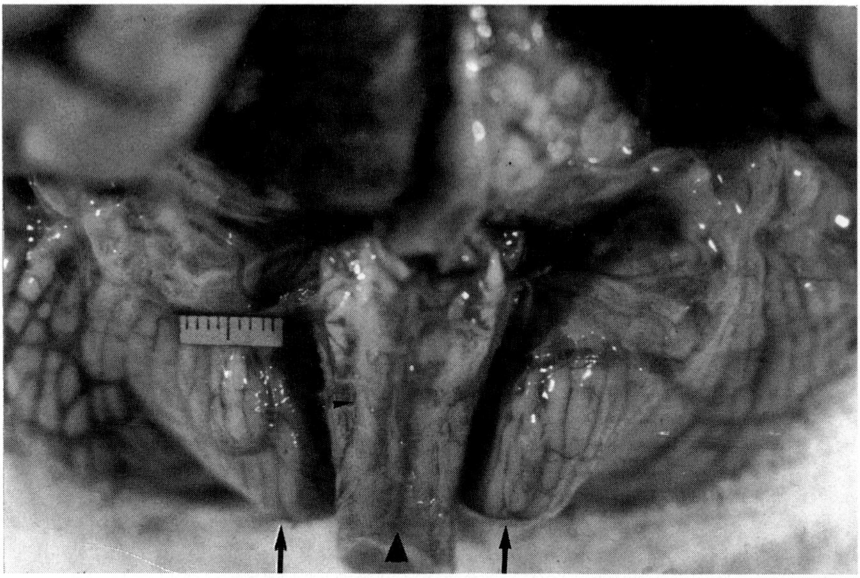

Figure 31 Cerebellar tonsillar herniation. Herniation of the cerebellar tonsils (arrows) is seen in response to mass lesions in the posterior fossa, or with massive focal or global cerebral edema. This photograph shows an anterior view of the brainstem. The herniated cerebellar tonsils (arrows) wrap around the posterior surface of the medulla (arrowhead). The pons, with prominent basilar artery, is present (just out of focus) at top of the photograph.

for regeneration. The PNS can be divided into three functional divisions: motor, sensory, and autonomic.

Motor nerves consist of the efferent fibers that exit the ventral horn of the spinal cord (and cranial nerve nuclei in the brainstem) and innervate peripheral or cranial muscular targets. Sensory nerves arise from peripheral receptors (i.e., mechanoreceptors, proprioceptors, nocireceptors) and travel back to the dorsal horn of the spinal cord (and cranial nerve nuclei in the brainstem). Unlike motor nerves, the cell bodies of sensory nerves lie outside the CNS within *dorsal root ganglia* (and cranial nerve ganglia). The one exception to this is the *trigeminal mesencephalic nucleus*, which contains the cell bodies for proprioceptive fibers from the jaw and lies within the upper pons. The autonomic nervous system consists of *parasympathetic* and *sympathetic* fibers. The peripherally located *parasympathetic* fibers arise from the brainstem and travel peripherally within the third, seventh, ninth, and tenth cranial nerves, and from the sacral spinal cord in the second and third sacral nerves. They synapse in

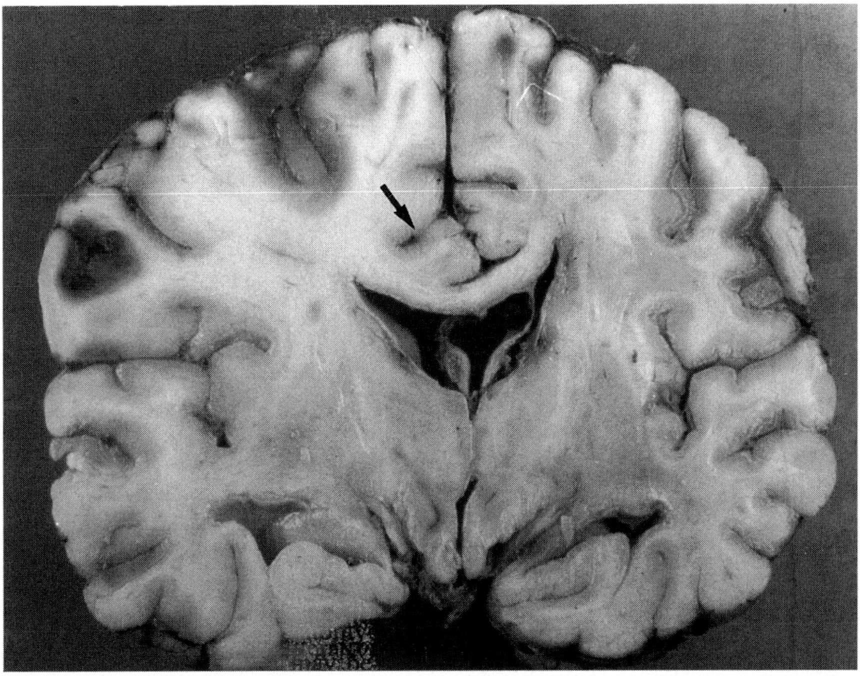

Figure 32 Subfalcine herniation. Massive edema of the left cerebral hemisphere has resulted in a shift of midline structures, with herniation of the left cingulate gyrus (arrow) beneath the falx cerebri (not seen since the brain has been removed from the skull prior to sectioning).

ganglia close to their peripheral targets. The *sympathetic* fibers arise from neurons in the intermediolateral gray cell column of the thoracic spinal cord and exit the spinal cord via the ventral roots. They travel a short distance before entering the sympathetic trunk and synapsing within the prevertebral and paravertebral ganglia.

Most peripheral nerves are actually composed of many nerve fascicles, each fascicle containing many axons. A peripheral nerve contains many circular nerve fascicles surrounded by connective tissue which surrounds and runs among the fascicles (Fig. 33). This connective tissue layer can be divided into three compartments: *epi*neurium, *peri*neurium, and *endo*neurium.

The epineurium consists of the dense connective tissue (mostly collagen with some elastic fibers) which surrounds all of the fascicles and merges with the adjacent fibrofatty connective tissues. The perineurium runs between nerve fascicles and consists of flat perineurial cells (modified fibroblasts) organized

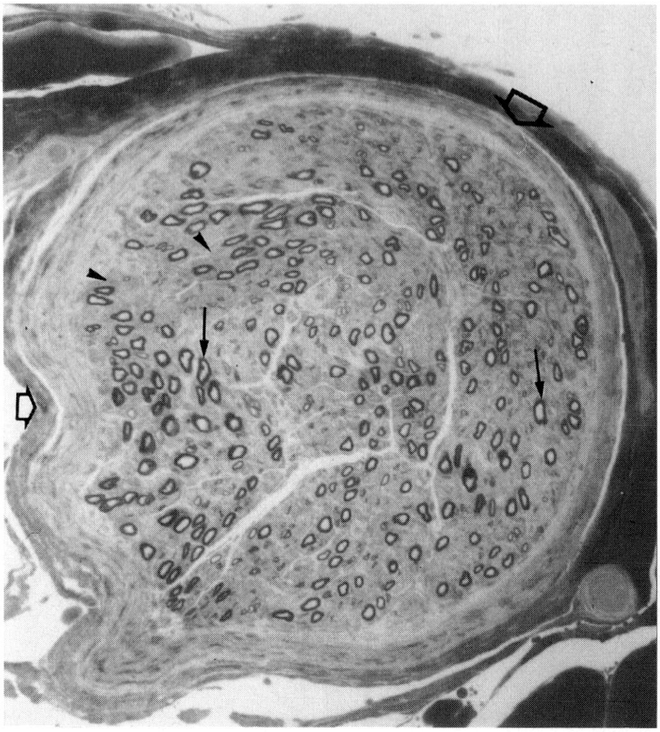

Figure 33 Peripheral nerve. Transverse section of the sural nerve examined in a plastic embedded section. Myelinated axons of various sizes are easily visible (arrows). The perineurium is the thick outer layer that surrounds the nerve (open arrow) and connects large nerve sheaths; the endoneurium (arrowhead) separates individual axons and Schwann cells within the nerve.

in a lamellar pattern. Collagen fibrils are interspersed between the perineurial cells. The perineurium has a role in maintaining structural integrity of the nerve fascicles and in forming the blood-nerve barrier (analogous to the BBB in the CNS). Endoneurium runs between the individual axons (and Schwann cells) within each fascicle. It contains fibroblasts, collagen, capillaries, and mast cells. A rich blood supply is present within peripheral nerves (vasa nervorum), and blood vessels can be seen within the epineurium, perineurium, and endoneurium.

Schwann cells are associated with both myelinated and unmyelinated axons. In a cross section of peripheral nerve, approximately 90% of the nuclei are those of Schwann cells. Multiple small unmyelinated axons can be ensheathed by a single Schwann cell, while a *single* Schwann cell produces the myelin sheath for a given segment of a *myelinated axon* (unlike in the CNS, where one oligodendrocyte produces the myelin sheath for multiple axons). Schwann cells are essential for the maintenance of axons and production of peripheral myelin. They are also capable of phagocytic activity, and their basement membranes (which are continuous in the form of a tube) are important for guiding regenerating axons following nerve damage.

Unmyelinated fibers in a peripheral nerve outnumber myelinated fibers by a ratio of approximately 2:1 or 3:1. A typical fascicle contains 7000 to 10,000 myelinated and 20,000 to 40,000 unmyelinated axons. The thickness of the myelin sheath is directly proportional to the axon diameter in mature fibers. Adjacent Schwann cells meet at the node of Ranvier. Although the adjacent myelin sheaths produced by consecutive Schwann cells are discontinuous, their basement membranes are continuous. Internodal distance can vary considerably, as the internodal length is directly proportional to fiber diameter (and therefore the myelin sheath thickness). Myelinated fibers range from 2 to 15 μm in diameter, while unmyelinated fibers are from 0.2 to 2.0 μm in diameter.

Renaut bodies are subperineurial cylindrical hyaline bodies, which are commonly encountered in normal peripheral nerve (Fig. 34). They are composed of randomly oriented collagen fibrils and glycosaminoglycans (which render them PAS-positive). They may appear either circular or as elongated cylinders when viewed, respectively, in cross or longitudinal section. Their function is unknown, although they may act as physical cushions. They are seen in normal nerve, but are increased in a number of neuropathies, especially those involving nerve compression.

Schmidt-Lanterman clefts/incisures are a frequent finding on routinely stained longitudinal sections of peripheral nerve (Fig. 35). They appear as arrow-shaped eosinophilic processes within myelinated axons. These clefts or incisures are fixed components of the myelin sheath, consisting of continuous spirals of Schwann cell cytoplasm seen at an oblique angle. The number of the clefts is directly proportional to axon diameter. Although deceptively dramatic in appearance, they are a normal finding.

Dorsal root ganglia (DRG) and cranial nerve ganglia have a characteristic appearance on histologic examination. They consist of numerous large, spherical neurons (ganglion cells) surrounded by satellite cells (Fig. 36). These satellite cells are also of neural crest origin, and bear a structural and functional similarity to Schwann cells. Satellite cells proliferate when DRG neurons disappear/die to produce typical "nodules of Nageotte."

B. Peripheral Nerve—Cellular Responses

Axons, and their cell bodies within the PNS (i.e., dorsal root ganglia and cranial nerve ganglia), are subject to the same cellular responses as seen in neu-

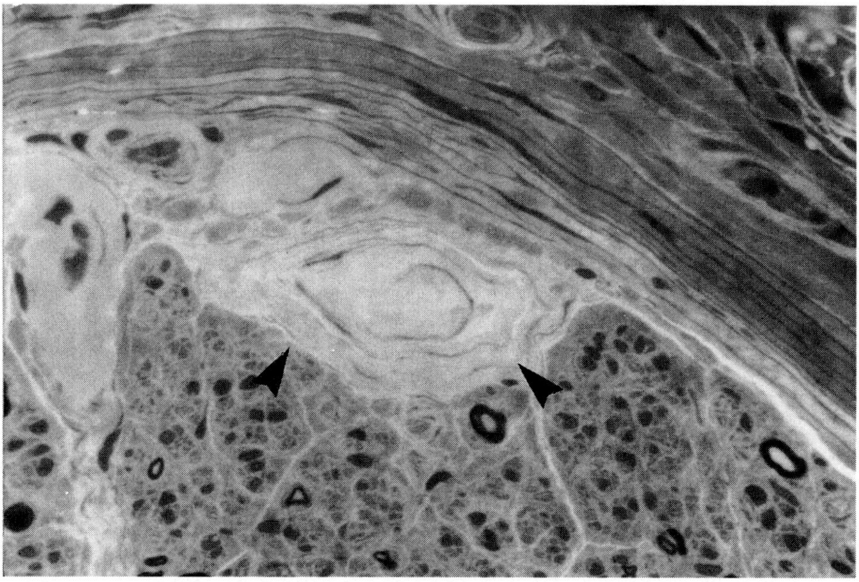

Figure 34 Renaut bodies. These subperineurial hyaline bodies (arrows) are seen in normal nerves. Note the appearance of a multilamellated structure composed of thin cells or cell processes that appear to displace myelinated fibers.

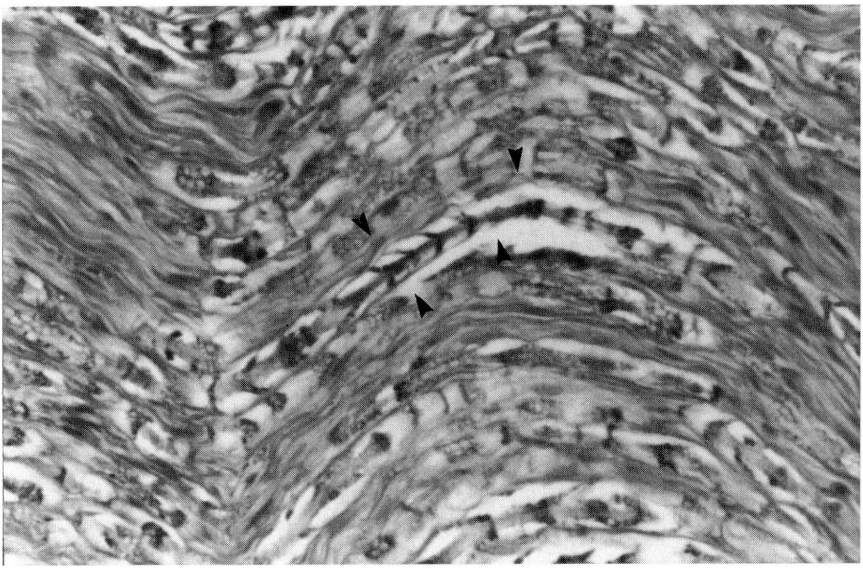

Figure 35 Schmidt-Lanterman incisures. These clefts are a frequent finding on routinely stained longitudinal sections of peripheral nerve, imparting an "arrowhead" appearance to the nerve.

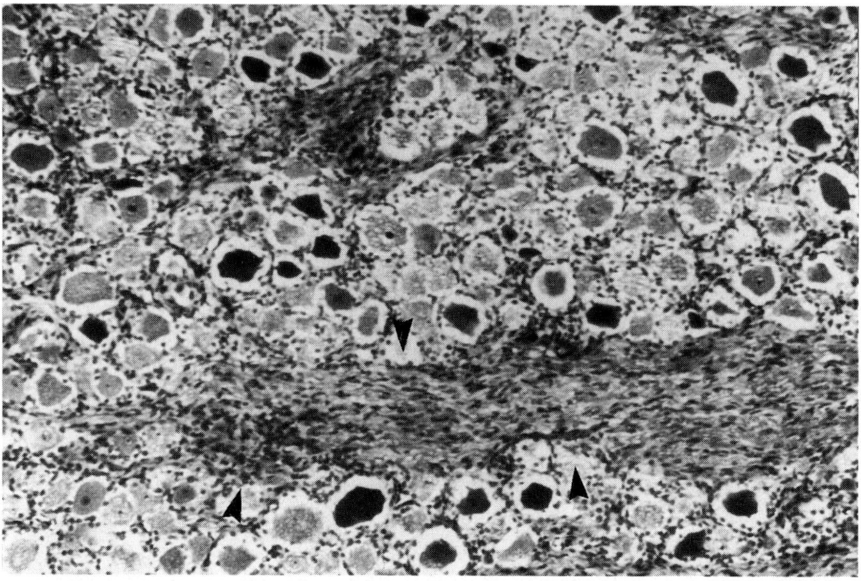

Figure 36 Dorsal root ganglion. Photomicrograph of dorsal root ganglion demonstrating the characteristic large ganglion neurons surrounded by numerous satellite cells. A nerve fascicle is noted to be passing through the ganglion (arrows). The variably light- or dark-staining properties of individual neurons represent an artifact.

ronal cell bodies and their axons in the CNS (as discussed above). Briefly this consists of chromatolytic change; neuronal necrosis, atrophy, and loss; Wallerian degeneration; retrograde degeneration; and focal axonal swelling. Secondary axonal injury in segmental demyelination, which is a frequent pathologic occurrence in peripheral nerves, will be discussed in Chapter 10.

Unlike the CNS, the PNS is capable of regeneration, and peripherally transected axons may undergo a slow and often incomplete regenerative process, usually with extensive formation of axon collaterals (terminal sprouting). Schwann cells proliferate and form columns (bands of Bungner) surrounded by basement membrane, providing a surface for the regenerating axon.

Segmental demyelination is the loss of a segment of the myelin sheath, usually due to direct injury to myelin or the Schwann cell. After demyelination, the original Schwann cell replicates, and the demyelinated segment of the axon is remyelinated by two or more Schwann cells. Recurrent cycles of demyelination with remyelination result in the formation of "onion bulbs" (accumulations of concentrically arranged Schwann cells) and an increase in total Schwann cell number (Fig. 37).

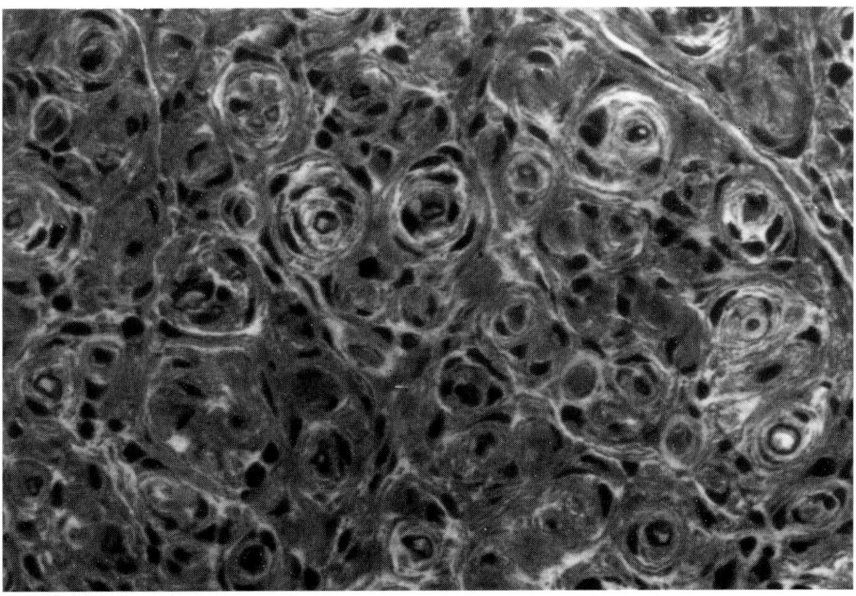

Figure 37 "Onion bulbs." These accumulations of concentric Schwann cells occur in the setting of recurrent cycles of peripheral nerve demyelination with remyelination seen in several chronic neuropathies and in "localized hypertrophic neuropathy."

REFERENCES

1. Alcolado R, Weller RO, Parrish EP, Garrod D. The cranial arachnoid and pia mater in man: anatomical and ultrastructural observations. Neuropathol Appl Neurobiol 1988; 14:1–17.
2. Barr ML, Kiernan JA. The Human Nervous System: An Anatomical Viewpoint. 6th ed. Philadelphia: J.B. Lippincott, 1993.
3. Burger PC, Scheithauer BW, Vogel FS. Surgical Pathology of the Nervous System and Its Coverings. 3rd ed. New York: Churchill Livingstone, 1991.
4. Cornford EM. The blood-brain barrier, a dynamic regulatory interface. Mol Physiol 1985; 7:219–260.
5. Dickson DW, Mattiace LA, Kure K, Hutchins K, Lyman WD, Brosnan CF. Microglia in human disease, with an emphasis on acquired immunodeficiency syndrome. Lab Invest 1991; 64:135–156.
6. Dohrmann GJ, Bucy PC. Human choroid plexus: a light and electron microscopic study. J Neurosurg 1970; 33:506–516.
7. Dyck PJ, Thomas PK, Griffin JW, Low PA, Poduslo JF, eds. Peripheral Neuropathy. 3rd ed. Philadelphia: Saunders, 1993.
8. Fedoroff S. Development of microglia. In: Kettenmann H, Ransom BR, eds. Neuroglia. New York: Oxford University Press, 1995:162–181.
9. Fuller GN, Burger PC. Central nervous system. In: Sternberg SS, ed. Histology for Pathologists. New York: Raven Press, 1992:145–169.
10. Hirano A. Neurons and astrocytes. In: Davis RL, Robertson DM, eds. Textbook of Neuropathology. 2nd ed. Baltimore: Williams and Wilkins, 1991:281–330.
11. Hulette CM, Downey BT, Burger PC. Macrophage markers in diagnostic neuropathology. Am J Surg Pathol 1992; 26:493–499.
12. Le Dourain NM, Smith J. Development of peripheral nervous system from the neural crest. Annu Rev Cell Biol 1988; 4:375–404.
13. Norenberg MD. Astrocyte responses to CNS injury. J Neuropathol Exp Neurol 1994; 53:213–220.
14. Okazaki H. Fundamentals of Neuropathology: Morphologic Basis of Neurologic Disorders. 2nd ed. New York: Igaku-Shoin, 1989.
15. Ortiz-Hidalgo C, Weller RO. Peripheral nervous system. In: Sternberg SS, ed. Histology for Pathologists. New York: Raven Press, 1992:169–193.
16. Pollock M. Nerve regeneration. Curr Opin Neurol 1995; 8:354–358.
17. Raine CS. Oligodendrocytes and central nervous system myelin. In: Davis RL, Robertson DM, eds. Textbook of Neuropathology. 2nd ed. Baltimore: Williams and Wilkins, 1991:115–140.
18. Rechthand E, Rapoport SI. Regulation of the microenvironment of peripheral nerve: role of the blood-nerve barrier. Prog Neurobiol 1987; 28:303–343.

19. Sarnat HB. Ependymal reactions to injury. A review. J Neuropathol Exp Neurol 1995; 54:1–15.
20. Stoll G, Griffin JW, Li CY, Trapp BD. Wallerian degeneration in the peripheral nervous system: participation of both Schwann cells and macrophages in myelin degradation. J Neurocytol 1989; 18:671–683.

2

Anoxic-Ischemic Change and Cerebrovascular Disease

I. PATHOPHYSIOLOGY OF ANOXIC-ISCHEMIC BRAIN DAMAGE

Although the terms hypoxia and ischemia are often used interchangeably, they have significantly different pathophysiology and sequelae in terms of producing brain injury. The term *ischemia* implies impairment of blood flow or supply to one or more regions of the brain (often producing ischemic stroke), whereas *hypoxia* describes events that follow a relative shortfall or deficiency of oxygenated blood to the CNS. Blood flow may be normal in the presence of severe hypoxic brain injury. Other important pathophysiologic differences between global ischemia and hypoxemic hypoxia include markedly decreased ATP and phosphocreatine and increased lactate in the former but not the latter, increased fatty acid and protein catabolism in the former, and selective neuronal necrosis and infarct with global ischemia but not necessarily hypoxemic hypoxia. It is well known that the density of capillaries, which (to some extent) determines the delivery of oxygen and nutrients to the brain varies regionally within the CNS; i.e., it is higher in the cortex than the white matter and is greatest in regions with the highest metabolic rates. Cerebral blood flow (CBF) is approximately 20 to 25 ml/100 g/min in white matter, and approximately 80 in gray matter, which averages out to 50 ml/100 g/min. CBF is determined by cardiac output and to a large extent, by cerebral metabolism, the phenomenon of "local autoregulation."

Respiration in the brain is dependent upon glucose as a fuel/substrate. Glucose is oxidized to CO_2 and H_2O by glycolysis (which yields 4 ATP molecules/glucose) or oxidative phosphorylation (which yields 38 ATP/glucose). Adult and developing (especially infant) brain tissues react differently to ischemic and hypoxic insults. Infants tend to be more resistant to hypoxia than adults, and hypoxic-ischemic lesions within the pediatric age group have a different distribution.

A. Clinical Features of Hypoxic Brain Damage

Hypoxic brain damage may occur in a hospital setting or "in the field." Clinical recovery is generally more optimal from hypoxemic hypoxia than ischemia; examples have been reported of excellent recovery from acute severe hypoxia so long as cardiac output was maintained. The long-term consequences of transient cerebral ischemia depend on factors such as the duration and completeness of the insult, blood glucose levels (elevated levels lead to a worse outcome), and CNS temperature (lower temperatures tend to be protective for the brain). Clinically, long-term sequelae may be difficult to gauge or predict in a given patient; careful patient observation over days or weeks following the insult is mandatory. It is known that the outcome from a comatose state after hypoxic brain damage, e.g., that which follows cardiac arrest, can be relatively good if pupillary light flexes, extraocular movements, and some response to pain are preserved during the initial neurologic examination while the patient is in the comatose state. Common clinical settings for hypoxic brain damage include events such as near drowning or respiratory arrest (which induces *hypoxemic* hypoxia), cardiac arrest with prolonged asystole or hypotension after a myocardial infarct or with major arrhythmia (which leads to *stagnant* hypoxia), exposure to chemicals such as cyanide, sulfide or CO (*histotoxic* hypoxia), and decompression sickness which results from nitrogen bubbles producing microinfarcts (e.g., in the spinal cord) when this gas comes out of solution following rapid decompression after an individual has dived to great depths. Anoxic-ischemic encephalopathy and head trauma are the commonest causes of the persistent vegetative state (PVS).

B. Neuropathologic Features

Despite the relatively (and somewhat artificially) straightforward clinical stratification of syndromes described above, gross and even microscopic features are extremely variable among patients who have suffered anoxic-ischemic insults. Lesions can, however, be considered acute/subacute or chronic. The gross characteristics of acute or subacute injury include a range of abnormalities from precursors of cystic infarct (e.g., in the watershed territories) to cortical laminar necrosis, to multifocal patchy gray discoloration of the cortex with blurring of

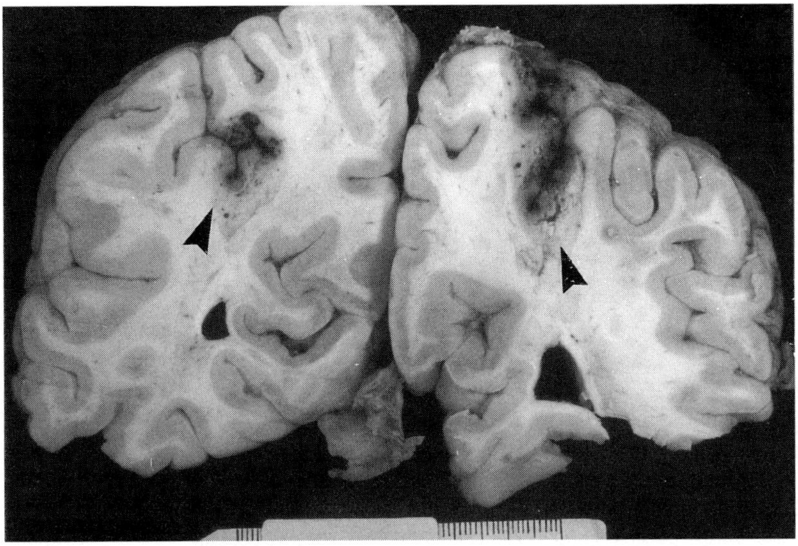

Figure 1 Watershed/borderzone infarcts in the parietal lobes. Regions of necrosis (arrows) are seen bilaterally in the ACA/MCA borderzone regions. Though different in size, both infarcts show a significant hemorrhagic component, probably resulting from reflow into a region of cortical necrosis. Patient had undergone orthotopic heart transplant with a stormy postoperative course that included sepsis and hypotensive episodes.

the cortex-white matter junction (i.e., appearances that resemble subacute infarct), to the appearance of "nonperfused brain," previously known inappropriately as "respirator brain." In the latter, the brain essentially begins to undergo autolysis and "softening" while in the cranial cavity. Indeed, no gross abnormality may be appreciated. In chronic anoxic-ischemic encephalopathy, gross findings in the affected brain may be relatively minimal, or might include one or more of the following: watershed infarcts (Fig. 1), cortical laminar necrosis (Fig. 2), or variable atrophy in the affected regions of cortex (Fig. 3). Most patients who have been in a PVS or coma will show some gross abnormalities (usually of this form) at the time of brain cutting. In the case of CO poisoning, there is characteristic cystic necrosis (usually symmetrical) of the globus pallidus, though this pattern is also occasionally noted without well documented CO exposure (Fig. 4). If there has been severe involvement of the hippocampus or cerebellar cortex (both regions vulnerable to hypoxia; see below), hippocampal (Fig. 5) or cerebellar atrophy may ensue.

Microscopic features of acute or subacute anoxic-ischemic encephalopathy include ischemic neuronal change, i.e., brightly eosinophilic neuronal cell

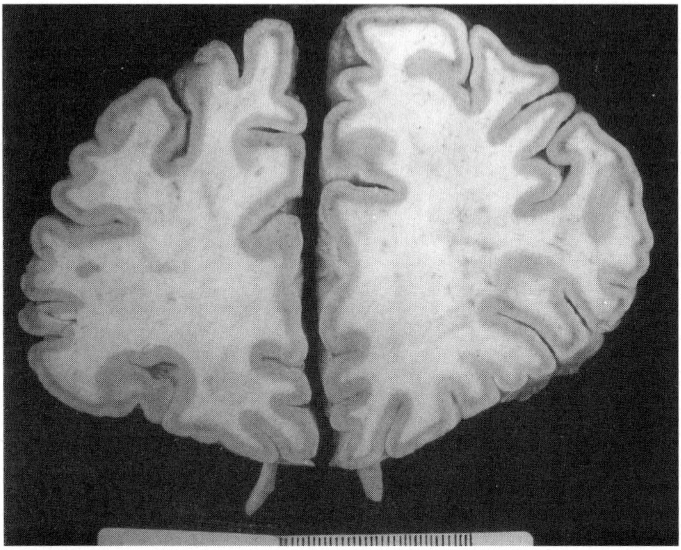

(A)

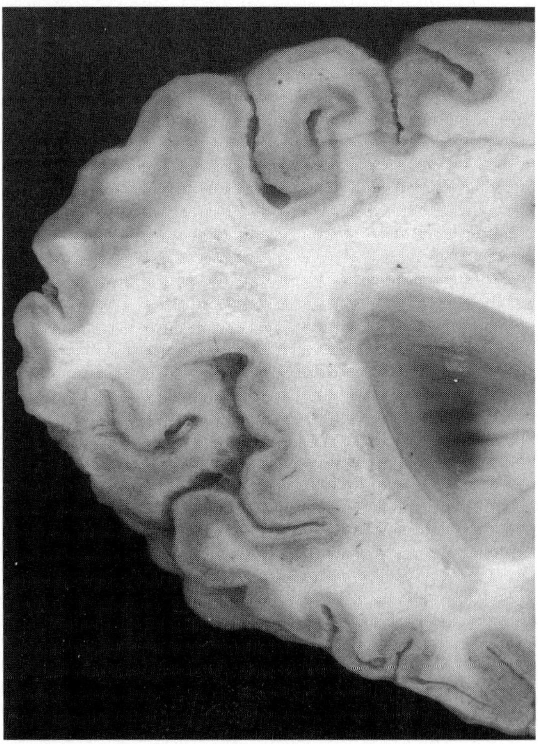

(B)

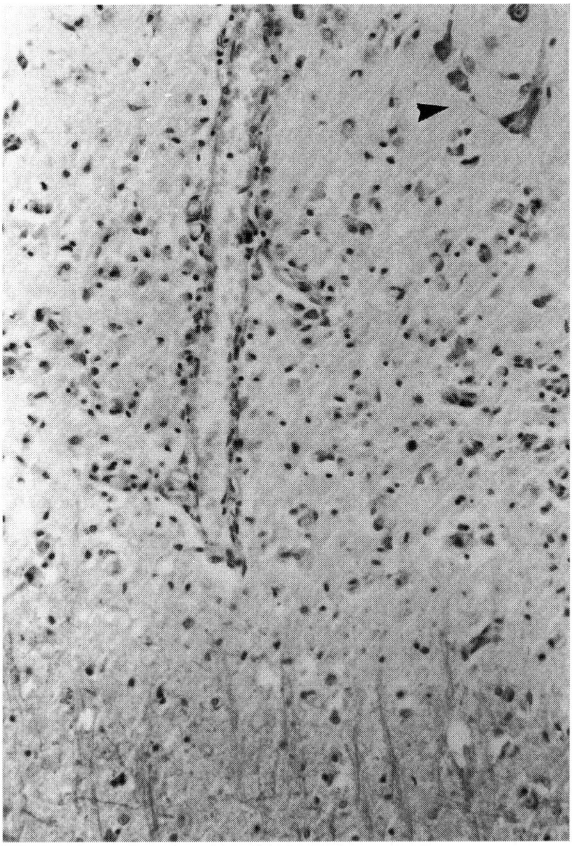

(C)

Figure 2 Cortical laminar necrosis. (**A,B**) Characteristic dark linear region of discoloration in a patchy distribution within deep cortex or at cortex–white matter junction, representing necrosis in these cortical layers. (**C**) Microscopic features of a subacute case, including increased cellularity (macrophages) in the deep cortex; note intact neurons (arrowhead) in the more superficial cortex. White matter is at bottom of the micrograph.

bodies with pyknotic nuclei, especially in anoxia-sensitive regions such as the cerebellar Purkinje cells (Fig. 6). Normal neurons may be seen adjacent to severely affected cell bodies, presumably reflecting differential susceptibility to anoxia. Corresponding ultrastructural features (most commonly observed in animal models of anoxic-ischemic encephalopathy) include those of cellular necrosis, with breaks in the nuclear and cell membranes and flocculent densities within mitochondria.

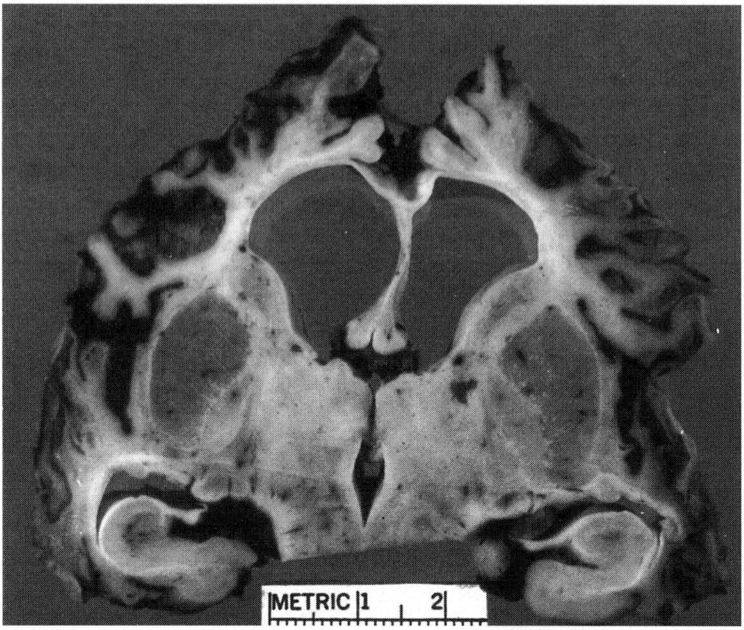

Figure 3 Chronic sequelae of anoxic-ischemic encephalopathy in an infant brain. Note profound cortical atrophy with mushroom-shaped gyri ("ulegyria"; see also Chap. 7). Ventriculomegaly is the result of profound loss of brain substance (hydrocephalus ***ex vacuo***). There is striking ***relative*** preservation of the hippocampi.

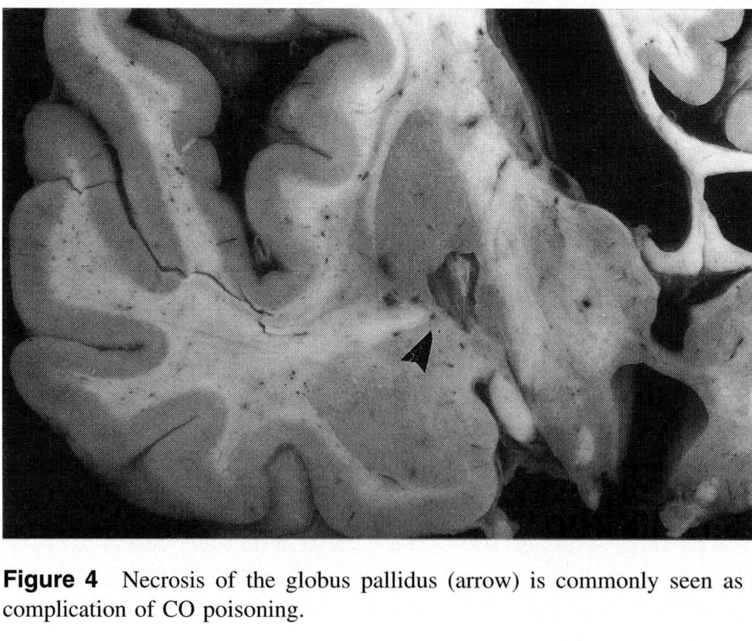

Figure 4 Necrosis of the globus pallidus (arrow) is commonly seen as a long-term complication of CO poisoning.

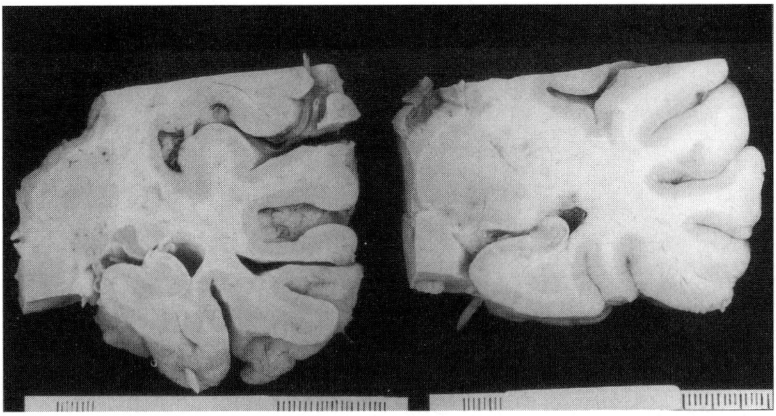

Figure 5 Relatively normal hippocampus (at left, coronal level of the lateral geniculate nucleus) compared to a severely atrophic hippocampus (at right) in a patient with a long history of alcoholic pancreatitis complicated by bowel obstruction and complex abdominal surgeries. The hippocampal atrophy was probably secondary to anoxia, though the precise causal "anoxic" incident could not be identified.

In chronic anoxic-ischemic encephalopathy, watershed infarcts (with typical appearances of cystic infarcts, to be described below) may be observed. Laminar necrosis usually affects the middle or deep cortical layers, though in extreme instances there may be pan-cortical necrosis rather than a laminar pattern (Fig. 2), a change that is accentuated in watershed/border zone arterial territories. In some regions, long-term anoxic-ischemic change may simply appear as focal neuron loss with pronounced reactive astrocytic gliosis. This appearance is particularly dramatic in the hippocampus, where certain regions of the pyramidal cell layer (e.g., the CA1 sector) show vulnerability to anoxic injury while others (CA2) are resistant (Fig. 7). A histologic distinction is often made between infarct and selective neuronal necrosis; in the latter, with the passage of time, neurons disappear with attendant astrocytic gliosis, while in the former, all cellular elements die and macrophages infiltrate the affected region of brain to remove cellular debris and residual neuropil. In practical terms, the two processes may be difficult to differentiate long after the inciting insult has occurred, though cystic change/encephalomalacia is clearly more common with ischemic infarcts.

Neuron loss may occur days after a global ischemic insult—i.e., the phenomenon of delayed neuronal death. This is particularly well documented in the hippocampus. *Nonperfused* (previously referred to as "respirator") *brain* gives an appearance of autolysis, with pale staining of the neuropil and neu-

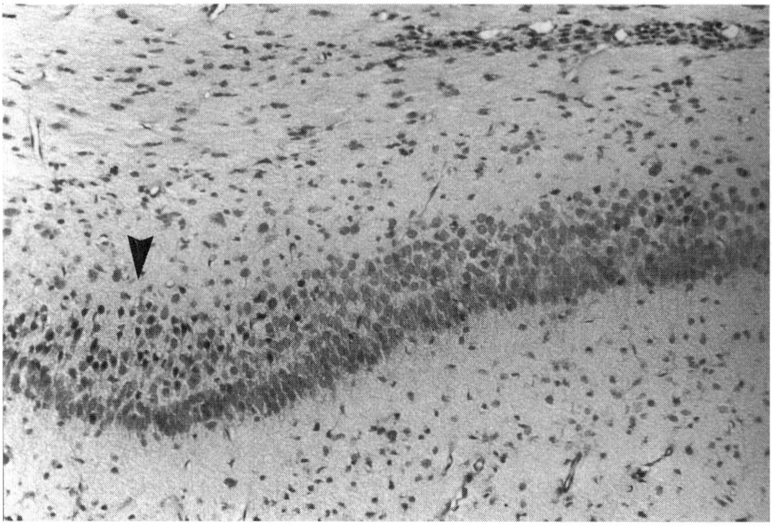

(A)

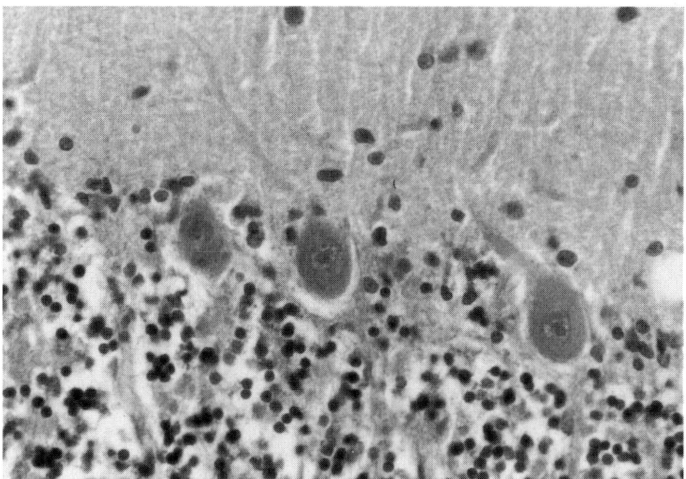

(B)

Figure 6 Hypoxic-ischemic neuronal change. (**A**) Hippocampus in a rat which was rendered acutely hypoxic. Arrow indicates dark pyknotic neurons in a field of otherwise intact and normal-appearing granule cell neurons. (**B**) Normal-appearing Purkinje cells, contrasted with (**C**) an acutely "anoxic" Purkinje cell (which was brightly eosinophilic) with pyknotic nucleus.

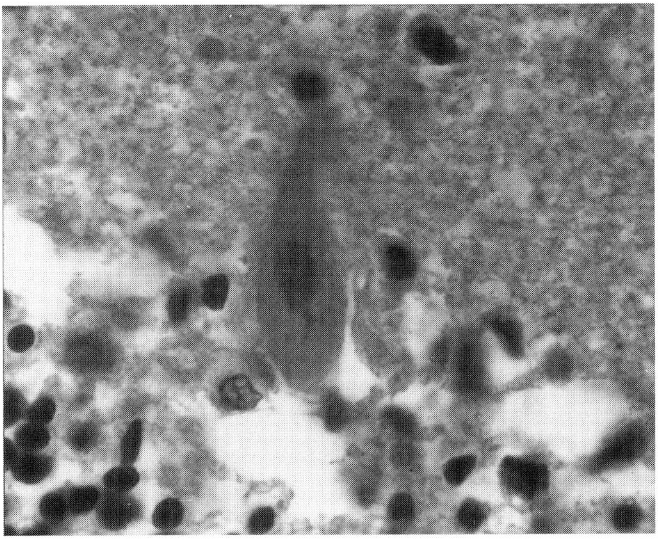

(C)

Figure 6 Continued

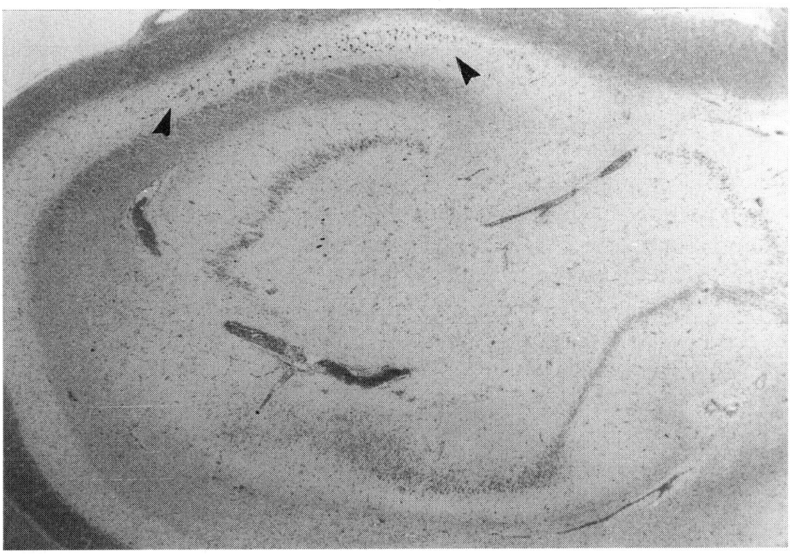

Figure 7 "Selective" neuronal necrosis in the hippocampus (hippocampal sclerosis) after anoxic-ischemic encephalopathy. Note preservation of the **CA2** neurons (indicated by arrowheads), with essentially total absence (disappearance) of cells in other portions of the pyramidal cell layer.

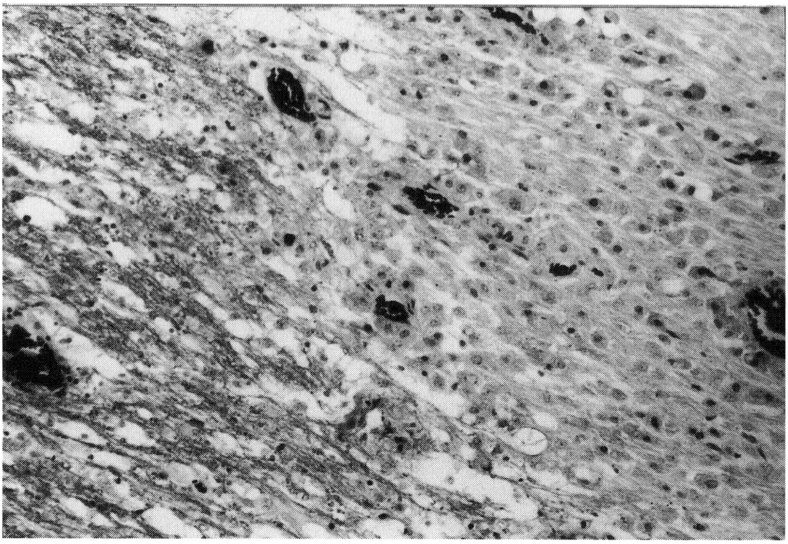

Figure 8 Rarely, white-matter tracts are affected by anoxic-ischemic encephalopathy, as in this case of a patient who developed severe neurologic dysfunction following complex vascular surgery (see also Chap. 5). Several white-matter tracts showed well-demarcated necrotic foci with abundant lesional histiocytes/gitter cells (at right), as illustrated in this micrograph from affected region in the corpus callosum. Preserved white matter is at left.

ronal cell bodies but an absence of inflammatory cell or macrophage infiltration. With nonperfused brain, anterior pituitary necrosis is common, and because severe brain edema has occurred (intracranial pressure exceeds cerebral perfusion pressure; hence the term nonperfused), there may be fragmentation of the cerebellum, cerebellar fragments being identified in the subarachnoid space surrounding the spinal cord. The morphoanatomic correlates of PVS include diffuse cortical injury, selective thalamic necrosis with restricted or multifocal cortical lesions, "anoxic *leuko*encephalopathy" (Fig. 8), a decidedly rare occurrence, or changes that are secondary to superimposed disease including seizures, the effects of infection, or medications.

C. Concepts of Selective Vulnerability and Excitotoxicity

These are fundamental to understanding anoxic-ischemic change within the brain. "Selective vulnerability" refers to the finding of regions of CNS that are especially likely to show injury after an anoxic-ischemic event. The most vulnerable regions in adult brain include cerebral and cerebellar cortex, hippocampus, thalamus, brainstem, hypothalamus, and spinal cord (in roughly descending order of susceptibility). In premature and term infants, the cortex is relatively *resistant* to anoxia while the brainstem and thalamus are more susceptible (see also Chap. 7). *Glutamate* receptor densities may, at least in part, explain why some neurons are more susceptible than others to anoxia-glutamate acts as an excitotoxic neurotransmitter upon a variety of receptor subtypes. "Excitotoxicity" is increasingly implicated in a variety of *chronic* neurodegenerative conditions as well. A discussion of determinants of selective vulnerability to neuronal necrosis (including excitotoxicity) is beyond the scope of this text but is covered in several excellent reviews (e.g., see Whetsell, 1996).

II. CEREBRAL/ENCEPHALIC INFARCTS

Infarcts are to be distinguished from focal or generalized anoxic-ischemic encephalopathy, which primarily affects neurons (see above), and from intracranial hemorrhage (see below). An infarct is defined as *a region of brain tissue in which all cellular elements undergo death or necrosis, usually as a consequence of the cessation of flow of oxygenated blood to this region.* The distinction between cerebral hemorrhage and infarct may not always be straightforward. Infarcts may become secondarily hemorrhagic and may thus mimic primary cerebral hemorrhage on both neuroimaging studies or at the time of brain cutting. Pathogenetic mechanisms, however, are usually quite distinct though risk factors that predispose to brain infarct (such as longstanding hypertension) also predispose to encephalic hemorrhage. The clinical term "stroke" describes a syndrome of *rapidly evolving or sudden onset, nonconvulsive, partly or completely irreversible neurologic deficit*, not a distinct clinicopathologic entity. For example, a stroke syndrome may be the presenting feature of a rapidly growing brain tumor or intracranial infection. By convention, however, the term stroke has come to describe either cerebral hemorrhage or infarct, and it will so be used in the ensuing discussion. Infarcts can be envisioned as resulting from *macrovascular* (large vessel arterial) disease, *microvascular* (small vessel arterial) disease, *emboli*, or *venous thrombosis*.

III. EPIDEMIOLOGY

Stroke in its various forms is a massive clinical problem, there being as many as 700,000 new strokes annually in the U.S. The American population also includes almost 3 million survivors of stroke, which is nationally the third most common cause of mortality, resulting in approximately 150,000 deaths per year. The incidence of stroke increases tremendously with age, from approximately 100/100,000 at age 45 to 54, to over 1,800/100,000 among individuals above the age of 85. Between 1979 and 1989, a declining mortality from stroke was observed together with declining mortality from other forms of cardiovascular disease, including coronary artery disease. Leading modifiable risk factors for stroke include cardiac disease, hypertension, diabetes, and cigarette smoking; less common risk factors include the use of oral contraceptives, various hematologic diseases, and cardiac valvular disease. Depending on the series of patients studied, *cerebral infarct* is approximately seven to 10 times more common than *intracerebral hemorrhage*, which in turn has approximately the same frequency as subarachnoid hemorrhage within the U.S. By contrast, some European (and virtually all Japanese) studies show a much higher relative incidence of intracerebral hemorrhage.

A. Arterial Disease

1. Large-Vessel Arteriopathy

a. Atherosclerosis. This is by far the leading systemic vasculopathy that produces cerebral infarcts, especially in elderly patients. Atherosclerosis may affect intracranial and/or extracranial large arteries. For excellent reviews of the pathogenesis and epidemiology of atherosclerosis and its impact on the brain, see Ross (1993) and the book edited by Barnett et al. (1992).

i. Clinical Features: Patients who have ischemic stroke related to atherosclerotic cerebrovascular disease usually have well-documented risk factors for (including a family history of) atherosclerosis, often premature atherosclerosis. The usual presentation is of a transient ischemic attack (TIA), i.e., a focal neurologic deficit that eventually (usually within 48 hours) resolves, the ischemic episode being referrable to the region of brain subserved by the vessel involved by severe atheroma. As an example, an atheromatous plaque which has become ulcerated in the right internal carotid artery (ICA) may produce transient right monocular blindness and left hemiparesis, while a symptomatic vertebral artery plaque may cause transient dizziness, vertigo, ataxia, and cranial nerve dysfunction. Patients who experience such TIAs are at high risk for developing a complete, or irreversible, stroke. Documentation of the location and severity of atheromatous plaques is by cerebral angiography, while CT or MRI scanning may be used to determine whether a completed infarct has occurred. The pathogenesis of cerebral ischemia is usually related to *hypoperfusion* secondary to an occlusive or severely stenotic (mural) thrombus, or an *artery-to-artery embolus* of platelet-fibrin material that has developed at the nidus of intimal ulceration, or of atheromatous material itself.

ii. Neuropathologic Features: A complete postmortem examination in a patient with stroke should include examination of the carotid and vertebral arteries throughout their full extent, which is more practically achieved for the carotid than the vertebral arteries. Atherosclerosis should be documented, if possible, by histologic sections of involved arteries. Atherosclerosis involving

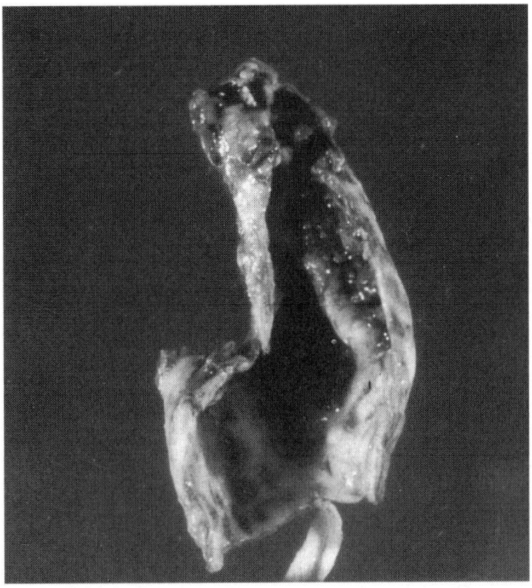

(A)

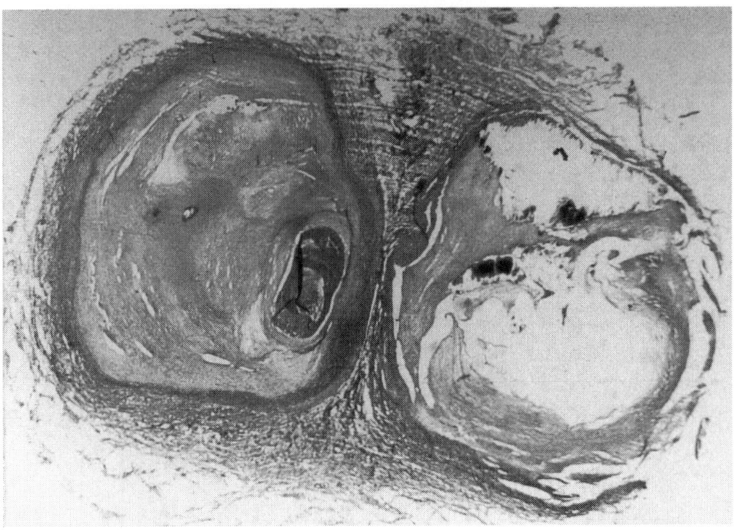

(B)

Figure 9 (**A**) Severe atherosclerosis at (common) carotid bifurcation. In this endarterectomy specimen, which has been "opened," common carotid a. atheromatous plaque is at bottom of the photograph, ICA at top. (**B**) Cross section at carotid bifurcation (autopsy specimen) shows severe atherosclerotic stenosis, with small residual lumen in branch at left, and severe calcified fractured atheroma in the branch at right.

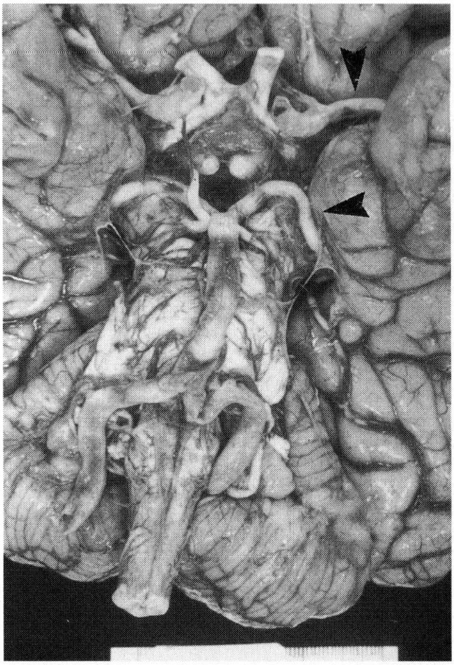

(A)

Figure 10 (A) Atherosclerosis of major branches of the circle of Willis; note especially pronounced involvement of the left PCA and MCA (arrowheads). (B) Severely atherosclerotic circle of Willis dissected free of the base of the brain.

the cerebral or *extracranial* feeding vessels is most often severe at the origins of the vertebral arteries, the carotid bifurcation (Fig. 9), and basilar artery, while *intracranial* atherosclerosis is usually most pronounced in major branches of the circle of Willis. The extent and topography of basal atherosclerosis is often best documented by removing the affected circle of Willis (and taking appropriate histologic sections) from the base of the brain (Fig. 10).

Microscopic features of atheroma (Fig. 11) are best demonstrated with stains that differentiate the various cellular elements present within atherosclerotic plaque, e.g. elastica van Gieson, or immunohistochemistry using primary antibodies to basement membrane elements or vascular smooth muscle actin. Complicated atheroma (usually the type that becomes clinically symptomatic) shows cholesterol clefts or foamy macrophages and evidence of old hemorrhage within the plaque itself, which may be calcified. Significant compromise of the vessel lumen may be present, often with ulceration and overlying mural or

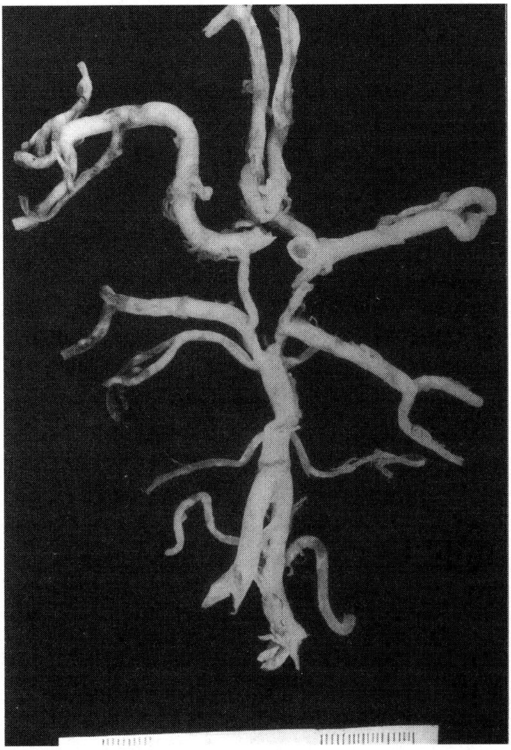

(B)

occlusive thrombus. The arterial circulation distal to a region of atherosclerotic stenosis or ulceration may show atherosclerotic change itself, sometimes extending into leptomeningeal arteries, or platelet-fibrin or atheromatous emboli (Fig. 12).

b. Fibromuscular Dysplasia (FMD). Compared to atherosclerosis, FMD is an extremely rare cause of ischemic stroke, but is particularly prone to occur in younger patients. By definition, it is an *idiopathic systemic vasculopathy characterized by nonatherosclerotic abnormalities of smooth muscle, fibrous and elastic tissue in small and medium-size arteries*. More common in women than men, it becomes symptomatic between the ages of 30 and 50. Its cellular pathogenesis is unknown, but FMD is associated with miscellaneous connective tissue disorders and α_1-antitrypsin deficiency. It is more often a radiographic than a pathologic diagnosis. FMD of the renal arteries is more common than

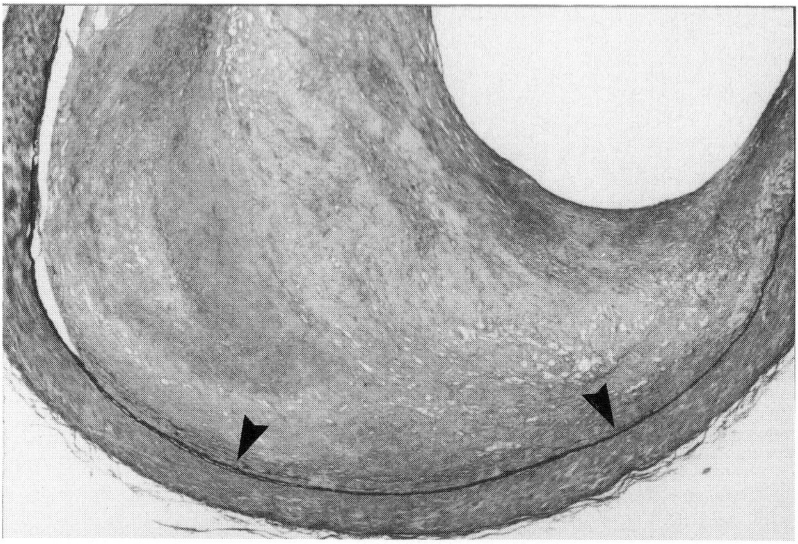

(A)

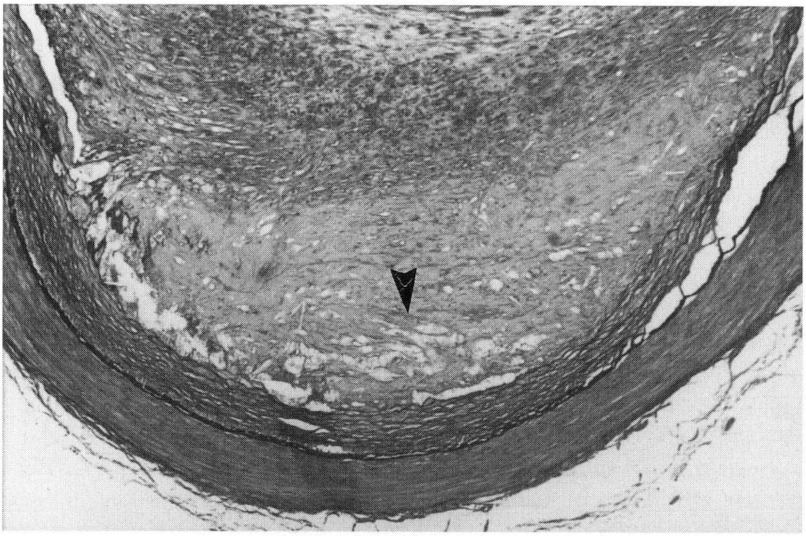

(B)

Figure 11 Sections of major branches of the Circle of Willis, including posterior cerebral artery (PCA, panel **A**) and left middle cerebral artery (MCA, panel **B**). Both sections, stained with a technique that highlights elastica (arrows, panel A), show pronounced eccentric intimal fibromuscular hyperplasia with stenosis of the lumen in each case. In panel B, cleftlike spaces may represent residual foci of cholesterol deposition; arrowhead indicates foamy histiocytes.

that involving the cephalic vessels, though 25% of FMD patients apparently show involvement of vessels feeding the brain, and cerebral arteries are the second most likely (after renal vasculature) to be affected. Among these vessels, the carotid arteries are much more commonly affected than the vertebral, with bilateral carotid artery involvement noted in over 50% of affected patients. Vessel wall involvement is usually medial (in over 90% of cases) or intimal (5% of cases)—very rarely adventitial. FMD may lead to ischemic cerebral infarcts secondary to vascular stenosis or (rarely) occlusion, and may also result in *arterial dissection* in the neck.

Pathologically, FMD is easily distinguishable from atherosclerosis (Fig. 13) by the absence of features of complicated atherosclerosis (see above) and the existence of smooth muscle cell hyperplasia or thinning, and destruction of the elastica, with fibrosis and general disorganization of the arterial wall components. Inflammation is usually negligible.

c. Moyamoya Disease. This is a rare condition that presents with idiopathic progressive stenosis and eventual occlusion of the basal intracranial arteries, with compensatory dilatation of the lenticulostriate arteries, giving a characteristic "misty" appearance or "blush" on cerebral angiography. The resultant or causal thrombotic lesions in the circle of Willis implicate abnormal thrombogenesis in the pathogenesis of this disorder; i.e., regions of intimal thickening may represent organizing thrombi. Initially identified in Japan, this disorder is now well documented in many other populations throughout the world. Presentation is with subarachnoid or intraparenchymal hemorrhage, cerebral infarct or TIA, seizures, or combined symptoms. The disorder may present in children or adults.

Pathologic features of the vasculature include thrombotic lesions throughout major branches of the circle of Willis in over half of affected patients. Most commonly involved vessels are the ICA, posterior communicating artery and the PCA. Microscopic features (Fig. 14) are those of severely stenotic, noncomplicated atherosclerosis with intimal fibromuscular hyperplasia but negligible inflammation, lipid deposition, or disruption of the elastica. Platelet-fibrin thrombi are often seen at the intimal surface.

d. Arterial Dissection. This rare entity affects women more commonly than men with vertebrobasilar involvement, but men more commonly than women with carotid involvement. Dissection may be of *intra*cranial or *extra*cranial arteries, and may involve any of the great vessels. Dissection may even occur simultaneously in several segments of an affected vessel, and appears to result from endothelial or intimal tears. Intramural hematoma in the vessel wall that results from dissection can be subendothelial (most commonly carotid) or medial (usually vertebral). The result of dissection is occlusion of the lumen with resultant ischemic infarct distally. Less commonly, dissection may extend to the

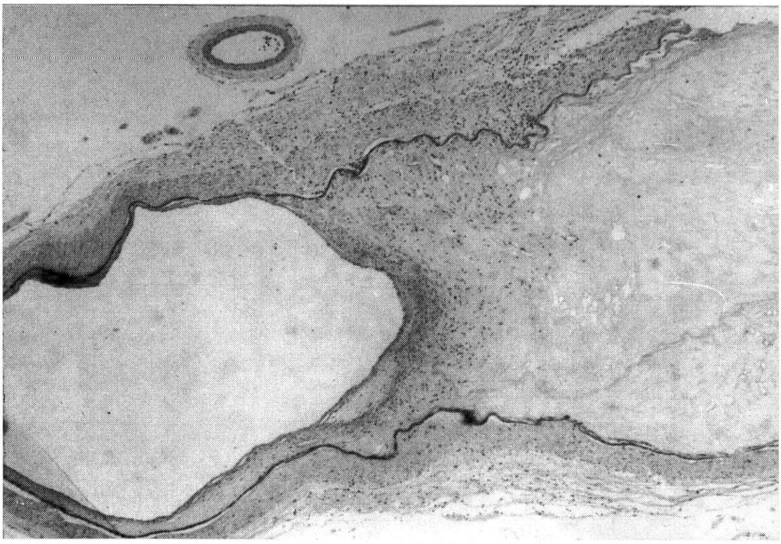

(A)

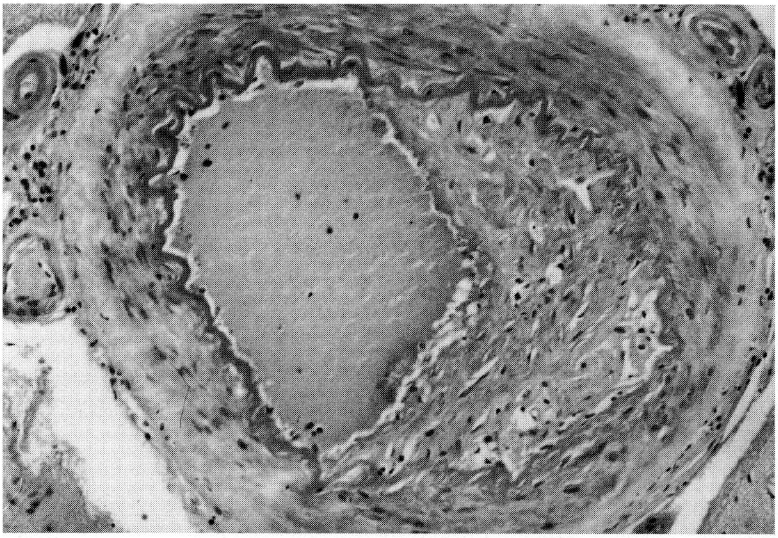

(B)

Figure 12 Atherosclerotic change in "distal" leptomeningeal branches of the circle of Willis, including **(A)** PCA adjacent to the hippocampus, and **(B,C)** superficial meningeal branches in another patient, (B) stained with H&E, (C) with a technique to demonstrate elastica. In each instance, note marked eccentric intimal (fibromuscular) hyperplasia superficial to the elastica.

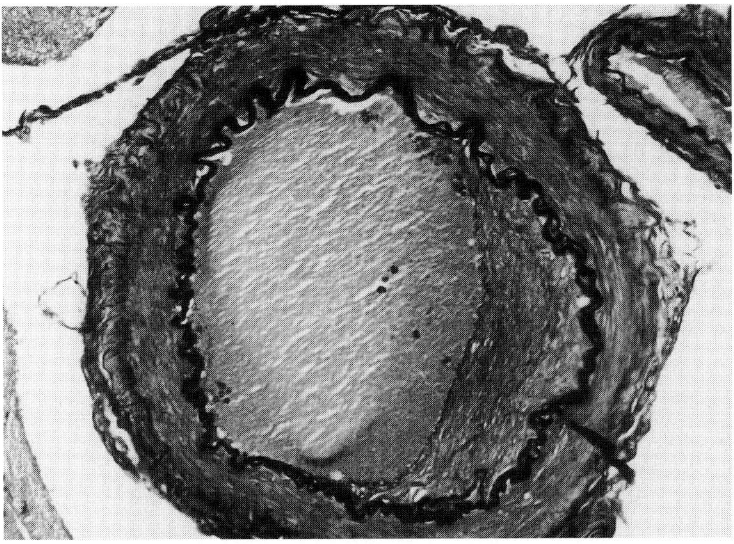

(C)

adventitia of an artery, resulting in subarachnoid hemorrhage. Etiologic factors are poorly defined but may include FMD, migraine, hypertension, "cystic medial necrosis," or even atherosclerosis.

Neuropathologic features include subarachnoid hemorrhage or ischemic infarct within the brain. Microscopically, the locus of dissection must be documented by complete examination of the intracranial and extracranial carotid and vertebral arteries, in one or more of which there will be an appearance of a subendothelial or intramural hematoma within the vessel wall (Fig. 15), usually acute, since survival with this arteriopathy is usually poor.

e. HIV-Associated Arteriopathies. These are among the more unusual complications of HIV infection, at least in adults. When stroke occurs in an AIDS/HIV-infected patient, its precise etiology may be difficult to define; i.e., many opportunistic infections frequently seen in AIDS patients may cause, contribute to, or even mimic cerebrovascular disease. However, as many as 5% to 10% of AIDS patients who come to autopsy may show evidence of significant cerebrovascular disease. In an AIDS patient who develops acute arterial occlusion causing a stroke, nonbacterial thrombotic (marantic) endocarditis (NBTE) must be considered and sought clinically at autopsy. Rarely, chronic basal meningitis and angiitis may result in cerebral ischemia. Cerebrovascular disease related to HIV infection is more common in children, almost one-quarter of whom may have evidence of cerebral hemorrhage or infarct.

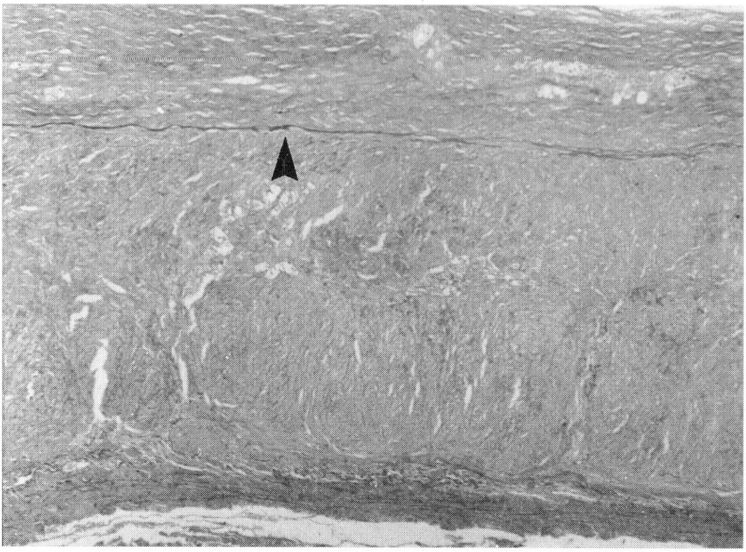

(A)

Figure 13 FMD associated with an extracranial ICA aneurysm. Attenuated internal elastic lamina is indicated by arrowhead **(A).** Note thickening of the vascular media with disorganized proliferation of fibromuscular elements. **(B)** Magnified view of one region; arrowhead indicates internal elastic lamina. (For details, see Miyauchi, Shionoya. **Eur J Vasc Surg** 1991; 5:587; case studied by courtesy of Drs. Miyauchi and Shionoya, Nagoya, Japan.)

The neuropathologic features of HIV-associated stroke are as varied as the neuropathologic spectrum of HIV-1 effects themselves. A characteristic HIV-associated arteriopathy is seen rarely, with intimal fibromuscular hyperplasia and aneurysmal dilatation of vessel walls in association with fragmentation or disruption of the internal elastic lamina, appearances consistent with healed arteritis (Fig. 16). HIV-infected cells—probably macrophages—have been found within affected arterial walls.

f. Cerebrovascular Disease Associated with Antiphospholipid Antibodies. Since the mid-1980s, there has been a growing interest in and documentation of antibodies that bind to phospholipids (aPLs), a phenomenon that is associated with various thromboembolic syndromes including recurrent venous and arterial thrombosis. The unique neuropathologic features of resultant ischemic infarct in the brain are poorly documented. However, an antiphospholipid syndrome must be suspected *clinically* in any young patient who develops an ischemic cerebral infarct.

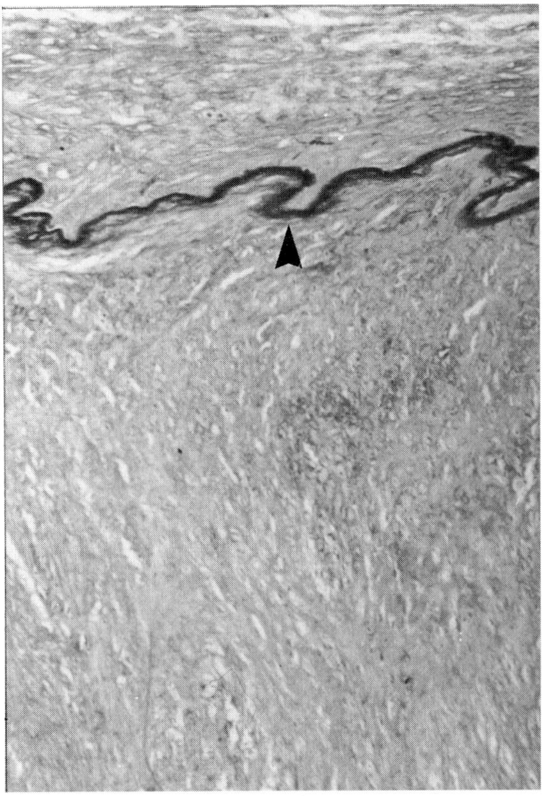

(B)

2. *Vasculitis/Angiitis Affecting Large Arteries*

Only two entities are of importance in this category, as follows:

a. Temporal Arteritis/Giant Cell Arteritis. The annual incidence of this condition is as high as 15 to 20/100,000 individuals over the age of 50 years. "Temporal arteritis" is somewhat of a misnomer, since this entity involves large and medium-size arteries and may affect the aorta, coronary arteries, or vessels supplying the brain. Its etiology is not fully understood, but it may represent an anomalous giant cell or granulomatous inflammatory response to the elastic component of arterial walls or another "inciting" vessel wall component. It may be related to Takayasu's arteritis and to primary CNS angiitis (see below). It occurs predominantly in elderly patients (over age 50) and often presents in the context of a systemic illness with generalized complaints of fever, malaise, weakness, and limb pain and tenderness. It is associated with polymyalgia rheu-

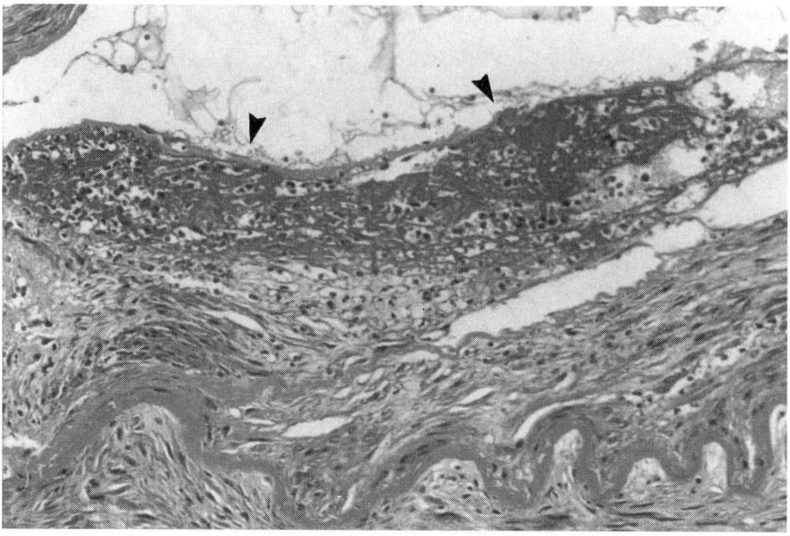

(A)

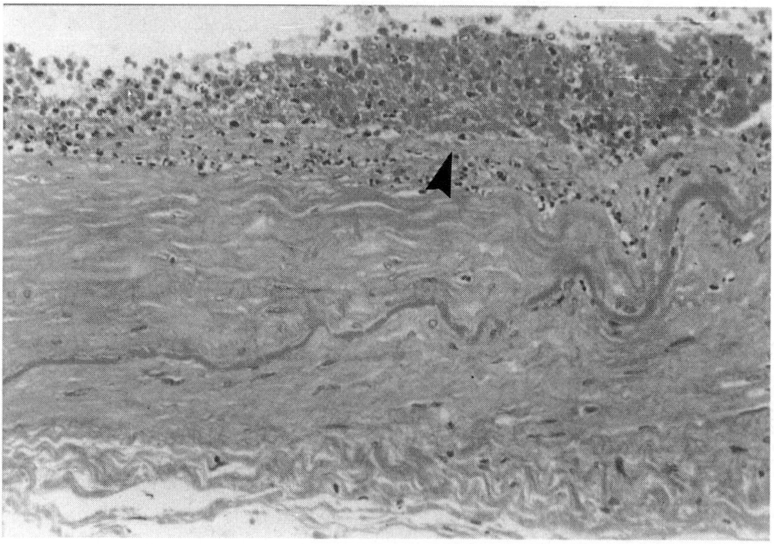

(B)

Figure 14 Moyamoya disease. Two different arterial lesions. Both show intimal fibrous thickening with platelet-fibrin thrombi at various stages of organization (arrows) at the luminal surface. (Micrographs generously provided by Drs. E. Ikeda and Y. Hosoda, Tokyo, Japan. For details, see Ikeda, Hosoda. **Clin Neuropathol** 1993; 12:44; micrographs reproduced with permission.)

matica. Headache and visual complaints are particularly common when the temporal artery is involved. A temporal artery biopsy may be diagnostic, but the presence of "skip lesions" within an affected artery means that a negative result in a segmental biopsy does not rule out the disease, and step cuts must often be made through the artery to document the presence of the arteritis. End-organ effects may include cerebral infarct. Neuropathologic features (Fig. 17) include widespread granulomatous inflammation of arterial walls, including especially the coronaries, aorta, carotid, and vertebral arteries, as well as their major branches. Fragments of elastica may be seen within the cytoplasm of multinucleated giant cells.

b. Aortic Arch Syndrome/Takayasu's Arteritis. This very rare disease of the aorta affects its main branches, including the cervical carotid arteries. Granulomatous inflammation is seen in the aortic wall with resultant scarring and destruction.

3. Arteriopathy Affecting Small Vessels (Microangiopathy)

The main noninflammatory components of this group, which usually (though not exclusively) affects small arteries (those less than 250 to 300 μm in cross-sectional diameter), include *arteriosclerosis/arteriolosclerosis*, *lipohyalinosis* (closely linked to arteriolosclerosis), and *congophilic/amyloid angiopathy* (CAA). Because these entities are more commonly associated with cerebral hemorrhage, they will be considered in the discussion of encephalic bleeds, to be found below.

a. Small-Vessel Angiitis/Vasculitis. Patients who experience ischemic infarcts or cerebral hemorrhages as a result of vasculitis usually have systemic as well as neurologic symptoms, so their presentation is distinct from stroke associated with nonvasculitic causes. Because of this, the differential diagnosis may be confusing; i.e., signs and symptoms may be masked as part of a clinical picture of multiorgan disease. This group of relatively unusual diseases can be subdivided into:

i. Those That Involve the CNS Exclusively—i.e., Primary Angiitis of the CNS (PACNS): Most cases of PACNS occur in older adults, men more commonly than women. The microvascular lesions show histopathologic similarities to *systemic* giant cell arteritis, with widespread granulomatous inflammation of vessel walls (within both leptomeninges and brain parenchyma) including branches of the circle of Willis (i.e., the disorder is not exclusively a microangiopathy). The presence of giant cells within vessel walls suggests that cell-mediated immune mechanisms are important in its pathogenesis. Fibrinoid necrosis of arterial walls is common. PACNS is probably multifactorial in origin, an unusual response to autoantigens, viral infection (varicella zoster has been implicated), or immune complexes. Rare examples of severe granulomatous inflammation have been identified in association with extensive CAA (Fig. 18).

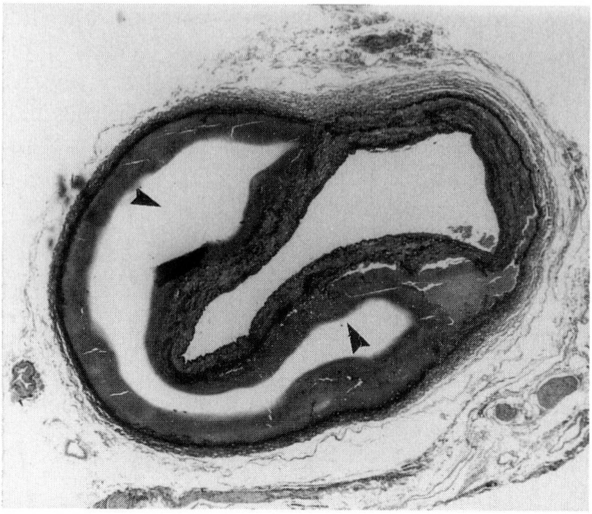

(A)

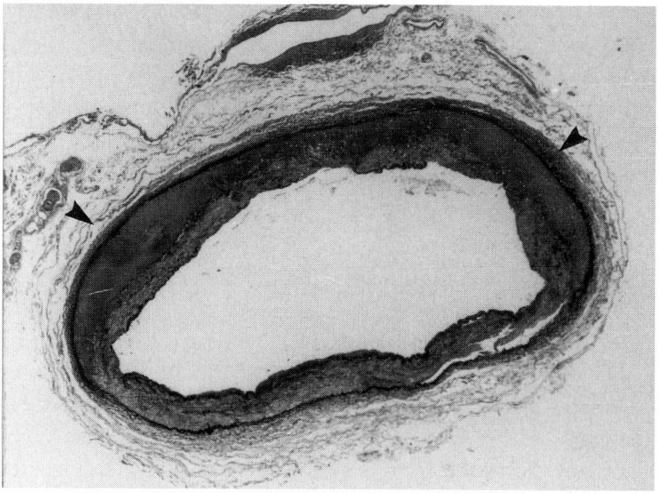

(B)

Figure 15 Arterial dissection. Vertebral a. dissection following chiropractic manipulation of the neck. Note variable degrees of medial dissection at two different levels of the artery, which has been stained with a technique to highlight elastica. In panels **A** and **B,** arrows indicate blood that has tracked into the arterial media. Panel **C** shows detail of the medial dissection.

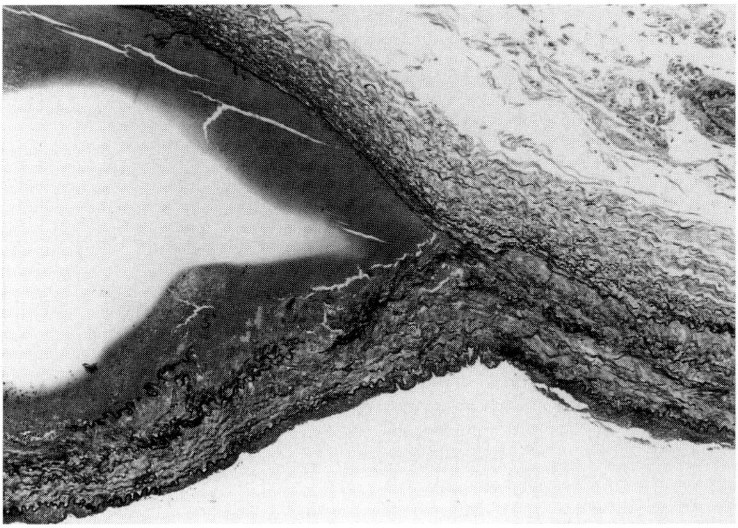

(C)

ii. Microvascular Angiitis/Vasculitis Occurring as Part of Systemic Vasculitis: Clinical presentation of these disorders may be extremely heterogeneous, but it usually includes a component of diffuse cortical dysfunction, encephalopathy, behavioral change, and seizures. The most important clinicopathologic entities are as follows:

1. Polyarteritis/periarteritis (PAN) nodosa. 20% to 40% of patients show CNS involvement in the context of a systemic necrotizing angiitis.
2. Allergic angiitis and granulomatosis (Churg-Strauss).
3. Hypersensitivity angiltis. 10% show CNS involvement.
4. Wegener's granulomatosis. 20% to 50% show CNS involvement (Fig. 19).
5. Lymphomatoid granulomatosis. 10% to 15% show CNS involvement. This is a controversial entity that appears to link vasculitis with primary CNS lymphoma (Fig. 20).

4. Microvasculopathy Associated with Dementia

a. Binswanger's Subcortical Arteriosclerotic Leukoencephalopathy (BSL). This controversial entity was first described over 100 years ago and appears to be a white-matter abnormality found most commonly in elderly hypertensive patients in association with dementia. Multiple pathogenetic factors have been implicated in its causation (including ischemia, hypoxia, and watershed infarct).

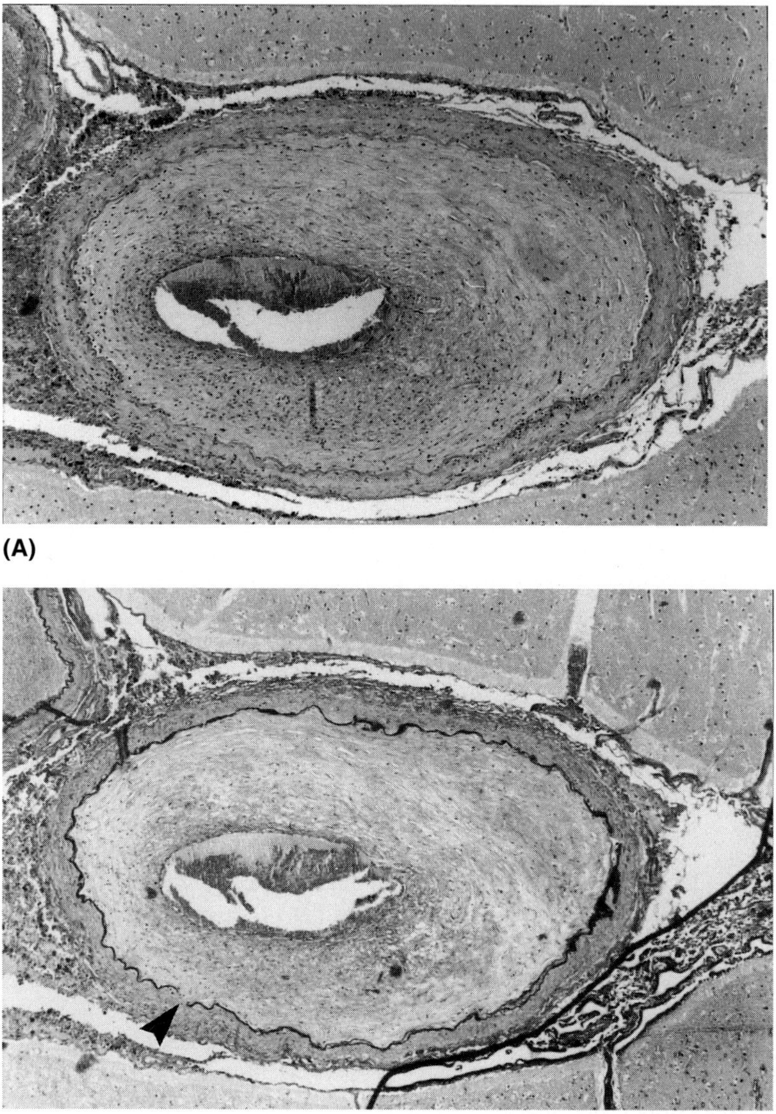

(A)

(B)

Figure 16 HIV-associated arteriopathy. The patient had experienced cerebral hemorrhage. **Panel A** stained with H&E; **panel B** with a stain to highlight elastica. Note pronounced eccentric intimal hyperplasia (i.e., superficial to the elastica), with focal discontinuities in the elastica (arrow, panel B) and elsewhere slight reduplication. No opportunistic viral/fungal pathogen could be demonstrated within the arterial wall.

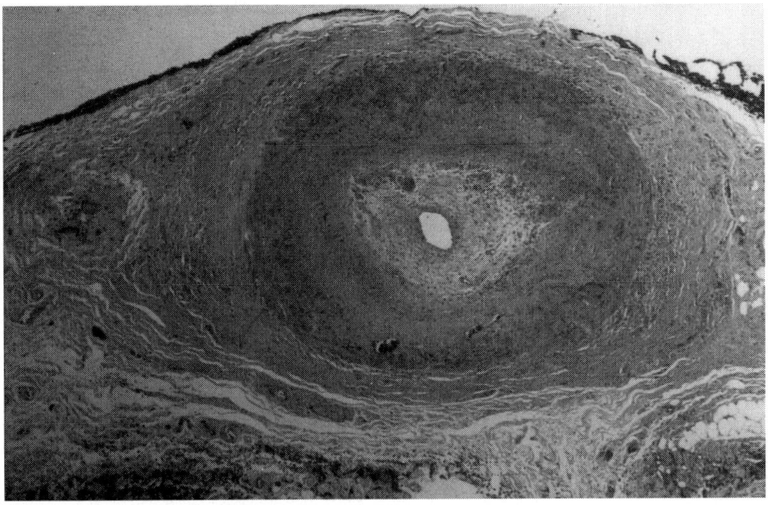

(A)

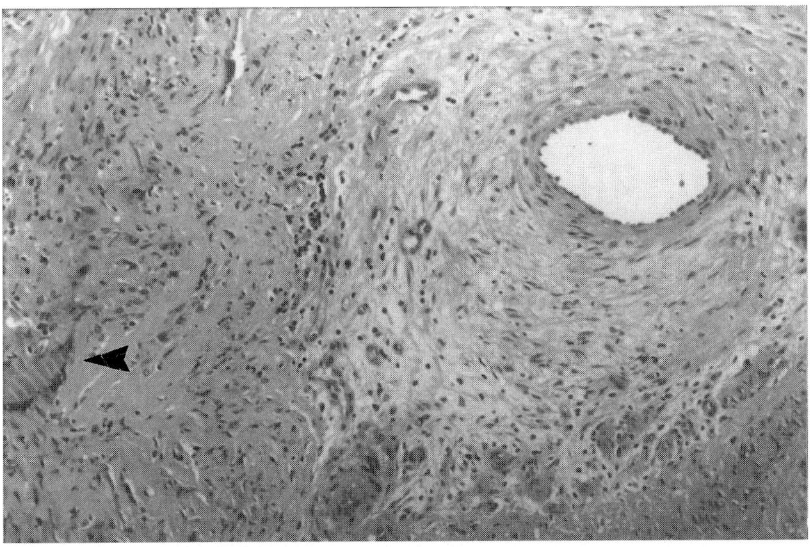

(B)

Figure 17 Temporal/giant cell arteritis. Temporal a. biopsy shows pronounced intimal hyperplasia, with severe stenosis of the arterial lumen. There is transmural granulomatous inflammation, best appreciated at higher magnification **(B).** A prominent multinucleated giant cell is indicated by arrowhead in panel B. (Micrographs courtesy of Dr. Benjamin Glasgow, UCLA Medical Center.)

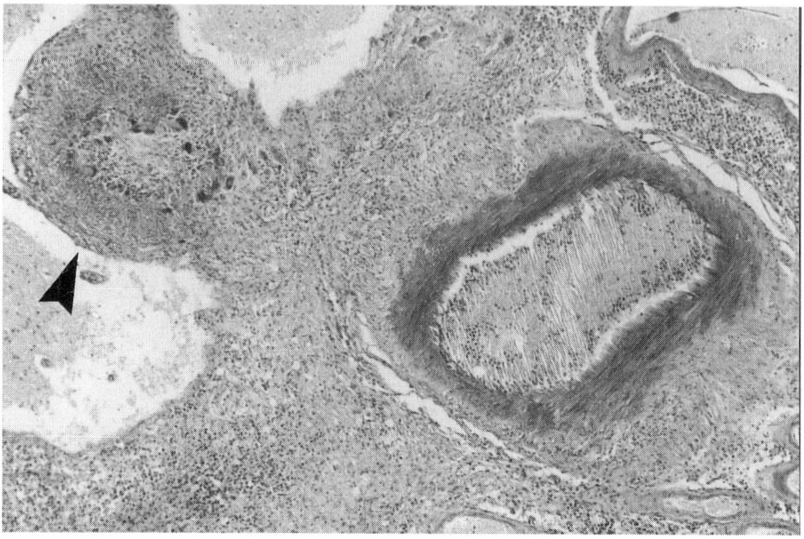

Figure 18 Granulomatous/giant cell arteritis associated with CAA. Parenchymal **and/or** leptomeningeal arteries may be involved. This section, of meningeal vessels, shows severe chronic inflammation within vessel walls, extending into the meninges. One small artery (arrow) shows obliteration of the vessel lumen with numerous multinucleated giant cells in the arterial wall.

Patients show slow evolution of disease, often with stepwise progression and partial recovery characteristic of cerebral infarcts. Disease onset is usually in the late 50s and disorders of memory, cognition, and mood are common. The MRI scan shows characteristic changes.

Neuropathologic features include diffuse myelin pallor, with or without well-defined larger or smaller subcortical infarcts (including lacunar infarcts), which are best appreciated on whole brain sections. Microscopic sections confirm multiple white-matter infarcts, usually with reactive change (Fig. 21). Microvascular changes are usually those of arteriosclerosis and lipohyalinosis, though not necessarily with thrombosis.

b. Cerebral Autosomal Dominant Arteriopathy with Subcortical Infarcts and Leukoencephalopathy (*CADASIL*). This recently characterized entity is similar to BSL but is distinguished by well-defined genetic and characteristic neuropathologic features. Disease pathogenesis involves small arteries and arterioles of the white matter and basal ganglia, which become fibrotic with medial destruction. There is usually a very strong family history. The responsible mutations appear to be in the *notch* 3 gene on chromosome 19p.

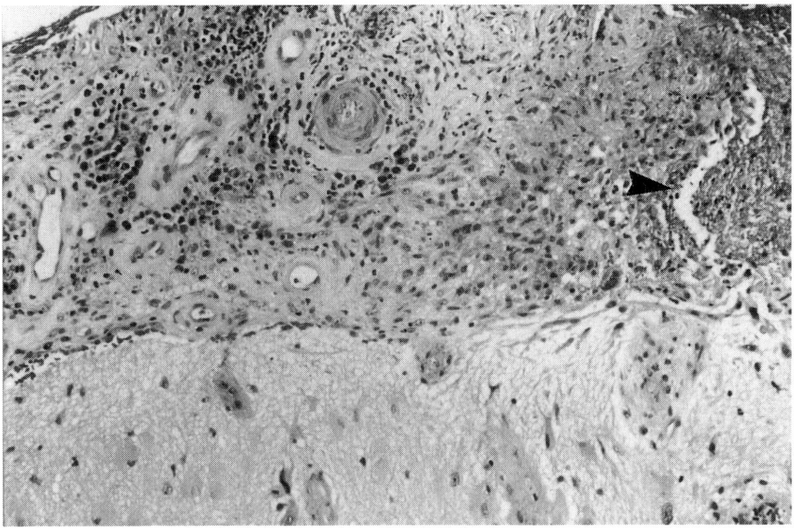

(A)

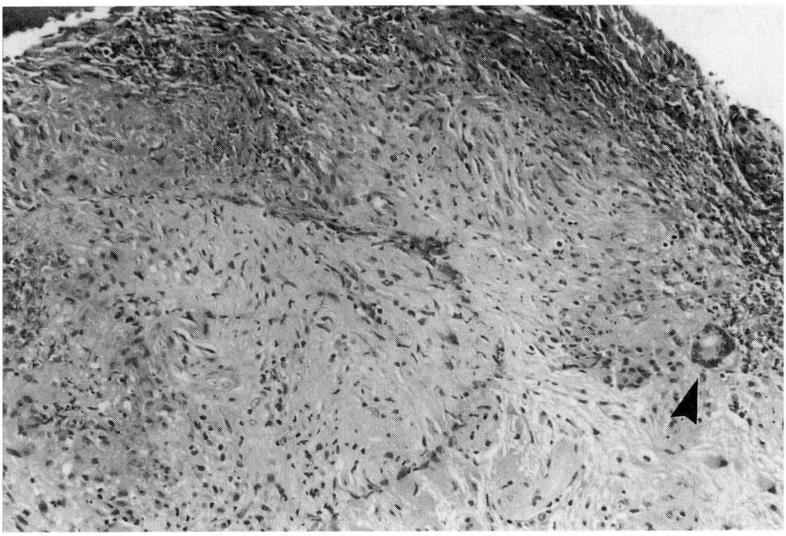

(B)

Figure 19 Wegener's granulomatosis in a 43-year-old male (biopsy specimen). Note dense meningeal inflammation centered on small blood vessels. Inflammatory cells included lymphocytes, plasma cells, and multinucleated giant cells (arrow, **B**). Arrow in **panel A** indicates a region of necrosis. Underlying brain parenchyma (A) shows pronounced reactive astrocytic gliosis.

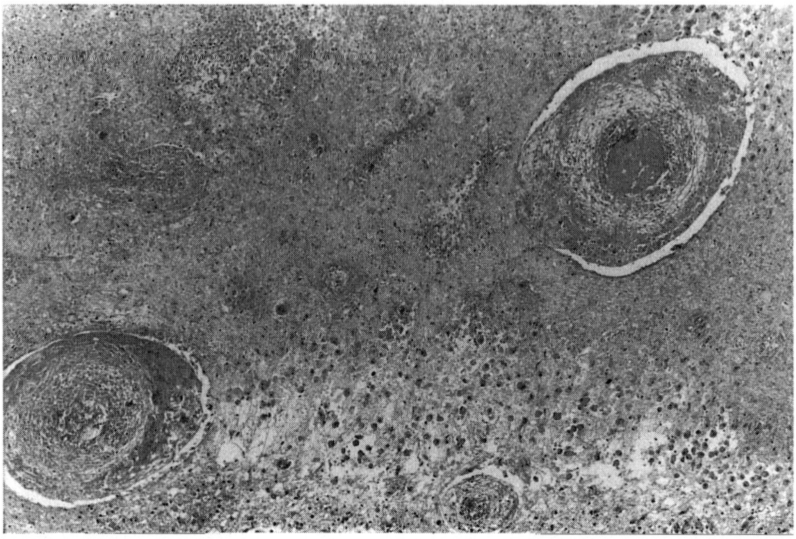

(A)

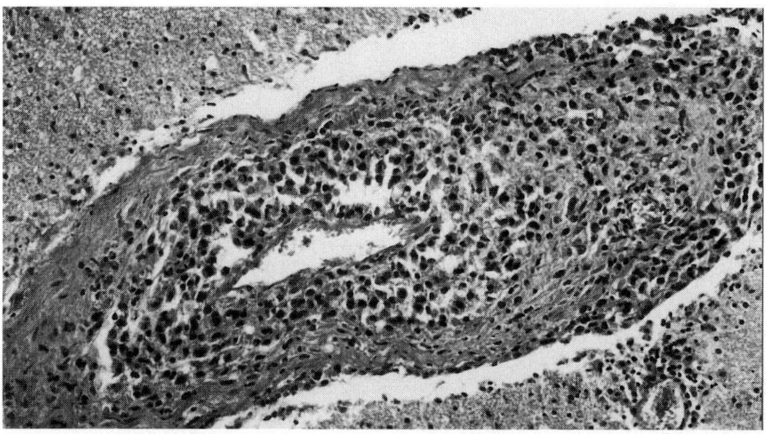

(B)

Figure 20 Lymphomatoid granulomatosis is a controversial entity that may affect the CNS. It shares features of a vasculitis and lymphoproliferative lesion (lymphoma). These two micrographs are from patients with HIV infection (for details, see Anders et al., **Hum Pathol** 1989; 20:326). Note angiodestructive nature of the process **(A)** with fibrinoid necrosis of arterial walls, and atypical though polymorphous inflammatory infiltrate in brain parenchymal vessel walls **(B).**

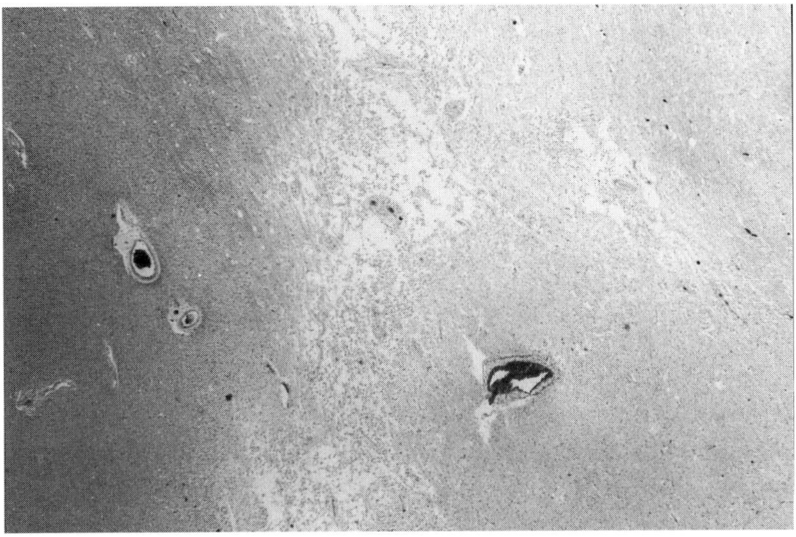

Figure 21 Binswanger's subcortical leukoencephalopathy. Brain from an elderly demented patient showed multiple regions of encephalomalacia within subcortical white matter, a representative example of which is illustrated (preserved white matter is at left). The distinction/interface between **BSL** and **multiple lacunar infarcts** that favor the subcortical white matter is controversial.

Neuropathologic features include cortical or subcortical atrophy with myelin loss, astrocytic gliosis, and lacunar infarcts in the subcortical white matter. Small arteries and arterioles show fibrosis and medial replacement by an eosinophilic, PAS-positive, Congo red-negative granular material which has a characteristic ultrastructural appearance (Fig. 22).

For a discussion of MELAS, see Chapter 9. Drug-induced cerebral microangiopathy is discussed with a consideration of cerebral hemorrhage below.

5. *Miscellaneous Microangiopathies*

Several very rare entities merit consideration in this category.

a. Systemic Lupus Erythematosus (SLE). As many as 5% to 6% of SLE patients are said to have stroke; infarcts are more common than hemorrhages. At least some examples result from hypertension associated with renal disease. Stroke in this population is multifactorial in etiology including those that result from endocarditis, disseminated intravascular coagulation, and infection sec-

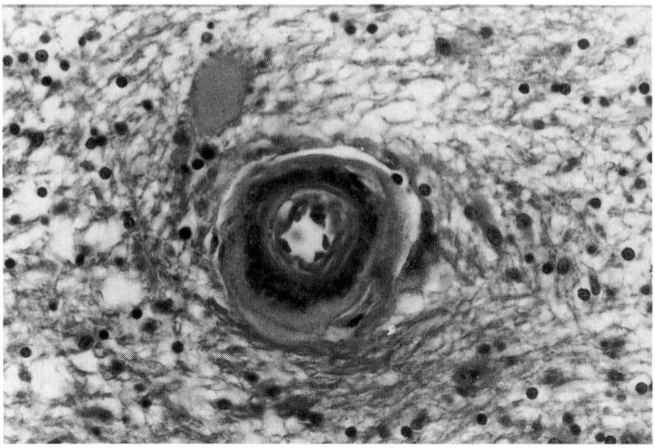

(A)

Figure 22 CADASIL. Light microscopic **(A)** and ultrastructural **(B)** features. Note small white matter arteriole (A) showing characteristic medial destruction with replacement by a (PAS-positive) granular material and adventitial fibrosis. Ultrastructural features (B) include coarse non-membrane-bound "globules" of electron-dense material. (For details, see Gray et al., **Neuropathol Appl Neurobiol** 1994; 20:22; micrographs kindly provided by Professor Françoise Gray, Paris, France.)

ondary to immunosuppression. Microinfarcts and hemorrhages are often seen at autopsy, but true angiitis is infrequently observed. A distinctive cerebral microangiopathy has not been described, though hyaline change, fibrinoid necrosis, and thrombosis of small arteries are sometimes observed.

b. Thrombotic Thrombocytopenic Purpura. TTP is a rare condition with extremely variable clinical manifestations. Widespread microvascular thrombosis (Fig. 23) leads to end-organ (including cerebral) ischemia.

c. Siderocalcinosis, or Ferruginization of Microvessels. This is arguably the most common form of cerebral microvasculopathy (Fig. 24) but is not consistently associated with any known clinical or metabolic abnormality. Small arteries, especially within the globus pallidus, develop calcium and iron deposits in their walls. Fahr's disease is a rare neurodegenerative disorder in the course of which pallidal and cerebellar dentate arteries show massive calcification that often extends into the brain parenchyma.

6. Embolic Infarcts

Any material that forms within the arterial circulation, that is introduced into the circulation, or that forms in the venous circulation and has a conduit to the arterial circulation may result in embolic stroke. Clinically, embolic infarcts are

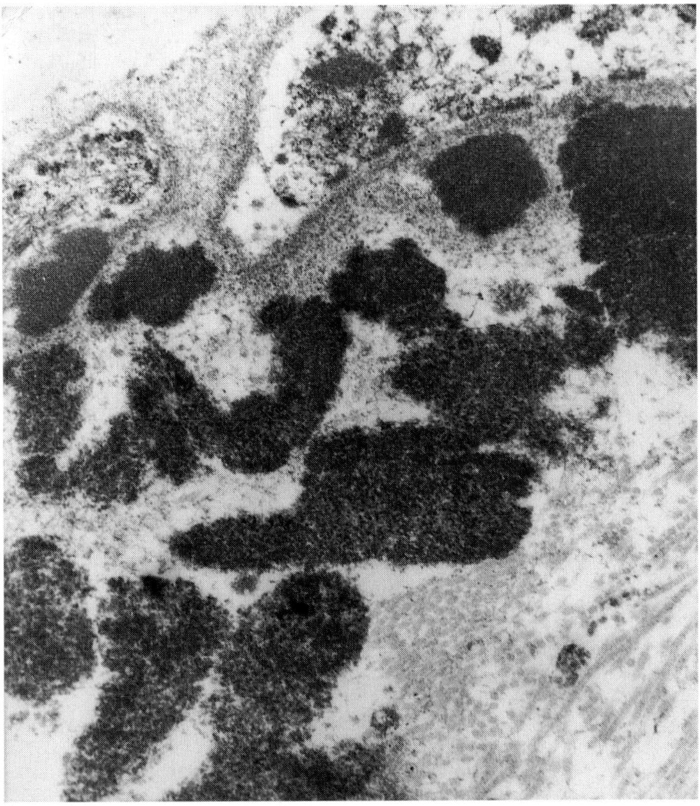

(B)

usually abrupt in onset because of the sudden cessation of flow in otherwise normal arteries, and result in infarcts that are usually hemorrhagic, possibly because of dissolution of the embolus with reestablishment of arterial flow into necrotic tissue. Some common forms of emboli include the following:

a. Atheroma. Foci of complicated atherosclerosis, especially when intimal ulceration is present (for example, in the carotid or vertebral arteries), can serve as the nidus for material that embolizes distally to produce cerebral or spinal cord necrosis. The lumina of blood vessels may show intravascular fragments of atheromatous plaque or platelet-fibrin material (Fig. 25).

b. Cardiogenic. Mural thrombi that form on the endocardial surface of the heart in patients with hypokinetic ventricular wall segments or ventricular aneurysms secondary to cardiomyopathy or old infarcts, in the left atrium secondary

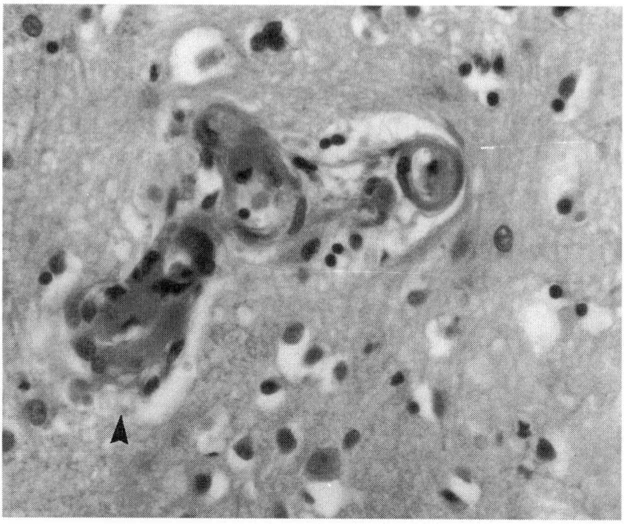

Figure 23 Thrombotic thrombocytopenic purpura (TTP) is characterized by patchy ischemic necrosis throughout the brain, centered on capillaries that show microvascular thrombi (e.g., arrow).

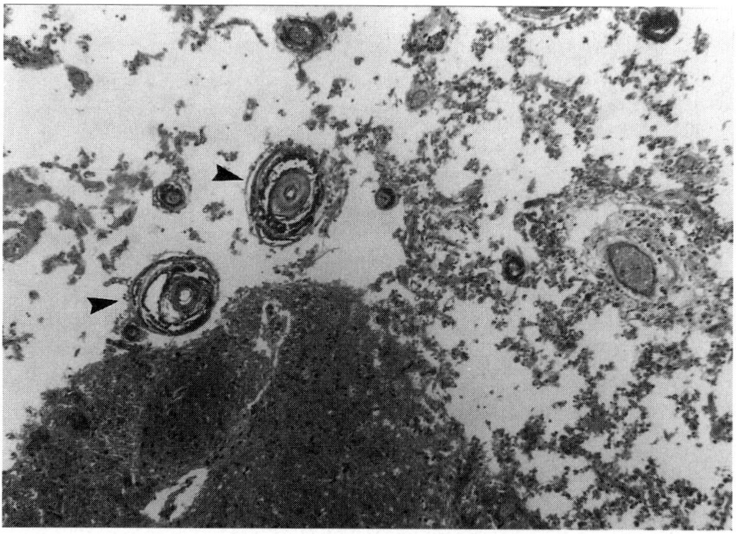

Figure 24 Severe ferruginization/siderocalcinosis of small arteries in the globus pallidus, indicated by arrowheads. Affected vessels were found in an area of necrosis which was probably **un**related to this vascular change—one commonly encountered in otherwise normal brains; it is especially common in the brains of patients with HIV infection.

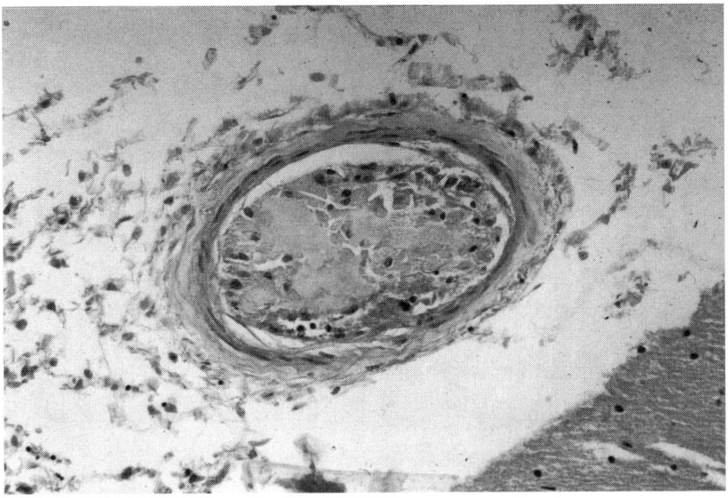

Figure 25 Embolus of atherosclerotic material. Patient had severe complicated carotid and vertebrobasilar atherosclerosis with multiple cerebral infarcts. Sections from many of the infarcts showed intraluminal atheromatous material—e.g., foamy macrophages shown in this leptomeningeal artery that probably originated in an atheromatous plaque, constituting an "artery-to-artery" embolus.

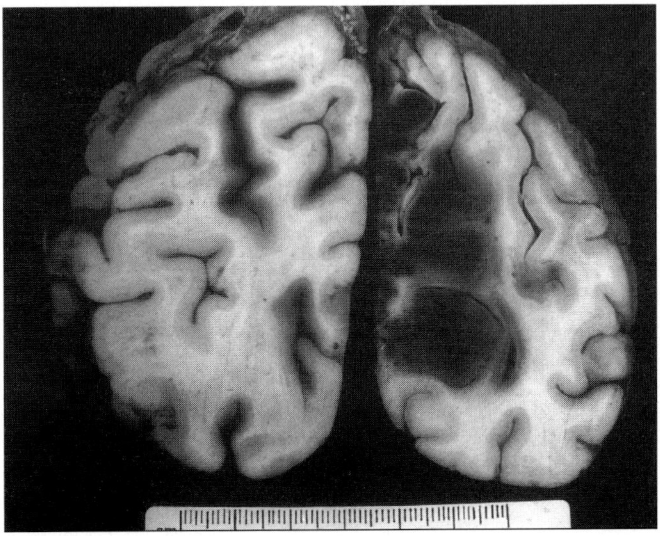

Figure 26 Brain section from a 75-year-old man with metastatic adenocarcinoma who experienced multiple (hemorrhagic) infarcts secondary to NBTE involving the mitral valve. This section shows a prominently hemorrhagic subacute right PCA territory infarct.

to atrial fibrillation, or on valves affected by rheumatic valvular disease or other degenerative changes may embolize distally to the brain (Fig. 26). The emboli that result can be sufficiently large to occlude major branch points in the circle of Willis—for example, the MCA bifurcation or trifurcation in the Sylvian fissure. Sections of affected blood vessels show bland platelet-fibrin thromboemboli with varying degrees of organization.

Infectious endocarditis (IE) and nonbacterial thrombotic (marantic) endocarditis (NBTE) (Fig. 26) may both result in cardiogenic emboli to the CNS. Endocarditis results in vegetations on cardiac valve surfaces, especially the mitral or aortic, or may involve prosthetic cardiac valves. Rheumatic valvular disease, seen infrequently in the 1990s, predisposes to IE. The resulting emboli may be infectious, containing abundant inflammatory cells (Fig. 27) and microorganisms (usually bacteria or fungi), or bland (platelet-fibrin) emboli in the case of NBTE. Miscellaneous valvular lesions that appear to predispose to thrombus formation on endocardial or valve surfaces include rheumatic valvular disease, mitral valve prolapse (myxomatous degeneration of the mitral valve), and calcific aortic sclerosis. Paradoxical emboli may result from venous thrombi passing through a right-to-left shunt such as occurs with a patent fora-

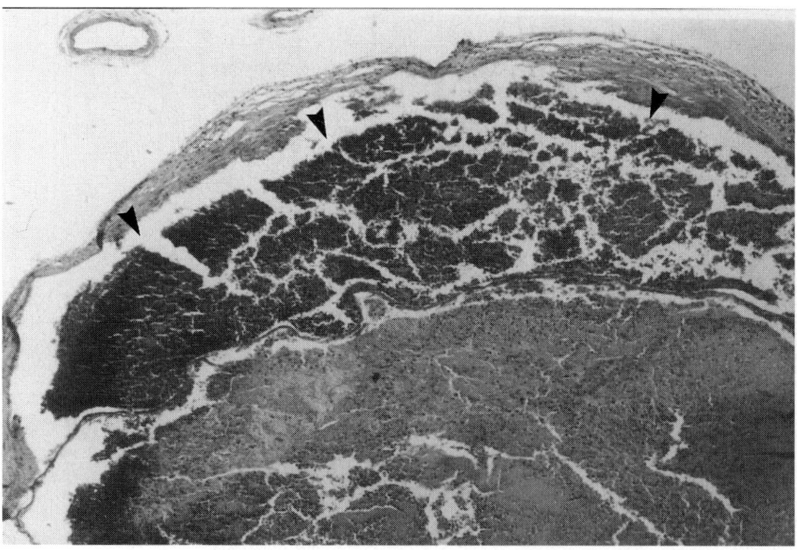

Figure 27 Section of MCA from an HIV-positive patient with *Streptococcus viridans* endocarditis and an MCA embolus. Note abundant acute inflammatory cells (arrowheads) extending into the arterial wall deep to the elastica which, had the patient survived, may have evolved into an infectious aneurysm (see below).

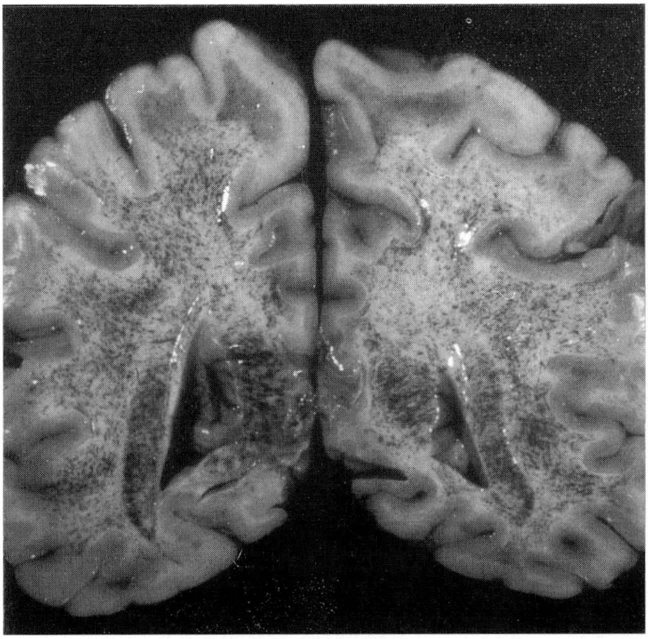

Figure 28 Fat emboli present a dramatic appearance on cut sections of the fresh or fixed brain, viz., as multiple petechial hemorrhages throughout the subcortical white matter. (Photograph courtesy of M.A. Verity, UCLA Medical Center.)

men ovale. Cardiac tumors, though extraordinarily rare (e.g., atrial myxoma), may either metastasize to the brain or produce tumor emboli in the cerebral circulation.

c. Fat Emboli. These constitute a rare form of embolization associated usually with fracture of long bones or the pelvis. The affected brain at autopsy shows petechial hemorrhages mainly within the subcortical white matter (Fig. 28). Fat emboli can be conclusively demonstrated *only* on appropriately stained frozen sections.

d. Miscellaneous. Miscellaneous (including iatrogenic) emboli include those produced by solid tumors that fragment and embolize through the arterial circulation to the CNS. Sometimes these may invade the arterial wall to produce weakening with microaneurysm formation (Fig. 29). Ova and parasites may embolize to the brain, and iatrogenic emboli can result from a variety of materials introduced into the arterial circulation during angiography or vascular surgery (Fig. 30). Rare examples have been reported of embolization to the spinal cord circulation of intervertebral disk material (Fig. 31).

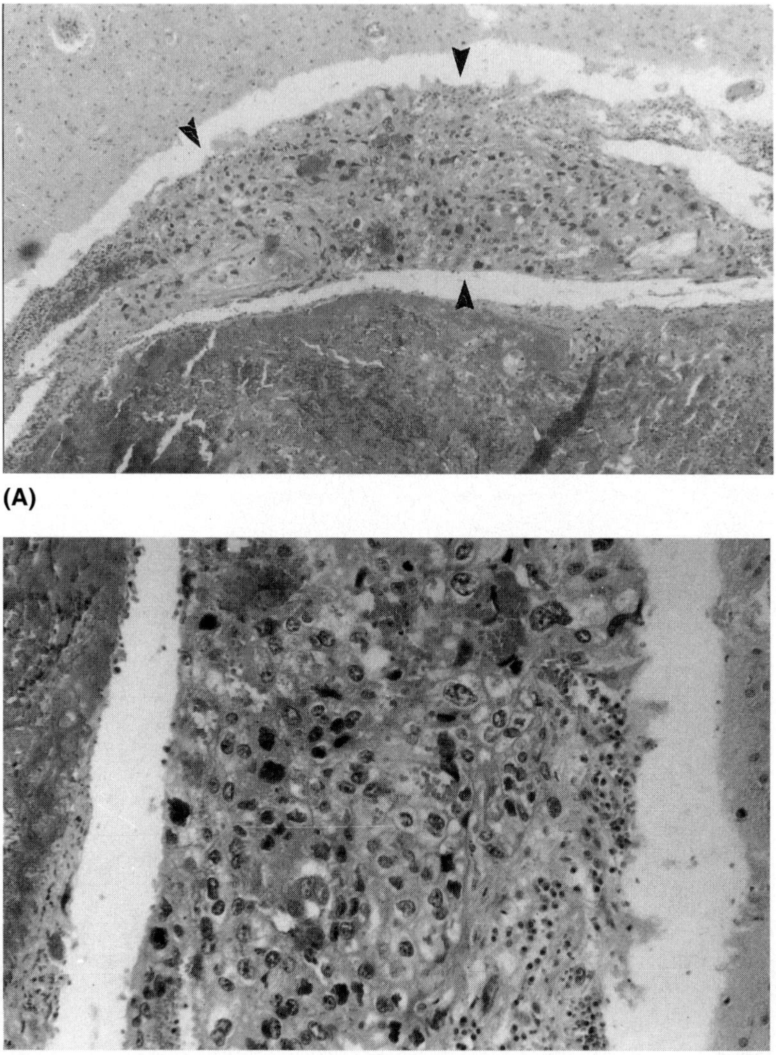

(A)

(B)

Figure 29 Tumor emboli. A woman developed multiple hemorrhagic brain metastases secondary to choriocarcinoma. Tumor had invaded many arterial walls, shown at low magnification (arrows indicate tumor) in **panel A** (lumen is at bottom of micrograph). Magnified view of tumor is shown in **panel B.**

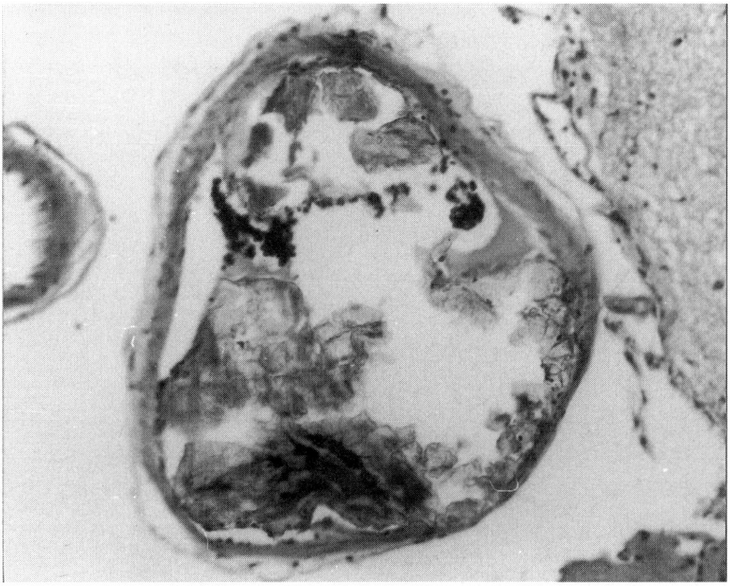

Figure 30 Particulate material may embolize into the cerebral circulation during open heart surgery, as in this example in a leptomeningeal artery—which was not associated with underlying cerebral ischemia. (Case studied by courtesy of Virginia M. Walley, Ottawa Civic Hospital and Ottawa Heart Institute, Ottawa, Canada.)

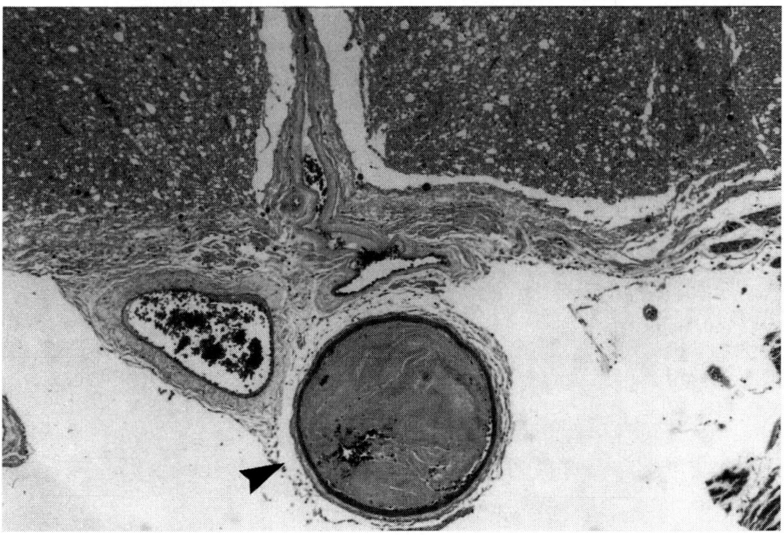

Figure 31 Intervertebral disk material may ***rarely*** embolize to the spinal cord arterial circulation, resulting in necrosis; note cartilaginous material in the anterior spinal a. (arrow). (For details, see D. F. Moorhouse et al., **Surg Neurol** 1992; 37:448.)

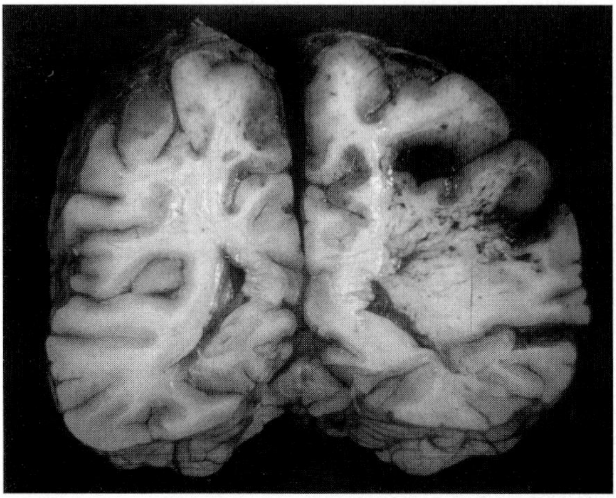

(A)

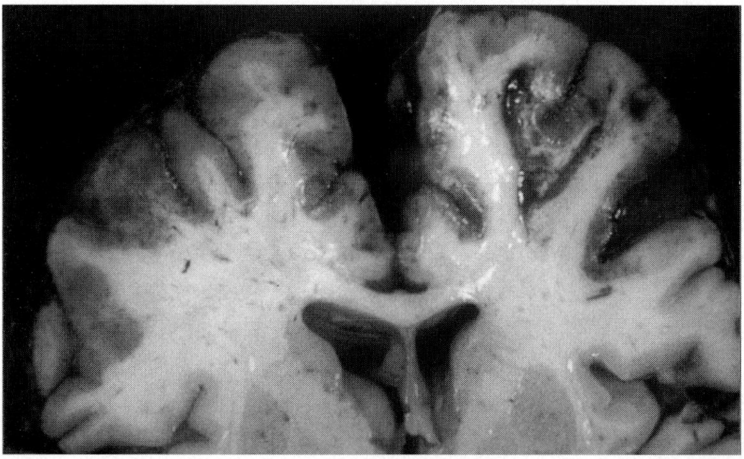

(B)

Figure 32 Sections of brain from a young woman who developed venous/sinus thrombosis, with rapid progression to coma and death. Multiple sections of brain **(all panels)** show bihemispheric regions of subacute severely hemorrhagic necrosis; in some areas, the lesions resemble intraparenchymal hematomas.

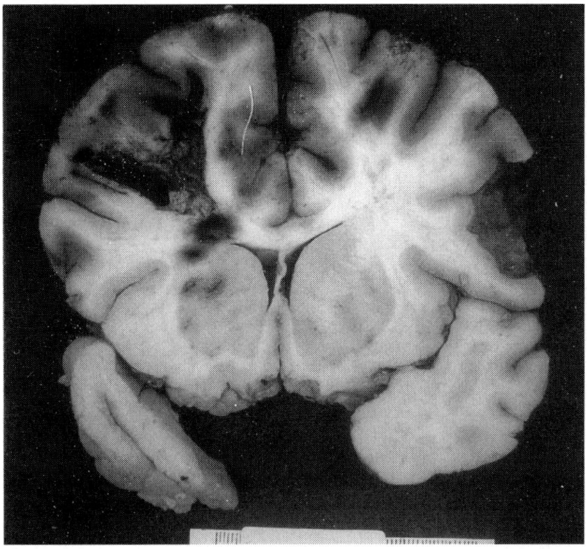

(C)

7. Venous Disease/Cerebral Venous Thrombosis (CVT)

This is a much less common cause of stroke than arterial disease, though autopsy series probably underestimate its true incidence. Studies from the United Kingdom in the 1960s suggested only 20 to 25 deaths per year attributable to CVT. As well, infection or sepsis—commonly associated with venous thrombosis—is becoming a relatively less important consideration in the modern era of widespread antibiotic use, though serious systemic infections have hardly been eradicated! *Cavernous sinus thrombosis* is the most common type of septic thrombosis. Etiologic factors associated with CVT include *local factors*, including infections, head injury, a neurosurgical procedure, or neoplasm; or *general etiologic factors* including (but not restricted to) the use of oral contraceptives, pregnancy and the puerperium, congenital heart disease, hematologic abnormalities (e.g., polycythemia, sickle cell disease), severe dehydration, and malignancy. Patients can present with a wide variety of symptoms, most commonly including severe headache, evidence of raised intracranial pressure, seizures, and obtundation progressing to coma.

Neuropathologic features include a variable appearance depending on the time after CVT that the brain is examined. The most consistent feature identified is severe and extensive hemorrhagic necrosis in the brain, often with evolution into parenchymal hematomas (Fig. 32). The thrombosed sinus is usually palpable and on cross section shows a distended appearance (Fig. 33). Micro-

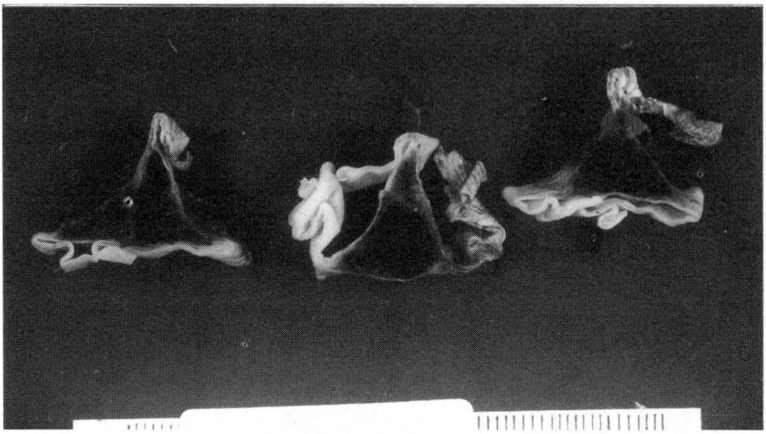

Figure 33 Sections of the superior sagittal sinus from patient whose brain is illustrated in Figure 32. Note distended sinus secondary to a recent thrombus, which, on microscopic sections, showed no evidence of organization; thrombi had propagated into superficial meningeal and cortical veins. Patient's only identifiable risk factor was use of oral contraceptives.

scopic features of the brain include hemorrhagic necrosis and, if a major septic component is present, microorganisms may be demonstrable among the inflammatory cells.

8. Neuropathologic Features of Infarcts

Any encephalic infarct examined at autopsy will show an appearance dependent on the length of time it occurred prior to death. "Timing" of infarcts using only gross and microscopic criteria is, however, relatively imprecise. Clinical history is important; often the neuropathologist assesses a cerebral infarct as being "consistent with" a given clinical history of stroke.

Acute infarcts, those that have occurred 5 to 8 hours prior to a patient's death, are almost by definition undetectable at gross inspection of the brain or at the time of brain cutting; indeed, even microscopic abnormalities in such brain might be minimal. Changes that develop and evolve within 8 to 36 hours include slight blurring of the cortex–white-matter junction, with a dusky discoloration of the cortex and underlying white matter and slight softening of the tissue on palpation. These changes are particularly easy to detect when (as is usually the case) they are confined to the territory of supply of a major cerebral artery (e.g., MCA, ACA, PCA).

Subacute infarcts, those that have occurred 2 to 4 days prior to death, show softening of the brain tissue with blurring of the cortex–white-matter

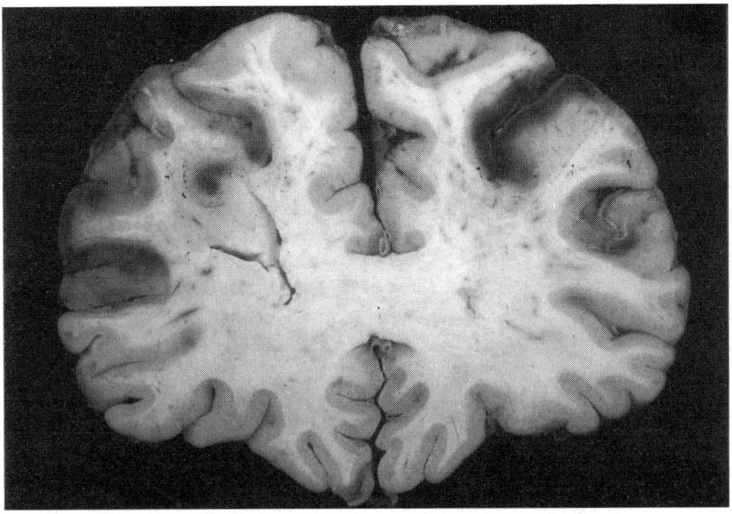

(A)

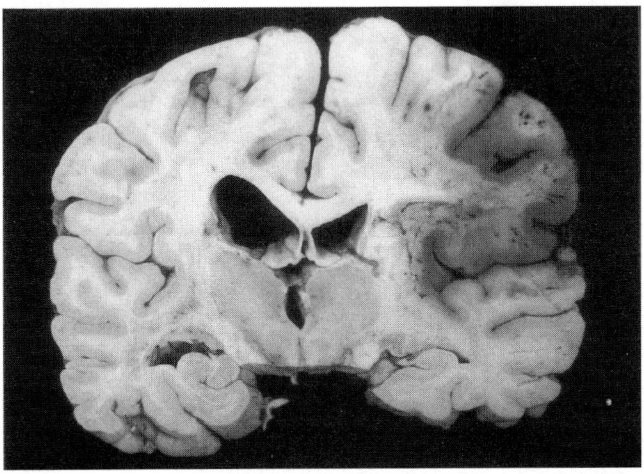

(B)

Figure 34 Recent cerebral infarcts. **(A)** Bihemispheric infarcts, in the left MCA territory and the right ACA/MCA watershed region. Note patchy grey discoloration in cortex and white matter; the watershed/borderzone infarct is hemorrhagic. **(B)** Subacute infarct confined to the right MCA territory.

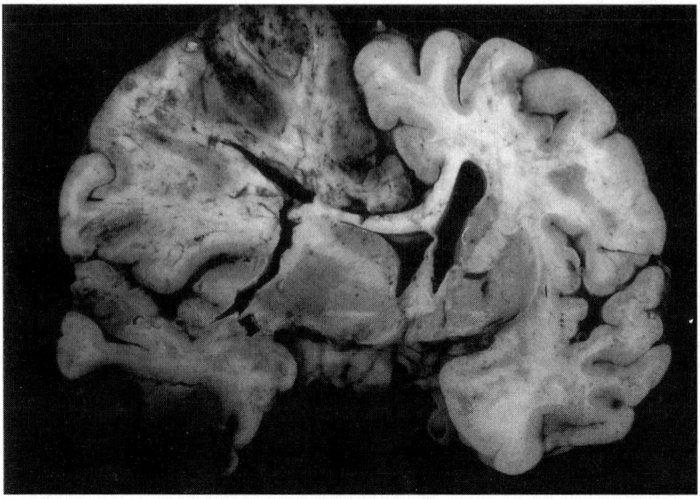

(A)

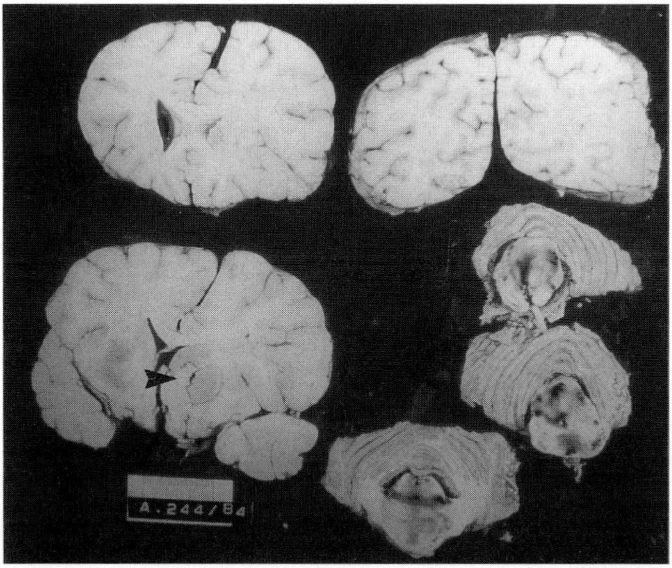

(B)

Figure 35 At 2 to 4 days following a large cerebral infarct, edema—usually confined to the infarcted hemisphere—predominates, as in these two examples. **(A)** Large left MCA and ACA territory, partly hemorrhagic infarct with "cracking" within the tissue and massive left-to-right shift of midline structures; severe compression of the ventricular system is noted. **(B)** shows large right MCA territory infarct (boundaries are difficult to appreciate at this magnification) with significant "cracking artifact" (arrowhead), right-to-left subfalcine herniation, and secondary (Duret) hemorrhages in the midbrain and pons, the result of severe cerebral edema.

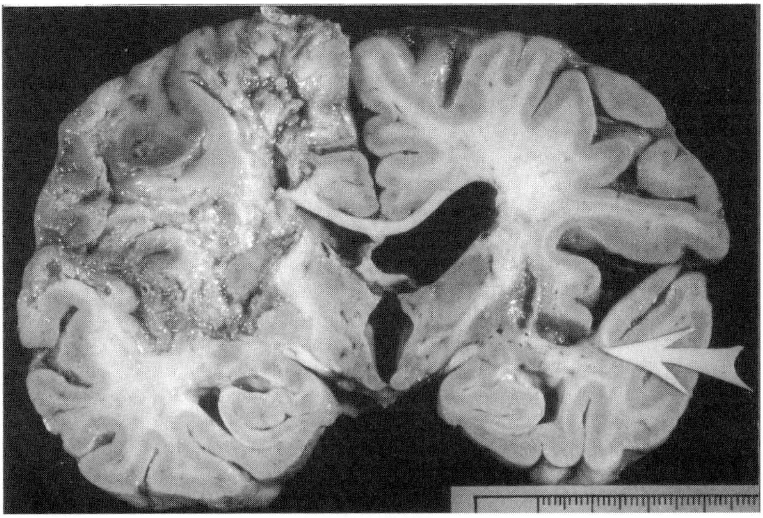

(A)

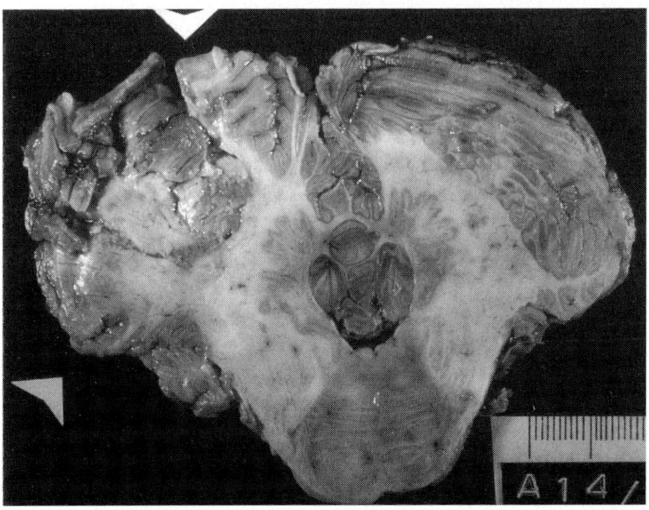

(B)

Figure 36 Several day-old infarcts (with liquefactive necrosis) in the left MCA territory (**A**) and the left cerebellum (arrows, **B**) of two different patients. Arrow in (**A**) indicates an old right-sided putaminal and insular infarct.

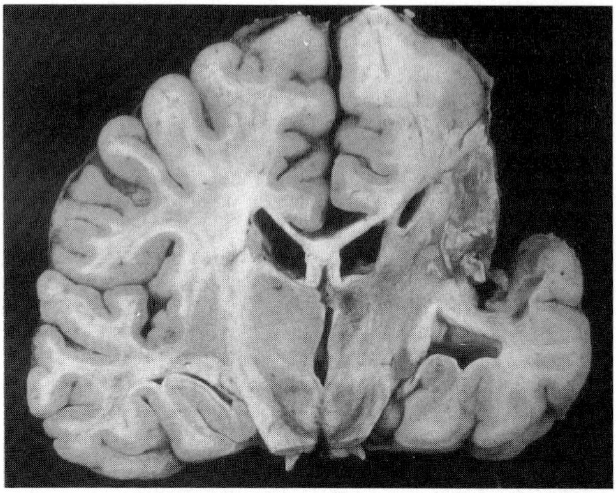

(A)

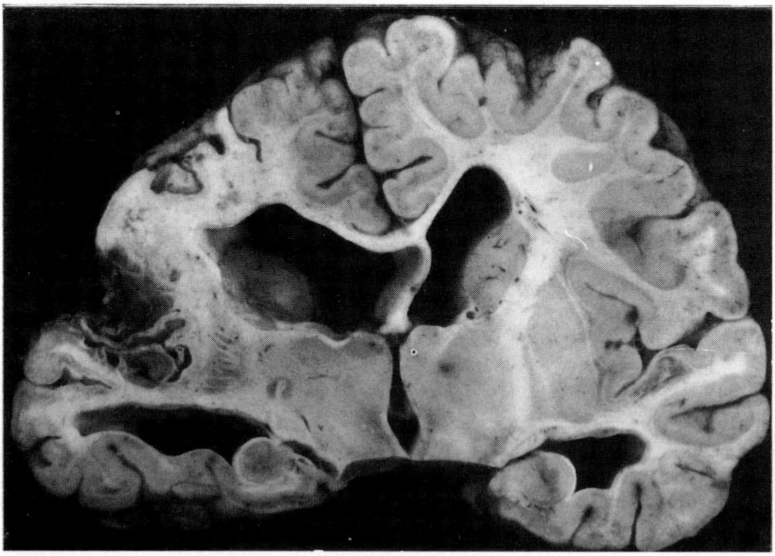

(B)

Figure 37 Characteristic appearances of old/remote cystic infarcts in **(A)** right MCA territory of an adult, **(B)** left MCA territory of a child, **(C)** a "branch" territory of the left MCA, and **(D)** cerebellum (arrow).

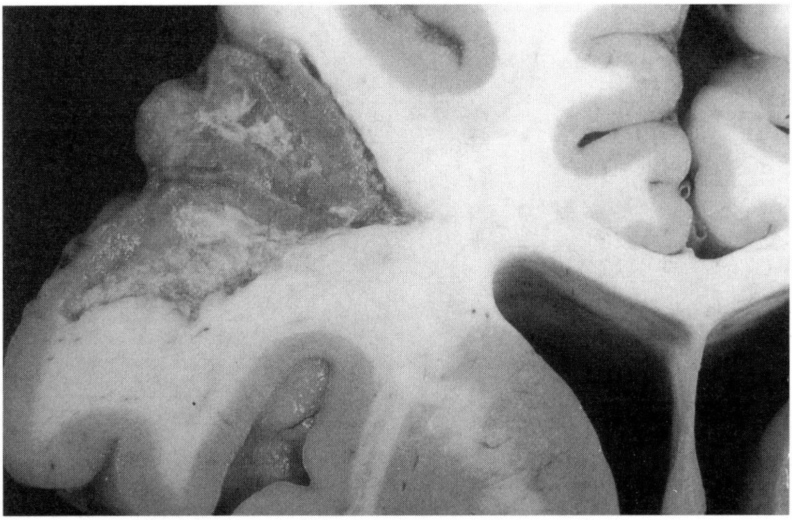

(C)

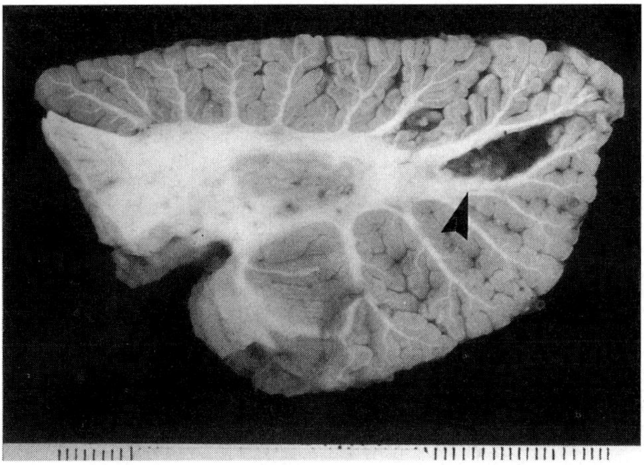

(D)

junction and dusky gray discoloration of both cortex and white matter (Fig. 34). At this stage, the most telling gross abnormality is cerebral swelling or edema (Fig. 35). The cortex may also separate from the underlying white matter, a phenomenon described as "cracking artifact." After edema has subsided, a subacute infarct evolves into the chronic phase, during which the brain tissue undergoes liquefactive necrosis, eventually leading to cavitation (Fig. 36). An

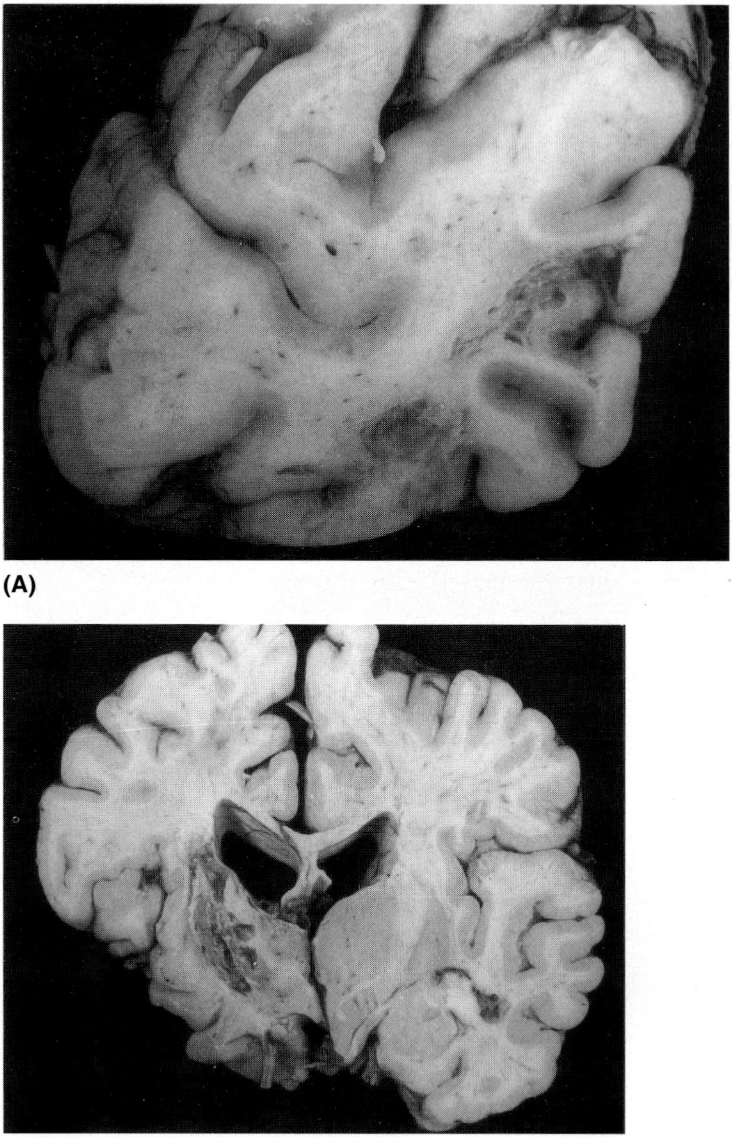

(A)

(B)

Figure 38 Not all old infarcts show large areas of cystic cavitation. In some instances, appearances are those of a "moth-eaten" region of cystic encephalomalacia, as in the left PCA territory **(A)** or the left internal capsule, basal ganglia, and thalamus **(B).**

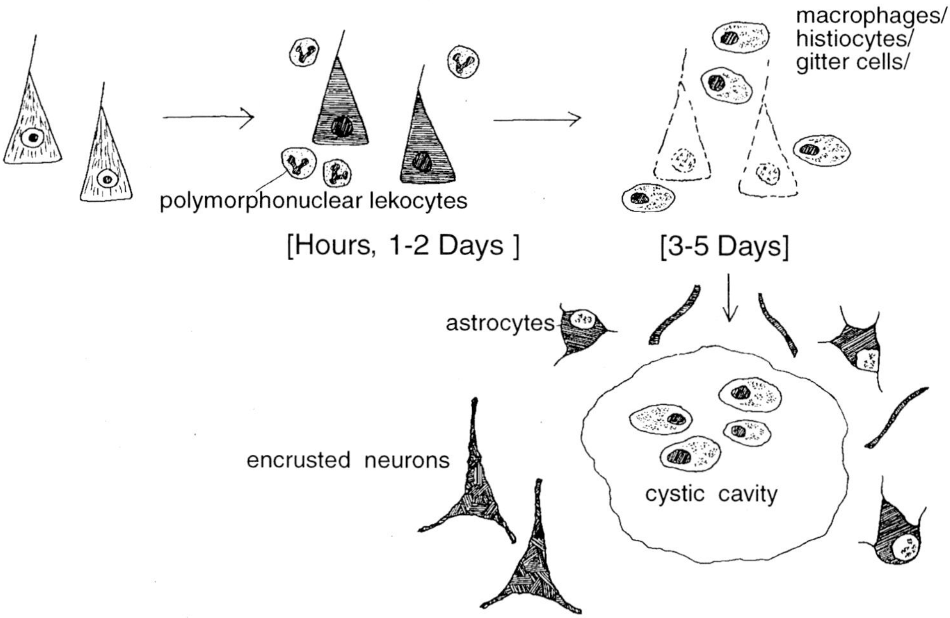

Figure 39 Schematic illustration of cellular events in the microscopic evolution of a cerebral infarct.

infarct that is weeks to years old appears as a cystic cavity within the brain substance, often with collapse of the surrounding cerebral tissue (Fig. 37). In some instances, a well-defined cavity does not form; rather there is a "moth-eaten" appearance to the region of encephalomalacia (Fig. 38).

The gross manifestations of cerebral infarct correspond to characteristic microscopic abnormalities (Fig. 39). In the acute phase, neuronal eosinophilia with pyknosis predominates, as in anoxic-ischemic encephalopathy. In the subacute phase, neuronal eosinophilia persists, with variable degrees of infiltration by polymorphonuclear leukocytes, often with necrotic microvessel walls. Early microglial activation occurs with the formation of foamy histiocytes or gitter cells by 3 to 5 days after an infarct has occurred (Fig. 40). At 1 to 2 weeks, endothelial proliferation with neovascularization, which is variable in extent, develops. In the chronic phase there is persistence of abundant gitter cells, often with hemosiderin in their cytoplasm. Thin-walled blood vessels can be seen passing through the infarct cavity. Abundant reactive astrocytes (including gemistocytes) are present around the infarct (Fig. 41). In a large cortical infarct, a characteristic pattern of preservation of the molecular layer (layer 1) of the

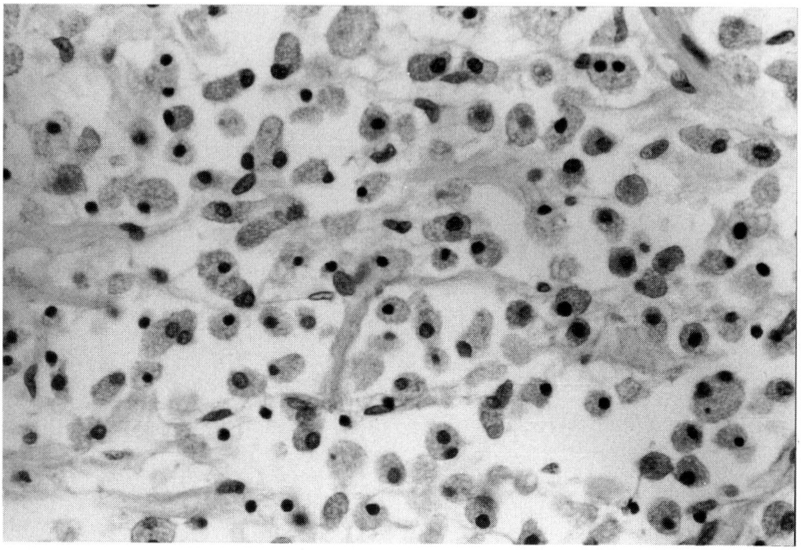

Figure 40 Foamy macrophages/"gitter cells" in a cystic infarct.

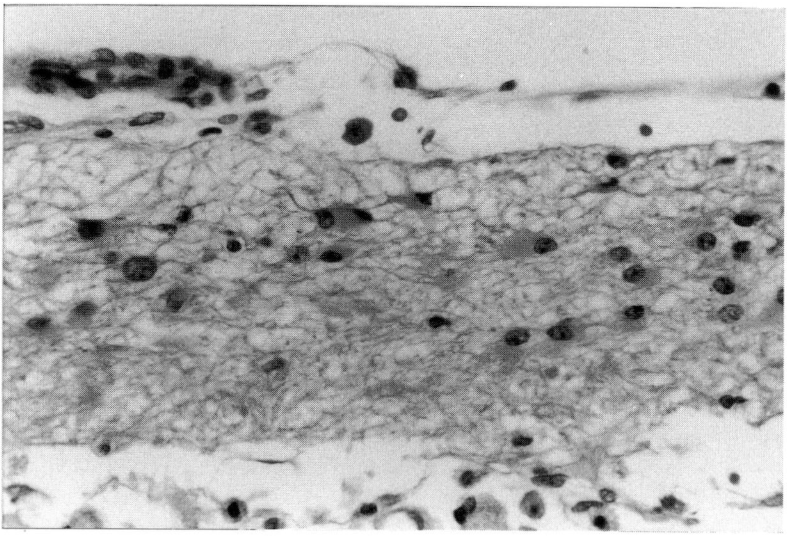

Figure 41 Reactive "gemistocytic" astrocytes at edge of an old/remote infarct. Contrast their appearance (glassy cytoplasm, coarse nuclear chromatin pattern) with that of gitter cells shown in Figure 40.

cortex, which usually contains abundant astrocytes, is seen (Fig. 42). Residual neurons or axons in and around an infarct may become encrusted with iron and calcium (Fig. 43). Thrombosed vessels are rarely encountered adjacent to a chronic infarct, though they are more easily discovered around an acute or subacute infarct (Fig. 42). Cerebral infarcts often occur in and may be confined to specific vascular territories, as illustrated in (Fig. 44). Infarcts in different vascular territories are associated with distinctive clinical syndromes; e.g., an MCA infarct in either hemisphere produces contralateral hemiparesis/hemiplegia, and an MCA territory infarct in the dominant hemisphere often leads to aphasia. A PCA territory infarct causes cortical blindness because of necrosis of the calcarine/visual cortex. An infarct in the vertebrobasilar system often produces ataxia, dizziness, cranial nerve abnormalities, and (eventually) coma because of damage to the reticular activating system.

Distinctive subtypes of infarct are also recognized:

Watershed or borderzone infarcts usually occur in elderly patients with significant atherosclerosis who experience a prolonged episode of hypotension or reduced blood flow (e.g., intraoperatively or after cardiac arrest). These are usually wedge-shaped, with their base at the pial surface (see Fig. 1). They may be symmetrical within the two cerebral hemispheres. Microscopically, atheroemboli may be encountered in the overlying (especially leptomeningeal) arteries.

Lacunar infarcts are usually small (less than 1 cm in maximal size) and occur deep within the brain (Fig. 45), e.g. in the deep central gray matter including thalamus and basal ganglia, or the subcortical white matter; they are also frequently encountered in the pons. They occur in regions where hypertensive microvascular disease is common (see below).

B. Cerebral/Encephalic Hemorrhage

The terms *intracerebral or cerebral hemorrhage* are often used as synonyms for *intracranial hemorrhage*. However, intracranial hemorrhage describes the extravasation of blood into the brain substance and/or regions defined and enclosed by the meninges, dura mater, and skull, as well as the ventricular cavities. "Cerebral hemorrhage" should be restricted to describing blood in the substance or parenchyma of the cerebral hemispheres, though by common usage and convention it has come to mean bleeding into any part of the brain parenchyma, including structures of the posterior fossa; a more global term to describe hemorrhage into any part of the brain substance is *encephalic/intraparenchymal hemorrhage*.

1. Extradural/Epidural and Subdural Hemorrhage (EDH, SDH)

Clinicopathologic features of these types of hemorrhage are reviewed in Chapter 3, since in most cases they are associated with craniocerebral trauma.

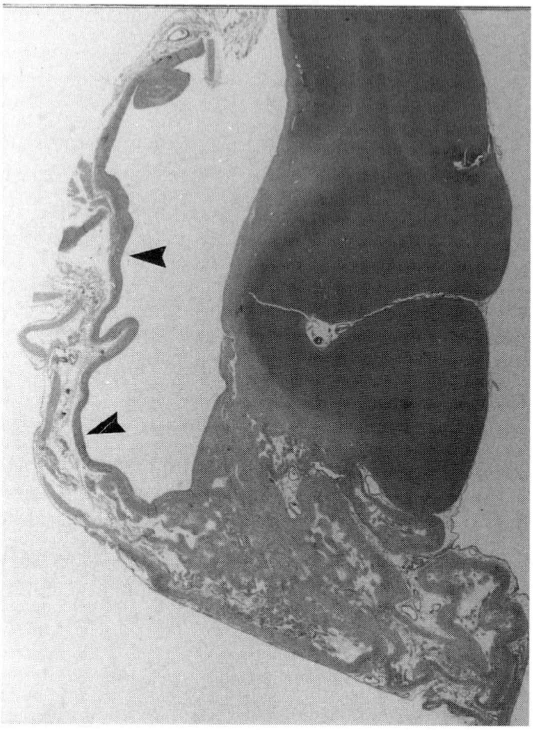

(A)

Figure 42 (**A**) Old cystic infarct adjacent to preserved cortex. Note that the cystic cavity, which has substantially collapsed, shows a thin rim of preserved subpial (layer I of cortex) tissue, indicated by arrowheads. (**B**) In old infarcts, the subpial, relatively "neuron-free" zone of cortex, is preserved though often heavily gliotic, while deeper cortical layers show typical cystic encephalomalacia (arrowheads) with foamy macrophages. In this instance, the occluded meningeal vessel that was presumed to have caused the infarct is identifiable at top of the micrograph.

2. *Subarachnoid Hemorrhage* (*SAH*)

This term describes an acute or chronic extravasation of blood into the cavity lined by the arachnoid membrane. Spontaneous SAH must be distinguished from SAH that often occurs with brain trauma. Spontaneous SAH is almost always the result of focal weakening and rupture of a cerebral vessel (usually an artery) involved by a pathologic process or vascular malformation at or near the surface of the brain. Specific patterns of SAH result from distinctive causal or etiologic lesions.

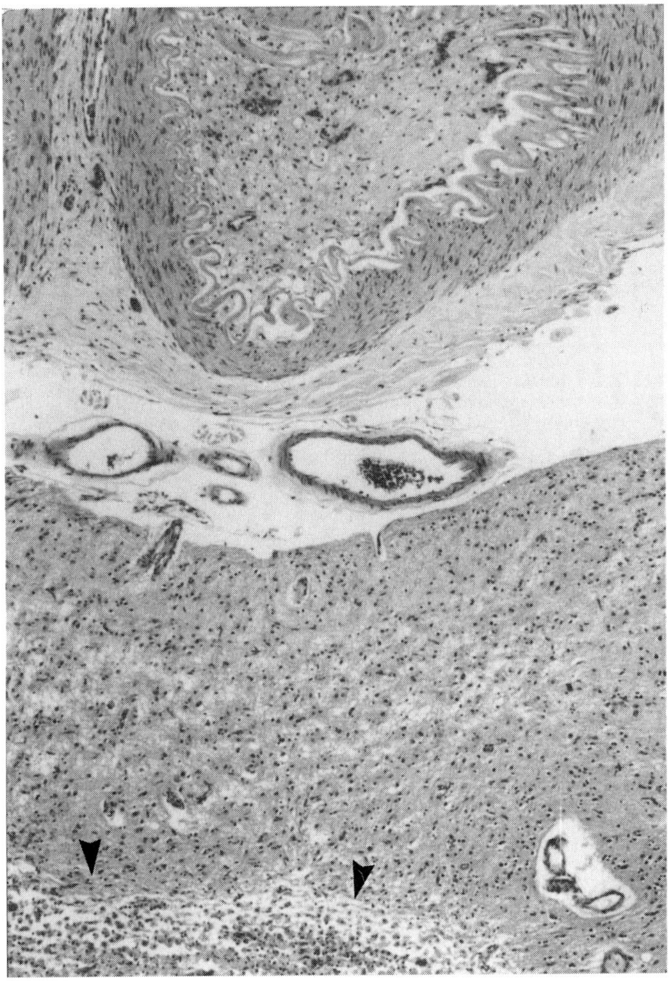

(B)

a. Saccular or Berry Aneurysms. Berry aneurysms are by far the commonest cause of spontaneous SAH. They are found as an incidental autopsy finding in as many as 2% to 3% of unselected postmortem examinations, usually with no history or pathologic features to suggest previous hemorrhage. The incidence of SAH is approximately 10 to 12/100,000 population, and increases with age, though the median age of SAH is in the mid-sixth decade of life. SAH due to berry or saccular aneurysm usually has devastating clinical consequences. It is

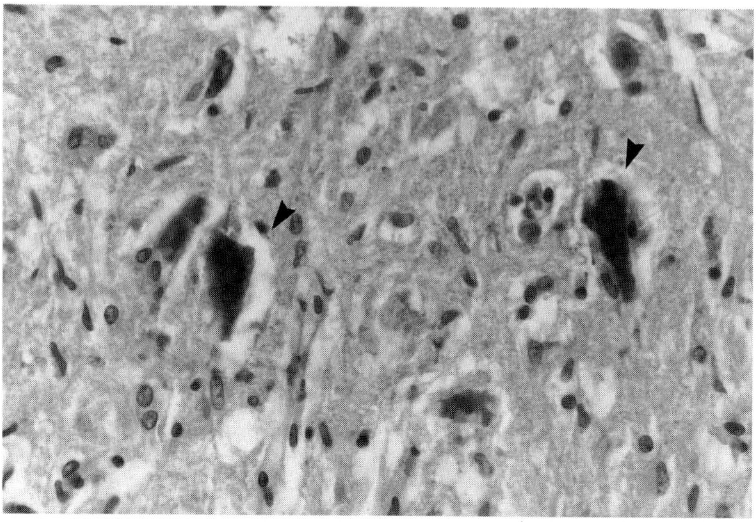

Figure 43 Residual neurons at the margins of an infarct often become encrusted or "mummified" with calcium and iron salts, giving them a characteristically basophilic appearance (arrowheads).

fatal or disabling in over two-thirds of patients; one-third die from the initial hemorrhage within 72 hours, and an additional one-third die or become significantly disabled secondary to the complications of SAH, the most important of which are vasospasm causing brain ischemia, hydrocephalus (acute or chronic, secondary to meningeal scarring/fibrosis), rebleeding, and complications of surgical intervention. However, patients who undergo successful surgical "clipping" or other treatment of the aneurysm with prevention of the major complications of SAH can lead a normal life. Whereas other forms of stroke due to brain hemorrhage or ischemia have declined over recent decades, the incidence of SAH due to saccular aneurysms has remained constant. General medical conditions such as *polycystic kidney disease* and *coarctation of the aorta* are associated with the development of berry aneurysms, possibly because both clinical conditions produce hypertension which by itself, however, is *not* a risk factor for saccular aneurysms. Very rarely, aneurysmal hemorrhage results from embolization of left atrial myxoma to cerebral vessels with resultant local weakening of the vessel wall. Defects of vascular collagen and elastic tissue may predispose to saccular aneurysms. While berry aneurysms are usually described as being "congenital," they are almost never found in infants or children. However, it is argued that certain segments of the vascular media—especially branch points on the Circle of Willis—are "at risk" for developing aneurysms later in life.

Many patients who have a major SAH experience warning symptoms, defined as a "sentinel leak" secondary to a small bleed, in the 2 to 3 weeks prior to overt SAH. This usually takes the form of a severe, sudden-onset headache, often during sexual intercourse, straining at stool, or spontaneously. The signs/symptoms and clinical course of a patient who has experienced SAH due to berry aneurysm are determined by its location (e.g., a posterior communicating artery aneurysm may cause compression of cranial nerve III), size of the initial hemorrhage, and intracranial regions into which hemorrhage extends (e.g., the brain parenchyma or substance, ventricular system). Nonfatal bleeds may produce prominent localizing signs and symptoms—hemiparesis, akinetic mutism, or lower limb paresis (with anterior communicating artery aneurysm). Aneurysms that bleed are usually smaller than 1 cm in size while approximately 10% to 15% are smaller than 5 mm. *Giant* aneurysms, those larger than 2.0 to 2.5 cm in maximal diameter, bleed less frequently and more commonly behave as a mass lesion within the CNS.

Neuropathologic features Abundant SAH is usually seen at autopsy (Fig. 46). However, in the less common circumstance in which the ruptured dome of an aneurysm is embedded in brain substance, a purely intraparenchymal bleed will result, with a negligible component of SAH. The prosector must be aware of this possibility when examining the brain of someone, especially a young person, who has died of an intracerebral hemorrhage of occult origin (Fig. 47). If a large amount of blood is identified at the base of the brain and the patient is suspected of having aneurysmal SAH, this blood must be gently dissected away until a single aneurysm or multiple aneurysms are discovered. This dissection should *not* under any circumstances be deferred until after the brain has fixed; fixed, unclotted blood is more difficult to handle and the source of bleeding more difficult to identify after brain fixation. More than one berry aneurysm or a combination of vascular lesions (most commonly berry aneurysm and arteriovenous malformation) should always be suspected. The responsible lesion that has produced subarachnoid or intraparenchymal hemorrhage is usually recognized by the proximity of abundant clotted blood and (in the case of a ruptured aneurysm) the tear or site of rupture in the aneurysm wall.

Aneurysms occur at major branch points on the circle of Willis, most commonly the "anterior circulation," especially the MCA bi/trifurcation in the sylvian fissure, the ICA/posterior communicating artery junction, and the ACA/anterior communicating artery junction (Fig. 48). Posterior circulation aneurysms (Fig. 49) constitute 10% to 30% of cases, and most aneurysms in this location are at the basilar artery tip or bifurcation. In patients who survive SAH by days or weeks, the prosector must document the extent of meningeal fibrosis

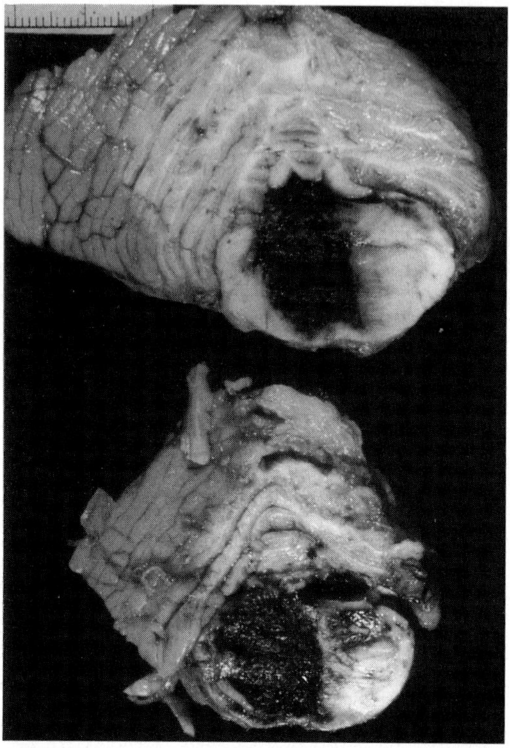

(A)

Figure 44 Hemorrhagic infarcts in **(A)** the basilar a. territory of the pons, and **(B)** the left PCA territory. The lesion illustrated in (A) mimics a primary brainstem hematoma, but is less well circumscribed and "expansile" than the latter (see below).

or scarring, the severity of hydrocephalus, ischemic lesions within the CNS that may result from vasospasm, and the location and status of any aneurysm clips that have been placed by the neurosurgeon (Fig. 50). Often an incidental aneurysm is discovered at autopsy in an elderly patient which may show superimposed atherosclerotic change within its walls. Rarely, a previously "clipped" aneurysm is found even when no history of such a clipping is available at the time of necropsy, usually because of the long duration of time that has elapsed between treatment and autopsy.

Microscopic features of an aneurysm (ruptured or intact) are best illustrated using a stain that highlights vessel wall components—e.g., an elastica stain. Aneurysms may be uni or multilobed. Characteristic features include at-

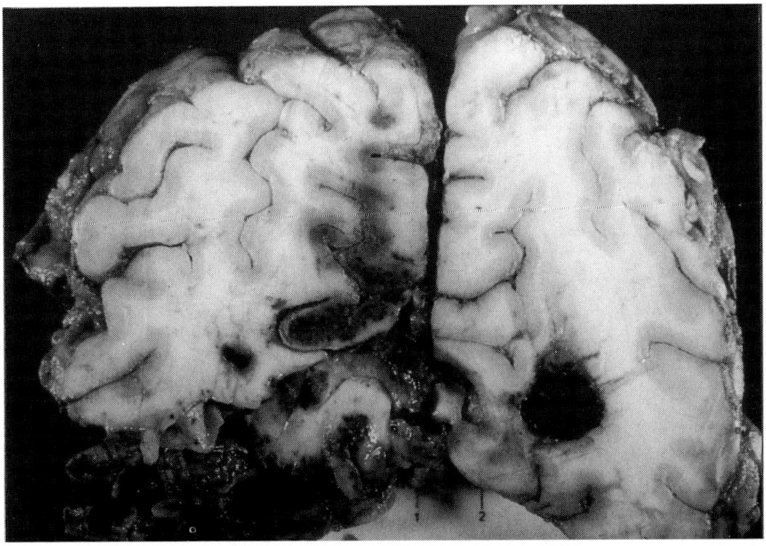

(B)

tenuation and focal loss of elastica and muscularis, generally most severe in the portion of the vessel underlying the site of rupture, with variable fibrosis in this region of the aneurysm wall, and variable degrees of superimposed atherosclerosis (Fig. 51). Microfoci of blood breakdown products in the vicinity may reflect previous hemorrhage. Giant aneurysms often show evidence of mural calcification, and thrombosis with or without recanalization (Fig. 52).

b. Infectious/Mycotic Aneurysms. The former term is preferable, since "mycotic" implies the presence of an etiologic fungal infection. These account for no more than 5% to 6% of intracranial aneurysms, and they result from bacterial or fungal colonization of a region of the arterial wall with associated inflammation and weakening leading to ectasia and eventually rupture. Bacterial infectious aneurysms have a lower mortality than fungal aneurysms. Infectious aneurysms may arise from arterial wall colonization by circulating microorganisms (e.g., associated with subacute endocarditis) or an extravascular source (e.g., meningitis, osteomyelitis). Among endocarditis patients, infectious aneurysms occur primarily in the young (second and third decades of life); 1% to 10% of patients with infectious endocarditis may develop infectious aneurysms.

Affected patients are often neurologically asymptomatic until the time of hemorrhage, though they may show symptoms of the underlying and predisposing disease (e.g., endocarditis). The presentation is usually with either subarach-

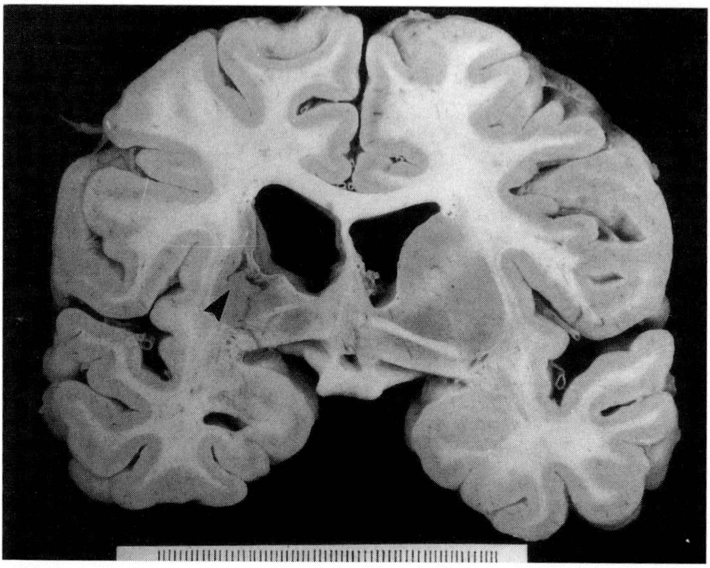

(A)

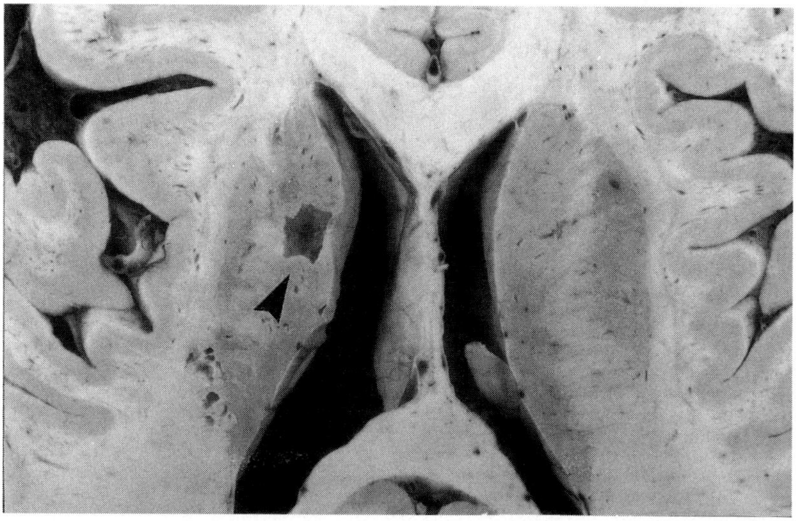

(B)

Figure 45 Lacunar infarcts. Arrowheads in each panel illustrate characteristic lacunar infarcts in **(A)** left putamen and internal capsule, with partial collapse of overlying lateral ventricle; **(B)** left caudate nucleus (horizontal brain section); and **(C)** pons—all common locations for these enigmatic lesions.

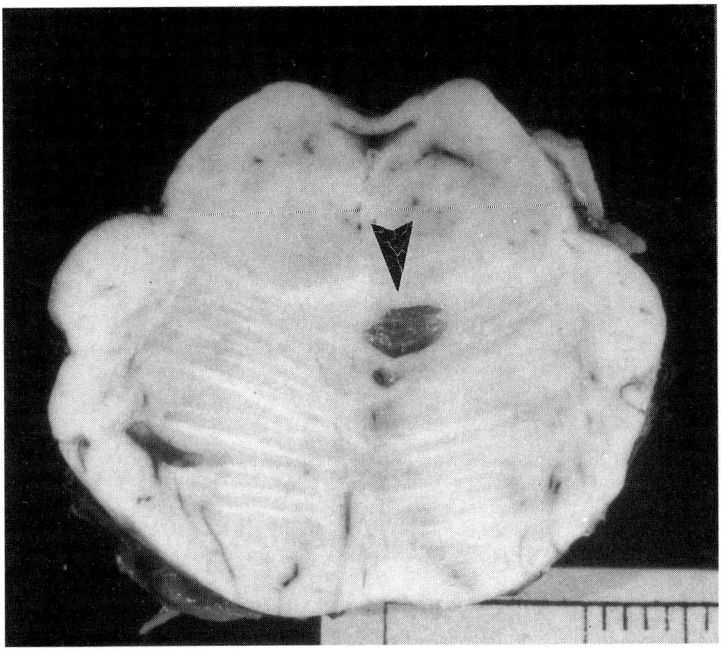

(C)

noid or intraparenchymal hemorrhage; less commonly, infarct or headache. The primary differential includes other causes of SAH; meningoencephalitis or brain abscess also needs to be considered, as affected patients may appear septic. Indeed, infectious aneurysms may coexist with brain abscess or meningoencephalitis.

Neuropathologic features: Infectious aneurysms usually occur distal to the main branch points on the circle of Willis. They are smaller than berry aneurysms, and may be difficult or impossible to identify grossly unless large; therefore, sections that incorporate small arteries from the edge of a hematoma are most likely to yield the finding of an infectious aneurysm. They can be identified in surgically resected clot evacuated from a patient at risk; clinical information on the patient from whom clot originates is important. Stains that highlight elastica, fungi, and bacteria are likely to show the extent of vessel wall damage and the causal organism in the vessel/arterial wall (Fig. 53).

c. *Fusiform Aneurysms.* These present as a tortuous, serpiginous, dilated, and ectatic artery, and may attain massive size. They usually occur in the vertebrobasilar system, especially the midportion of the basilar artery, less often in

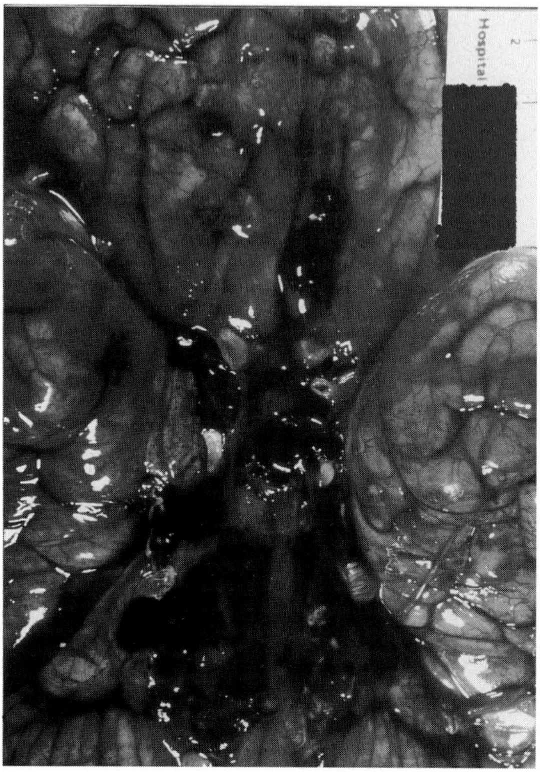

(A)

Figure 46 Subarachnoid hemorrhage secondary to berry/saccular aneurysm. Patient died following a severe sudden-onset headache with rapid progression to coma. Note abundant fresh blood in the basal cisterns **(A).** Panel **B** shows the responsible ant. communicating a./ACA aneurysm—note the tear in the aneurysm wall. No other aneurysms or vascular malformations were discovered within the brain.

the intracranial ICA. Except in children (where they occur very rarely), fusiform aneurysms are associated with severe complicated atherosclerosis in the involved arterial wall. Affected patients usually present with brainstem or cranial nerve compression when a fusiform aneurysm is on the basilar artery, ischemia (secondary to thrombosis), or hemorrhage.

Neuropathologic features: Major features include effects of the aneurysm on brain parenchyma (e.g., compression, ischemia, acute or remote hemorrhage) and histologic components of the aneurysm itself—usually those of severe complicated atherosclerosis including foamy histiocytes, evidence of old

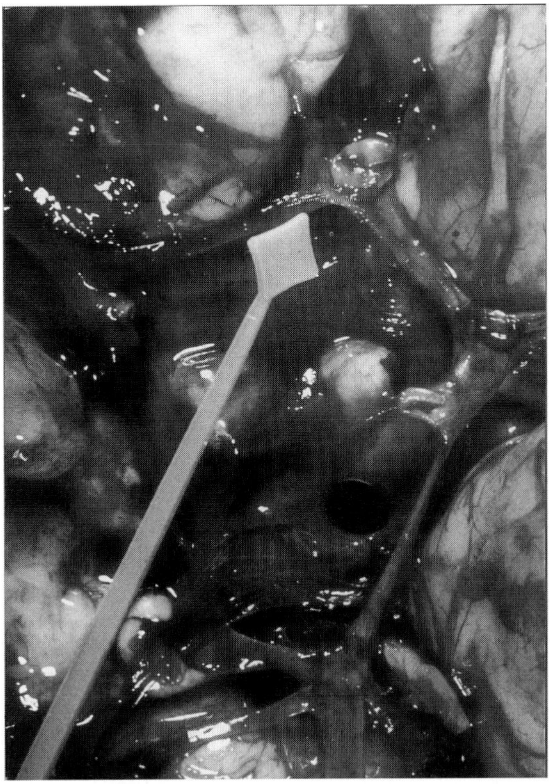

(B)

intraplaque hemorrhage, calcification, and thrombosis. Variable degrees of inflammation may be seen, and acute subarachnoid hemorrhage may be present.

d. Miscellaneous Causes of SAH. Small to moderate-size SAH of unknown origin is commonly encountered at autopsy, especially in thrombocytopenic patients or those with a coagulopathy. Rare causes of SAH include neoplastic aneurysms, especially originating in occlusive emboli from cardiac myxoma or choriocarcinoma that invade multiple foci in the distal vasculature to produce ectasia with focal rupture, and traumatic aneurysms, which are in reality false aneurysms. The cause of a given SAH remains clinically "occult" in approximately 15% to 20% of patients, who have a better overall prognosis than patients who suffer SAH due to a ruptured aneurysm. Hypothesized causes of bleeding in these patients, which may represent a special challenge to the neuropathologist performing the necropsy in such an individual, include clinically undiscovered bleeding diathesis; rupture of a small, angiographically unde-

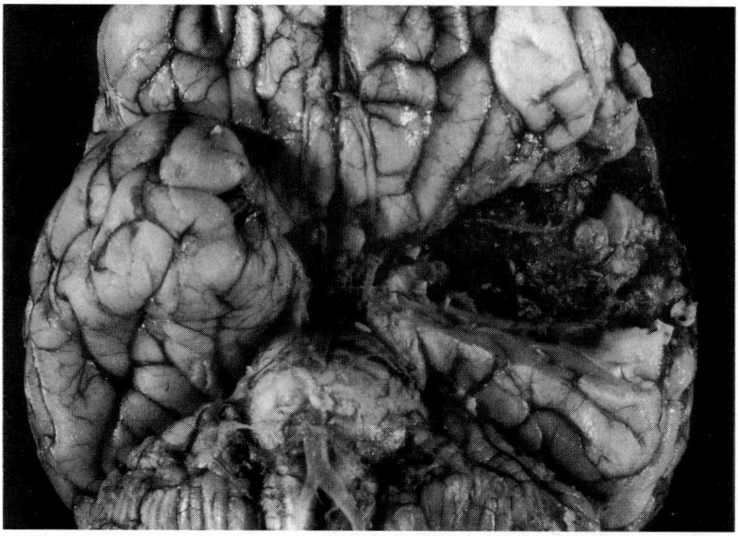

(A)

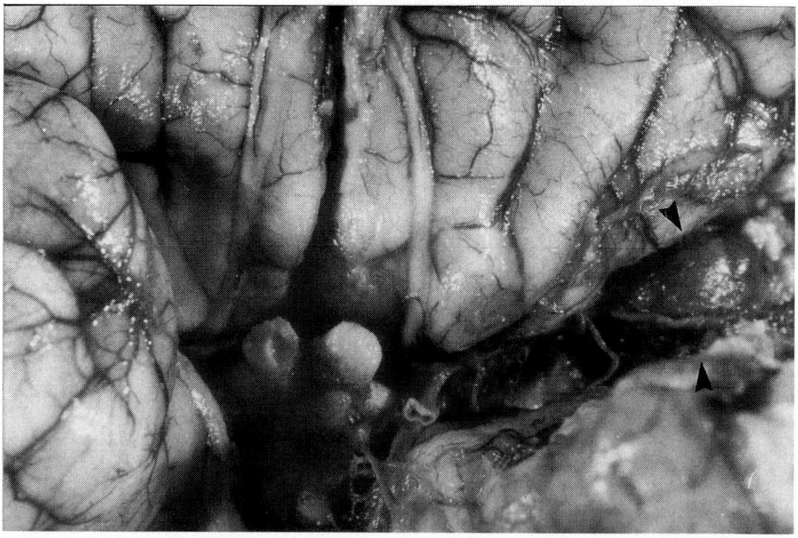

(B)

Figure 47 A young man developed severe headaches and right hemiparesis, with rapid progression to coma and death. **(A)** Large amount of clotted blood in the left Sylvian fissure (temporal tip has been cut away). **(B)** Close-up view of the left Sylvian fissure—a large berry aneurysm (arrowheads) is just visible. **(C)** Large left MCA bi/

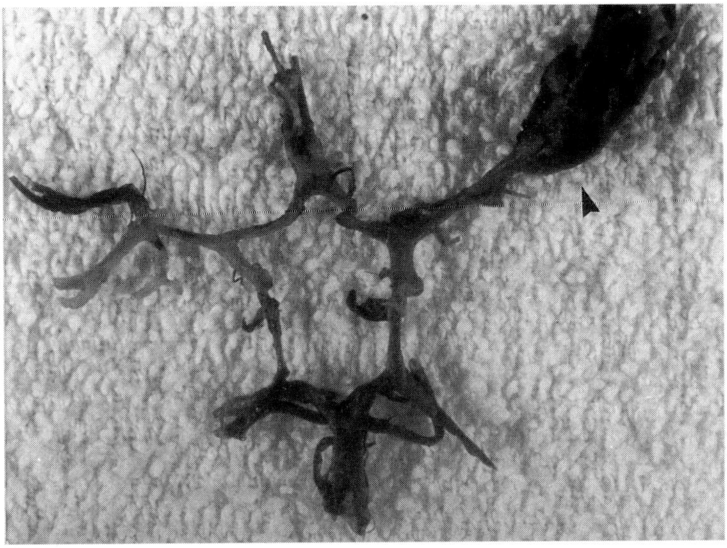

(C)

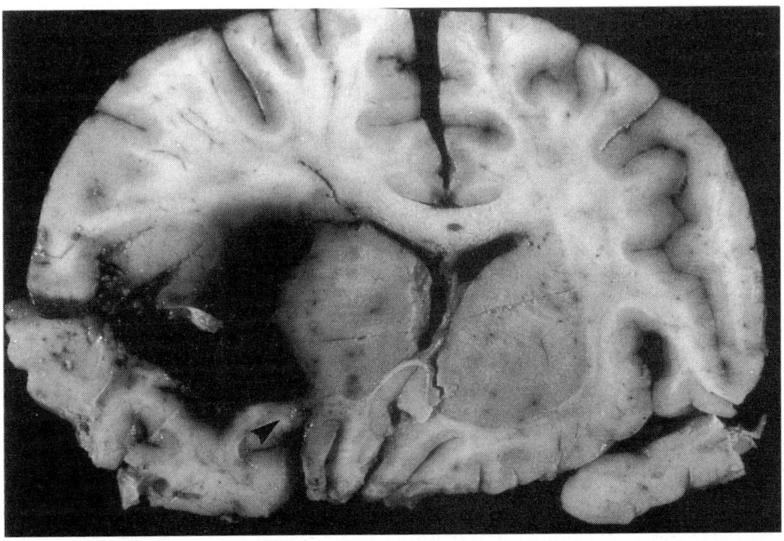

(D)

trifurcation aneurysm (arrow) on the circle of Willis, which has been dissected away from the fixed brain. **(D)** Coronal section of fixed brain; note clotted blood in the left cerebral hemisphere in and adjacent to the basal ganglia. Arrowhead indicates likely site of entry of blood into brain parenchyma.

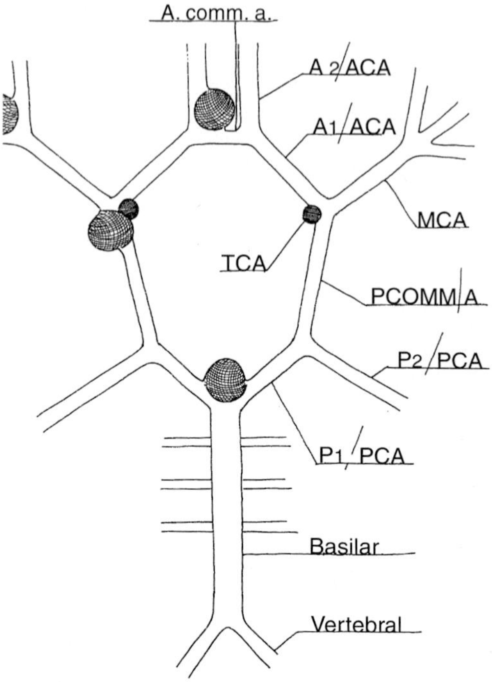

Figure 48 Common sites of berry aneurysms on the circle of Willis. Approximately 70–85% of such aneurysms occur in the "anterior" circulation—i.e., anterior to the post. communicating arteries. ACA = anterior cerebral a; PCA = posterior cerebral a; P. comm. a. = posterior communicating a; A. comm. a. = anterior communicating a; ICA = internal carotida.

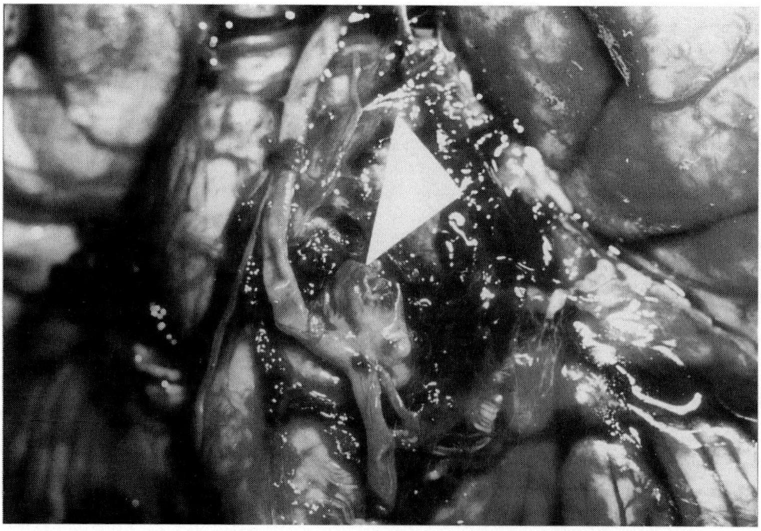

Figure 49 **Vertebral a.** aneurysm (arrow) which had ruptured to produce extensive acute SAH in the posterior fossa surrounding brainstem and cerebellum (visible in the background).

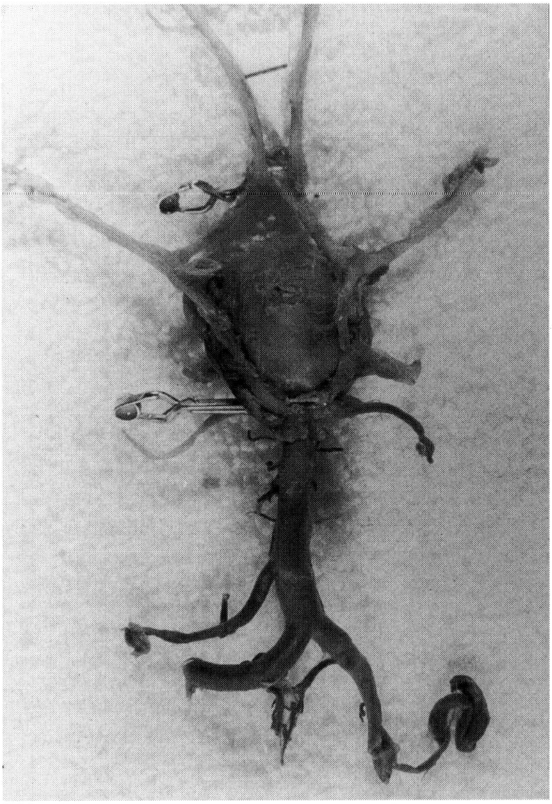

Figure 50 Berry aneurysms are frequently "clipped" as a therapeutic measure. In this patient, note two clips—one on a small (not visible) ant. communicating a. aneurysm (top of photograph), the other on a large basilar tip aneurysm.

tected vessel or vascular malformation; and rupture of a partly thrombosed berry aneurysm.

3. Intracerebral/Intraparenchymal Hemorrhage (ICH)

This term defines "extravasation of blood into the brain substance or parenchyma." Because in common usage, it is also used to describe bleeding into the cerebral hemispheres, brainstem, and cerebellum, the adjective *encephalic* is more accurate and inclusive than *intracerebral*; in practical terms, the two are synonyms. Although a hematoma may originate within brain substance, blood may commonly extend into the ventricles, meninges, and basal cisterns, producing secondary subarachnoid or intraventricular hemorrhage. There are many etiologies for encephalic hemorrhage, and hemorrhage is attributed to these different causes with varying frequency among tertiary medical centers, depending on their areas of interest and specialization. For instance, a geriatric hospital would more likely have comparatively large numbers of ICH secondary to cerebral amyloid angiopathy, whereas a cancer hospital would encounter a disproportionately large number of hematomas related to thrombocytopenia or blood dyscrasias. In general, cerebral infarcts are five to 10 times more common than ICH, except in Asian populations.

a. Hypertension. As hypertension became recognized as a major risk factor for both large and small vessel disease affecting the viscera and brain, its control and prevention have become a major public health challenge—one met with remarkable success. As a result, hypertensive ICH has declined by as much as 50% from the years 1945 to 1960 to the late 1980s. However, it continues to account for 40% to 50% of ICH. Microvascular events leading to ICH are described by various terms, one of the most popular being "lipohyalinosis." The distinction or relationship between *lipohyalinosis* and *arteriolosclerosis* (which affects arteries in the range of 50 to 250 μm diameter) is not clear, and they may represent different parts of a spectrum.

Such hemorrhages present in patients who have a documented history of hypertension or, if the bleed is fatal, evidence of hypertension is found at autopsy (e.g., left ventricular [cardiac] hypertrophy, arteriolonephrosclerosis). Hemorrhages most commonly occur in the lateral basal ganglia (especially the putamen), thalamus, cerebellum, pons, and subcortical white matter.

Neuropathologic features: These depend largely on the duration and location of the hematomas; most are commonly found in one of the locations described above. Hypertensive bleeds tend to be single. An acute hematoma has an appearance of "red currant jelly"—a variably sized clot of blood distinct from brain parenchyma that may fall away from the fixed brain during cutting of the specimen (Fig. 54). Hypertensive hemorrhages frequently extend into the ventricular system and very rarely dissect directly into the subarachnoid space, though blood may reach the subarachnoid region secondarily after passage through the ventricular system. Cerebral herniations often result and may be

---

Figure 51 Berry aneurysm, microscopic features. **(A)** Trilobed aneurysm with variable fibromuscular hyperplasia and pronounced focal thinning throughout its lobes. Note that elastica, which is easily identifiable in the "parent" artery (at bottom), is almost totally absent from the aneurysm. **(B)** Rupture site of a berry aneurysm. Blood emanating from the aneurysm "dome" is seen at right; aneurysm lumen is at bottom of the micrograph. Thin/attenuated portion of the aneurysm wall has "folded back" over itself after yielding to blood. In this section, stained for elastica, none is visible.

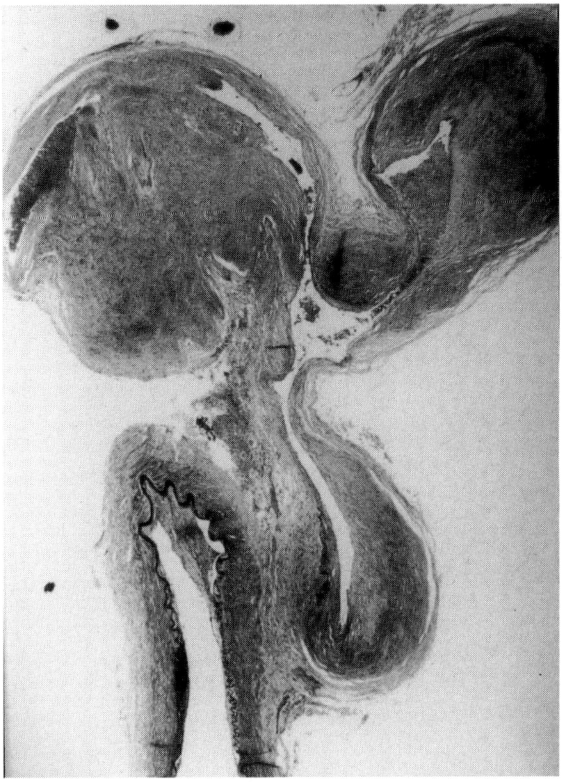

(A)

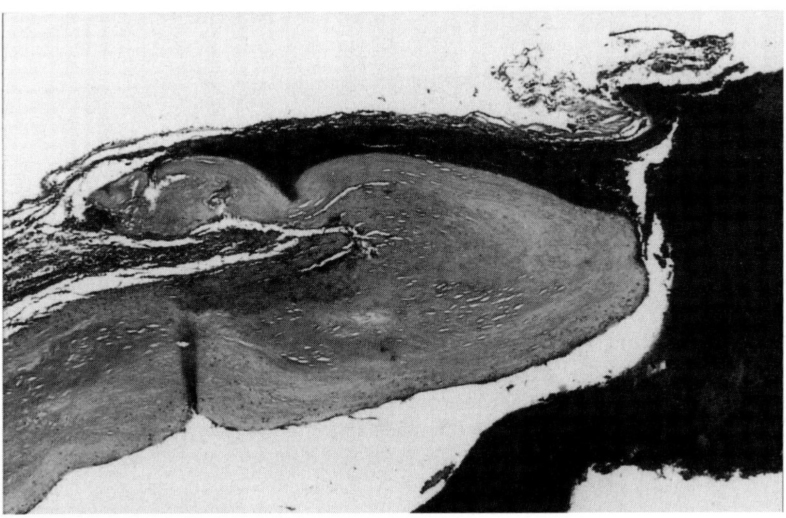

(B)

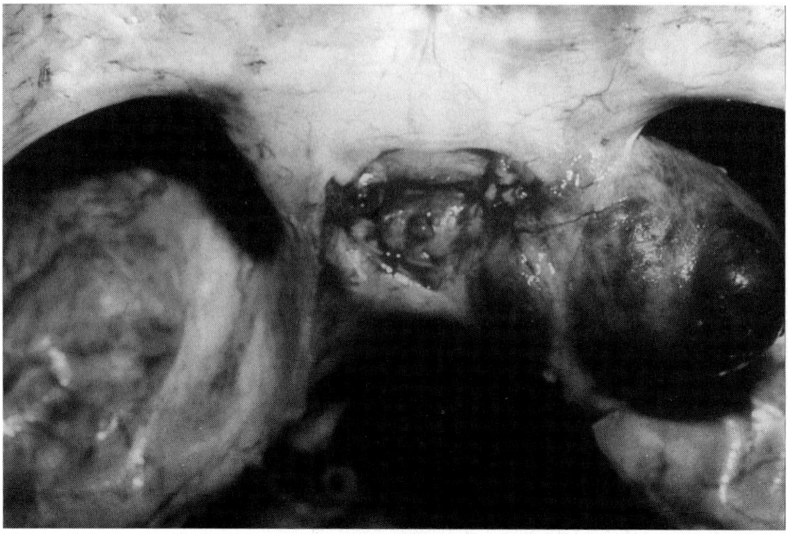

(A)

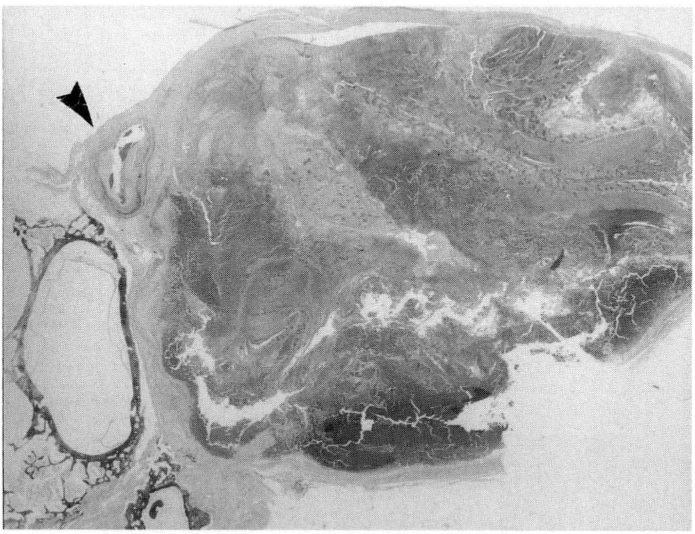

(B)

Figure 52 Giant internal carotid (cavernous segment) aneurysm discovered in an 81-year-old man who came to necropsy as part of a dementia study protocol. Aneurysm had caused extensive compression of the optic n. and oculomotor n. Gross appearance at autopsy shows aneurysm bulging massively in the right middle fossa **(A)**; sella turcica with pituitary gland is at center of the photograph. **(B)** Whole mount of the aneurysm (ICA indicated by arrow) with extensive thrombosis. (Figures kindly provided by Robert Hammond, University Hospital and University of Western Ontario, London, Ontario, Canada.)

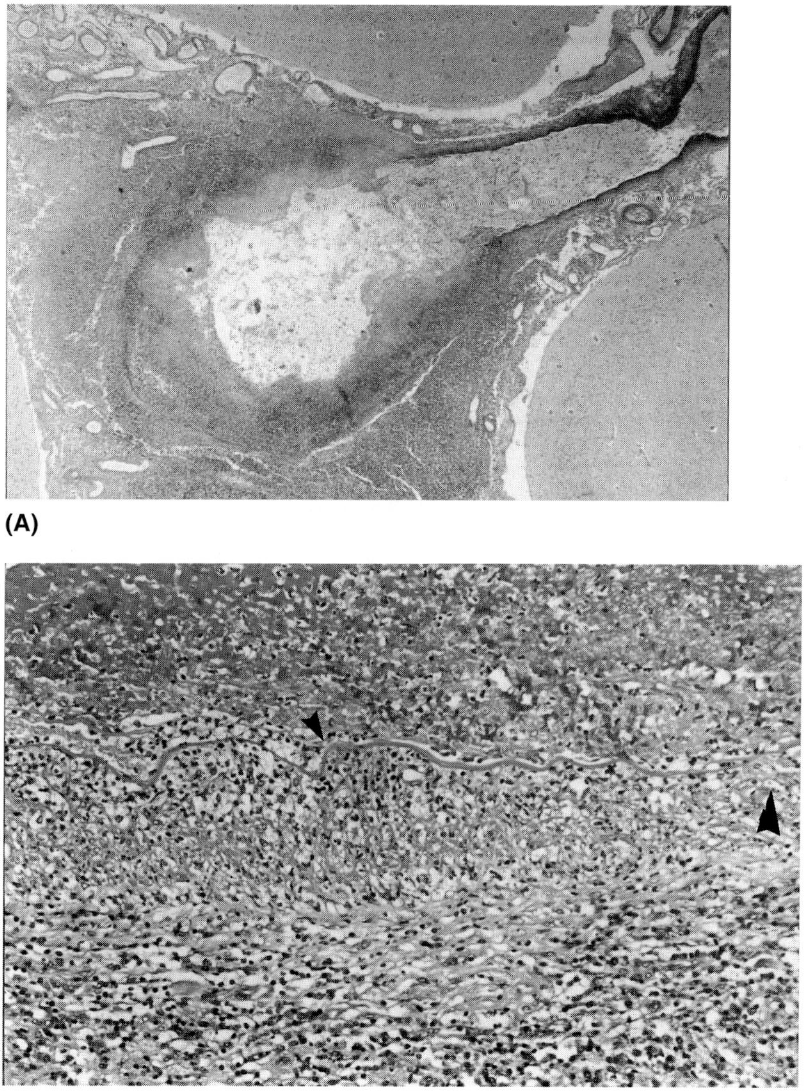

(A)

(B)

Figure 53 Infectious aneurysms (IAs). **(A)** Meningeal artery, in a section stained for elastica, shows abrupt loss of elastica and expansion of the arterial wall into a goblet-shaped enlargement. Patient had undergone orthotopic liver transplant and had widespread *Aspergillus* infection, including meningitis; fungal organisms were identified in the affected segments of arterial wall. Widespread cerebral hemorrhage had occurred. **(B)** An 87-year-old man with lung carcinoma and cerebral abscesses. Some parenchymal arteries showed transmural infiltration by polymorphonuclear leukocytes (as in this micrograph) with early destruction of the elastica (indicated by arrows).

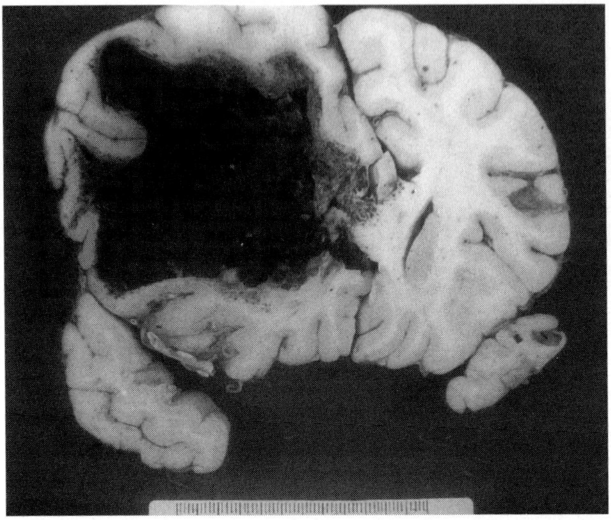

(A)

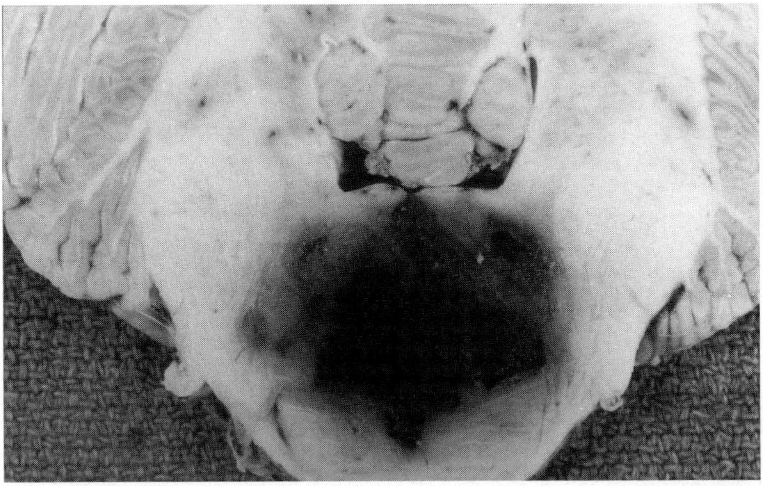

(B)

Figure 54 Hypertensive ICH. (**A**) A left cerebral hemorrhage, probably originating in the basal ganglia, fills and expands the white matter of the adjacent centrum semiovale, with intraventricular extension and massive left-to-right shift of midline structures. (**B**) Pontine hematoma of several weeks' duration shows early organization at its edges.

fatal. Older hematomas may resorb, producing a cystic cavity within brain lined by orange-brown material representing altered blood pigment (Fig. 55). This appearance may mimic that of an old cystic infarct; however, an area of "remote" cerebral hemorrhage may be distinguished from an infarct by *location* (hypertensive hematomas are usually not confined to a major vessel territory), and the *amount of altered pigment* that remains at the margin of the cavity; this is usually more plentiful after ICH than in an infarct, except a prominently hemorrhagic infarct. If a hematoma is longstanding, the expected Wallerian degeneration will occur within affected long tracts (Fig. 55).

Microscopically, acute bleeds show fresh blood where it has dissected through tissue planes or along tracts; there may be variable numbers of inflammatory cells including polymorphonuclear leukocytes and (if at least 2 or 3 days have elapsed between the hemorrhage and death) macrophages and gitter cells. Older hematomas show margination by hemosiderin-laden macrophages, non-hemosiderin-laden macrophages, cytoid bodies, and variably dense collections of astrocytes (Fig. 56). Microvascular lesions vary; the affected vessels are usually in the size range of 50 to 250 μm in diameter. There may be onion-skin-type thickening, particularly at loci in which hypertensive bleeds are common (Fig. 57). Lipohyalinosis, with thickening of the vessel wall by hyaline (nonamyloid) material and lipid-bearing macrophages may occur, with resultant compromise or even obliteration of the lumen. Microaneurysms (Charcot-Bouchard type) may be seen as outpouchings that originate in an abnormal vessel wall (Fig. 58). The aneurysm lumen may be partly or entirely obliterated and/or surrounded by recent hemorrhage or altered blood pigment. Though Charcot-Bouchard aneurysms are said to be of pathogenic importance in causing hypertensive hemorrhage, in practice they are observed rather infrequently and may be seen with other forms of microangiopathy (e.g., amyloid angiopathy; see below). Fibrinoid necrosis may be present in arteriolar walls and is consistently present with hypertensive encephalopathy of malignant hypertension. Attempting to define the microvessel(s) from which hemorrhage originated may be frustrating and counterproductive, since in some cases this site is almost certainly obliterated in the course of the bleeding.

b. Cerebral Amyloid/Congophilic Angiopathy (CAA). In many series, this is now described as the second most common cause of primary nontraumatic ICH, accounting for as many as 10% to 15% of all ICHs. The most common form of CAA is strongly (but not exclusively) associated with Alzheimer's disease (AD) and brain aging; indeed, CAA has long been recognized as one of the microscopic defining lesions of AD, the only one that consistently involves AD brain microvasculature. CAA results from replacement of the media of brain parenchymal microvessels (mainly arterioles) by skeins of filamentous material of 7 to 10 nm thickness which show tinctorial properties of amyloid. CAA can involve meningeal and parenchymal (usually cortical) arterioles. ICH usually

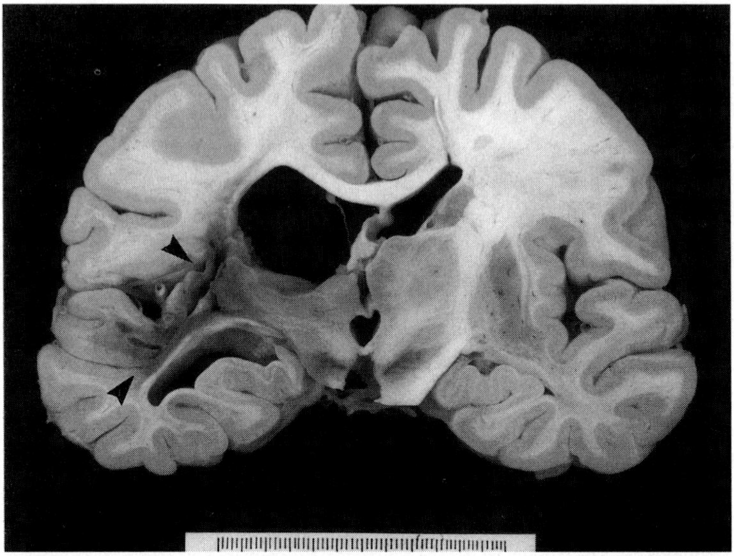

(A)

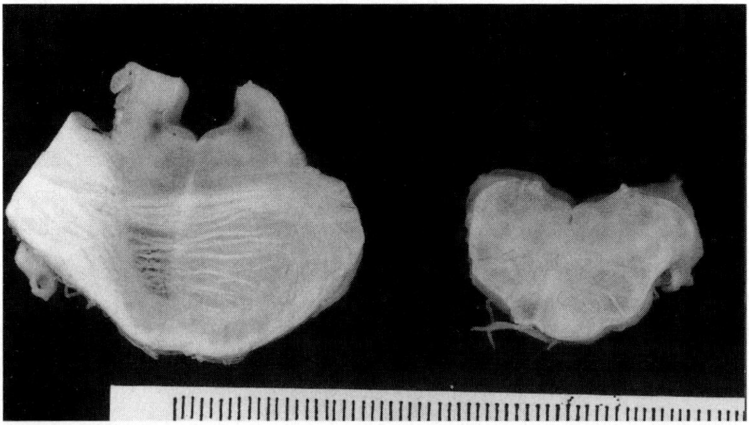

(B)

Figure 55 Old/remote hypertensive ICH which had occurred years prior to the patient's death. (**A**) Note residual cystic cavity in the left cerebral hemisphere (indicated by arrowheads); at time of brain cutting, the cavity was surrounded by orange-brown material representing residua of old hemorrhage (the gray region surrounding the cavity in this B&W photograph). Note atrophy of surrounding brain parenchyma with massive dilatation ("hydrocephalus ***ex vacuo***") of left lateral ventricle. (**B**) Severe Wallerian degeneration, as expected, was noted in ipsilateral corticospinal tracts in the pons and medulla.

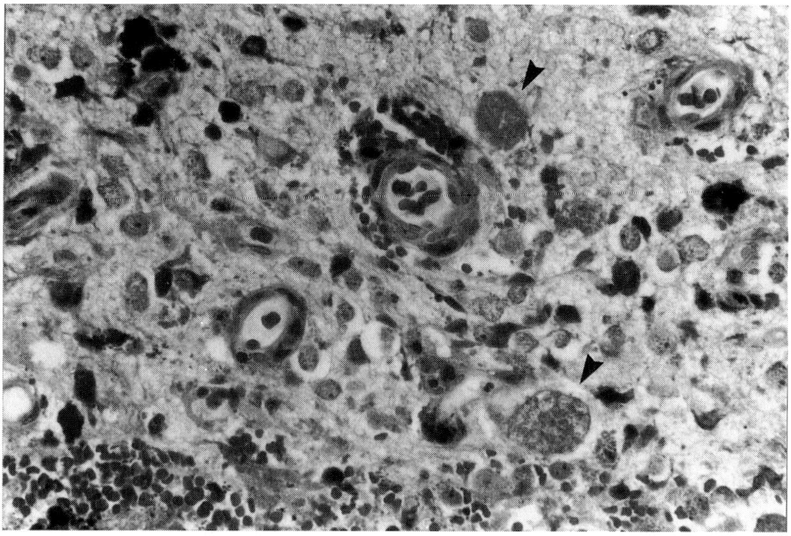

Figure 56 Microscopic histologic findings at margin of an "old" cerebral hemorrhage are relatively uniform **regardless** of the etiology of the hemorrhage. Typically, abundant hemosiderin-laden macrophages are seen, and cytoid boides (arrows) are plentiful, as are reactive astrocytes.

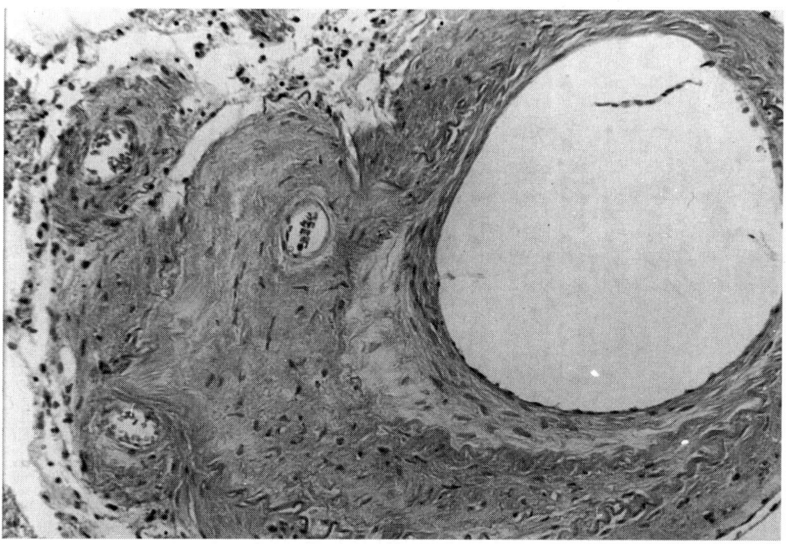

Figure 57 Arteriosclerotic microvascular disease. A small parenchymal artery shows intimal hyperplasia—i.e., fibromuscular thickening of the vessel wall superficial to the elastica.

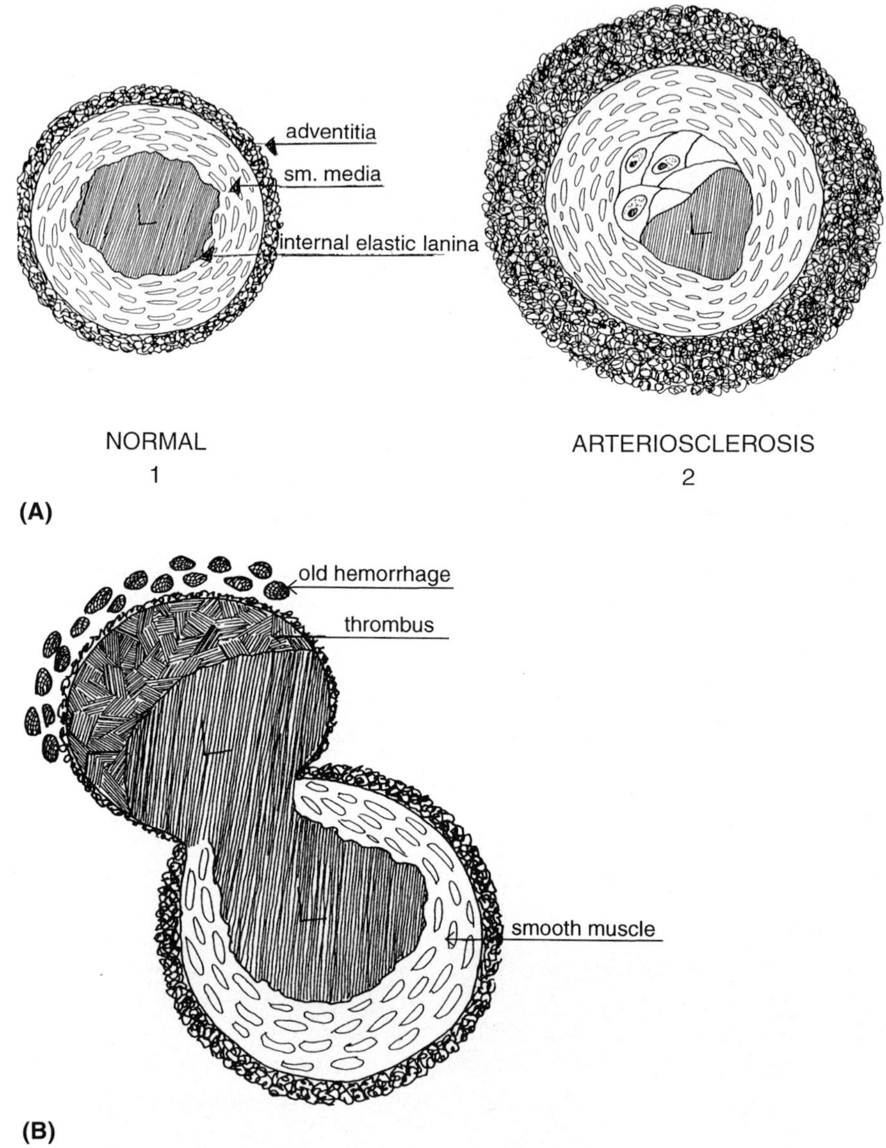

Figure 58 One scenario for "progression" of intraparenchymal arteriosclerotic change from "normal" vessel to severe arteriosclerosis and (sometimes) formation of Charcot-Bouchard-type microaneurysms. Oval cells pictured adjacent to the lumen (L) in (2) represent lipid-laden macrophages. The distinction between ***arteriosclerotic*** change and ***lipohyalinosis*** is not always clear; many authors use the terms interchangeably.

results from rupture of *parenchymal* vessels. The recognition that CAA was a microscopic hallmark of AD led initially to isolation of CAA-affected microvessels from AD brain, with amyloid purification and its preliminary chemical characterization by Glenner's group in 1984. This form of CAA has been biochemically characterized as resulting from deposition within the vessel wall of the AD β/A4 protein, a roughly 4-kDa peptide which derives from a larger precursor protein, the A4 or amyloid precursor protein (APP). Within AD brains, A4 deposits within cortical parenchyma as senile plaques, and in microvessel walls as CAA (see Chap. 8). Two regionally important familial forms of CAA have also been characterized:

i. Icelandic CAA. This is inherited as an autosomal-dominant trait, associated with ICH in young adult or middle-aged patients in this country. It is biochemically distinct from A4 CAA, and is characterized by microvascular deposition of a mutant form of cystatin C-γ trace, a cysteine proteinase inhibitor. A single nucleotide substitution occurs in codon 68 of the gene that encodes the protein. This form of cerebral hemorrhage is now widely referred to as *hereditary cystatin C amyloid angiopathy* (*HCCAA*), or hereditary cerebral hemorrhage with amyloidosis—Icelandic (HCHWA-I).

ii. Dutch CAA. Also inherited as an autosomal-dominant trait, described by the term *hereditary cerebral hemorrhage with amyloidosis—Dutch* (*HCHWA-D*). In this geographic region and condition, amyloid deposition occurs in brain arterial walls leading to hemorrhage in middle-aged and older patients. Amyloid and amyloid precursor protein are also deposited within brain parenchyma, but less extensively than in AD, though patients frequently become demented prior to the development of cerebral bleeding. The vascular amyloid is related to β/A4 and results from a mutation at codon 693 of APP.

CAA-related hemorrhages are almost always *lobar* intraparenchymal hematomas occurring (except in Icelandic and Dutch forms) in elderly individuals, especially those with clinical or neuroimaging features consistent with an AD type of dementia. Hematomas may be multiple, occurring sequentially over a period of months or years. Such hemorrhages may dissect into the subarachnoid space and/or ventricles (Fig. 59). Hematomas seen with HCCAA or HCHWA-D are similar to lobar bleeds seen with AD-related CAA and are defined by their geographic, genetic, clinical, and neuroimaging features.

Neuropathologic features: Identification of a lobar cerebral hemorrhage (Fig. 60), particularly in an elderly individual, suggests CAA as the etiology. Cortex and subcortical white matter are frequently involved, often with direct extension of hemorrhage into the subarachnoid space. Unlike hypertensive hematomas, CAA-related bleeds are rarely cerebellar and are virtually never found in the brainstem. Other appearances of the hematoma depend on its duration prior to the patient's death. Microscopically, brain changes reactive to the presence of intraparenchymal blood are as described for hypertensive bleeds;

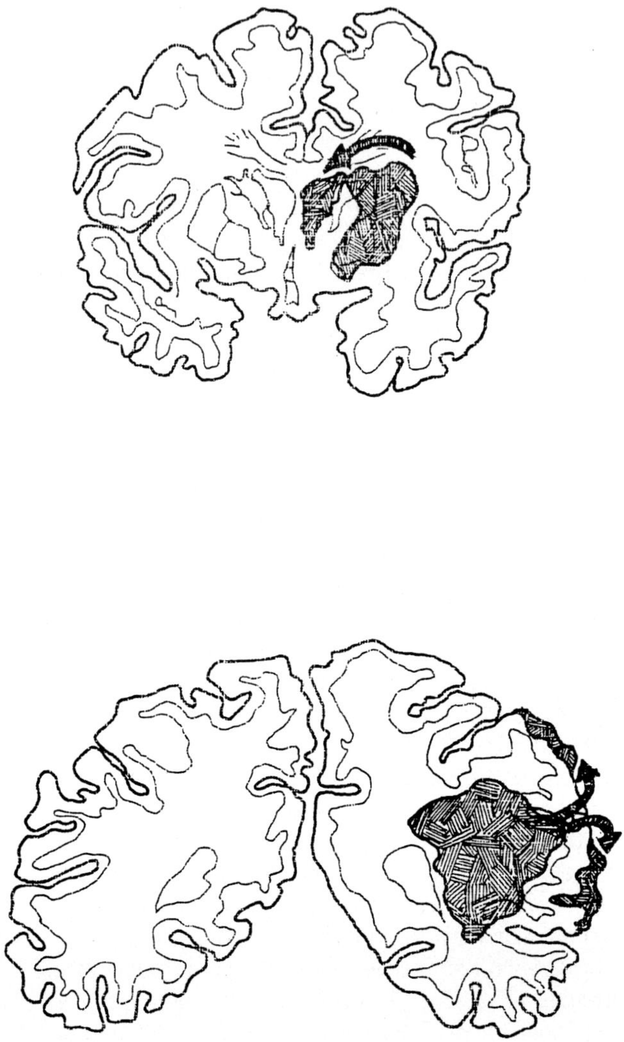

Figure 59 Whereas hypertensive cerebral hemorrhages are usually "central" and tend to dissect into the **ventricular cavities** (top panel), CAA-related hematomas are usually lobar and dissect directly into the **subarachnoid space** (lower panel).

Figure 60 CAA-related cerebral hemorrhage. **(A,B)** Characteristic hematomas in two different individuals. The hematoma in **(B)** shows early organization at its edges; other regions of this patient's brain showed cystic cavities representing resorbed CAA-related bleeds that had occurred months or years prior to death.

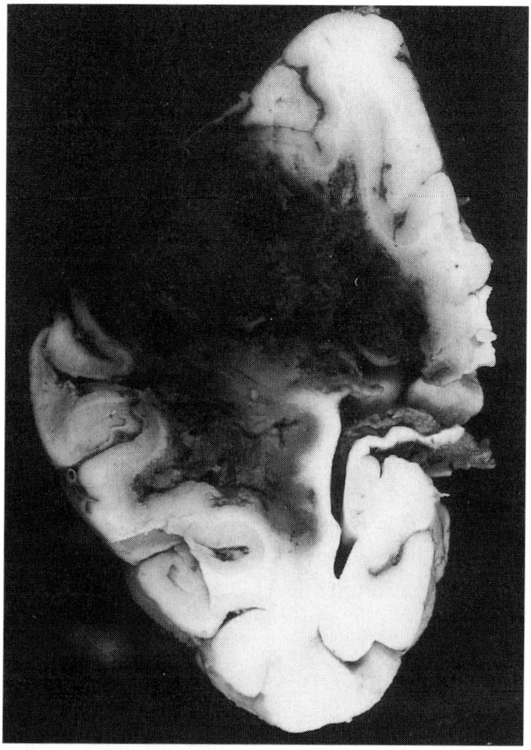

(A)

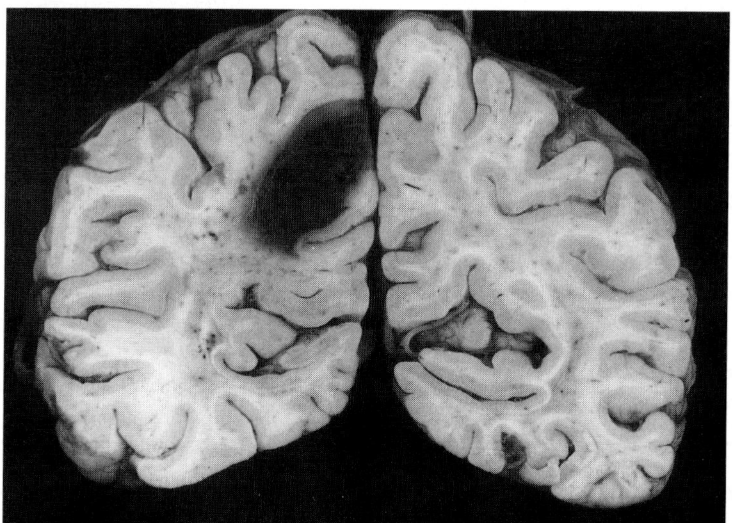

(B)

rarely, severe CAA may be seen in regions of encephalomalacia, though its relationship to ischemic lesions is not well defined. CAA (of all biochemical varieties) is demonstrable by stains that are used to highlight the presence of amyloid (Fig. 61). However, biochemical CAA subtypes can be demonstrated using specific anti-β/A4 immunohistochemistry or anticystatin C antibodies (Fig. 62). CAA-associated microangiopathies include microaneurysm formation (essentially indistinguishable from Charcot-Bouchard aneurysms seen with hypertension), hyalinosis, variable degrees of inflammation (including granulomatous angiitis), fibrinoid necrosis, and (rarely) thrombosis.

c. Vascular Malformations. Here, we will consider vascular malformations other than berry aneurysms (see above). They are considered here for convenience, though all do not necessarily present with ICH; many forms are most commonly encountered as an incidental finding at autopsy. The pathogenesis of all subtypes is unknown. Often erroneously described as "congenital," these lesions (with the exception of vein of Galen aneurysms) are almost never found in infants. They may result, however, from a poorly defined congenital propensity to develop later in life, but the biologic substrate of this tendency has yet to be defined. As a group, they probably account for 4% to 5% of ICH; Figure 63 schematically illustrates their characteristic morphologic features. They include the following subtypes:

i. Arteriovenous Malformation (AVM): This is the most commonly symptomatic variety of vascular malformation and the most common type of vascular malformation encountered among surgical specimens. It may present with ICH, subarachnoid hemorrhage, or focal ischemia, the last due to a "steal" of blood from normal brain leading to a progressive neurologic deficit. These are rarely familial and rarely multiple, but may be associated with berry aneurysm on an artery that "feeds" the AVM. They are slightly more common in men than women, and can occur at any age but are most common in the third and fourth decades. AVM-related brain hemorrhage is different from hemorrhage related to berry aneurysm in that the former rarely leads to vasospasm. Angiographically, AVMs are defined as having a nidus, "feeding" arteries, and draining veins.

These lesions often extend from the brain parenchyma into the subarachnoid space and are often in the MCA territory. They contain arteries, veins, and intermediate vascular forms, sometimes described as "arterialized veins" with thick walls lacking elastica. Vessels are of markedly variable caliber, wall thickness, and lumen diameter (Fig. 64). The vessel walls and surrounding brain parenchyma often show varying degrees of calcification. Intimal cushions resulting from fibromuscular hyperplasia that impinge on the lumen, and vessel wall hyalinization are prominent features within AVMs. Surrounding brain often shows major reactive changes including old hemorrhage, cytoid bodies, Rosen-

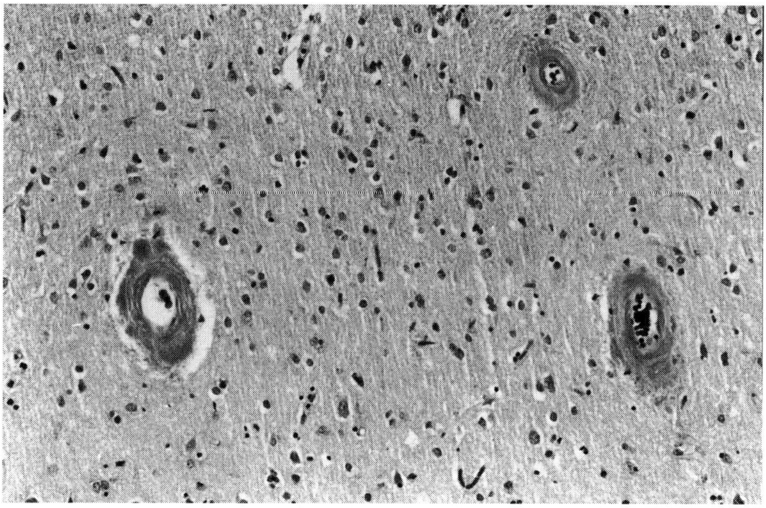

(A)

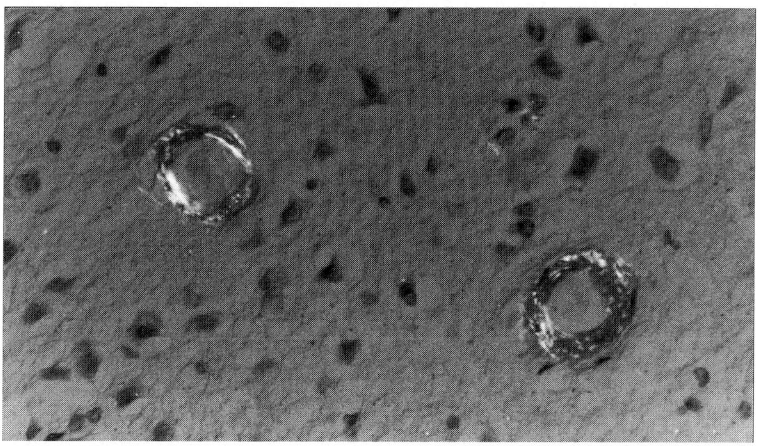

(B)

Figure 61 CAA is recognized on routine stains as an effacement of the normal arteriolar wall with replacement of the medial smooth muscle by eosinophilic hyaline material **(A).** The amyloid often (as in this case) appears to extend into the brain parenchyma (see also Chap. 8). When a section is stained with Congo red and examined under polarized light **(B),** characteristic (yellow-green) birefringence is noted in the affected vessel walls.

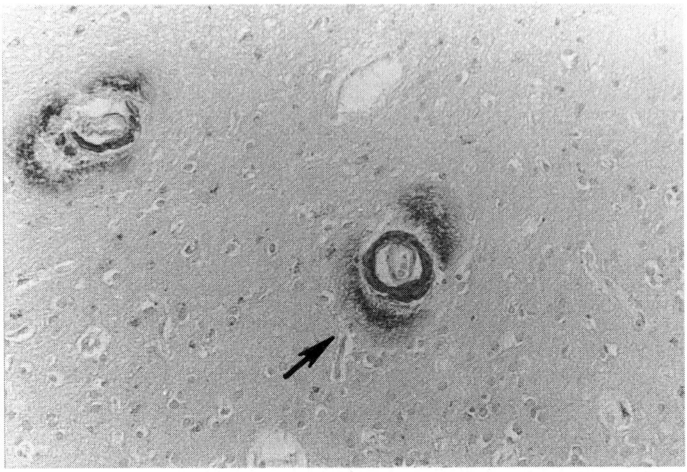

Figure 62 CAA can be highlighted using antibodies to amyloid proteins; in this case AD-related CAA is demonstrated by immunohistochemistry using primary antibodies to the Alzheimer β/A4 protein. β/A4 immunoreactive ***parenchymal*** material (arrow) is also seen surrounding affected arteries.

thal fibers, and astrocytic gliosis. Current therapy for AVM often includes iatrogenic embolization with various substances that are meant to induce thrombosis, but may also cause a pronounced inflammatory (including foreign body giant cell) reaction in the lumen and adjacent vessel walls (Fig. 65).

ii. Cavernous Hemangioma: These are not infrequently familial and, when familial, may be multiple. They present with cerebral hemorrhage, focal signs or seizures.

Neuropathologic characteristics include (grossly) a mulberrylike appearance, like a small, circumscribed hematoma within brain parenchyma. Microscopically, these lesions are tightly arrayed collections of hyalinized vessels lacking intervening brain parenchyma (Fig. 66) surrounded by abundant old hemorrhage and reactive astrocytic gliosis.

iii. Venous Angioma: Hemorrhage from these lesions is rare, except when they occur in the cerebellum. They are usually identified as an incidental finding at necropsy. Neuropathologic features include (grossly) the appearance of petechial or slightly larger hemorrhages, especially in the subcortical white matter of the cerebral hemispheres. Microscopically, these lesions are thin-walled, slightly ectatic, or dilated vascular channels lying within otherwise unremarkable brain parenchyma (Fig. 67).

iv. Telangiectases: These are almost always an incidental finding in the brainstem (especially the pons) at autopsy and virtually never produce

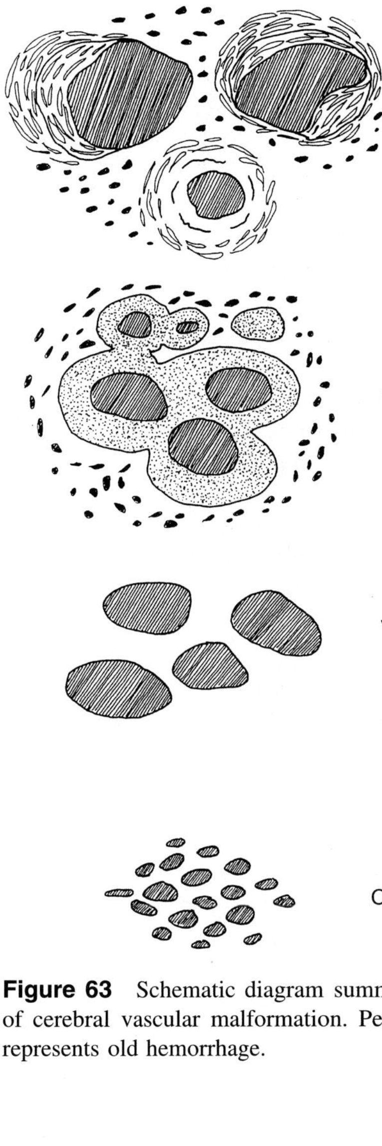

Figure 63 Schematic diagram summarizing key features of the most common types of cerebral vascular malformation. Perivascular "granular" material in top two panels represents old hemorrhage.

symptomatic hemorrhage. Neuropathologic features closely mimic the appearances of petechial hemorrhage. Microscopically, these lesions appear as collections of small-caliber, very thin-walled channels surrounded and encompassed by unremarkable CNS parenchyma, which the vessels do not appear to disturb (Fig. 68).

v. Arteriovenous Fistula: Strictly defined, this is not a vascular malformation but rather a "fistula," often a lesion resulting from aneurysmal rupture

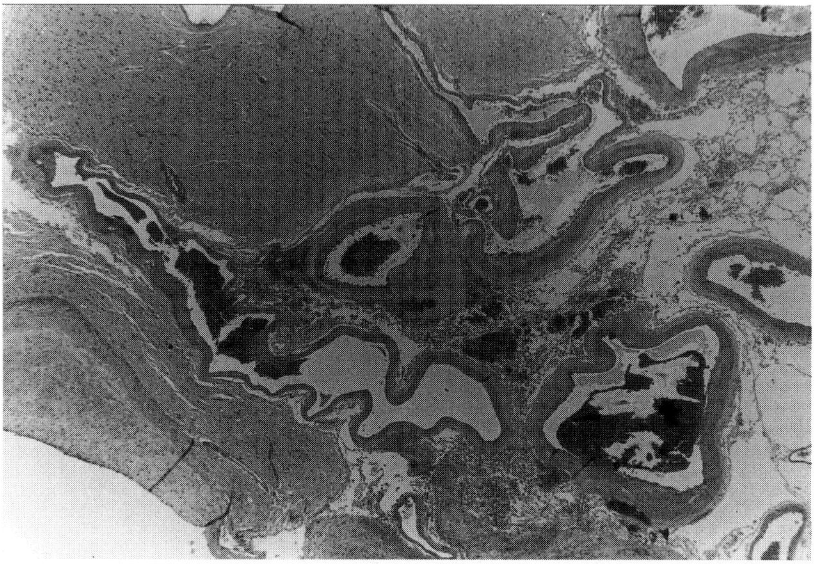

(A)

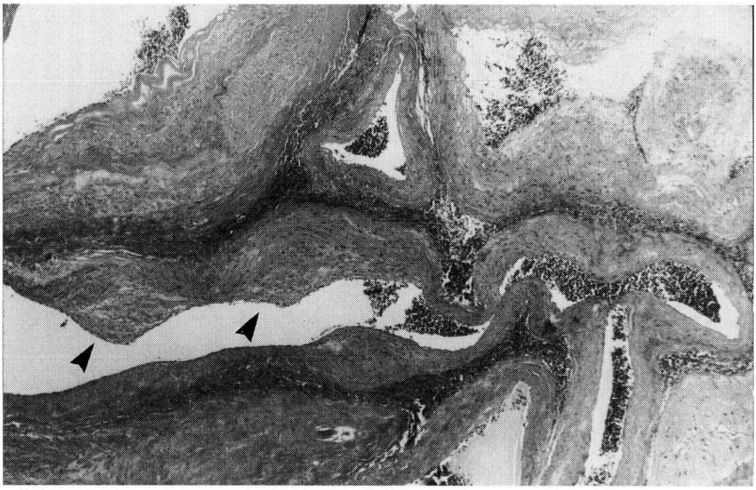

(B)

Figure 64 AVM, histologic features. AVMs consist of turtuous enlarged vessels of varying caliber and wall thickness; the "rupture" site in an AVM that has bled is frequently difficult/impossible to identify, **unlike** in a berry aneurysm. **(A)** AVM that extends from brain parenchyma (upper left) into the subarachnoid space (lower right). **(B)** Pronounced intimal hyperplasia (arrows) that "extends" into the vessel lumen.

into a venous sinus (e.g., carotid-cavernous fistula). This group includes the rare but clinically important congenital vein of Galen aneurysm (really an arteriovenous fistula) usually discovered in infants and children (Fig. 69).

d. ICH Secondary to Systemic/Medical Illness, Therapy, or Drug Treatment. This heterogeneous group of disorders encompasses conditions of diverse etiology. In some tertiary medical centers, this group may overall represent the commonest cause(s) of ICH. Pathologic features do not distinguish them from other types of ICH described above, except that microscopic examination fails to yield evidence of the type of microangiopathy seen with, for instance, CAA or hypertension. An etiologic diagnosis is usually made by association with the clinical condition together with laboratory documentation. Resultant hematomas are often multiple, and locations can be similar to those seen with cerebral hematomas noted with hypertension and CAA.

The most common causes of ICH in this group are:

1. Leukemia, with very high peripheral WBC count or thrombocytopenia secondary to treatment (or both); pancytopenia noted in patients prior to or after undergoing therapeutic bone marrow transplantation (Fig. 70).

2. Coagulopathy, either induced by iatrogenic anticoagulation (as many as 1% of these patients experience ICH), or secondary to hepatic disease or orthotopic liver transplantation (Fig. 71).

3. Administration of thrombolytic agents—e.g., streptokinase, urokinase, tissue plasminogen activator; these can also increase the tendency to ICH from primary microvascular disease—e.g., CAA.

e. ICH Secondary to Illicit Drug Use. Particularly in urban environments, where recreational drug use is common, this is becoming an increasingly observed phenomenon. However, the neuropathologic substrate and even pathogenesis of ICH in these patients are unclear. Drugs with which ICH is commonly encountered include cocaine (especially "crack"), amphetamines, phencyclidine, and phenylpropanolamine. ICH may result from sudden rises in blood pressure or from drug-associated vasculitis, which has rarely been documented pathologically but is often suggested by a characteristic (though not specific) "beading" appearance on angiography in affected patients. Neuropathologic features of drug-related ICH are otherwise not unique; thus many resemble classic hypertensive or CAA-related hematomas. Knowing the clinical context in which they occur is crucial. ICH related to ethanol abuse is probably multifactorial. Putative etiologic mechanisms include hepatic dysfunction with abnormal coagulation factors, and low platelet counts. Intraparenchymal hemorrhage may be associated with intraventricular and subarachnoid extension.

f. ICH Secondary to "Nonvascular" Causes. It is important to remember that all hemorrhagic lesions in the brain are not necessarily vascular. As noted elsewhere in this volume, both neoplasms and infections (e.g., with *Aspergillus*)

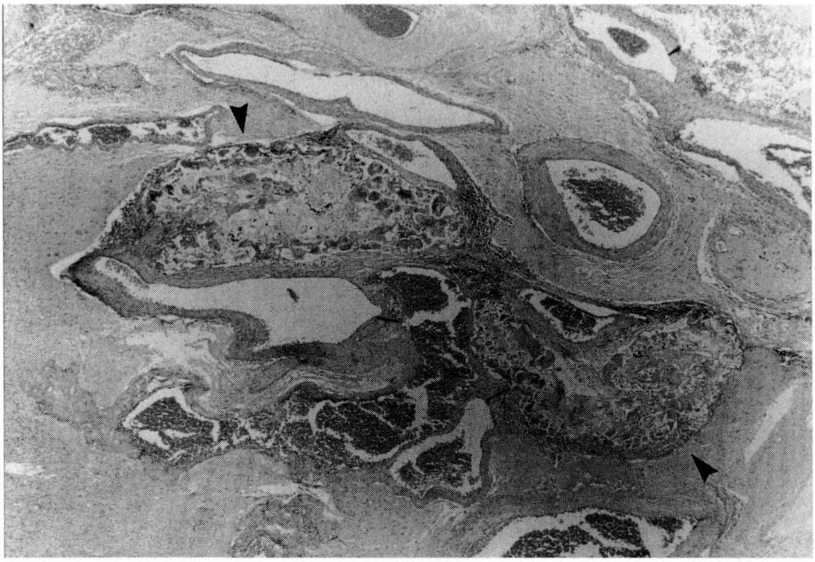

(A)

Figure 65 AVMs that underwent therapeutic embolization months prior to resection. Note partly or totally occluded lumina (arrowheads) containing multinucleated/foreign-body giant cells and peripheral clusters of lymphocytes that surround (barely discernible) residual particulate material **(A). (B)** Particulate material (together with reactive cells; arrow) that has become "incorporated" into an AVM vessel wall.

of various types may present with ICH. Among neoplasms, oligodendroglioma, glioblastoma, metastatic melanoma, and choriocarcinoma are notorious for occasionally "presenting as" ICH (Fig. 72). In the case of metastatic neoplasms, this may occur even before the primary tumor has declared itself. Knowledge of this masquerade leads to an important warning to all pathologists: *Carefully examine clot material that is resected in the course of surgical evacuation of an ICH*! Not only may a clinically occult neoplasm be discovered, but a vascular cause for the hemorrhage may be found (e.g., vasculitis, portion of a vascular malformation, evidence of CAA).

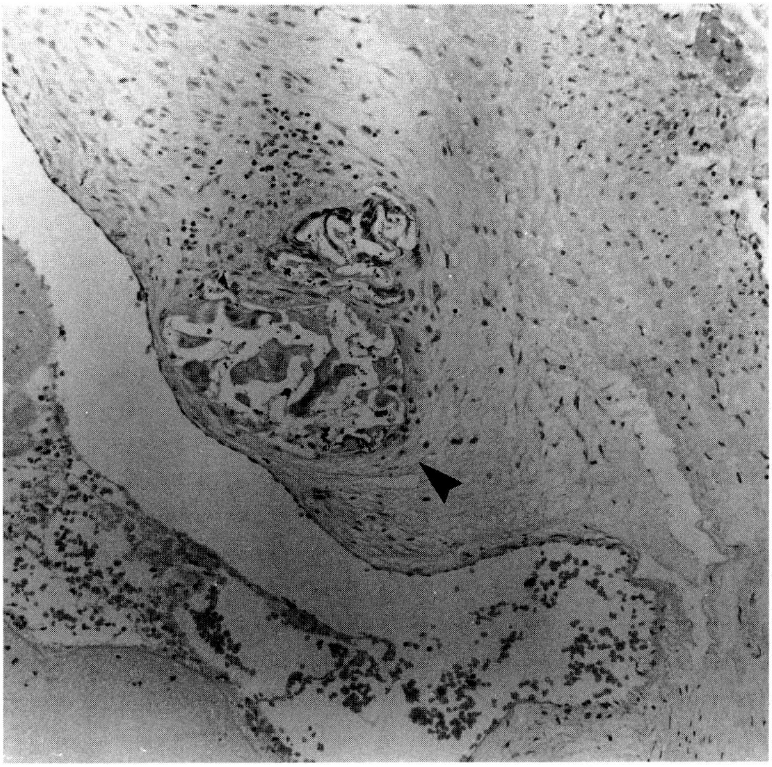

(B)

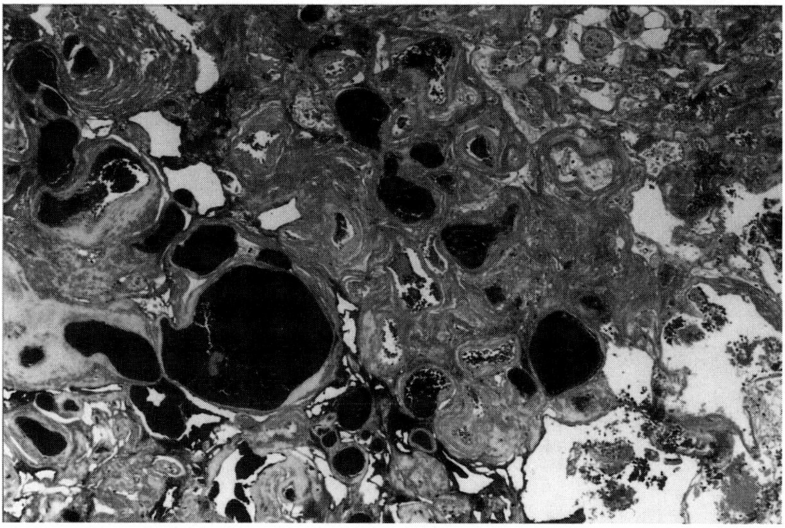

Figure 66 Cavernous hemangioma (Masson trichrome stain). Note variably dilated vascular channels with thick, hyalinized walls and **no** intervening brain parenchyma **between** the channels.

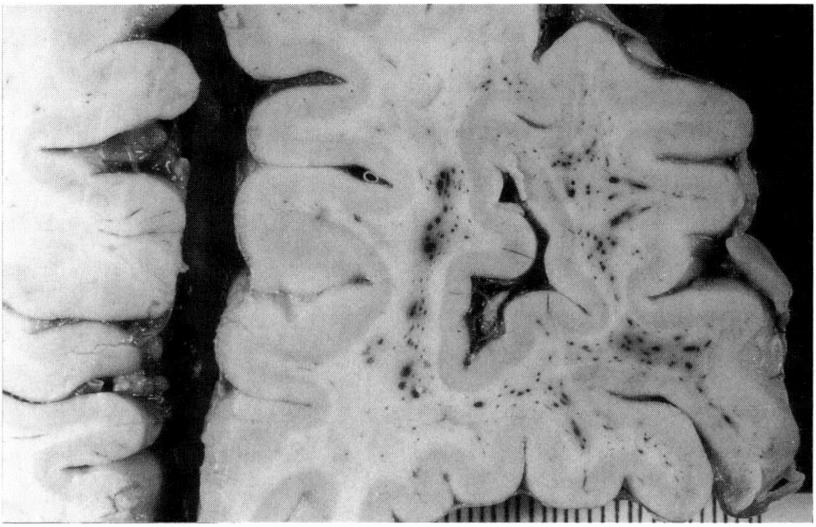

(A)

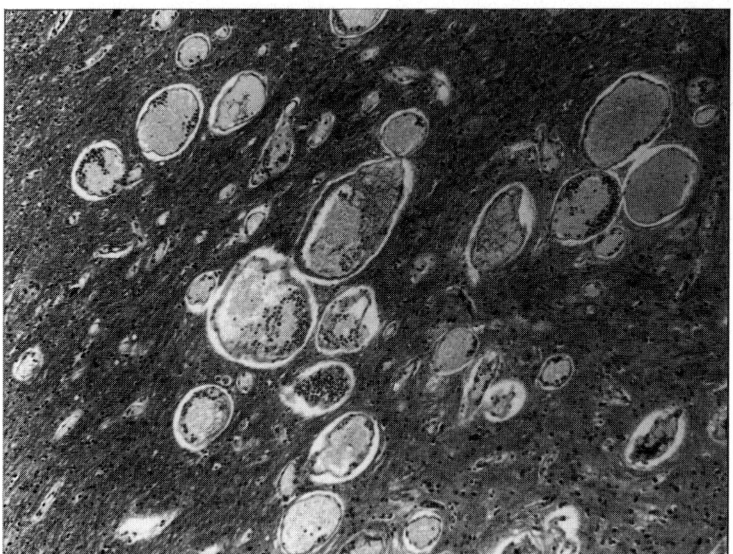

(B)

Figure 67 Venous angioma. These are often detected as an "incidental finding" at brain cutting, as for the example illustrated in **panel A. Panel B** shows typical microscopic findings. Note thin vessel walls with negligible reactive change (and **no** evidence of old hemorrhage) in the surrounding brain parenchyma.

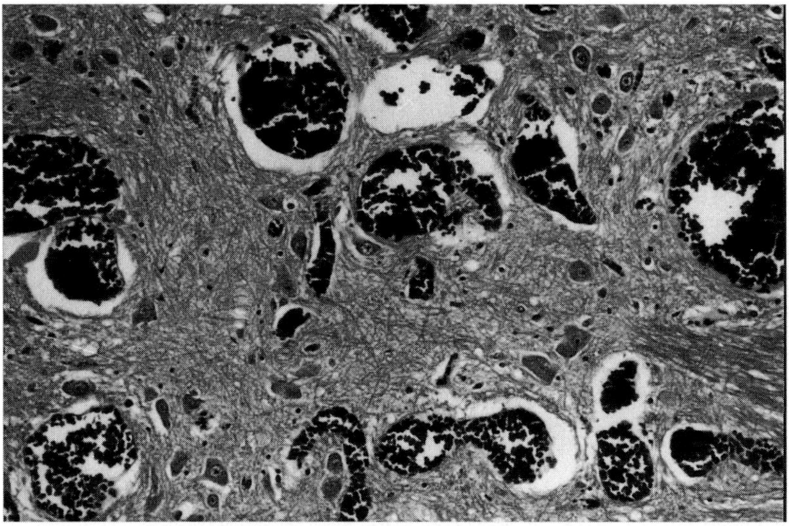

Figure 68 Capillary telangiectases. An incidental finding in the basis pontis. Small caliber of the prominent (and excessive) vascular channels can be appreciated by comparing their sizes to those of surrounding neuronal cell bodies.

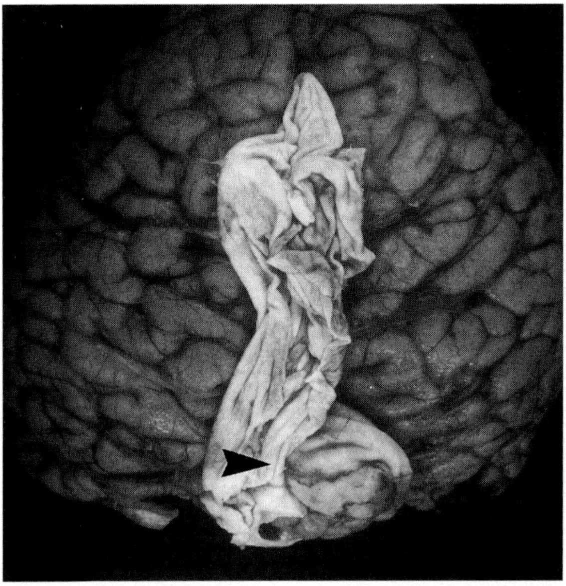

(A)

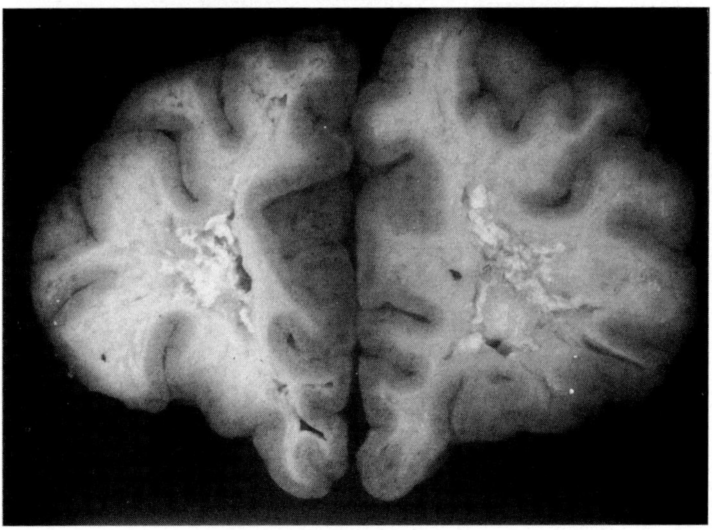

(B)

Figure 69 Vein of Galen aneurysm. (**A**) View from the cerebral convexities. Note large bulbous aneurysmal dilatation adjacent to the falx, indicated by arrowhead. (**B**) Cerebral damage in patients with this lesion often results from a "steal" of blood from normal brain secondary to the large arteriovenous shunt. Coronal sections of frontal lobes from this patient illustrate extensive leukomalacia.

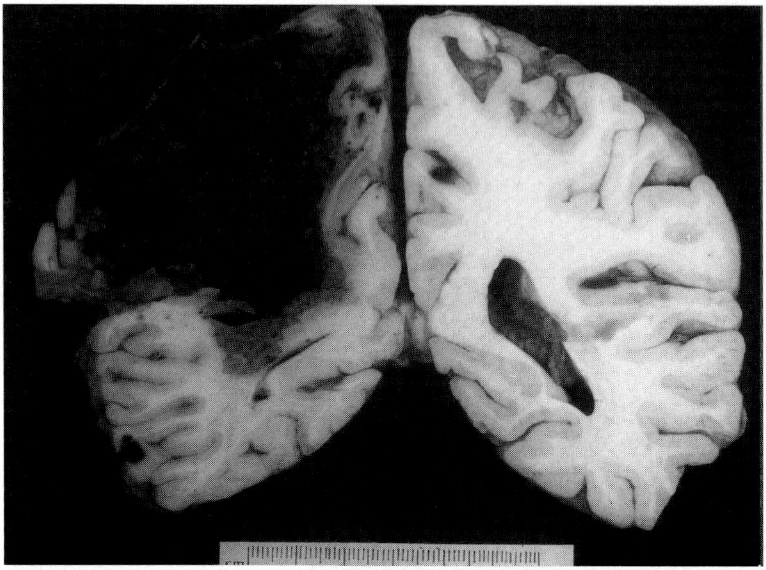

(A)

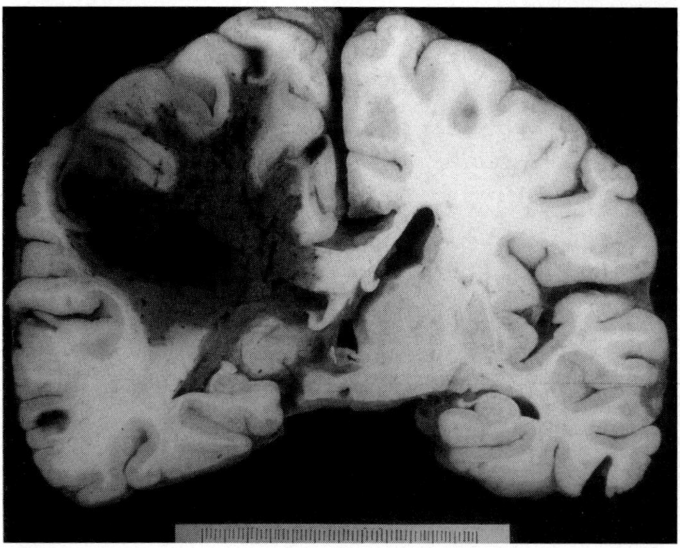

(B)

Figure 70 ICH associated with leukemia/bone marrow transplanatation (BMT). **(A,B)** Large lobar hemorrhage in a 10-year-old child who had recently undergone BMT; note similarities to CAA-related cerebral hemorrhage. **(C)** Left ganglionic hematoma in a man with acute myelogenous leukemia who had undergone BMT. Note similarities to hypertensive hemorrhage. Hematoma extends into the lateral ventricle.

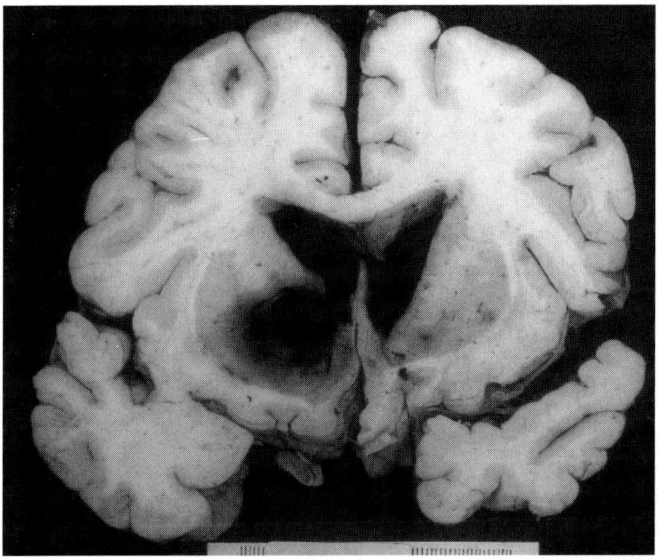

(C)

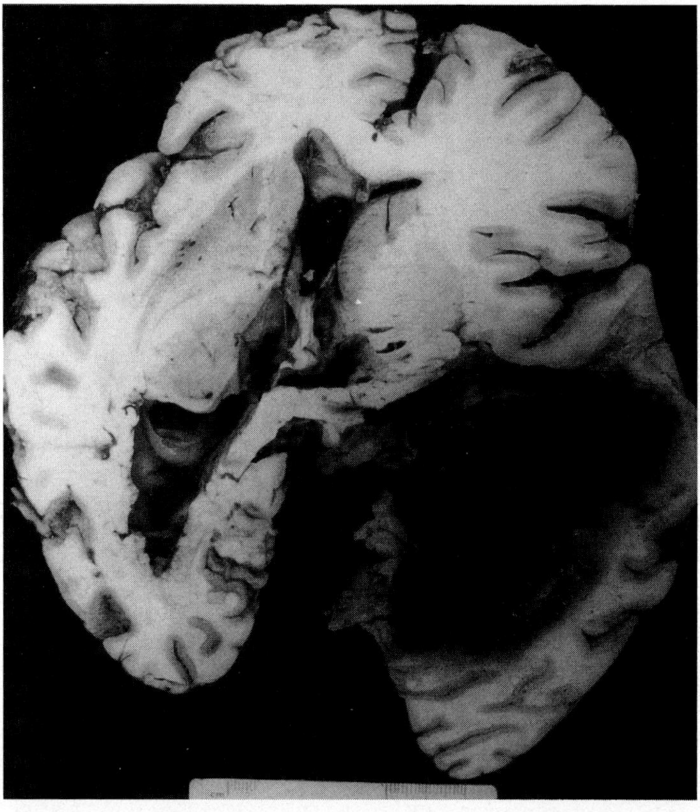

Figure 71 Horizontal brain section shows massive right parietotemporal hematoma in a patient who had undergone two orthotopic liver transplants (for chronic heptatitis) approximately 3 months prior to death, with a subsequent coagulopathy. Note massive right-to-left shift of midline structures and extension of clot into the ventricular system.

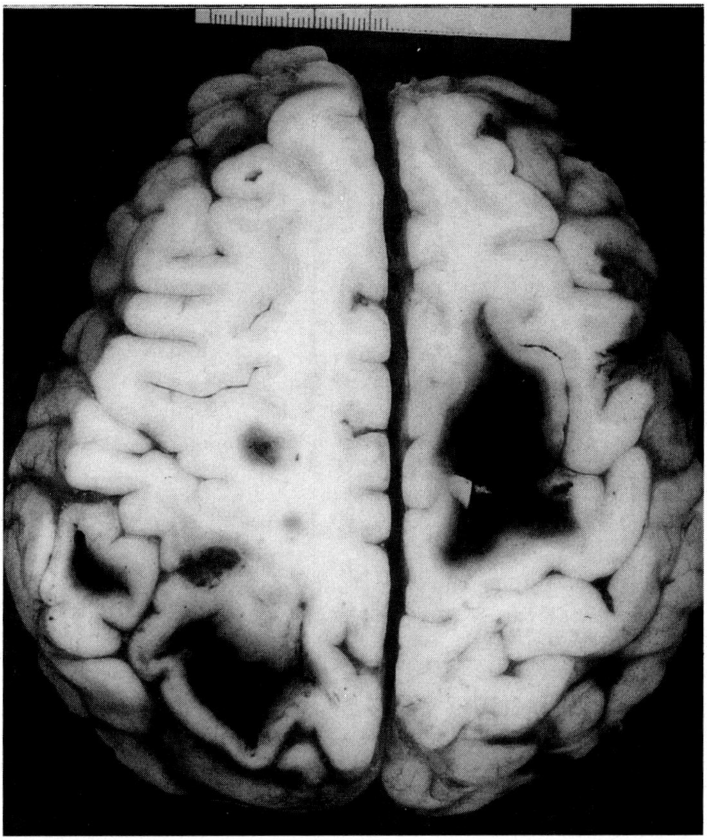

Figure 72 Metastatic choriocarcinoma to the brain in a 33-year-old female. Parenchymal metastases were found within regions of hemorrhage, as were foci of choriocarcinoma infiltrating some cerebral arterial walls (see also Fig. 29).

REFERENCES

1. Adams JH, Brierley JB, Connor RCR, Treip CS. The effects of systemic hypotension upon the human brain. Clinical and neuropathological observations in 11 cases. Brain 1966; 89:235–268.
2. Albin RL, Greenamyre JT. Alternative excitotoxic hypotheses. Neurology 1992; 42:733–738.
3. Anders KH, Latta H, Chang BS, Tomiyasu U, Quddusi AS, Vinters HV. Lymphomatoid granulomatosis and malignant lymphoma of the central nervous system in the acquired immunodeficiency syndrome. Hum Pathol 1989; 20:326–334.
4. Auer RN, Benveniste H. Hypoxia and related conditions. In: Graham D, ed. Greenfield's Neuropathology. 6th ed. New York: Oxford University Press, 1996:263–314.
5. Auer RN, Siesjö BK. Biological differences between ischemia, hypoglycemia, and epilepsy. Ann Neurol 1988; 24:699–707.
6. Babikian V, Ropper AH. Binswanger's disease: a review. Stroke 1987; 18:2–12.
7. Barnett HJM, Eliasziw M, Meldrum HE. Drugs and surgery in the prevention of ischemic stroke. N Engl J Med 1995; 332:238–248.
8. Barnett HJM, Mohr JP, Stein BM, Yatsu FM, eds. Stroke. Pathophysiology, Diagnosis, and Management. 2nd ed. New York: Churchill Livingstone, 1992.
9. Beal MF, Williams RS, Richardson EP Jr, Miller Fisher C. Cholesterol embolism as a cause of transient ischemic attacks and cerebral infarction. Neurology 1981; 31:860–865.
10. Berger JR, Harris JO, Gregorios J, Norenberg M. Cerebrovascular disease in AIDS: a case-control study. AIDS 1990; 4:239–244.
11. Bogousslavsky J, Van Melle G, Regli F. The Lausanne Stroke Registry: analysis of 1,000 consecutive patients with first stroke. Stroke 1988; 19:1083–1092.
12. Carter LP, Spetzler RF, Hamilton MG, eds. Neurovascular Surgery. New York: McGraw-Hill, 1995.
13. Castaigne P, Lhermitte F, Gautier JC, et al. Arterial occlusions in the vertebrobasilar system. A study of 44 patients with post-mortem data. Brain 1973; 96:133–154.
14. Challa VR, Moody DM, Brown WR. Vascular malformations of the central nervous system. J Neuropathol Exp Neurol 1995; 54:609–621.
15. DiNubile MJ. Septic thrombosis of the cavernous sinuses. Arch Neurol 1988; 45:567–572.
16. Estol CJ, Pessin MS, Martinez AJ. Cerebrovascular complications after orthotopic liver transplantation. A clinicopathologic study. Neurology 1991; 41:815–819.
17. Farrell MA, Gilbert JJ, Kaufmann JCE. Fatal intracranial arterial dissection: clinical pathological correlation. J Neurol Neurosurg Psychiatry 1985; 48:111–121.
18. Fisher CM. Binswanger's encephalopathy: a review. J Neurol 1989; 236:65–79.
19. Fisher CM, Gore I, Okabe N, White PD. Atherosclerosis of the carotid and vertebral arteries—extracranial and intracranial. J Neuropathol Exp Neurol 1965; 24:455–476.

20. Fisher M. Clinical Atlas of Cerebrovascular Disorders. London: Mosby-Wolfe, 1994.
21. Freytag E. Fatal hypertensive intracerebral haematomas: a survey of the pathological anatomy of 393 cases. J Neurol Neurosurg Psychiatry 1968; 31:616–620.
22. Garcia JH, Ho K-L. Carotid atherosclerosis. Definition, pathogenesis, and clinical significance. Neuroimag Clin North Am 1996; 6:801–810.
23. Ginsberg MD, Hedley-Whyte ET, Richardson EP Jr. Hypoxic-ischemic leukoencephalopathy in man. Arch Neurol 1976; 33:5–14.
24. Gray F, Robert F, Labrecque R, et al. Autosomal dominant arteriopathic leukoencephalopathy and Alzheimer's disease. Neuropathol Appl Neurobiol 1994; 20:22–30.
25. Hachinski V, Norris JW. The Acute Stroke. Philadelphia: F.A. Davis, 1985.
26. Hart RG. Vertebral artery dissection. Neurology 1988; 38:987–989.
27. Ikeda E, Hosoda Y. Distribution of thrombotic lesions in the cerebral arteries in spontaneous occlusion of the circle of Willis: cerebrovascular Moyomoya disease. Clin Neuropathol 1993; 12:44–48.
28. Kase CS, Robinson RK, Stein RW, et al. Anticoagulant-related intracerebral hemorrhage. Neurology 1985; 35:943–948.
29. Kinney HC, Samuels MA. Neuropathology of the persistent vegetative state. A review. J Neuropathol Exp Neurol 1994; 53:548–558.
30. Levy DE, Caronna JJ, Singer BH, Lapinski RH, Frydman H, Plum F. Predicting outcome after hypoxic-ischemic coma. JAMA 1985; 253:1420–1426.
31. Masuda J, Yutani C, Ogata J, Kuriyama Y, Yamaguchi T. Atheromatous embolism in the brain: a clinicopathologic analysis of 15 autopsy cases. Neurology 1994; 44:1231–1237.
32. Mettinger KL. Fibromuscular dysplasia and the brain. II. Current concept of the disease. Stroke 1982; 13:53–58.
33. Mohr JP. Lacunes. Stroke 1982; 13:3–11.
34. Moody DM, Bell MA, Challa VR, Johnston WE, Prough DS. Brain microemboli during cardiac surgery or aortography. Ann Neurol 1990; 28:477–486.
35. Moore PM, Fauci AS. Neurological complications of vasculitis. Ann Neurol 1983; 14:155–167.
36. Park YD, Belman AL, Kim T-S, et al. Stroke in pediatric acquired immunodeficiency syndrome. Ann Neurol 1990; 28:303–311.
37. Pia HW, Langmaid C, Zierski J, eds. Spontaneous Intracerebral Haematomas. Berlin: Springer-Verlag, 1980.
38. Rhodes RH, Madelaire NC, Petrelli M, Cole M, Karaman BA. Primary angiitis and angiopathy of the central nervous system and their relationship to systemic giant cell arteritis. Arch Pathol Lab Med 1995; 119:334–349.
39. Rinkel GJE, van Gijn J, Wijdicks EFM. Subarachnoid hemorrhage without detectable aneurysm. A review of the causes. Stroke 1993; 24:1403–1409.
40. Ross R. The pathogenesis of atherosclerosis: a perspective for the 1990s. Nature 1993; 362:801–809.
41. Shokunbi MT, Vinters HV, Kaufmann JCE. Fusiform intracranial aneurysms. Clinicopathologic features. Surg Neurol 1988; 29:263–270.

42. Siesjö BK. Hypoglycemia, brain metabolism, and brain damage. Diabetes/Metab Rev 1988; 4:113–144.
43. Stehbens WE. Pathology of the Cerebral Blood Vessels. St. Louis: C.V. Mosby, 1972.
44. Southwick FS, Richardson EP Jr, Swartz MN. Septic thrombosis of the dural venous sinuses. Medicine 1986; 65:82–106.
45. Torvik A, Jörgensen L. Thrombotic and embolic occlusions of the carotid arteries in an autopsy material. Part 1. Prevalence, location and associated diseases. J Neurol Sci 1964; 1:24–39.
46. Trouillat R, Bogousslavsky J, Regli F, Uske A. Hémorragies intracérébrales supratentorielles. Schweiz Med Wschr 1990; 120:1056–1063.
47. Ueda K, Hasuo Y, Kiyohara Y, et al. Intracerebral hemorrhage in a Japanese community, Hisayama: Incidence, changing pattern during long-term follow-up, and related factors. Stroke 1988; 19:48–52.
48. Vinters HV. Cerebral amyloid angiopathy. A critical review. Stroke 1987; 18:311–324.
49. Vinters HV. Interactions between the heart and brain. In: Silver MD, ed. Cardiovascular Pathology. 2nd ed. New York: Churchill Livingstone, 1991:1029–1071.
50. Vinters HV, Lundie MJ, Kaufmann JCE. Long-term pathological follow-up of cerebral arteriovenous malformations treated by embolization with bucrylate. N Engl J Med 1986; 314:477–483.
51. Walley VM, Stinson WA, Upton C, et al. Foreign materials found in the cardiovascular system after instrumentation or surgery (including a guide to their light microscopic identification). Cardiovasc Pathol 1993; 2:157–185.
52. Weisberg LA. Alcoholic intracerebral hemorrhage. Stroke 1988; 19:1565–1569.
53. Welch KMA, ed. Cerebrovascular diseases: eighteenth Princeton conference. Stroke 1993; 24 (suppl 1).
54. Whetsell WO Jr. Current concepts of excitotoxicity. J Neuropathol Exp Neurol 1996; 55:1–13.

3

Craniocerebral and Spinal Trauma

I. INTRODUCTION

Head injury is the primary cause of death and disability under 35 years of age, but the importance of head injury in the elderly and the young must not be underestimated. Clinical recognition of the severity of a head injury may be difficult at the extremes of life. The majority of head injuries are usually uncomplicated and unassociated with loss of consciousness or with any long-term sequelae. The difficulty faced by the physician caring for a patient with a suspected head injury is to try to predict which patients will develop raised intracranial pressure with the possibility of death and which patients will recover completely without loss of consciousness. In situations where the clinical history is unclear or blurred by the presence of alcohol or drugs, there is the possibility that beneath what appears to be an apparently trivial head injury, a process has begun that will give rise to series of intracranial events that may result in fatal brain swelling and death. A goal in the management of head injury is the early recognition and treatment of secondary and potentially fatal intracranial events occurring in the context of a relatively minor head injury, together with the prevention of further brain damage in patients with established moderate or severe head injuries. Intracranial events such as swelling, hemorrhage, ischemia, hypoxia, and increasing intracranial pressure may develop with frightening rapidity.

II. ETIOLOGY

Falls and motor vehicle accidents are the leading causes of head injury in the industrialised world, but gun-shot and nonpenetrating injuries caused by physical assault are dominant in larger urban centers, particularly in North America. Domestic, industrial, and sports-related accidents account for an increasing number of head injuries. Nonaccidental injury in childhood, in spite of an increased awareness of the social factors leading to its occurrence, is still common.

III. ANNUAL INCIDENCE

Incidence figures for head injury partly reflect the degree of mechanization in a particular society and vary widely. Even within a particular society there may be considerable variations in head injury incidence between various social and ethnic groups. As many as 15,000/100,000 of the British population report to the emergency room each year with a suspected head injury, but just under 2% of patients in this group are actually admitted to the hospital. Five percent of patients requiring hospitalization will ultimately receive treatment in a specialized neurosurgical unit. From this it can be seen that the majority of head injuries are relatively minor and are usually treated in general hospitals by nonspecialist physicians and surgeons. Nevertheless, head injury is the most common cause of death and long-term disability under the age of 50.

IV. KEY CLINICAL POINTS IN RELATION TO BRAIN INJURY

Patients with head injuries frequently have other potentially life-threatening injuries which may be overlooked in the presence of a dramatic injury of the scalp and face. Extreme injury of the brain and spinal cord is possible with little or no disruption of overlying tissues, and conversely dramatic injury of the superficial tissues may be associated with little or no damage to the underlying nervous system. The importance of preventing further injury to a traumatized brain by maintenance of a clear airway and blood pressure (to maintain cerebral perfusion) cannot be overstated. Constant monitoring of patients with head injury is essential to ensure early recognition and treatment of developing mass lesions and increasing intracranial pressure.

V. CLASSIFICATION OF CRANIOCEREBRAL TRAUMA

Head injuries are traditionally classified into penetrating and nonpenetrating, or closed. Penetrating head injuries usually result from gunshot or stab wounds and in the majority of cases are fatal. The neuropathologic findings in gunshot depend on several factors including the proximity of the gun muzzle to the head and the caliber, velocity, and trajectory of the bullet. Interpretation of neuropathologic findings is usually done by forensic pathologists and will not be considered further. In closed head injuries, the nature and severity of the injuries to the scalp, skull, and brain will be determined by the relative contributions of direct blunt force and the rate of acceleration/deceleration of the head. In the discussions that follow, consideration is given only to head injuries that have resulted in gross or microscopic lesions of the brain or its surrounding coverings. Traditionally, patients with concussion do not exhibit structural lesions, although there is increasing evidence from animal models of subtle cerebral electrochemical disturbances in concussion.

VI. MECHANISMS OF BRAIN INJURY

The circumstances surrounding each head injury are unique. Additionally, there are differences in the brain's response to injury in childhood and adulthood which will be reflected in the underlying pathology. Primary brain injury, which occurs at the moment of impact, differs from secondary brain injury caused by subsequent complicating factors such as hypotension, hypoxia, infection, and herniations due to brain swelling.

A. Blunt Force Injury

Following moderate to severe blunt force injury, there is invariably evidence of contact phenomena in the scalp, skull, and brain in the form of bruising and lacerations, fractures, and contusions, respectively. Each of these will be dealt with separately. It is necessary to consider the location of contusions on the brain surface in relation to the primary contact injury. When the moving head comes to a stop against a hard or resistant object, contusions are usually located opposite to the point of impact, so-called *contrecoup* contusions. These are most frequently found in the inferior frontal and anterior temporal lobes. When an object strikes a head that is not moving but is free to do so, contusions are usually found immediately beneath the point of impact—i.e., *coup* contusion. If the force is sufficient to cause a depressed fracture of the skull, contusions may be found on the brain surface beneath the skull fragment.

Many theories have been proposed to explain *contrecoup* phenomenon. The most easily understood suggests that as the head accelerates toward the ground, for example in a fall, the brain (because of its relative inertia) lags behind the skull and is displaced toward the trailing edge of the skull (Fig. 1). In this location CSF is displaced from the space between the brain surface and skull. In contrast, a cushion of CSF accumulates between the advancing edge of the skull and the brain. Thus when the head hits the ground, the accumulated CSF at the advancing surface acts as liquid buffer for the brain. At the trailing

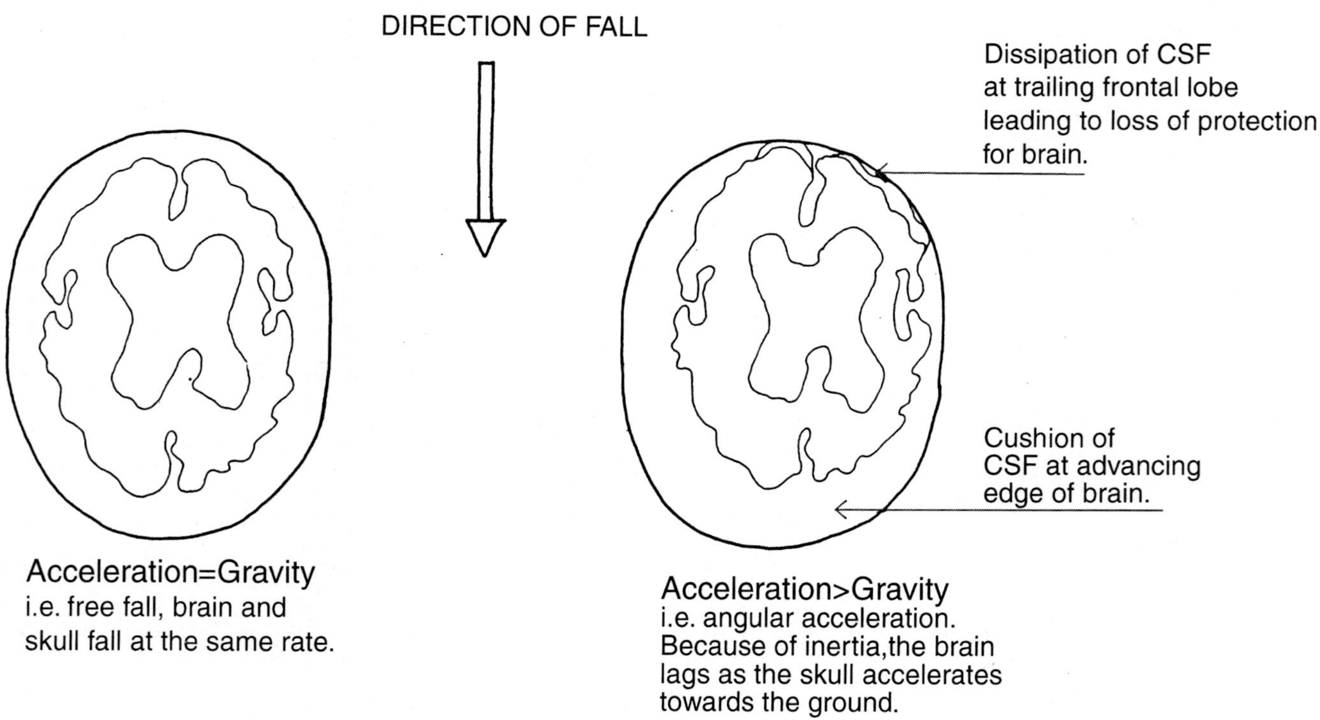

Figure 1 When the rate of acceleration is greater than that due to gravity alone, the brain tends to lag behind the skull, with the result that a cushion of CSF collects at the advancing edge and is conversely dissipated from the trailing edge. Consequently, on impact, the advancing lobes of the brain are relatively protected by CSF from the effects of direct impact. Most of the brain injury occurs at the trailing edge.

surface, i.e., that remote from the point of skull impact with the ground, where a CSF cushion does not exist, the brain will impact with force against the rough inner periosteum at cessation of the head's movement. Unprotected by CSF, the impact of brain against skull results in contusions, the number and extent of which will depend on the force of impact.

B. Acceleration-Deceleration Injury

A controversial but important primate experiment in which the effects of rapid changes in velocity of the head were studied, has demonstrated that the delivery of acceleration loads of increasing magnitude to the brain will result in a variety of changes ranging from concussion to prolonged unconsciousness. Neuropathologic examination of the brains of these animals demonstrated shearing injuries to subdural veins and axons. Such changes were induced in the absence of any contact force being applied to the skull. The changes are identical to those observed in patients with diffuse axonal injury (DAI), a carefully characterized clinicopathologic condition which is recognized as the most frequently encountered form of primary brain injury and which is the most important cause of long-term neurologic disability following closed head injury. In practice, the intracranial consequences of most head injuries usually result from a combination of blunt force trauma, which induces contact or focal injuries, and acceleration-deceleration, which leads to a diffuse shearing injury. The relative contributions of each will depend on the nature of the injury—whether high velocity as in a motor vehicle accident, or low velocity as in a fall.

VII. CLASSIFICATION OF HEAD INJURY PATHOLOGY

Head injuries are traditionally divided into focal and diffuse (Table 1). Injuries may occur to any of the structures of the head either singly or in combination.

A. Scalp

The scalp is extremely vascular and can bleed copiously when lacerated and quickly lead to hypovolemic shock. Avulsion injuries are likely to occur when hair is entangled in machinery or when the head is dragged along a road surface by a moving vehicle. Nonavulsed scalp injuries heal well. In contrast, facial soft-tissue injuries may result in scarring and disfigurement which may cause considerable long-term psychological problems.

B. Skull

The skull is a major protector of the brain and serves to dissipate the energy of blows to the head—if necessary, through fractures. The relationship of skull to

Table 1 Craniocerebral Trauma—A Classification

Focal	Diffuse
Scalp/facial lacerations	Hypoxic-ischemic brain injury
Skull fractures	Diffuse axonal injury
	Cerebral edema
Hematoma—Extradural	
—Subdural	
—Intracerebral	
Contusions	

brain is similar to that of an eggshell to a hard-boiled egg in that it is possible to shatter the skull without causing significant brain injury. Conversely, as many as 31% of patients with fatal head injuries do not have a skull fracture. Thus the presence or absence of a skull fracture should have little bearing on the immediate management of a head injury, nor should the *absence* of a skull fracture give rise to any sense of reassurance about intracranial events. Fractures may be of four types: linear or fissure type; depressed with one edge forced deeper into the head; compound in which there is an associated laceration of scalp or extension to involve a sinus; and penetrating in which there is a tear of the underlying dura. Fractures of the skull base, remote from the initial point of impact, usually imply dissipation of major impact energy through the skull base. Complications of skull fractures include persistent leakage of CSF with a significant risk of meningitis, contusions to the underlying brain if the fracture is depressed, damage to cranial nerves (especially from skull base fractures), and, most importantly, damage to major vessels such as the middle meningeal artery. Additionally there may be considerable hemorrhage from skull base fractures and blood may track through the nasopharyngeal wall into the upper airway and into the distal tracheobronchial tree. Airway obstruction from this source is underestimated and is frequently diagnosed only at autopsy.

C. Fractures of Facial Bones

While a detailed discussion of mandibulofacial fractures is beyond the scope of this chapter, they are also important in terms of producing airways obstruction either from fracture-related hemorrhage or from occlusion of the oropharyngeal region, particularly when the mandible is fractured.

D. Traumatic Intracranial Hematoma Formation

In this section traumatic hemorrhage into the extradural, subdural, and intracerebral locations is considered. Traumatic subarachnoid hemorrhage rarely if ever occurs in isolation and in the acute phase is not associated with clearly defined clinicopathologic syndromes. In the longer term, the presence of blood in the subarachnoid space may give rise to meningeal fibrosis and resultant obstructive hydrocephalus. Isolated traumatic intraventricular hemorrhage is exceptional, though repetitive "head bopping," as occurs with certain forms of contemporary dance, may result in shearing of the choroid plexus with resultant intraventricular hemorrhage.

1. Extradural Hemorrhage/Hematoma

Hemorrhage in the cranial extradural space typically occurs when an associated skull fracture results in laceration of a dural arterial vessel (Figs. 2, 3). Fracture of the thin squamous temporal bone with tearing of the middle meningeal artery is the most common occurrence. On occasion, the fracture may be tiny and involve only the inner periosteal table but nevertheless cause an arterial injury. Rarely, the arterial injury may occur in the absence of a fracture. Blood from the leaking vessel causes an expanding hematoma between the dura and the inner periosteal table. The parietal convexity is the most favored site, but extradural hematomas may occur in the middle, anterior, or posterior cranial fossae.

Patients with extradural hematomas typically have a posttraumatic period of normal consciousness followed by a decline in the consciousness level which may be rapid. If the hematoma is not removed, death will ensue. Such patients

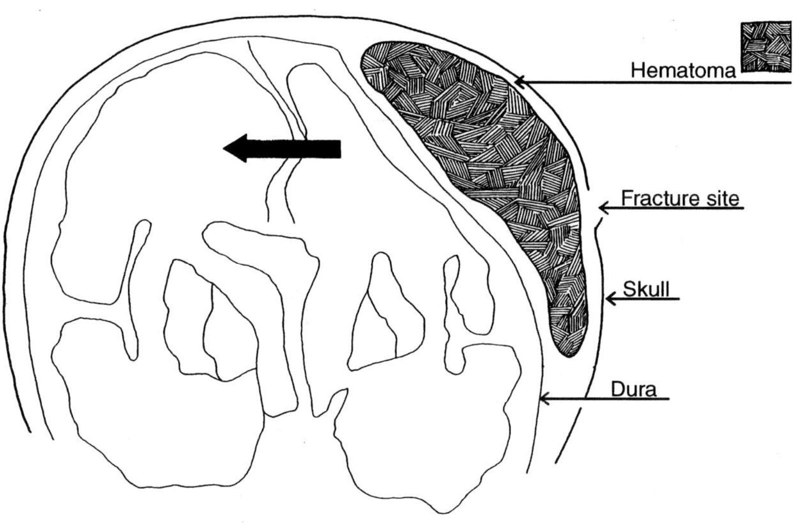

Figure 2 Extradural hematomas are invariably associated with a fracture of the squamous temporal bone. The collecting hematoma causes midline shift and subfalcine and transtentorial herniation (not illustrated).

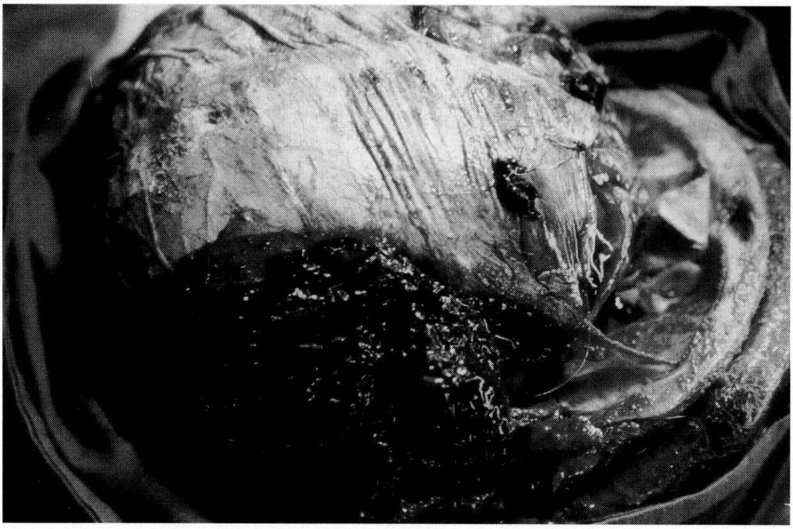

Figure 3 A large extradural hematoma has collected on the right side of the head. The calvarium (previously removed) demonstrated a tiny fracture in the squamous temporal bone which traversed the groove of the middle meningeal artery.

are said to have "talked and died." Retention of a patient's ability to talk following onset of a head injury that eventually causes death is interpreted as evidence that the brain has not suffered significant injury at the moment of impact and that secondary events such as swelling and hemorrhage have not yet occurred. Failure to recognize that such a patient is at risk for the development of, or is already harboring an expanding extradural hematoma, usually results in tragedy for patient and doctor. A high index of clinical suspicion based on detailed history of the circumstances of the head injury is essential, especially when coupled with the realization that the middle meningeal artery is vulnerable when there is a fracture of the squamous temporal bone.

2. *Subdural Hemorrhage/Hematoma*

Subdural haematomas (SDHs) may be acute or chronic. The pathogeneses of acute SDH and chronic SDH differ. In both, the blood accumulates between between the inner aspect of the dura mater and the arachnoid (Figs. 4, 5). In acute SDH, the blood may arise from two possible sources. Bridging veins that extend between dura and brain surface may be torn during rapid acceleration or deceleration as the brain moves inside the skull. Alternatively, if there are contusions of the brain with tearing of the overlying pia, blood will seep from the contused and lacerated brain surface into the subdural space. The majority

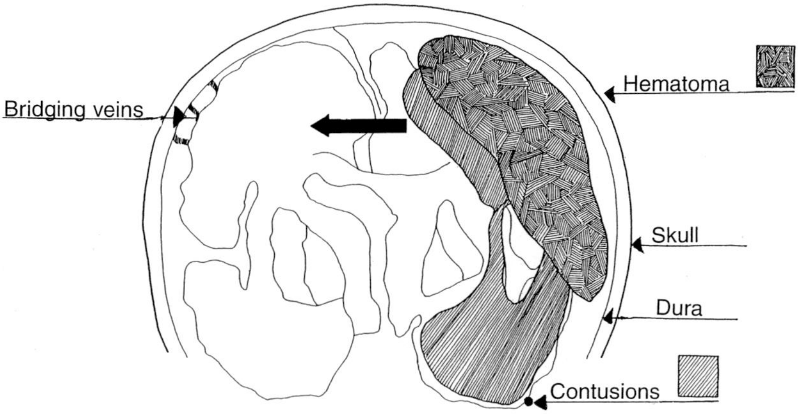

Figure 4 Diagrammatic illustration of an acute subdural hematoma, which is invariably associated with contusions of the underlying brain.

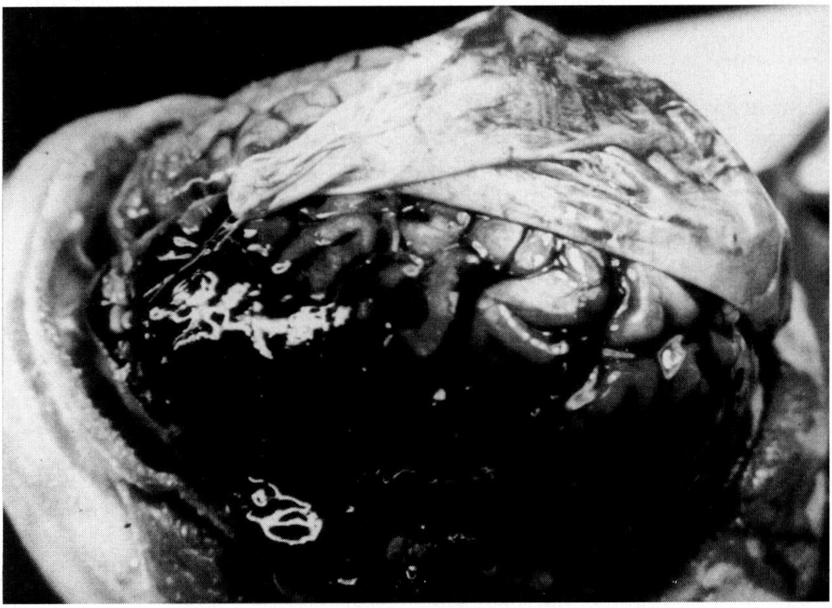

Figure 5 The dura has been reflected at autopsy to reveal a massive collection of subdural blood. Note the bridging veins stretching from the dura to the surface of the brain.

of acute subdural hematomas are associated with severe underlying brain injury in the form of either contusions or diffuse axonal injury. Although the acute subdural hematoma may be evacuated with a resultant fall in intracranial pressure, the patient's survival and ultimate outcome will be determined by the severity of the underlying injuries to the brain.

Chronic subdural hematomas typically occur in the elderly. There is usually only a vague prior history of trauma. Indeed, the initiating injury may be so trivial as to be overlooked. When there is cerebral atrophy as in the elderly (with or without dementia), the bridging veins that extend from the brain surface to dura must traverse a widened subdural space. Consequently, the veins are vulnerable to tearing even with minor injury. There is usually no injury to the brain. Blood slowly leaks from the torn veins and may become partly encapsulated by a membrane composed of granulation and fibrous tissue. The hematoma slowly increases in size over weeks or months until it becomes sufficiently large to produce a focal neurological deficit or increased intracranial pressure. Chronic subdural hematomas may be bilateral. The surrounding membrane of richly vascularized connective tissue may also bleed and cause a new, acute hemorrhage into a preexistent chronic subdural hematoma. If recognized early and removed, the prognosis for survival is excellent, but any underlying cerebral pathology will obviously have a bearing on the patient's survival.

3. *Traumatic Intracerebral Hematoma*

Pure intracerebral hematomas (not in contact with the brain surface) are uncommon in head injuries. They usually imply a severe shearing injury to the intracerebral vessels and are often associated with diffuse axonal injury. Sometimes the onset of traumatic intracerebral hemorrhage is delayed for a few days after the head injury. The mechanism of so-called delayed posttraumatic intracerebral hemorrhage is unknown, though a trauma-related coagulopathy may be relevant. The outcome in a patient with a traumatic intracerebral (N.B. *intracerebral* is not synonymous with *intracranial*) hematoma is invariably fatal.

E. Contusions

These are the most common findings in nonmissile head injury and are defined as areas of bruising on the surface of the brain (Figs. 6, 7). If the pia-arachnoid is torn, the contusion is defined as a laceration-contusion. Contusions are usually located on the crests of gyri and are most frequent on the subfrontal and anterior temporal cortical surfaces. They are caused by impact of the moving brain against the inner rough surface of the skull base. Contusion severity and distribution is determined by mobility of the head at impact (the immobilized head will show contusions at the point of impact—coup injury), whereas the mobile head will show contusions on the side of the brain opposite the point of impact (*contrecoup*). Contusions may also be seen immediately beneath a frac-

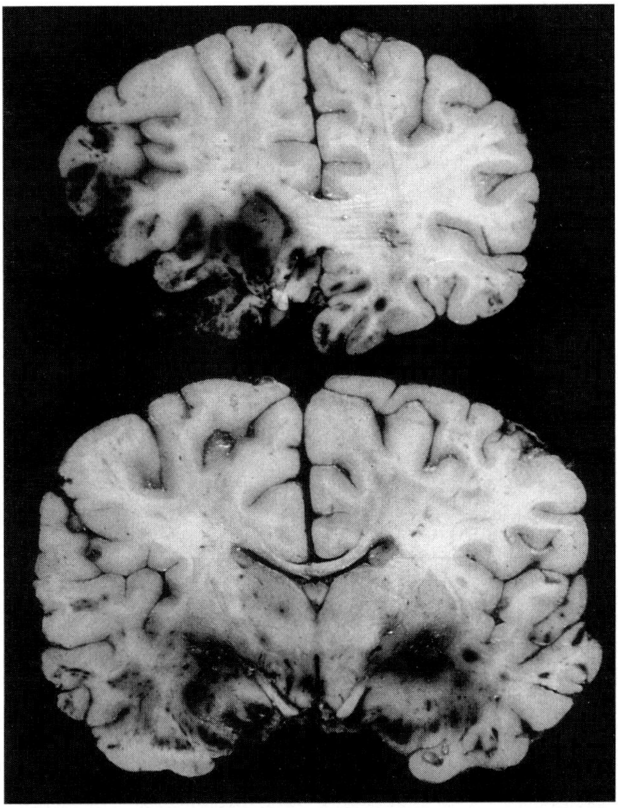

Figure 6 Coronal section of brain, which demonstrates extensive basal contusions extending into the frontal region on the left.

ture site (so-called fracture contusions). Gliding contusions are located in the deep white matter of the parasagittal parietal regions and are considered to result from a shearing injury rather than from contact of brain with skull (Fig. 8).

In general, there is good correlation between the extent of contusional injury and the likelihood of developing brain swelling due to hemorrhage and edema at the contusion sites. If the pial surface is torn, blood will seep into the subdural space and give rise to subdural hematoma. If the patient survives long enough for healing to take place, the contusions will be replaced by a yellow-orange gliotic scar (*plaque jaune*). Depending on the extent and location of the contusions, a surviving patient may develop posttraumatic behavioral distur-

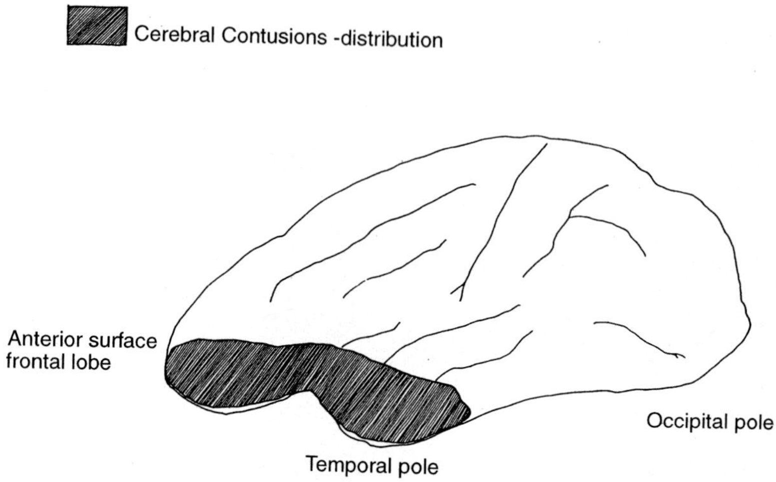

Figure 7 Diagram illustrates frontotemporal distribution of contusions.

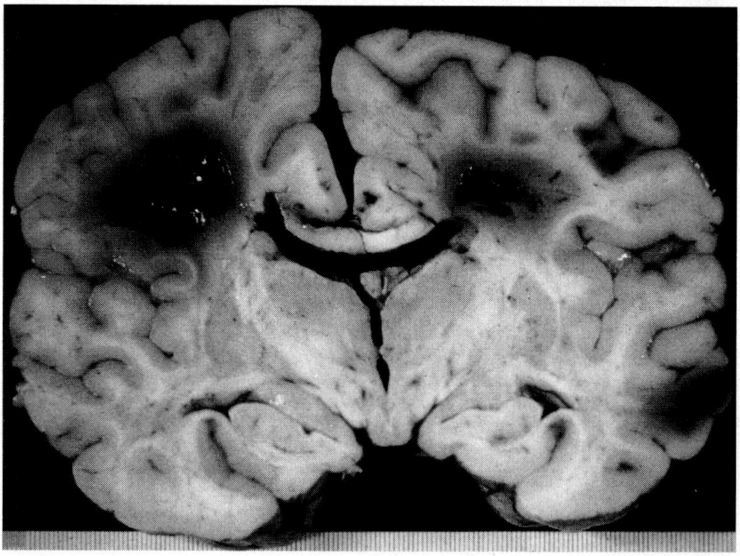

Figure 8 Gliding contusions in the parasagittal parietal white matter. Apart from a small contusion in the right middle temporal gyrus, there is little evidence of direct trauma to the brain. Gliding contusions result from shearing of intracerebral vessels.

bances or focal neurological deficits. Additionally, the healed contusions may become a pathologic substrate for posttraumatic epilepsy.

F. Diffuse Axonal Injury

Diffuse axonal injury (DAI) is the commonest cause of long-term morbidity from head injury and is present at autopsy in as many as 42% of patients with fatal head injury. DAI is a diffuse shearing injury of nerve fibers that occurs at the moment of impact and is a feature of acceleration-deceleration injury. The classical lesions of DAI are best seen in the areas where rotation is greatest. Typically, the gross appearances are those of hemorrhage in the corpus callosum and superior cerebellar peduncles (Figs. 9, 10). Rotation is maximum at

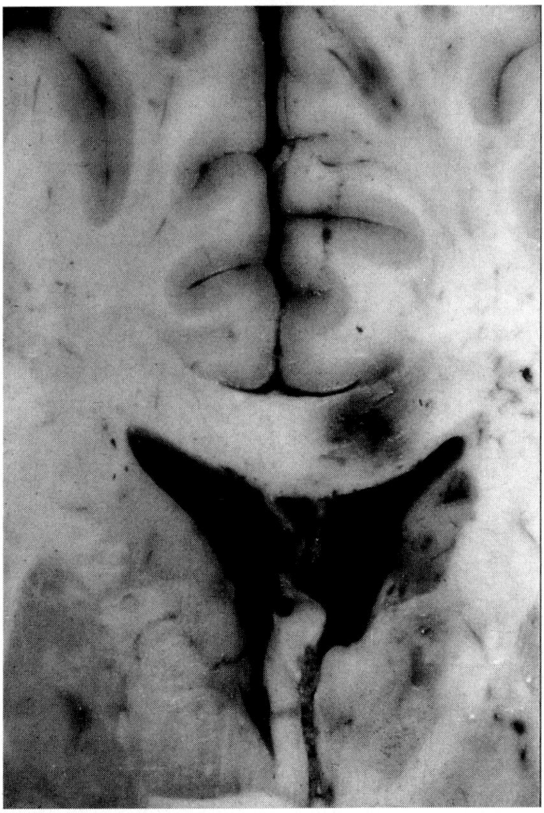

Figure 9 A small hemorrhage in the corpus callosum to the right of midline is indicative of diffuse axonal or shearing injury.

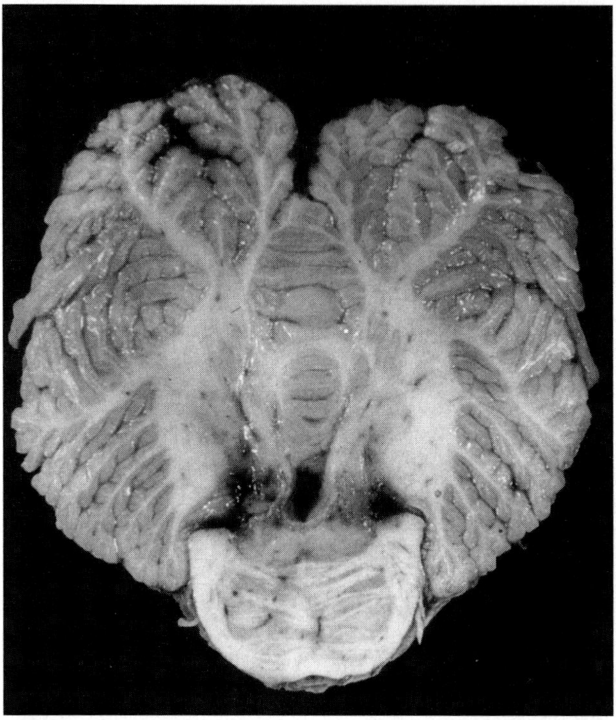

Figure 10 Symmetrical areas of hemorrhage and necrosis located in the superior cerebellar peduncles, indicative of diffuse axonal injury and caused by rotation of the cerebellum in relation to the brainstem during a high-velocity head injury.

these sites, but all areas of white matter may be affected, especially if severe. The microscopic changes will depend on the duration of the patient's survival. The earliest change (excluding hemorrhage) is axonal spheroid formation due to extrusion of axoplasm from the severed end of the axon (Fig. 11). Microglial scars form around the extruded axoplasm. Distally, the axons undergo Wallerian degeneration with resultant tract degeneration and progressive loss of white matter (Fig. 12). Such patients will ultimately develop hydrocephalus ex vacuo.

Although axonal regeneration may take place following DAI, it is usually inadequate for a return of useful neurologic function. Effectively, patients with DAI have irreversible disruption of connections between cerebral cortex and the deep central gray matter and spinal cord. In its severest form, DAI may cause a patient to remain in a persistent vegetative state after the initial brain injury. Less severe forms of DAI are associated with morbidity that may include major cognitive impairment together with motor, sensory, speech, and visual impairment.

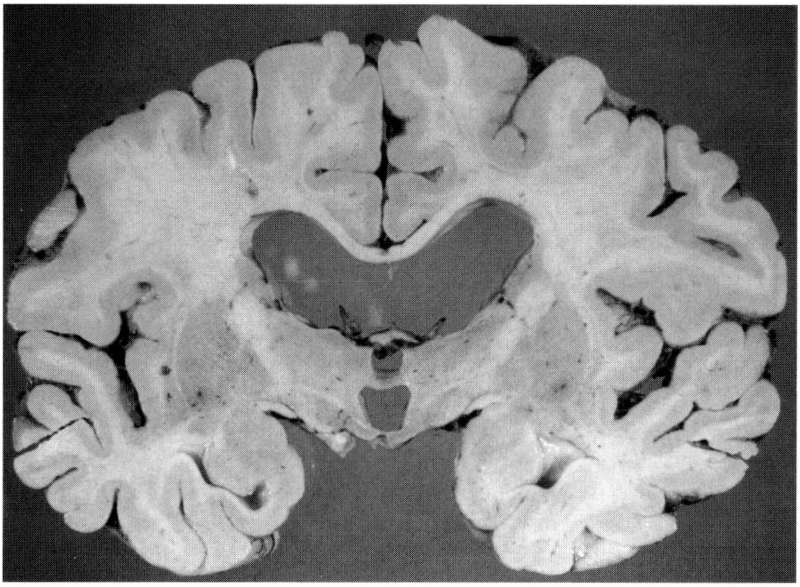

Figure 11 Hydrocephalus ex vacuo occurring as a consequence of diffuse axonal injury. Note the extreme thinning of the corpus callosum. This patient remained in a vegetative state for 8 years following a high-velocity head injury.

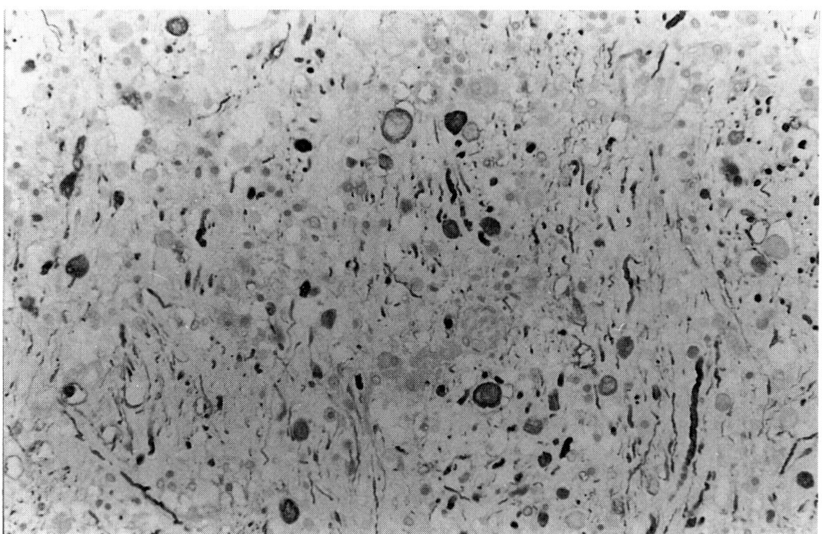

Figure 12 Section of corpus callosum immunostained with an antineurofilament antibody to demonstrate extruded axoplasm or neuroaxonal spheroids. This patient died 6 days following a closed head injury and had small hemorrhages in the corpus callosum.

Clinically, patients with DAI are unconscious from the moment of impact, but there is increasing recognition of less severe forms of DAI not necessarily associated with coma. Diagnosis is established when all other causes of persistent coma have been excluded. Computed tomography (CT) is unable to demonstrate DAI, but the white matter changes may be demonstrated by magnetic resonance imaging (MRI).

G. Hypoxic-Ischemic Brain Injury

Hypoxic-ischemic brain injury is present in up to 80% of all fatal head injuries. In contrast to DAI, hypoxic-ischemic brain damage usually occurs after the initial injury and is related to events that occur either at the roadside or en route to hospital. The most important preventable events are airways obstruction and hypovolemic shock. The polytraumatized patient is at major risk of developing both hypoxia and ischemia. Although there are major differences in the mechanisms of hypoxic and ischemic neuronal injury, for practical purposes their effects on an already traumatised brain may be regarded as similar, hence the term hypoxic-ischemic encephalopathy (HIE). The response of the traumatized brain to an hypoxic-ischemic insult is not comparable to that of a normal brain. In a situation of raised intracranial pressure and possible falling mean arterial blood pressure, the cerebral perfusion pressure may be significantly reduced. The areas of the brain most remote from arterial supply (junction or "watershed" between major vascular territories) are most at risk from ischemic brain damage (Fig. 13); the more recently developed areas of the brain such as neocortex are most at risk from hypoxia.

Hypoxia and ischemia are the most important manifestations of secondary brain injury and are considered good indicators of potentially avoidable brain injury. Good correlation exists between the prevalence of HIE and previous antemortem hypotensive episodes. The demonstration of HIE in up to 80% of patients dying from a closed head injury should not be taken as a reflection of the quality of emergency or neurosurgical care. Inevitably there is a period of several hours between formal certification of brain death and cessation of life support systems, and in this interval HIE may continue to develop in the brain. It is probable that there is a certain minimal level of histologic postmortem HIE that was not clinically relevant during life.

Hypoxic-ischemic change occurring in a regional vascular territory is usually, though not always, attributable to compression of a major artery during intracranial shifts. The posterior cerebral artery may be compressed during transtentorial herniation, and the supraclinoid portion of the internal carotid artery may be compressed when there is extensive right-to-left midline shift. Similarly the anterior cerebral artery may be compressed during subfalcine herniation. However, regional vascular ischemia occurring in the distribution of a major vessel may occur in head injury in the absence of obvious vascular com-

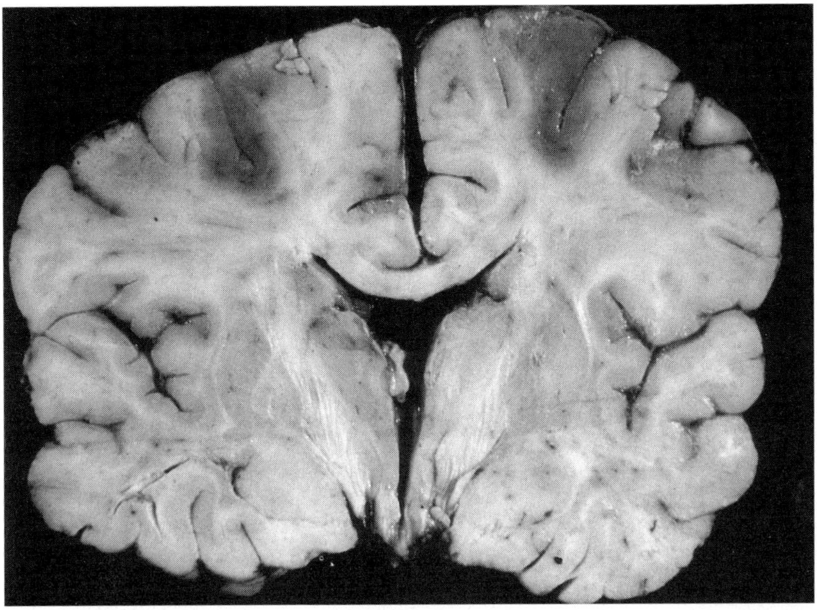

Figure 13 Bilateral symmetrical areas of necrosis in the watershed regions of the parietal cortex. This patient was involved in a motor vehicle accident and was thought to have had a head injury to account for his coma, but in fact died as a result of hypovolemic shock due to a ruptured spleen. The only evidence of a primary head injury was a skull fracture.

pression. Such cases might be due to spasm induced by the presence of blood in the subarachnoid space. For the pathologist, it is important to ensure, through histologic timing of the area of the infarction (to the limited extent this is possible), that the patient did not suffer an ischemic infarct which caused a fall *during which* the patient developed a head injury.

VIII. OTHER FORMS OF CRANIAL INJURY

A. Repetitive Non-Coma-Producing Head Injury

Although dementia pugilistica has been recognized as a distinct clinicopathologic entity for many years, there is still controversy relating to the likelihood of any individual boxer developing long-term neurologic disability. MRI studies carried out before and after boxing bouts have failed to demonstrate any microhemorrhages in the brain. Although prospective investigations of the cognitive effects of amateur boxing have failed to demonstrate evidence of significant neuropsychological dysfunction at 2-year follow-up, a much longer follow-up period is required. In spite of the paucity of neuropsychological data to show that boxing is

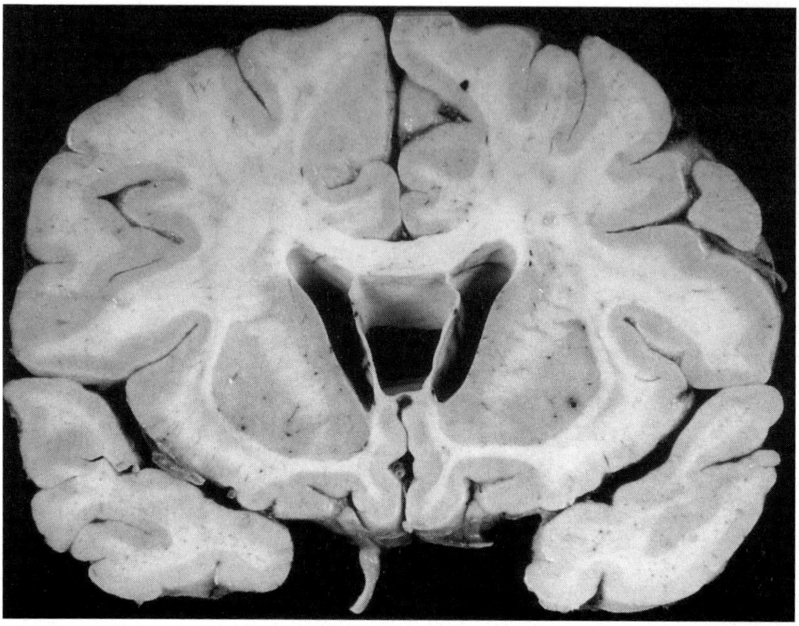

Figure 14 A large cavum septum pellucidum in the brain of a middleweight boxer.

detrimental, there are many studies of boxers' brains in which striking and relatively stereotyped neuropathologic findings have been described. Brain atrophy as depicted by CT was present in 6.5% of 338 active professional boxers, but those with abnormal scans did not differ from those with normal scans in relation to number of bouts or professional record. Brain atrophy occurred more frequently in those with a large cavum septum pellucidum (Fig. 14). Accumulation of ubiquinated neurofibrillary tangles in superficial cortex has also been described. Typically, in the cortex of a patient with dementia pugilistica there are few neuritic plaques. Changes indistinguishable from Alzheimer's disease have also been described in the brains of boxers and include τ-immunoreactive tangles and amyloid β-protein-positive neuritic plaques.

B. Nonaccidental Brain Injury in Childhood (NAI)

Battered children, in addition to suffering injuries of the skeleton and soft tissues, may sustain severe head injuries. Through vigorous shaking, punching, dropping and being swung against a hard object by the legs, severe craniocerebral trauma may occur. Typically the children have retinal hemorrhages together with subdural and subarachnoid hemorrhage. In general, however, the neuropathologic findings are not dissimilar from those that occur in association with true accidental injuries such as falls and motor vehicle accidents. However, evidence of previous craniocerebral trauma, retinal hemorrhages, and contusional tears in the subcortical white matter should raise the possibility of NAI in the minds of the clinician and pathologist. Such tears may be difficult to see but are best observed at the interface between gray and white matter and when present are highly pathognomonic of NAI. Retinal hemorrhages in the bipolar and nerve fiber layers must always be considered the result of child abuse until proven otherwise.

C. Pontomedullary Transection

In some high-velocity injuries, particularly motorcycle accidents, hyperextension of the neck may result in a partial separation of the pons from medulla (Fig. 15). Such injuries are usually associated with instantaneous death. This type of injury may be easily missed at autopsy, but careful examination of the ventral pontomedullary surface should reveal the tear or a few small petechial hemorrhages.

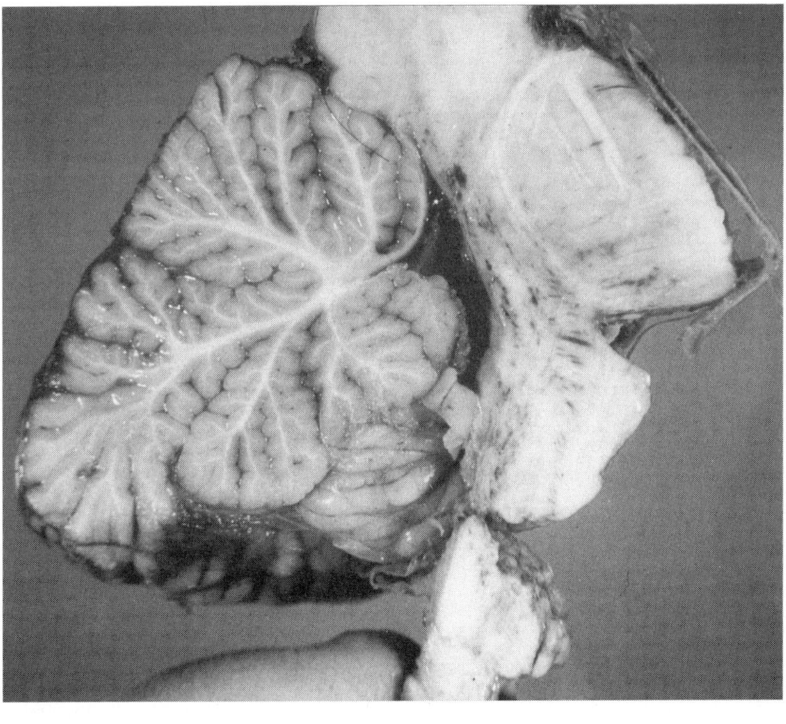

Figure 15 Parasagittal section of the brainstem which demonstrates incomplete pontomedullary and cervicomedullary transection. This patient was involved in a high-speed motorcycle accident during which the bike hit a wall at over 100 mph. It is likely that there was massive hyperextension of the neck.

D. Vascular Injury

Traumatic dissection of the cranial vessels (either intracranial or extracranial or both) is well described. Traumatic dissection of the cervical segment of the carotid artery may result when an improperly positioned seat belt impacts against the lateral aspect of the neck in sudden deceleration. Similarly, hyperextension or hyperflexion injuries of the neck may result in traumatic dissection of a vertebral artery (Fig. 16). Dissections of the major neck vessels may result in delayed neurologic deterioration after a head injury. Thrombosis of the dissected vessel may not be complete for a few days. Sometimes the dissection may extend through to the adventitia and result in traumatic subarachnoid hemorrhage, especially in the posterior fossa, from a vertebral artery dissection. During postmortem examination, it may be necessary to examine the intraosseous portion of the vertebral artery to locate the adventitial tear.

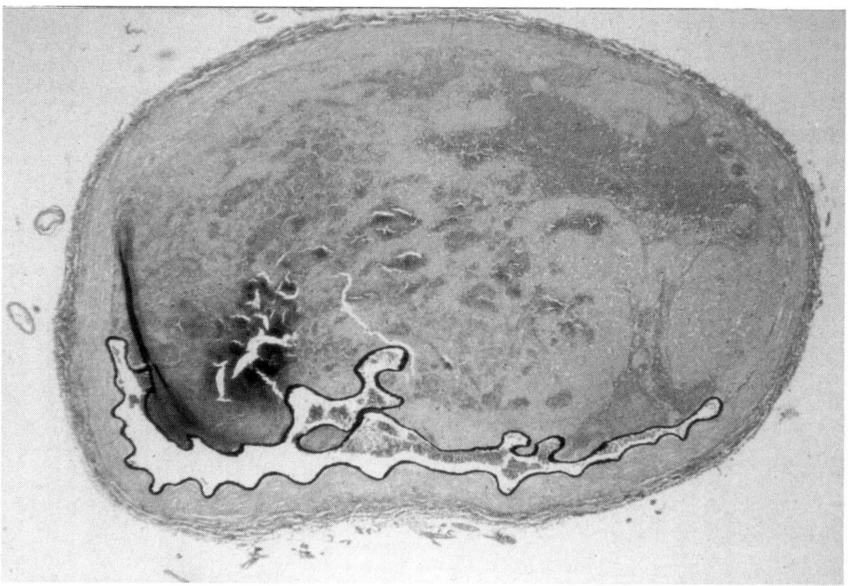

Figure 16 Transverse section of the cervical segment of the vertebral artery which demonstrates an intramural hematoma. Hyperextension injury of the neck resulted in an intimal tear, as a result of which blood dissected beneath the internal elastic lamina, causing it to separate from the media and occlude the vessel lumen.

IX. SPINAL INJURIES

Approximately 2.6% of patients entered into a major trauma outcome study in North America from 1982 to 1989 had spinal cord injuries. The majority of these patients had multiple other injuries. The most frequent causes of spinal cord injuries are motor vehicle accidents (40%), falls (20%), and gunshot wounds (13.6%). Over 90% of patients with isolated spinal cord injury survive, as do the majority of patients in whom spinal cord injury is associated with other injuries. Such patients have varying degrees of neurologic disability, but the majority remain either paraplegic or tetraplegic. MRI studies have contributed much to our understanding of spinal cord injuries. As with brain injury, the concept of primary and secondary cord injury is widely accepted. Although direct compression of the spinal cord at the time of injury is still the most important cause of neurologic dysfunction, there is increasing evidence of the importance and potential avoidability of secondary spinal cord injury.

A. Primary Spinal Cord Injury

Primary spinal cord injury usually results from either hyperextension or hyperflexion of the vertebral column. In hyperflexion, compression of a vertebral body will result in extrusion of bone fragments, blood, disk material, or ligamentous fragments into the spinal canal with resultant cord compression. Hyperextension, particularly in the cervical region, will result in considerable narrowing of the canal with resultant cord compression. In this instance the cord compression may be transient. If the bony injury is sufficiently severe to dislocate the vertebral column, traction on the spinal cord may result in a pial tear and complete cord transection. In childhood, a time when the bony elements are more flexible, the vertebral column may remain intact with little or no evidence of any continuing cord compression. However, even in such circumstances, the degree of acute cord compression with or without an associated vascular compression may have been sufficient to cause massive spinal cord injury. Direct penetrating injuries of the spinal cord, particularly with stiletto-like objects, may cause complete transection of the cord without any associated bone injury.

B. Secondary Spinal Cord Injury

Hypotension, whether due to associated neurogenic shock or to hypotension caused by other injuries, will have an obvious detrimental effect on the existing spinal cord injury and may contribute significantly to the worsening or increasing extent of that injury. There is growing evidence that local vascular factors such as vasospasm of the spinal arteries induced by blood, bony, or other tissue fragments may also result in secondary spinal cord injury. It is reasonable to assume that edema of the spinal cord confined by an intact pia will result in ongoing and continuing axonal compression. The response of some spinal cord injuries to large doses of steroids supports the possibility of edema as a causative factor in spinal cord injury. The most important concept in spinal cord injuries is that although a patient may show complete loss of neurologic function, the spinal cord may be structurally intact with a variable degree of underlying injury, some of which may be reversible and some of which may be due to continuing spinal cord compression.

C. Neuropathologic Findings in Spinal Cord Injury

In general, descriptions of the neuropathologic findings in spinal cord injury are heavily weighted toward those cases in which death ensues. Such injuries are likely to be of the most severe type and to involve the cervical region. The neuropathologic findings will be dictated to a large extent by the duration of survival following injury. In the initial stages of a severe spinal cord injury (where the cord is still in continuity), there is usually a central area of softening involving gray matter which becomes hemorrhagic. The degree of hemorrhage may increase over the following few days. There is invariably tearing of the adjacent motor and sensory roots. Transected axons in the cord will continue to extrude axoplasm which will accumulate in the form of neuroaxonal spheroids, or "axon retraction balls." Macrophages infiltrate the traumatised area and will become filled with myelin degradation products. Edema is usually a prominent feature.

With time the cellular infiltrate subsides, astrocytes proliferate (though not to the same extent as in cerebral infarction), and it may be possible to see regenerating axons. With time, the hemorrhagic-necrotic-inflammatory process recedes. The macrophage infiltrate subsides. Cavitation will inevitably result, though the size and location of the cavity will vary enormously from case to case. On occasion the cavities may reach a sufficiently large size to constitute a syrinx. Posttraumatic syringomyelia is present in up to 20% of patients with severe traumatic spinal cord injury. Progressive enlargement of a syrinx is an important cause of deterioration in neurologic function in a patient with a long-standing spinal cord injury. Such deterioration may be sufficient to cause a patient to lose upper-limb function or to become ventilator-dependent. Posttraumatic arachnoiditis may hasten syrinx formation. Adhesions may form between the dura and arachnoid, and there may be intense fibrosis and scarring of the spinal cord. Schwann cells in roots may proliferate and migrate along the intraspinal segments of the nerve roots, where their accumulation may be sufficiently extensive to form an intraspinal schwannoma. A less severe form of intraspinal migration of Schwann cells is referred to as schwannosis.

Neuropathologic details of less severe forms of spinal cord injury can be gleaned from MRI studies which have attempted to correlate MRI appearances with neurologic status and outcome. Patients with MRI evidence of intraspinal cord blood are considered to have severe lesions and show little or no neurologic improvement. Patients in whom the MRI does not demonstrate intraspinal blood but who are thought to have intraspinal edema, show some clinical improvement. However, there is no pathologic correlate of what constitutes edema in these patients. Though there is histologic evidence that axons may survive at the periphery of an area of hemorrhagic necrosis in traumatized spinal cords, there are insufficient data to determine whether or not these axons are capable of sustaining any useful neurologic function.

The major research thrust in spinal cord injury is directed toward the prevention of secondary spinal cord injury together with the development of biomechanical devices which, through insertion of intramuscular or intraneural electrostimulators, can be used to cause synchronized contraction and relaxation of lower-limb muscle groups. Such devices have already been used successfully to allow paraplegic patients to stand and take some steps.

REFERENCES

1. Adams CW, Bruton CJ. The cerebral vasculature in dementia pugilistica. J Neurol Neurosurg Psychiatry 1989; 52:600–604.
2. Adams JH, Doyle D, Ford I, Gennarelli TA, Graham DI, McLellan DR. Diffuse axonal injury in head injury: definitions, diagnosis and grading. Histopathology 1989; 15:49–59.
3. Adams JH, Doyle D, Graham DI, Lawrence AE, McLellan DR. Deep intracerebral (basal ganglia) haematomas in fatal non-missile head injury in man. J Neurol Neurosurg Psychiatry 1986; 49:1034–1043.
4. Adams JH, Doyle D, Graham DI, et al. The contusion index: a reappraisal in man and experimental non-missile head injury. Neuropathol Appl Neurobiol 1985; 11:299–308.
5. Bennett M, O'Brien DP, Phillips JP, Farrell MA. Clinicopathologic observation in 100 consecutive patients with fatal head injury admitted to a neurosurgical unit. Irish Med J 1995; 48:111–116.
6. Berney J, Froidevaux AC, Favier J. Paediatric head trauma: influence of age and sex. I. Epidemiology. Childs Nerv Syst 1994; 10:509–516.
7. Berney J, Froidevaux AC, Favier J. Paediatric head trauma: influence of age and sex. II. Biomechanical and anatomo-clinical correlations. Childs Nerv Syst 1994; 10:517–523.
8. Bracken MB, Shepard MJ, Collins WF, et al. A randomized, controlled trial of methylprednisolone or naloxone in the treatment of acute spinal cord injury. Results of a second national acute spinal cord injury study. N Engl J Med 1990; 322:1405–1411.
9. Burney RE, Maio RF, Maynard F, Karunas R. Incidence, characteristics and out-

come of spinal cord injury at trauma centers in North America. Arch Surg 1993; 128:596–599.
10. Chesnut RM, Marshall LF, Klauber MR, et al. The role of secondary brain injury in determining outcome from severe head injury. J Trauma 1993; 34:216–222.
11. Cogbill TH, Moore EE, Meissner M, et al. The spectrum of blunt injury to the carotid artery: a multicenter prospective. J Trauma 1994; 37:473–479.
12. Davis SJ, Khangure MS. A review of magnetic resonance imaging in spinal trauma. Australasian Radiol 1994; 38:241–253.
13. Dawson SL, Hirsch CS, Lucas FV, Sebek BA. The contrecoup phenomenon—reappraisal of a classic problem. Hum Pathol 1980; 155–166.
14. Doberstein CE, Hovda DA, Becker DP. Clinical considerations in the reduction of secondary brain injury. Ann Emerg Med 1993; 22:993–997.
15. Farrell MA, Gilbert JJ, Kaufman JCE. Fatal intracranial arterial dissection: clinicopathological correlation. J Neurol Neurosurg Psychiatry 1985; 48:111–116.
16. Graham DI, Adams JH, Doyle D. Ischaemic brain damage in fatal non-missile head injuries. J Neurol Sci 1978; 39:213–234.
17. Graham DI, Adams JH, Nicoll JAR, Maxwell WL, Gennarelli TA. The nature, distribution and causes of traumatic brain injury. Brain Pathol 1995; 5:397–406.
18. Gennarelli TA. Animal models of human head injury. J Neurotrauma 1994; 11:357–368.
19. Haglund Y, Eriksson E. Does amateur boxing lead to chronic brain damage? A review of some recent investigations. Am J Sports Med 1993; 21:97–109.
20. Hof PR, Bouras C, Buee L, Delacourte A, Perl DP, Morrisson JH. Differential distribution of neurofibrillary tangles in the cerebral cortex of dementia pugilistica and Alzheimer's disease cases. Acta Neuropathol 1992; 85:23–30.
21. Holzgraefe M, Lemme W, Funke W, Felix R, Felten R. The significance of diagnostic imaging in acute and chronic brain damage in boxing. A prospective study in amateur boxing using magnetic resonance imaging (MRI). Int J Sports Med 1992; 13:616–620.
22. Jaspan T, Narborough G, Punt JA, Lowe J. Cerebral contusional tears as a marker of child abuse—detection by cranial sonography. Pediatr Radiol 1992; 22:237–45.
23. Jellinger K. Neuropathology of cord injuries. In: Vinken PJ, Bruyn GW, eds. Handbook of Clinical Neurology, Amsterdam: North-Holland Publishing Co, 1976:43–121.
24. Jennett B, MacMillan R. Epidemiology of head injury. Br Med J 1981; 282:101–104.
25. Jordan BD, Jahre C, Hauser WA, et al. CT of 338 active professional boxers. Radiology 1992; 185:509–512.
26. Kawamata T, Katayama Y, Hovda DA, Yoshino A, Becker DP. Lactate accumulation following concussive brain injury: the role of ionic fluxes induced by excitatory amino acids. Brain Res 1995; 674:196–204.
27. Kondo T, Saito K, Nishigami J, Ohshima T. Fatal injuries of the brain stem and/or upper cervical spinal cord in traffic accidents: nine autopsy cases. Sci Justice 1995; 35:197–201.
28. Kraus JF, McArthur DL, Silberman TA. Epidemiology of mild brain injury. Semin Neurol 1994; 14:1–7.

29. Levy ML, Masri LS, Levy KM, et al. Penetrating craniocerebral injury resultant from gunshot wounds: gang-related injury in children and adolescents. Neurosurgery 1993; 33:1018–1025.
30. Marshall LF, Toole BM, Bowers SA. The National Trauma Coma Data Bank II. Patients who talk and deteriorate: implications for treatment. J Neurosurg 1983; 59:285–288.
31. Miller JD. Head injury. J Neurol Neurosurg Psychiatry 1993; 56:440–447.
32. Rakier A, Guilburd JN, Soustiel JF, Zaaroor M, Feinsod M. Head injuries in the elderly. Brain Injury 1995; 9:187–93.
33. Riffenburgh RS, Sathyavagiswaran L. Ocular findings at autopsy of child abuse victims. Ophthalmology 1991; 98:1519–24.
34. Roberts GW, Allsop D, Bruton CJ. The occult aftermath of boxing. J Neurol Neurosurg Psychiatry 1990; 53:373–378.
35. Shimura T, Nakazawa S, Takahashi H, et al. Neuropathological study of battered child syndrome: eight autopsy cases. No Shinkei Geka Neurol Surg 1994; 22:23–28.
36. Silberstein M, Hennessy O. Implications of focal spinal cord lesions following trauma: evaluation with magnetic resonance imaging. Paraplegia 1993; 31:160–167.
37. Simpson DA, Blumbergs PC, Cooter RD, Kilminster M, McLean AG, Scott G. Pontomedullary tears and other gross brainstem injuries after vehicular accidents. J Trauma 1989; 29:1519–1525.
38. Sosin DM, Sniezek JE, Waxweiler RJ. Trends in death associated with traumatic brain injury, 1979 through 1992. Success and failure. JAMA 1995; 273:1778–1780.
39. Stein SC, Young GS, Talucci RC, Grenbaum BH, Ross SE. Delayed brain injury after head trauma: significance of coagulopathy. Neurosurgery 1992; 30:160–165.
40. Stewart WF, Gordon B, Selnes O, et al. Prospective study of central nervous system function in amateur boxers in the United States. Am J Epidemiol 1994; 139:573–588.
41. Squier MV, Lehr RP. Post-traumatic syringomyelia. J Neurol Neurosurg Psychiatry 1995; 58:1095–1098.
42. Sung JH, Mastri AR, Chen KTK. Aberrant peripheral nerves and neuromas in normal and injured spinal cords. J Neuropathol Exp Neurol 1981; 40:551–565.
43. Tator CH. Review of the secondary injury theory of acute spinal cord trauma with special emphasis on vascular mechanisms. J Neurosurg 1991; 75:15–26.
44. Tator CH. Update on the pathophysiology and pathology of acute spinal cord injury. Brain Pathol 1995; 5:407–413.
45. Valsamis MO. Pathology of trauma. (Review.) Neurosurg Clin North Am 1994; 5:175–183.
46. Willis BK, Greiner F, Orrison WW, Benzel EC. The incidence of vertebral artery injury after midcervical spine fracture or subluxation. Neurosurgery 1994; 34:435–441.

4

Infections

I. INTRODUCTION

Infectious and inflammatory disorders of the central nervous system (CNS) and even the peripheral nervous system (PNS) are a major cause of neurologic morbidity and mortality. Even as the advent of powerful new antibiotics has allowed for the effective treatment of many bacterial and fungal infections of the CNS, new viral agents—and even transmissible agents with little similarity to conventional viruses—have emerged or become recognized as significant pathogens in the causation of both fulminant and slowly progressive diseases of brain and spinal cord. Whereas at the turn of the last century rabies was the only known form of viral encephalitis, numerous RNA and DNA viruses with a myriad of biological capabilities are now known to produce a host of neurologic disorders. Viral pathogens are *suspected* as the cause of some CNS diseases with a chronic inflammatory component, especially demyelinating diseases (see Chap. 5).

One viral disorder that has emerged as a major epidemic in the final two decades of this millenium, viz. acquired immunodefiency syndrome (AIDS) caused by infection with human immunodeficiency virus type 1 (HIV-1), not only results in opportunistic viral, fungal, and parasitic infections of the nervous system, but may result in a dementia that is caused by direct HIV-1 invasion of CNS cells (though probably *not* neurons). Iatrogenic therapies associated with aggressive cancer treatment, bone marrow transplantation, and the transplantation of solid organs (liver, lungs, and heart) predispose patients to opportunistic infections that often involve the CSF and brain or spinal cord parenchyma.

Several issues of terminology are important with reference to CNS infections. Regardless of the specific causal organism that produces CNS disease (or even when a specific pathogen has *not* been identified), the resultant inflammation can generally be thought of as being "compartmentalized," affecting the leptomeninges, meninges, *and* brain (or spinal cord) parenchyma, or the CNS parenchyma *only*. When inflammation is confined to the meninges, it is described as a meningitis; when it affects both CNS parenchyma and CSF, it is more correctly described as a meningoencephalitis, meningocerebritis (when in the brain and adjacent coverings), or meningomyelitis (when involving spinal cord). When inflammation is present only in the CNS parenchyma, it is termed encephalitis, cerebritis, or myelitis (Fig. 1). A disorder that begins as a relatively "pure" encephalitis or cerebritis may, with disease progression, extend into the subarachnoid space producing meningoencephalitis. Conversely a meningitis can, by various mechanisms, eventually involve the CNS parenchyma and thus become a meningoencephalitis. However, it is relatively unusual for a pure meningitis to develop into a pure encephalitis.

Inflammatory/infectious disorders that involve the brain and its coverings are usually classified by the predominant inflammatory cell present—e.g., in the meninges or brain/spinal cord parenchyma (Fig. 2). In the case of a *purulent* (pyogenic, suppurative) meningitis or meningoencephalitis, the inflammatory exudate contains primarily neutrophils or polymorphonuclear leukocytes (PMNs).

Purulent/suppurative meningitis is usually caused by "conventional" bacteria and some fungal organisms. When the predominant inflammatory infiltrate is composed of histiocytes/macrophages, the meningitis is described as *granulomatous*. A granulomatous meningitis need not show the presence of multinucleated giant cells, though these are frequently encountered. The most common causes of granulomatous meningitis in humans include tuberculosis, some fungi (especially *Coccidioides immitis* and *Cryptococcus neoformans*), and sarcoidosis, for which no causal organism has been definitively proven. Granulomatous meningitis can also occur as part of a foreign body reaction to "foreign" proteins in the CSF—the most dramatic example may be that of a ruptured epidermoid cyst which sheds keratin into the subarachnoid space, potentially causing a brisk granulomatous meningitis.

The third common type of leptomeningitis is that categorized as *lymphocytic*. Lymphocytic meningoencephalitis is usually caused by (conventional) viruses and may be seen in neurosyphilis. Lymphocytic infiltrates are also encountered in the meninges of patients with leukemia, (systemic) lymphoma, some collagen-vascular diseases, and lymphocytic choriomeningitis. Necropsy experience with most forms of lymphocytic meningitis is minimal, since this is usually a self-limited and reversible disorder.

Each of these three types of inflammation—purulent, granulomatous, or lymphocytic—rarely manifests with the presence of only one cell type in the infiltrate. The different subtypes are defined by the *predominant* cell type present and should guide the pathologist or clinician in seeking a likely causal microorganism. This is done by the judicious use of culture of the cerebrospinal fluid (CSF) (or brain parenchyma) at biopsy or autopsy, and/or appropriate use

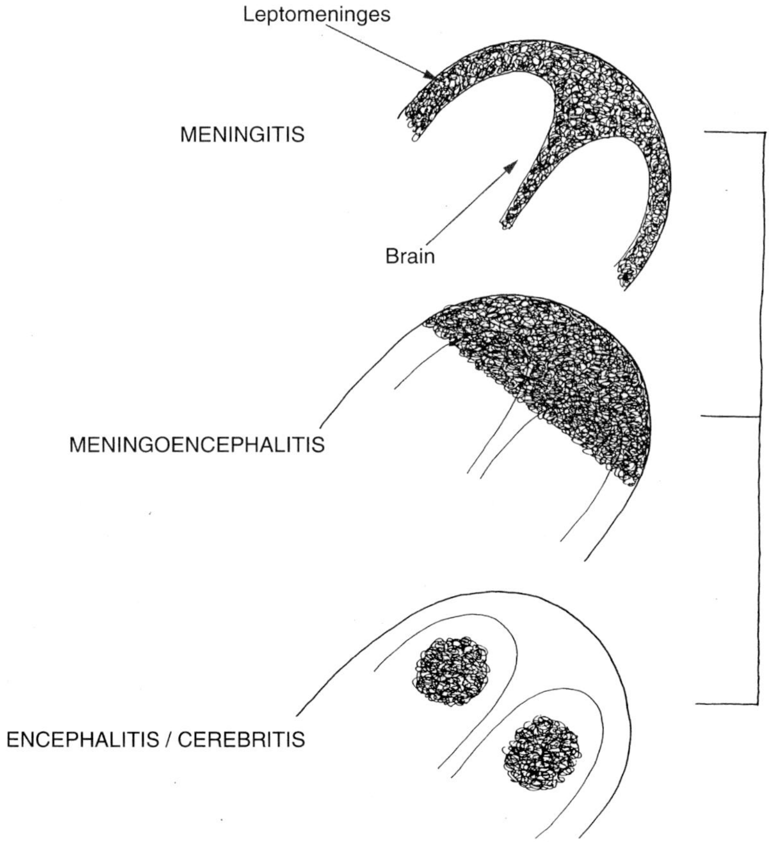

Figure 1 Terminology used to describe infectious/inflammatory disorders of the CNS, based on compartmental localization of the inflammatory infiltrate (i.e., meningeal vs. parenchymal). Either a "pure" meningitis or encephalitis may evolve into a meningoencephalitis. Evolution of a pure meningitis into a pure encephalitis (or the reverse) is a relatively rare occurrence.

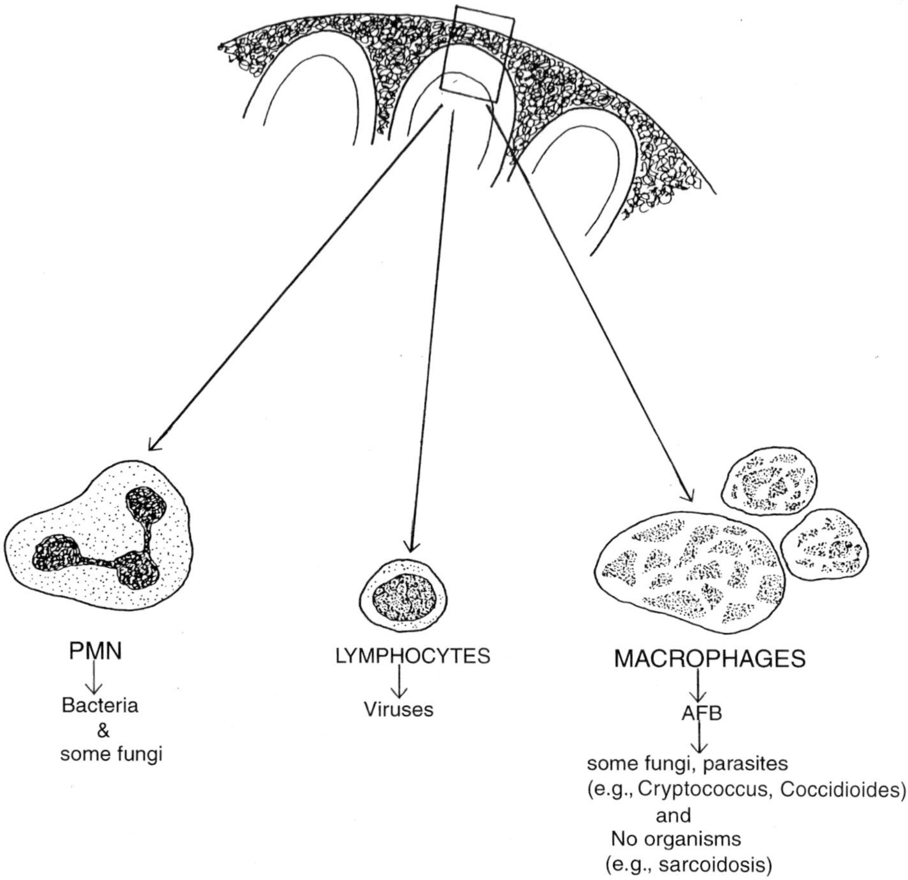

Figure 2 Classification of CNS inflammatory/infectious disorder (in this case simplified as a meningitis) based on the primary inflammatory cell type present. Though different types of meningitis are defined by the *major* cell type present, it is rare for each to be characterized exclusively by the one inflammatory component. PMN = polymorphonuclear leukocyte, AFB = acid fast bacillus.

of special stains to demonstrate the presence of specific pathogens (Gram stain and acid-fast for bacteria, PAS and methenamine silver for most fungi), immunohistochemistry, or in situ hybridization using probes for bacterial, fungal, viral, or parasitic organisms on tissue sections. The diagnostic approach to infections of the CNS/CSF has been augmented by the development, over the past 10 to 15 years, of molecular diagnostic aids that allow for extremely detailed characterization of CNS pathogens—e.g., using the methodology of genomic fingerprinting (which incorporates restriction-endonuclease analysis and Southern blot hybridization) and polymerase chain reaction (PCR) amplification of pathogen-specific DNA and/or RNA. PCR technology is so sensitive that it may be used to detect and identify previously "unculturable" pathogens. A note of caution: PCR may also detect small quantities of a "bystander" virus that has nothing to do with a given infectious disorder.

Whereas the anatomical pathologist encounters these inflammatory processes in the context of a brain or leptomeningeal biopsy or at necropsy, the different forms of meningitis also produce characteristic CSF changes, which can be detected by a clinician in the course of examining such fluid obtained from a lumbar puncture. Purulent/suppurative meningitis is associated with abundant PMNs in the CSF, markedly elevated protein, and diminished glucose, whereas lymphocytic meningitis causes elevated protein but a relatively modest (if any) decrease in CSF glucose.

The brain and CSF are, under normal circumstances, free of infectious organisms. If an infectious disorder is discovered within the CNS or CSF (or both), a clinician must be suspicious of how and why microorganisms have traversed the usually obstructive barriers that protect these compartments. Microorganisms can enter the CNS/CSF via the cardiopulmonary system, nasopharynx, sinuses, or middle ear; in the course of traumatic skull lesions (including neurosurgical procedures) (Fig. 3); and along nerve axons that communicate with cutaneous or neuromuscular structures. Patients who have circulating microorganisms in the blood are also at risk for these organisms' "seeding" into the CSF and brain. Immunosuppressed individuals are particularly susceptible to developing overwhelming CNS infections, including those caused by organisms that normally do not produce significant disease in immunocompetent individuals.

II. PURULENT/SUPPURATIVE INFECTIONS

Purulent infections of the CNS can result in meningits, meningoencephalitis (Fig. 1), or cerebritis, the last usually leading to brain abscess (discussed in section VI below). As indicated above, the predominant inflammatory cell type in such an infection is the PMN. Purulent meningitis is usually caused by conventional (i.e., non-acid-fast) bacteria, though some fungi may also produce this type of inflammation. Causes of this type of meningitis differ depending on whether it occurs in the neonatal period, childhood, or adulthood. Regardless, its clinical evolution is usually rapid and dramatic, and it constitutes both a diagnostic and a therapeutic emergency. This is all the more important since suppurative meningitis caused by bacteria in an immunocompetent individual can be remarkably amenable to appropriate antibiotic therapy.

Suppurative meningitis classically presents with the rapid onset and progression of pyrexia, severe headache, vomiting, photophobia, and signs of me-

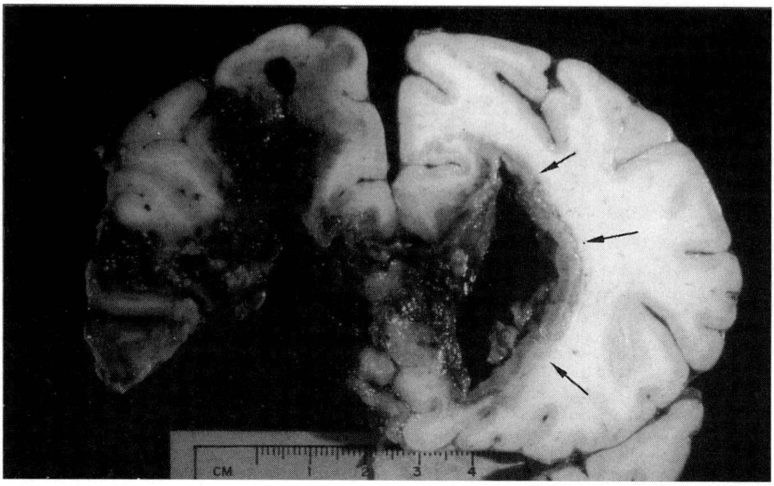

Figure 3 Dramatic example of one way in which microorganisms (in this case bacteria) may gain access to the (usually) sterile environment of the brain. Patient had suffered a self-inflicted gunshot wound to the left side of the face, with resultant avulsion of the left frontal lobe. The wound had produced a direct open conduit between ambient bacterial flora and the CSF which was difficult to "close" because of extent of the wound. Antibiotic therapy was also ineffective because of size of the wound. The patient eventually expired because of massive meningo-cerebro-ventriculitis. Arrows indicate ventricular lining that was covered with a thick layer of pus.

ningeal irritation. Obtundation and coma may ensue with remarkable rapidity, due to raised intracranial pressure. In the neonatal period, presentation may be with less specific symptomatology which may include poor feeding, diarrhea, and lethargy progressing to coma; nuchal rigidity may be accompanied by the finding of a bulging fontanelle.

No matter at which age purulent meningitis occurs, histopathologic findings are relatively consistent and dramatic. The subarachnoid space is generally filled with PMNs, many of which may be undergoing nuclear fragmentation (Fig. 4). In severe (and especially, untreated) purulent meningitis, inflammatory cells frequently extend into the adjacent brain parenchyma to produce meningoencephalitis (Fig. 5). Vessels entrapped in the inflammatory infiltrate may undergo thrombosis, leading to superimposed necrosis (with eventual cavitation) of the underlying brain parenchyma. Cranial nerve elements traversing the inflammatory exudate can undergo scarring, and cranial nerve dysfunction is a potential long-term consequence of severe purulent meningitis. Depending on the stage at which this form of meningitis is discovered and treated, significant scarring may also occur in the meninges, leading to subsequent meningeal fibrosis, which in turn can result in hydrocephalus. On gross inspection of the brain of a patient who has died of purulent meningitis, it may show significant edema with herniations, and a meningeal exudate is sometimes identified grossly (Fig. 6). In the case of purulent meningitis caused by conventional bacteria, exudate may be present over the cerebral convexities and at the base of the brain, whereas granulomatous meningitis tends to be much more prominent in the basal meninges.

In the neonatal period bacterial meningitis most commonly results from infection with group B *Streptococcus* and *E. coli*. Other microorganisms implicated include (among gram-positives) *Staphylococcus aureus* and *Listeria monocytogenes* and (among gram-negatives), *Citrobacter* spp., *Klebsiella*, and *Pseudomonas*. Most cases of purulent meningitis in children between the ages of 1 month and 5 years are the result of infection by *Haemophilus influenzae* and *Neisseria meningitidis*, the latter also known as meningococcus. Rarely, subdural effusion (progressing to subdural empyema) may occur as a complication of pediatric meningitis. In adults, the most commonly observed pathogen is *S. pneumoniae*. Patients who develop meningitis caused by *H. influenzae* or *S. pneumoniae* usually give a history of an antecedent upper

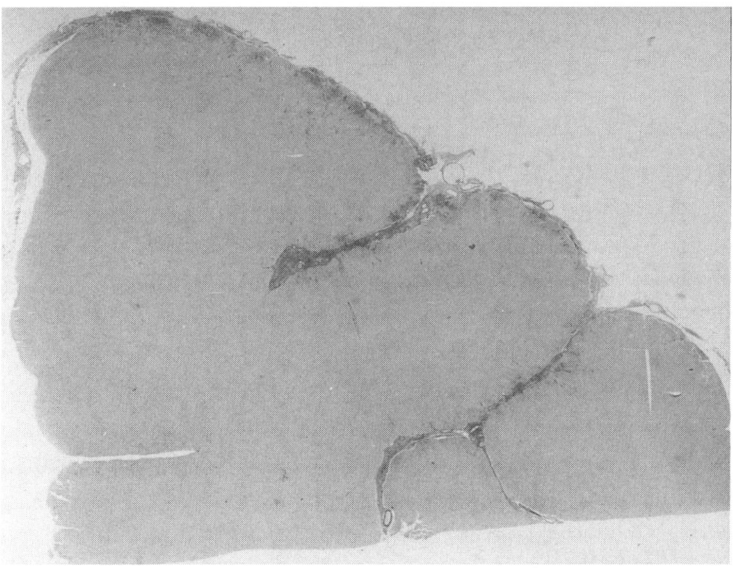

Figure 4 Purulent/suppurative meningitis. The subarachnoid space, normally a "potential" space devoid of any inflammatory cells, is (in this case) packed with a dense exudate of (acute) inflammatory cells (PMNs), which show multifocal extension into the brain substance.

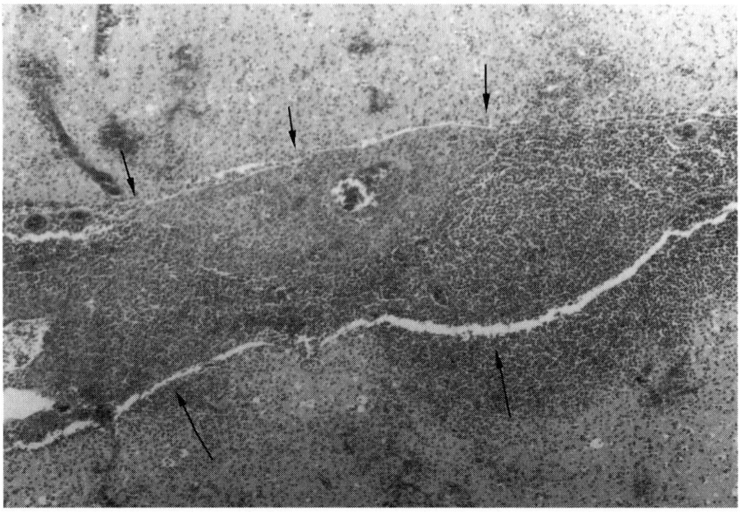

Figure 5 Meningoencephalitis probably originating from a meningitis. The subarachnoid space (arrows) is filled with an exudate which (at higher magnification) was seen to be overwhelmingly composed of PMNs. Inflammatory cells clearly extend into the surrounding brain parenchyma. Note entrapped blood vessels, which are at risk for undergoing thrombosis, in the meningeal exudate.

respiratory tract or middle-ear infection. Meningococcal meningitis tends to occur in outbreaks or epidemics, particularly among individuals in regions with substandard hygiene and poor public health, and is accompanied by a severe petechial rash. Meningitis that complicates neurosurgical procedures is commonly caused by gram-negative bacilli. Among children, neurologic sequelae of bacterial meningitis—including hearing impairment, developmental delays, mental retardation, and seizures—are found in as many as 10% to 30% of survivors.

III. GRANULOMATOUS INFECTIONS

These are usually caused by acid-fast bacteria (especially mycobacteria), some fungi, or (unusually) an intense foreign body-type granulomatous response to a "foreign" substance in the subarachnoid space (SAS)—e.g., keratin from a ruptured epidermoid cyst—or by no identifiable inciting/causal agent—e.g., the case of sarcoid meningitis.

Tuberculous meningitis may occur as a complication of initial bloodborne dissemination of primary pulmonary infection by the bacterium (i.e., in the course of miliary disease). Primary infection with *Mycobacterium tuberculosis* is less common in third-world countries than in North America or Western Europe; i.e., primary infection with the causal microbe may occur in "Western" populations at any age, whereas in poor nations it is more likely to occur in infancy or childhood.

Epidemiologic evidence suggests a resurgence of tuberculosis (TB), largely as a function of active pulmonary TB among AIDS patients and residents of inner cities, with concomitant emergence of multi-drug-resistant strains of this acid-fast bacterium. Growth and progression of *M. tuberculosis* after initial bloodborne spread is generally arrested as a consequence of cell-mediated immunity. However, viable bacilli may persist in either the CNS or extra-CNS sites. These tubercles can be reactivated to produce active tuberculosis (including tuberculous meningitis) at any time. If a tubercle localized within brain ruptures, widespread TB meningitis or even meningoventriculitis can result. TB meningitis in the context of miliary TB has high rates of morbidity and mortality.

Neuropathologic features of tuberculous meningitis, the quintessential granulomatous meningitis, show some similarities to purulent/suppurative meningitis. A prominent meningeal exudate is often found on gross inspection of the brain at necropsy, though in granulomatous meningitis this is more likely to be predominantly basal (sometimes extending into the Sylvian fissures and around the spinal cord) and more firm or "fibrotic" to palpation. Because granulomatous meningitis is, by the nature of the cellular infiltrate, composed of densely cohesive inflammatory infiltrates with a major component of macrophages (and, almost invariably, multinucleated giant cells), the exudate may appear more "nodular" than that of a purulent meningitis, in which PMNs extend freely throughout the SAS. On microscopic examination, typical features of granulomatous inflammation are found: caseating granulomas scattered throughout the SAS, sometimes with extension of granulomatous inflammation into the adjacent brain parenchyma (Fig. 7).

Foci of tuberculous meningitis that involve the adventitia of meningeal vessels can cause intimal proliferation, sometimes resulting in occlusion of leptomeningeal vessels with necrosis in the underlying brain parenchyma. TB can also present as a mass lesion (tuberculoma) in the brain, and is in the broad differential of *any* space-occupying CNS mass—especially in high-risk patients. Microscopic sections of tuberculoma show solitary or confluent granulomas with central caseous necrosis surrounded by lymphocytes, Langhans'-type multinucleated giant cells and macrophages, collagen, and fibroblasts.

Any patient found (at autopsy or biopsy) to have granulomatous meningitis, with or without associated necrosis, must have tissue studied (by culture and stains for microorganisms) with the likelihood in mind that the meningitis has resulted from mycobacterial or fungal infection. Granulomas with necrosis, though especially common in TB, are also seen in some fungal granulomatous meningitides—e.g., those due to coccidioidomycosis (especially common in the

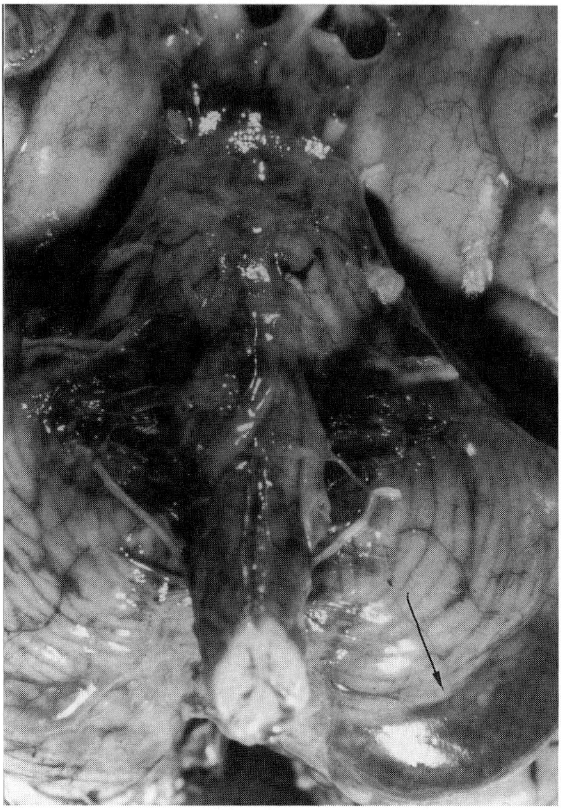

(A)

Figure 6 Suppurative meningitis, gross appearance of brain. (A) View of basal meninges overlying brainstem, cerebellum, and mesial temporal lobes, which are moderately opacified secondary to the meningeal infiltrate. Purulent fluid shows loculation at base of left cerebellar hemisphere (arrow). (B) A young immunocompromised patient with an especially hemorrhagic meningitis secondary to *Pseudomonas.*

southwestern U.S.) and even (rarely) cryptococcosis (Fig. 8). Coccidioidomycosis is especially adept at producing an endarteritis that can lead to extensive necrosis. If—and only if—a causal microorganism is effectively and conclusively ruled out as an etiologic agent, can the patient be given the (more likely) diagnosis of sarcoid meningitis. Modern diagnosis of mycobacterial infection also incorporates not just appropriate/routine CSF staining and culture, but molecular diagnostic techniques that include restriction fragment length polymor-

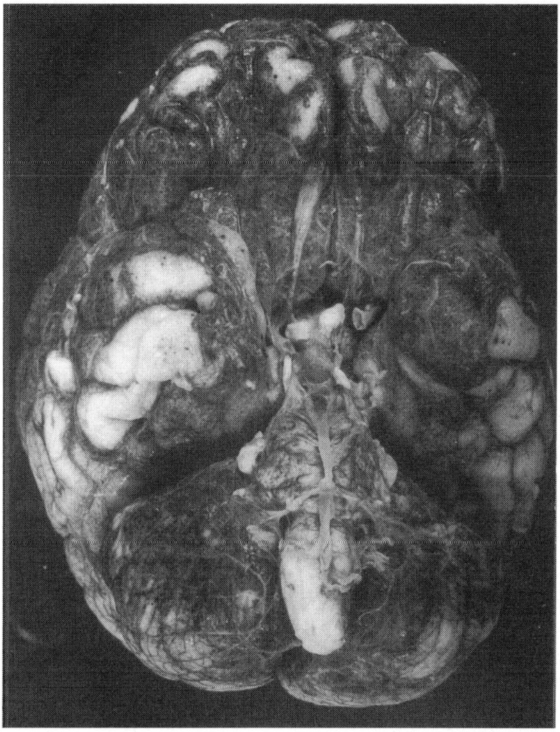

(B)

phism (RFLP) fingerprinting of distinctive TB strains, and diagnosis of the bacterium in fluids using PCR-based methods.

IV. LYMPHOCYTIC MENINGITIS

In autopsy material, this is rarely encountered as the cause of death; however, patients with a (fatal) viral encephalitis frequently have lymphoid cells in the SAS as a manifestation of meningeal extension of the cerebritis—e.g., in patients with herpes simplex encephalitis. The diagnosis of lymphocytic meningitis is more commonly encountered by clinicians as a self-limited infection caused by a relatively mild viral meningitis. As well, when a clinician encounters a lymphocytic meningitis (sometimes also referred to as aseptic meningitis) in the course of studying the CSF of a patient with neurologic symptoms, he or she must decide if the lymphoid cells encountered are "reactive" or "neoplastic"—the latter in particular posing a challenge for the cytopathologist. The

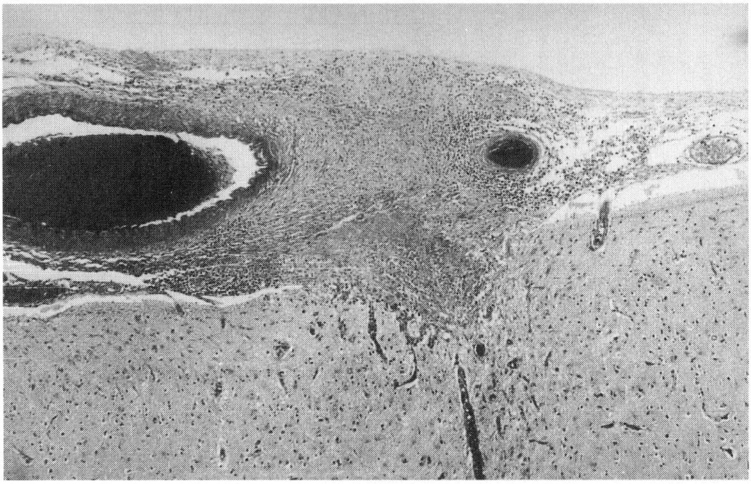

(A)

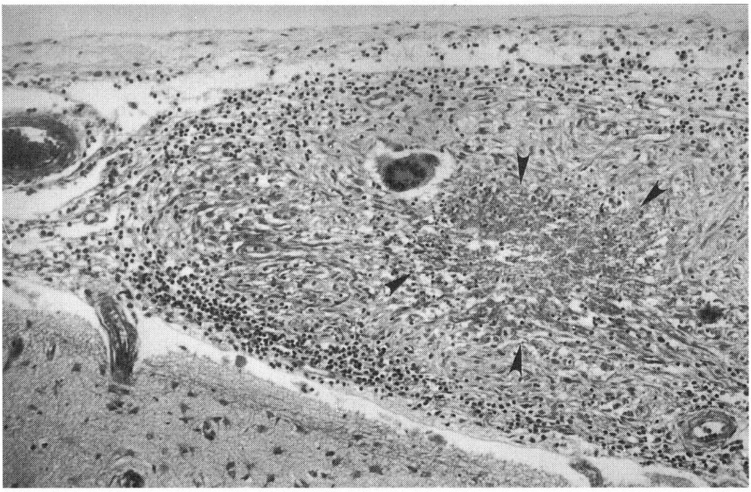

(B)

Figure 7 Tuberculous meningitis, the classic example of granulomatous meningitis. Note nodular inflammatory infiltrate in the subarachnoid space (A) extending into brain parenchyma. It is composed of macrophages, lymphocytes, and Langhans'-type giant cells (B). Caseating necrosis (arrowheads) may be present.

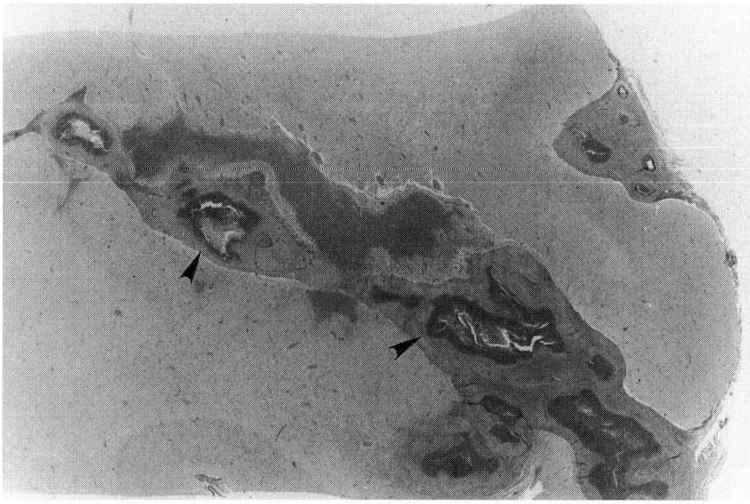

(A)

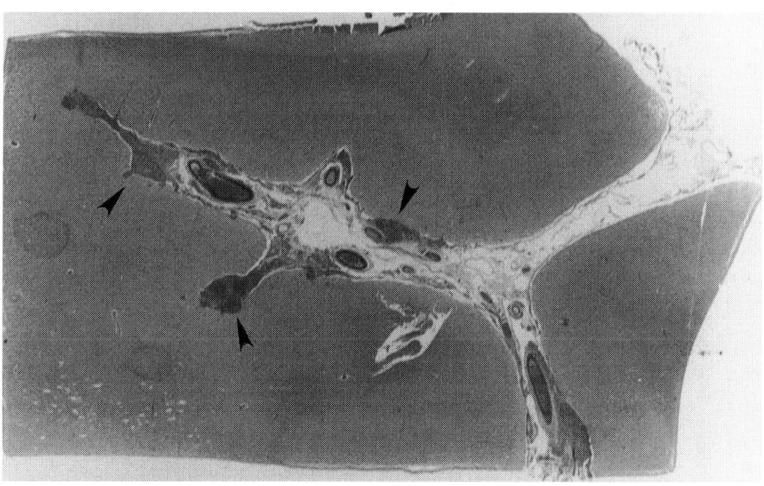

(B)

Figure 8 Granulomatous meningitis caused by cryptococcosis (A), illustrated by a PAS-stained section in patient with an intact immune system and coccidioidomycosis (B) in a patient with AIDS. Note dense inflammatory infiltrates that fill and distend the subarachnoid space (A) or are nodular (arrowheads, B). In both examples, clusters of inflammatory cells extend into the subpial brain parenchyma. In (A), necrotic regions are present in the meningeal infiltrate (arrowheads).

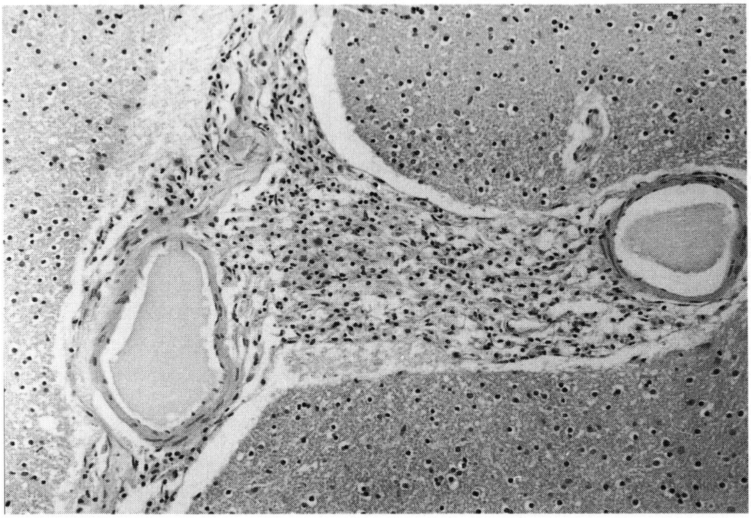

Figure 9 Lymphocytic meningitis in a patient with AIDS. CNS showed evidence of primary brain infection by HIV-1 as well as opportunistic infection (OI) with CMV. The lymphocytic meningitis may be secondary to HIV infection (of the brain *or* CSF) or to the widespread brain CMV infection.

differential becomes particularly important for a patient who has had a history of a leukemia/lymphoma which may spread to the SAS/CSF without significant brain involvement, even when there is minimal evidence of systemic disease.

Lymphocytic/aspetic meningitis, often caused by viruses such as enteroviruses (e.g., Coxsackie A or B), mumps virus, measles, and adenovirus, is also encountered frequently in the brains of patients with systemic HIV-1 infection (Fig. 9). In immunosuppressed individuals, some of these viruses (e.g., mumps, adenovirus) have been shown to cause a severe necrotizing encephalitis as well. A rare form of chronic/recurrent aseptic meningitis (Mollaret's) is now believed, based on PCR data, to result from herpes simplex viral infection.

V. NEUROSYPHILIS

Syphilis, a relatively rare condition in recent decades after the advent of effective antibiotic therapy, has made a comeback in the era of AIDS. Affected patients may develop active infection of the CNS by the causal organism (*Treponema pallidum*) after CNS invasion by the spirochete in the course of early syphilis. CSF abnormalities may occur in asymptomatic patients, manifest as pleocytosis, decreased glucose level with increased protein, and a positive

VDRL serologic test. In meningovascular syphilis, leptomeningeal and/or CNS parenchymal small arteries may show endarteritis with intimal hyperplasia that can cause microfoci of CNS parenchymal necrosis. The meninges may show a prominent lymphoplasmacytic inflammatory infiltrate that mimics lymphocytic meningitis (see above). Parenchymatous neurosyphilis has two manifestations: tabes dorsalis (demyelination of the spinal cord dorsal columns, dorsal roots, and their adjacent dorsal root ganglia); and general paresis, characterized by widespread (cortical) neuron loss and microglial proliferation secondary to brain invasion by the spirochete.

VI. ABSCESS AND EMPYEMA

Brain abscesses occur in well-defined populations of at-risk patients, may be single or multiple, and present and behave as mass lesions (brain abscess is almost always in the differential diagnosis of patients who have single/multiple space-occupying lesions in the brain) with the added feature that patients with brain abscess(es) usually have one or more manifestations of an infectious illness—though these may be surprisingly mild. Patients most likely to develop brain abscess are summarized in Table 1. The prognosis of cerebral abscess has improved remarkably since the mid-1970s, primarily for two reasons: 1. Mod-

Table 1 Causes/Predisposing Factors for Cerebral Abscess

1. Contiguous cranial meningeal site of infection
   - Middle ear, mastoid air cells, paranasal sinuses
   - Dental abscess/instrumentation
   - Craniofacial osteomyelitis
   - Purulent/suppurative meningitis
2. Compound skull fracture, other deep cranial injury
3. Complication of neurosurgical/interventional procedure
4. Pleuropulmonary disease
   - Lung abscess, bronchiectasis
5. Hematogenous source
   - Cyanotic congenital heart disease, with right-to-left shunt (esp. tetralogy of Fallot)
   - Infectious endocarditis
   - Septicemia
6. Immunosuppression
   - Iatrogenic (chemotherapy for malignancy, organ, or bone marrow transplant)
   - Acquired immunodeficiency syndrome (AIDS)
   - Congenital immunodeficiency
   - Poorly controlled diabetes mellitus

ern neuroimaging techniques (which have flourished since the late 1970s) allow for timely detection and accurate localization of abscesses; and 2. currently used techniques in diagnostic microbiology allow for the precise isolation and characterization of causal bacteria, especially anaerobes, with more appropriate and targeted effective antibiotic therapy. Brain abscesses have an estimated annual incidence of approx. 4/1 million/year and occur especially in young males; in children, the peak incidence is between 4 and 7 years of age. Their treatment focuses on the dual approach used to treat abscesses elsewhere: drainage of pus and antibiotic administration. Increasingly, treatment with antibiotics alone is found to be effective in a growing number of patients.

Approximately half of brain abscesses arise by spread of infection from a contiguous cranial site. The obvious implication of this fact is that treatment of a potential site of origin for an abscess represents optimal preventive medicine. Spread of infection from an adjoining site to CNS tissue occurs either by direct spread across bone and dura or by way of blood vessels, in the form of a septic thrombophlebitis or arteritis. The zone of affected brain is adjacent to the region of primary infection; e.g., abscess resulting from a middle ear infection or mastoiditis is likely to be in the temporal lobe or cerebellum (the cerebellum is a favored site in children). Pleuropulmonary disease is the commonest cause of metastatic brain abscess (indeed, usually multiple abscesses) in adults.

Hematogenous spread of infectious organisms leading to brain abscess also occurs in patients with cyanotic congenital cardiac disease with a right-to-left shunt. As many as 2% of these patients may develop this complication, and as many as 25% of children with brain abscess have congenital heart disease. Tetralogy of Fallot is the commonest abnormality with which this occurs. Infectious endocarditis more commonly produces *micro*abscesses that probably originate in septic microinfarcts.

Bacterial flora found in brain abscesses most commonly include streptococci (including *milleri, viridans,* nonhemolytic streptococci), and enterococci, members of the *Bacteroides* family (found in up to 25% to 60% of patients), Enterobacteriaceae (e.g., *Proteus* spp. and *E. coli*), and *Staphylococcus aureus*. Two or more bacteria may be isolated from over half of brain abscess patients. Immunosuppressed patients develop abscesses more likely to be caused by unusual organisms such as *Nocardia asteroides* and (especially, given the high frequency of T-cell abnormalities) fungi (see also sections VIII and IX below). In patients who have received bone marrow or liver transplants, abscesses caused by *Aspergillus* and *Candida* are especially common, whereas AIDS patients more commonly develop cryptococcal meningitis and may rarely show "cryptococcomas" of the brain parenchyma.

Neuropathologic features of a given brain abscess reflect the length of time it has been present within CNS tissue. Evolution of a brain abscess is through the following stages:

1. Acute cerebritis (lasting 1 to 3 days) that occurs by inflammatory cells infiltrating a zone of necrosis (probably the initiating event of an abscess), with surrounding edema.
2. Subacute or late cerebritis (4 to 9 days) with early capsule formation and endothelial proliferation ("neovascularization") at the edge of the abscess.
3. Early capsule formation by fibroblasts with shrinkage of the necrotic center and an abundance of macrophages (10 to 13 days).
4. Late capsule formation (2 weeks on) at which time the abscess takes on a chronic appearance, with a well-delineated necrotic center, peripheral inflammatory cells (acute and chronic), macrophages, a dense collagen-containing capsule, and outside of this reactive astrocytes with variable (but often severe) edema.

Selected microscopic features of CNS abscess are illustrated in Figure 10. Gross features of an evolving and "established" cerebral abscess are illustrated in Figure 11, which dramatically highlights the observation that such an abscess may be associated with a severe overlying (though relatively focal) meningitis. Any suspected abscess reviewed by the surgical pathologist must be stained for microorganisms and sent for bacterial and fungal culture.

Epi-/extradural abscess is a rare occurrence that may result from distant or local infection (e.g., related to trauma or surgical intervention). *Subdural empyema*, defined as a pyogenic/suppurative infectious/inflammatory disorder confined to the subdural space, while much less common than brain abscess, carries a high morbidity. A disorder most likely to occur in young males in the second decade, the most common predisposing factors for subdural empyema are sinusitis and trauma (including the iatrogenic/surgical variety). Causal bacteria are usually anaerobic strains and streptococci.

VII. "CONVENTIONAL" VIRAL INFECTIONS IN IMMUNOCOMPETENT HOSTS

The genesis in our understanding of (and appreciation for) the role of viruses in causing neurologic disease has almost directly paralleled the development of sophisticated techniques enabling one to study them. From crude inferences based on examination of "filterable agents" at the turn of the last century, the subspecialty of neurovirology has progressed through techniques that allow viruses to be studied in culture, ultrastructurally, biochemically, and immunocytochemically, to the modern era in which viral "footprints" (even ones that are extraordinarily faint) can be detected in nervous system tissue using in situ hybridization, polymerase chain reaction (PCR), or the combined methodology of in situ PCR.

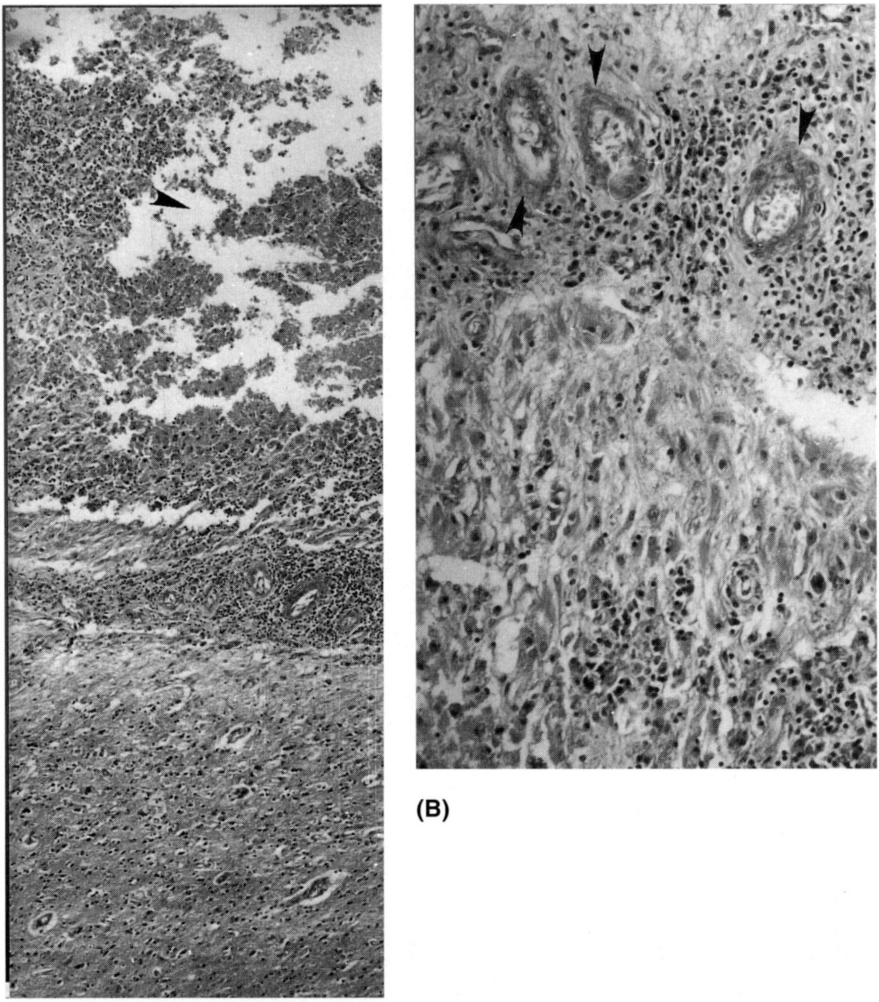

(A) (B)

Figure 10 Cerebral abscess, microscopic features. Note necrotic center (arrow, panel A) associated with histiocytes and PMNs. At junction with surrounding brain parenchyma (B), there is neovascularization (arrowheads), evidence of more chronic inflammation, and (in the CNS itself) reactive astrocytic gliosis.

Unfortunately, these elegant and powerful techniques sometimes provide information on the existence of viruses in neural tissue that may not be of pathogenetic relevance for a disease under study. The role of the neuropathologist in resolving issues of viral neuropathogenesis will thus continue to be pivotal.

Viral infections in the immunocompetent host are characterized by several unifying and distinctive microscopic findings—indeed, the presence of a combination of such histopathologic abnormalities in CNS tissue from a patient with an illness of unknown etiology strongly suggests that it might be caused by a viral pathogen. (The specific examples of Rasmussen encephalitis and paraneoplastic encephalomyelitis will be briefly discussed below and in Chap. 8.) These features include:

1. Chronic inflammation with or without necrosis of CNS parenchyma (including infiltration by mononuclear inflammatory cells, prominent among which are microglia/macrophages).
2. Perivascular cuffing by mononuclear inflammatory cells (especially lymphocytes).
3. Death of individual neurons, often surrounded by microglia—the phenomenon of neuronophagia (Fig. 12).

Each of these abnormalities may be seen in a variety of neuropathologic entities, but, assuming they are present in combination, the search for a specific causal viral agent must be undertaken using the ancillary techniques already described, several of which will be illustrated. Viruses in the CNS may cause cell (especially neuron) destruction—known as "lytic infection"—more indolent or gradual cell dysfunction leading to chronic cell injury and/or death (which may be mediated in part by immune/inflammatory mechanisms), or no apparent cell damage as persistent infections. The role of viruses in the causation of human CNS/PNS neoplasms is as yet unproven, though (for instance) Epstein-Barr virus may have a major role in the causation of primary CNS lymphoma. Several specific viral diseases will now be considered.

A. Herpes Simplex Encephalitis and Neurologic Disease Due to Other Herpesviruses

Encephalitis caused by herpesviruses (especially herpes simplex, HSV) represents the most common, and arguably the most devastating, form of human viral encephalitis. In adults, HSV encephalitis (HSVE, caused by HSV-1) is rare, with an estimated incidence in developed nations of 1 to 2 per million per year—probably an underestimate since the correct diagnosis is "easy to miss." Caused by a large enveloped double-stranded DNA virus (a feature shared by all human herpesviruses), HSVE presents with some combination of headache, pyrexia, drowsiness, meningismus, and seizures. The causal virus is identical to

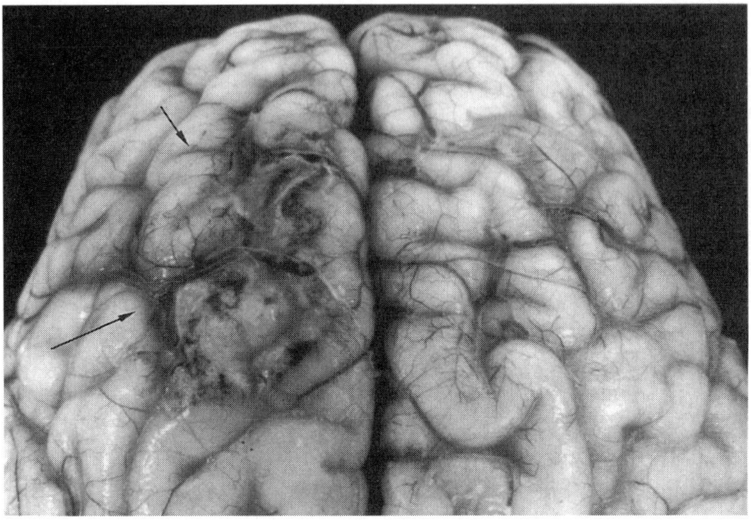

(A)

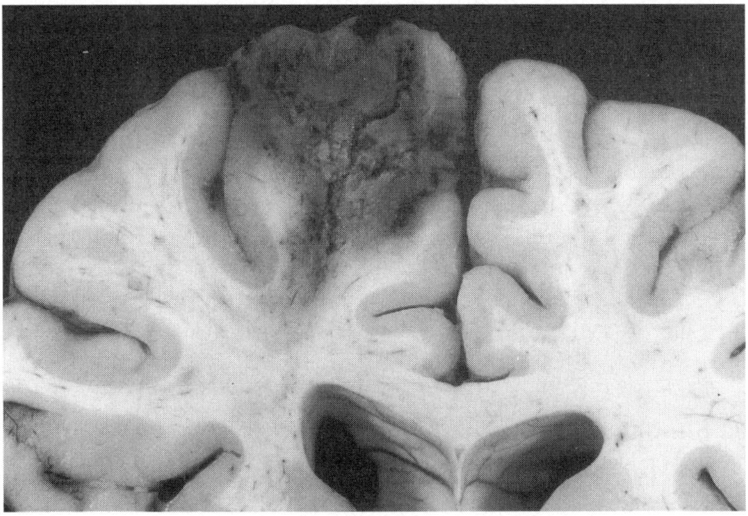

(B)

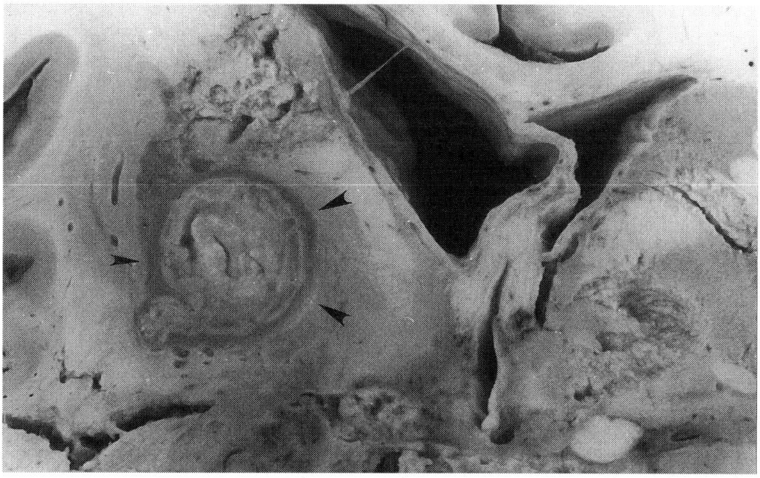

(C)

Figure 11 Cerebral abscess, in early stage of evolution (subacute) secondary to fungal infection in an immunosuppressed patient. View of brain from the convexities (A, opposite page) shows a relatively well-demarcated zone of purulent meningitis (arrows) which overlies an abscess shown in coronal section in (B). Had this patient undergone lumbar puncture (not a recommended procedure in a patient with a mass lesion!) PMNs and microorganisms may have been present secondary to communication of the abscess with the subarachnoid space. (C) Chronic brain abscess in an AIDS patient. Note necrotic center surrounded by a dense capsule.

HSV-1 that causes cold sores of the lip. Primary infection by the virus is thought to occur in the lip or buccal mucosa, from which locus virus spreads by retrograde axonal transport to trigeminal ganglia. Latent HSV infection persists in the ganglionic neurons (in an estimated half to three-quarters of the adult population), though it can be reactivated to cause recurrent cold sores (following anterograde viral transport back to labial skin).

Much less commonly, virus "moves" to the brain by mechanisms not fully understood, or is reactivated there from latent infection analogous to that within trigeminal ganglia, to produce HSVE. This condition is often fatal without treatment and still has high morbidity and mortality with appropriate therapy that includes antiviral agents, especially acyclovir. The role and potential value of brain biopsy (as weighed against its complications) in the diagnostic workup of individuals with suspected HSVE continues to be the subject of considerable debate. One argument in favor of diagnostic biopsy is the large number of (infectious and noninfectious) diseases, many of them treatable

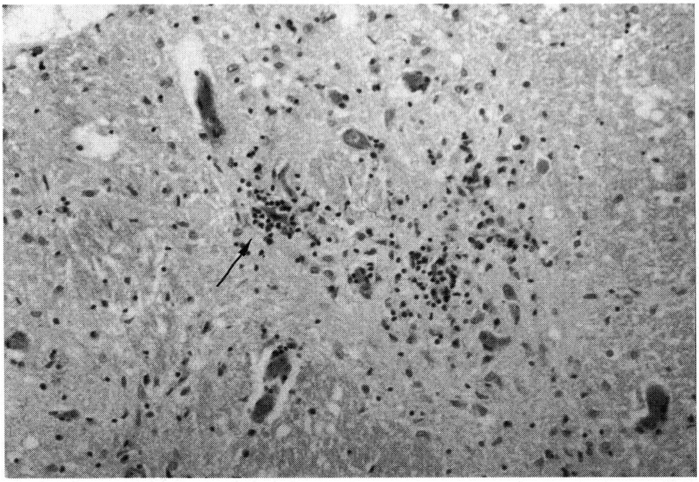

(A)

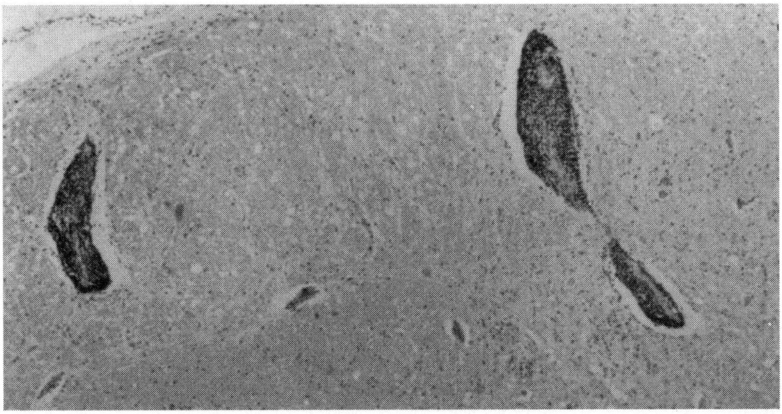

(B)

Figure 12 Microscopic features strongly suggestive of (conventional) viral infection. (A) Infiltration of CNS parenchyma by mononuclear cells, which often show immunohistochemical features of microglia/macrophages; arrow indicates a neuron surrounded by such cells, in the process of undergoing neuronophagia. (B) Perivascular cuffing by mononuclear inflammatory cells. Surrounding brain parenchyma also shows patchy mild chronic inflammation. (C) Perivascular cuffing in another patient (shown at higher magnification) highlights the cytologic uniformity of the cells.

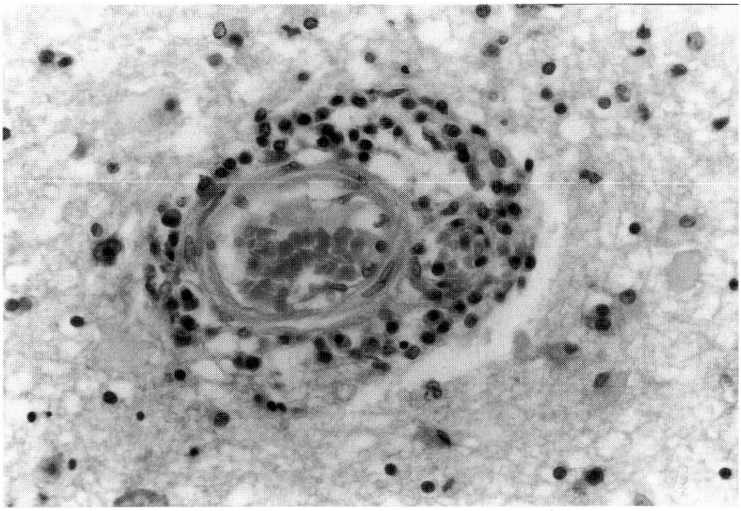

(C)

(though not with antiviral agents!), that can mimic HSVE clinically and on neuroimaging investigations.

Neuropathologic features of acute or subacute adult HSVE are characteristic of severe acute necrotizing and extensively hemorrhagic encephalitis. Grossly the brain is edematous and shows hemorrhagic necrosis in areas of predilection, including temporal and orbital frontal cortex (Fig. 13), insular regions, and the cingulate gyri, though often with marked right/left asymmetry in the extent and severity of lesions. Appearances may mimic those of a hemorrhagic infarct, the difference being that HSVE lesions are not confined to a vascular territory. Patients who die after a lengthy course of the illness (months/years) show appearances of cystic encephalomalacia in affected lobes of the brain (Fig. 14). Microscopic features typically include (as predicted from the gross appearance) regions of hemorrhagic necrosis sometimes centered on microvessels, the walls of which may show fibrinoid necrosis and their lumina thrombosis (Fig. 15).

Features characteristic of the viral encephalitides (see above) including perivascular cuffing, microglial nodules, and foci of neuronophagia may all be present, and overlying meninges usually show a lymphocytic infiltrate. Characteristic intranuclear inclusions (Cowdry type A)—i.e., dense eosinophilic round or vaguely polygonal structures surrounded by a clear space or halo between the inclusion and the nuclear membrane—are easier to identify in acute than in chronic

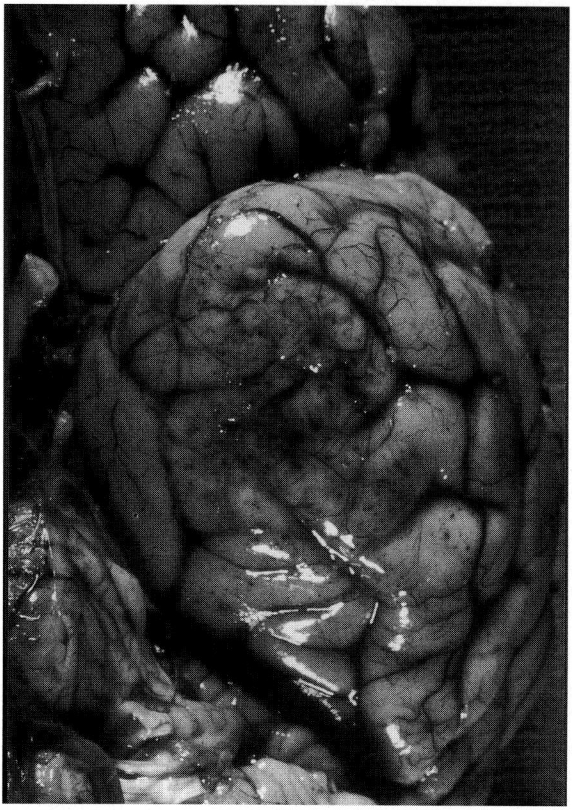

(A)

Figure 13 HSV-1 encephalitis (HSVE) in an adult. (A) Basal view of brain shows poorly demarcated area of hemorrhagic necrosis on undersurface of the left temporal lobe. Without clinical history, the differential diagnosis would include contusion secondary to a traumatic brain injury, and hemorrhagic infarct within the left PCA territory. (B) Coronal section from brain of a patient with HSVE shows patchy hemorrhagic necrosis within both white matter and cortex (arrow), and several areas in which cortex–white matter junction is indistinct.

cases (Fig. 16). Presence of the etiologic agent can be confirmed by immunohistochemistry using anti-HSV antibodies, in situ hybridization, and/or PCR carried out using HSV-1-specific primers on DNA extracted from the tissue (Fig. 17). PCR methodology can be utilized to detect HSV-specific DNA in suspected cases of HSVE that come to autopsy even years after the onset and "resolution" of clini-

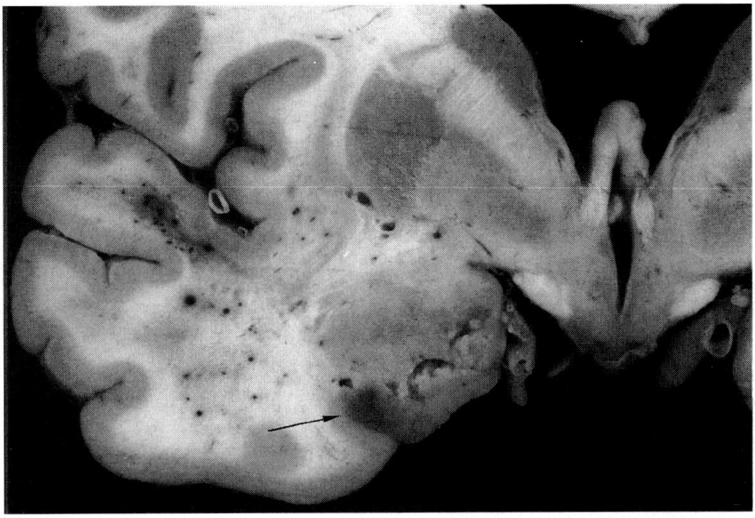

(B)

cal disease, when only extensive tissue destruction with astrogliosis and scant inflammation may remain as histologic markers of the original infection.

HSVE can also occur in newborn infants, among whom approx. four-fifths of cases are secondary to infection by HSV-2, which establishes latent infection in the sacral dorsal roots rather than trigeminal ganglia (usually as a consequence of maternal genital herpes). The infection can be acquired in utero, at the time of delivery, or shortly after birth. Microscopic neuropathologic features are as for HSVE in adults; the distribution of lesions is, however, far more widespread throughout the cerebral hemispheres. Both HSV-1 and HSV-2 can also produce a necrotizing myelitis, which is extraordinarily rare.

Varicella zoster virus (VZV), the causal virus for chickenpox, can subsequently establish latency in the dorsal root ganglia or trigeminal ganglia and periodically emerge on the skin to produce "shingles." Other complications of VZV infection include meningoencephalitis, a (usually self-limited) cerebellitis, and vasculopathy secondary to viral infection of cells of arterial walls, leading to thrombosis with resultant devastating stroke. Manifestations of CNS VZV infection in the immunocompromised host will be discussed in connection with AIDS (see below). The other major human herpesviruses (especially cytomegalovirus/CMV and Epstein-Barr virus/EBV) are of major significance as pathogens in immunocompromised patients, where their neuropathologic features will be more appropriately considered. Indeed, severe widespread CMV and

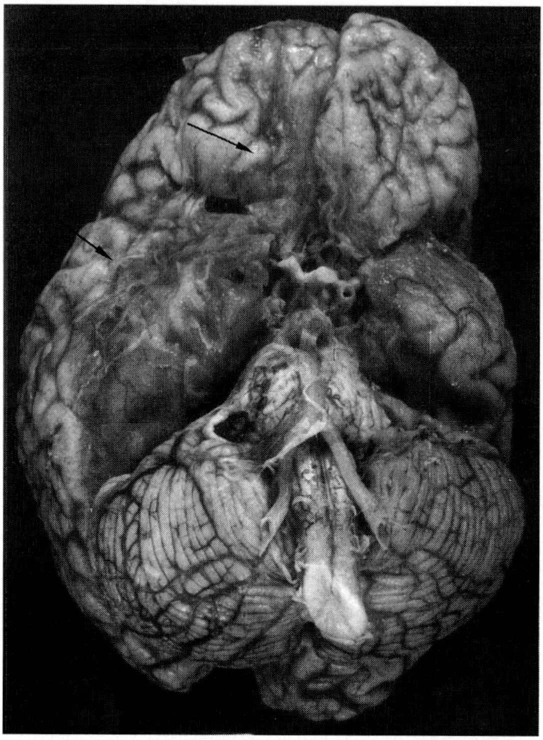

Figure 14 "Chronic" HSVE in a patient who survived for many months after symptom onset. Note asymmetric regions of cystic encephalomalacia involving both temporal lobes (involvement on the right [lower arrow] more severe than on the left) and the right mesial orbital frontal cortex (upper arrow).

VZV encephalitis are, in the 1990s, encountered almost exclusively in this unique and growing patient population. However, EBV infection of the brain has been known to mimic adult HSVE, and CMV infection is associated with Guillain-Barré syndrome or ascending polyradiculoneuropathy (see Chap. 10). Neuropathologic features of infection with human herpesvirus 6 (HHV-6) are not well characterized.

B. Arbovirus Infection

Arboviruses are small ARthropod-BOrne (hence their name) RNA viruses (size range 50 to 120 nm) that are encountered infrequently by most pathologists. They are subdivided into several families (e.g., Togaviridae, Bunyaviridae, Reo-

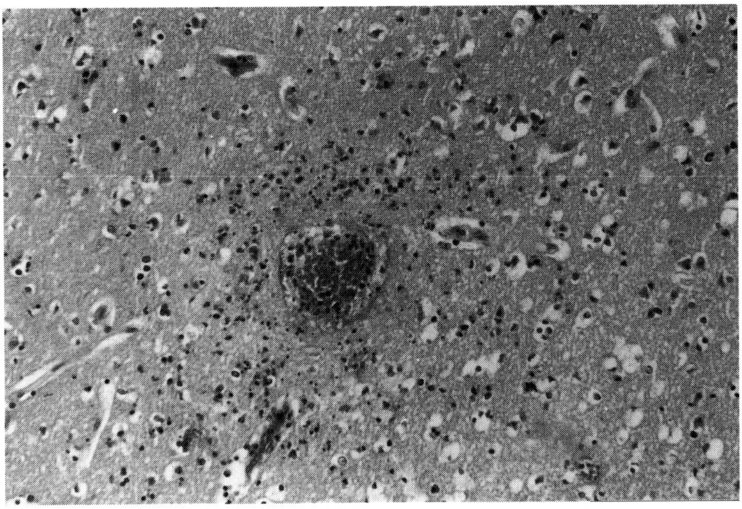

(A)

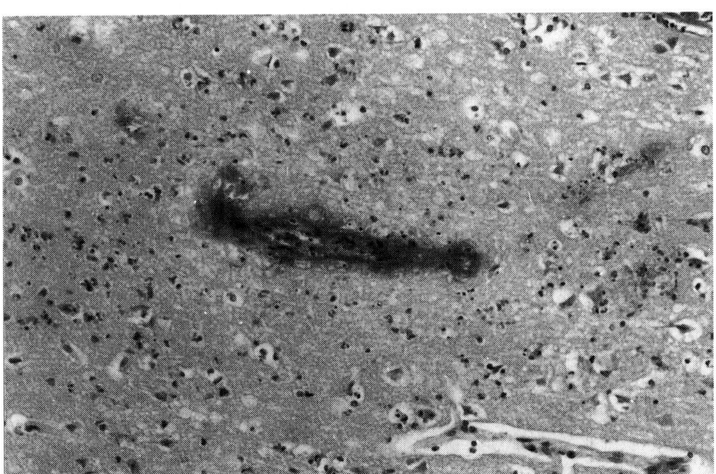

(B)

Figure 15 Herpes simplex encephalitis (subacute) in an adult. The diagnosis was clinically unsuspected until the time of autopsy. (A) Region of acute necrosis centered on a small blood vessel. Note a corona of inflammatory cells surrounding this vessel. (B) Vessel that has undergone fibrinoid necrosis, also surrounded by fragmented inflammatory cells.

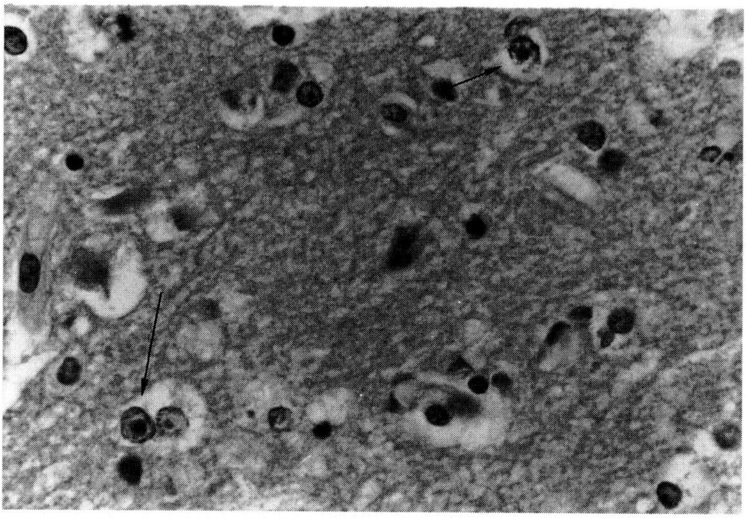

(A)

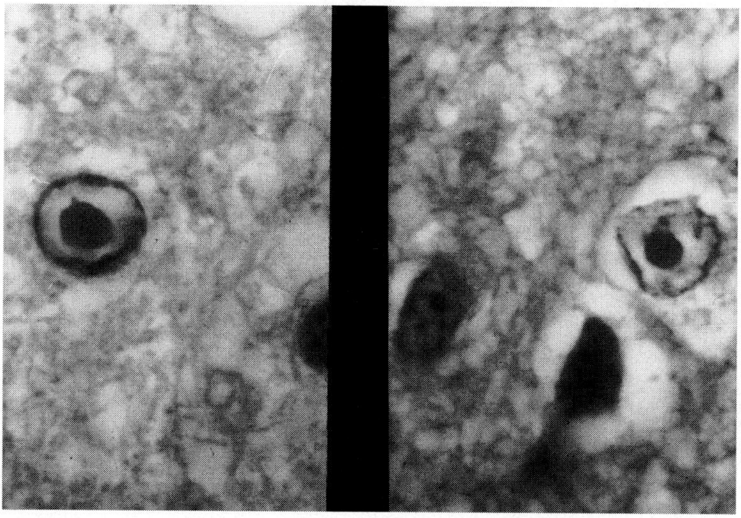

(B)

Figure 16 Intranuclear (Cowdry A) inclusions typical of HSVE. (A) At intermediate magnification, vacuolated neurons are present and scattered cells (arrows) show typical intranuclear inclusions. Note relative paucity of inflammation in this region. (B) Two typical inclusions shown at high magnification, the one on the right adjacent to a pyknotic neuronal cell body. Phenotype of the infected cells is, as in this case, often not apparent.

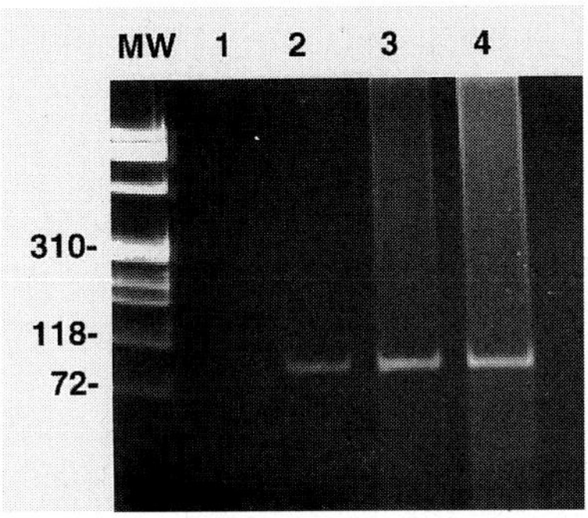

Figure 17 PCR used to demonstrate HSV genome in DNA extracted from a case of HSVE. PCR was carried out on DNA from autopsy brain. Figure shows a gel on which PCR products have been electrophoresed, stained with ethidium bromide and photographed under UV light. Bands on this gel (lanes 3 and 4) represent presence (within brain samples) of the "target" DNA. Molecular weight standards (BP) are in the far left lane, and negative and positive controls are shown, respectively, in lanes 1 and 2. Similar studies can be done to verify presence of VZV, CMV, or EBV DNA in tissue samples. Caution must be exercised in interpreting the results of such studies, since small amounts of viral genes may also be present in "bystander" cells that have little to do with the tissue alterations or even (rarely) in entirely normal brain tissue. In this case, presence of characteristic distribution of tissue changes with positive PCR results supports the diagnosis of HSVE.

viridae); representative examples from each family cause human disease, including encephalitis. Arboviruses are capable of replication in both vertebrate and invertebrate hosts. The vector by which infection is transmitted to humans is the mosquito or tick. Most arboviruses are found predominantly in certain regions of the world, which is sometimes implicit in their name—e.g., Far Eastern and Central European tickborne complex in those regions; Venezuelan equine encephalitis virus in South and Central America, Florida, and the southwestern U.S.; St. Louis encephalitis widely distributed throughout the Americas. There is marked seasonal variation in the numbers of cases encountered; considering the vectors, summer and early fall are times during which most infections are found. Outbreaks of some arbovirus infections occur in cycles; e.g., St. Louis encephalitis epidemics are seen about every 10 years. Japanese encephalitis may occur in as many as 10,000 to 20,000 patients annually in the Far East. Some arboviruses favor patients in a characteristic age range; e.g., western equine encephalitis virus usually infects infants.

Disease-causing virus is "injected" by the bite of a tick or mosquito, with primary viremia which causes a febrile illness and ends with a macrophage response and antibody production. Secondary viremia occurs with viral replication remote from the primary inoculation site. Though systemic infection does not always lead to involvement of the brain and/or spinal cord, CNS infection may occur following passage of virus into the cerebral capillary endothelium, or by direct (olfactory) spread to the brain. Arboviruses vary markedly in their neuroinvasiveness and neurovirulence; e.g., eastern equine encephalitis virus is more "neurovirulent" than its western counterpart. The full range of CNS cell types infected by arboviruses is not well characterized.

Clinical features are relatively nonspecific though they may be devastating. Typical features include disorientation, altered level of consciousness sometimes leading to coma, headache, seizures, and paralysis. Some arboviruses may produce only an aseptic meningitis. Residual morbidity and mortality are variable among the specific viruses—e.g., they are high for eastern equine encephalitis, relatively low for western equine encephalitis. The diagnosis is established by serology and virus isolation from the CSF, which usually shows a lymphocytosis (50 to 500/mm^3) and slightly elevated protein level. Molecular diagnostics (e.g., using reverse transcriptase PCR) are being developed.

Neuropathologic features, on both gross and microscopic inspection of the brain, are characteristic but nonspecific. Vascular congestion with punctate/petechial hemorrhages and cerebral edema may be present. Histologic sections show perivascular cuffing by mononuclear inflammatory cells (especially lymphocytes), microglial nodules and neuronophagia, or microfoci of necrosis (Fig. 18). Larger regions of necrosis may be present, sometimes around thrombosed microvessels. No typical viral inclusions are helpful in establishing a specific etiologic diagnosis, though culture of (e.g., biopsy-derived) brain tissue and electron microscopy may be diagnostic. The corollary of this is that, when a nonspecific encephalitis is encountered at brain biopsy or autopsy, inclusions are absent, and immunohistochemistry and probe studies (e.g., for herpesviruses) are negative, arbovirus encephalitis should be suspected.

C. Enterovirus Infection

Some members of this group of small RNA viruses (e.g., Coxsackievirus A and B) are responsible for lymphocytic/aseptic meningitis. The most feared member of this family, poliovirus and the disease it causes, poliomyelitis, are now, thanks to the prophylactic Salk and Sabin vaccines introduced in midcentury, encountered by clinicians only rarely, and then usually in groups who have refused or not had access to vaccination. Clinical features include nonspecific "flulike" symptoms during primary viremia, within a week of primary infection. Coxsackievirus also commonly produces a severe myocarditis, sometimes in conjunction with encephalomyelitis. A small percentage of affected patients develop CNS manifestations in the course of secondary viremia. These include paralysis referable to affected regions of the spinal cord and brainstem.

Neuropathologic (microscopic) abnormalities include acute and chronic inflammation (with typical viral encephalitic features). The defining hallmark of polioencephalomyelitis is loss of infected anterior horn cells or motor neurons within the pons, medulla, and deep cerebellar nuclei, which early in the disease may show neuronophagia with prominent surrounding microglia and macrophages. No typical viral inclusions are found within surviving neurons or other neuroectodermal elements. In a patient who comes to autopsy years after the acute illness, as one might expect, neuropathologic features resemble those of MND/ALS (see Chap. 8), though without corticospinal tract degeneration.

D. Rabies Virus Infection

This biologically fascinating and deadly viral CNS infection is one rarely encountered by Western neuropathologists; it is more common in third-world nations. Only one or two human cases are identified in the U.S. annually, a significant decline from the 50+ cases per year seen prior to 1940. The etiologic agent is a rod-shaped, RNA-containing rhabdovirus with dimensions of approx. 75×180 nm. Its envelope contains a glycoprotein (essential for pathogenicity) and a matrix protein. Initial infection (usually from the bite of an infected animal—e.g. bat, dog, or cat—though most cases in the U.S. occur without a history of such exposure) is of the bitten muscle, where the virus replicates and subsequently moves into the nervous system through muscle spindles or neuromuscular junctions. From these loci, rabies virus makes use of axonal transport mechanisms to reach the CNS, resulting in clinically apparent CNS abnormalities that may set in as long as 3 months after initial virus exposure. Clinical manifestations include a flulike illness with pain or paresthesiae referable to the initial site of inoculation. Later, patients become apprehensive, anxious, irritable, and depressed and eventually become encephalopathic prior to lapsing into coma. These undesirable and almost invariably fatal consequences of rabies virus infection can be prevented in an exposed patient by thorough cleansing of the wound site, postexposure vaccination, and administration of a hyperimmune globulin.

Neuropathologic features include perivascular cuffing by lymphocytes and typical microglial nodules, which in this disorder are named Babes nodules (though they possess no unique identifying markers) and are found in all parts of the CNS, though disease seems to begin in the diencephalon, hippocampus, and brainstem. A less common paralytic variant of the illness mimics polioencephalomyelitis, both clinically and pathologically. Two types of neuronal inclusions occur:

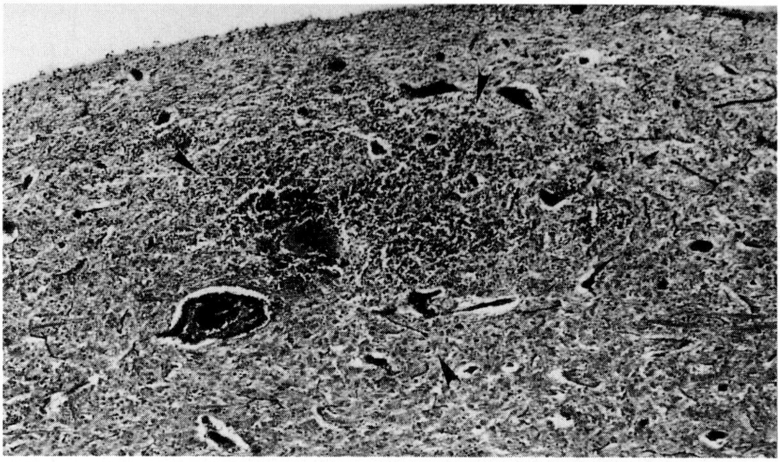

(A)

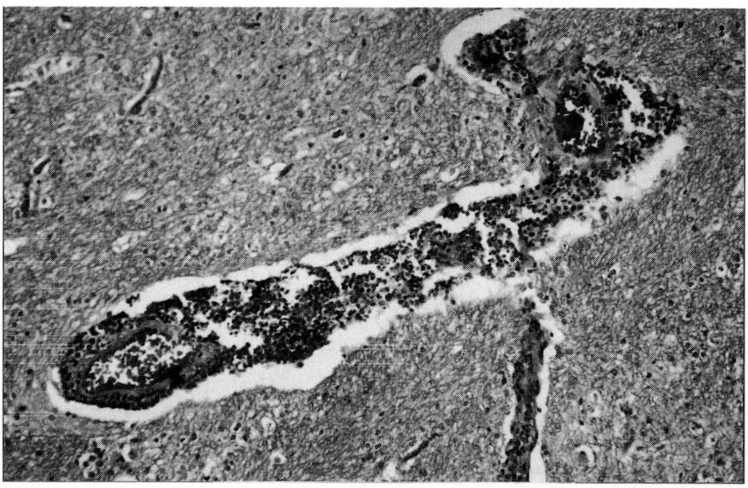

(B)

Figure 18 Arbovirus encephalitis. (A) Venezuelan equine encephalitis. Note a region of hemorrhagic necrosis (arrows) centered on clusters of acute and chronic inflammatory cells. (B) Eastern equine encephalitis. Brain tissue shows only prominent perivascular lymphocytic cuffing. In neither case are cytoplasmic/nuclear inclusions identified. Precise etiologic diagnosis rests on culture/ultrastructural/molecular identification of the viral pathogen. (Tissue studied, courtesy of Dr. R. V. Jones and Bruce H. Williams, Armed Forces Institute of Pathology, Washington, D.C.)

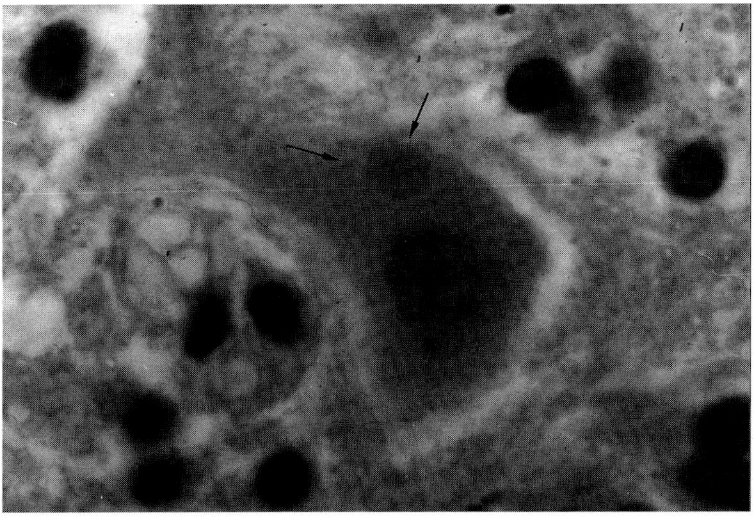

Figure 19 Negri body in Purkinje cell cytoplasm of a patient who died of rabies encephalitis. Note its well-defined hyaline appearance (arrows); Negri bodies are eosinophilic and are to be distinguished from lyssa bodies, which are also intracytoplasmic but less consistently round/oval in shape.

1. Negri bodies, well-defined, round eosinophilic cytoplasmic structures (Fig. 19)
2. Lyssa bodies, irregular eosinophilic cytoplasmic inclusions that may be seen in any neuron but tend to be easiest to find in the hippocampal pyramidal cells or Purkinje cells of the cerebellum.

The presence of viral antigen can be demonstrated by immunofluorescence or immunoperoxidase techniques—immunoreactivity is seen within neuronal cytoplasm and dendrites, not just the diagnostic inclusions. Further details pertinent to rabies pathogenesis are to be found in the excellent review of Mrak and Young (1994).

VIII. HUMAN IMMUNODEFICIENCY VIRUS AND RELATED RETROVIRUSES

Human immunodeficiency virus type 1 (HIV) is a retrovirus first recognized as the cause of the pandemic of acquired immunodeficiency syndrome (AIDS) in the early 1980s. By the early 1990s over 11 million people worldwide were known to be infected with HIV, of whom 10% to 15% had AIDS. By the year 1996, over 6 million deaths worldwide had been attributed to AIDS. In some geographic zones (e.g., urban areas of California), AIDS is the leading cause of death among men aged 25 to 44 years. AIDS is a clinical syndrome associated with HIV-1 infection. The Centers for Disease Control (CDC) definition of AIDS patients (since January 1993) has been the following:

All HIV-infected persons with CD4+ T-lymphocyte counts of less than 200 cells/μl OR a CD4+ percentage of less than 14%. Patients MUST ALSO HAVE one of 23 specific (AIDS-associated or defining) illnesses, e.g. cryptosporidiosis, Kaposi sarcoma, various fungal/viral infections [other than HIV itself], HIV encephalopathy/dementia, wasting syndrome or pulmonary tuberculosis, recurrent pneumonia, or invasive cervical cancer.

Transmission of HIV occurs by vaginal/anal intercourse (three-fourths of cases), intravenous drug injection, transmission from an infected mother to her child (5% to 10% of cases each), or blood transfusion (at most, 3% to 5% and declining, as careful surveillance of blood supplies for HIV is now widely practiced). Infection by the agent is detected using serology or PCR assay of the blood. Factors that determine progression from "simple" HIV infection to the syndrome of AIDS are under investigation, and the time interval between the two events may be measured in years. Once a patient is infected by this retrovirus, clearance from the bloodstream does not occur except perhaps in very rare circumstances, though combination therapy that includes protease inhibitors can substantially reduce viral burden in the blood; whether it also has this effect on neural tissue remains to be seen. Neurologic disease in HIV-infected patients occurs as a complication of:

1. Direct HIV infection of the CNS.
2. Opportunistic infections (OIs) and neoplasms (lymphoma) that result from HIV-related immunosuppression.
3. Miscellaneous abnormalities including "stroke," some of which probably relate to systemic factors that include wasting/cachexia, hypoxia, and metabolic derangements.

A. HIV Infection of the Central Nervous System

Syndromes that result from this unfortunate occurrence have received many names, including AIDS dementia complex (ADC), HIV-related cognitive-motor deficit, subacute AIDS encephalitis or HIV encephalitis (HIVE), and AIDS/HIV-related encephalopathy. The reported frequency of the disorder varies among centers in part because its various descriptors reflect some confusion as to the nature of the nosologic entity itself. Some patients who are thought to have HIV/AIDS encephalopathy during life are found to have OI(s) or CNS lymphoma at necropsy.

Nevertheless, dementia caused by HIV in the brain can be the presenting or dominant feature of HIV infection in a given patient. This appears to result, in some cases, from neurotropic strains of HIV, though these are not *neurono*-tropic variants of virus but rather ones that infect mainly (perhaps exclusively) microglia and macrophages within brain. Infected cells can in turn produce immunomodulatory and/or neurotoxic molecules, among which are included cytokines, nitric oxide, superoxide anion, and quinolinic acid; some of these may be mediators of the associated neuropathologic change (see below).

Clinically, AIDS/HIV encephalopathy patients present with a dementing illness that shows prominent features of *sub*cortical degeneration. Early in the AIDS epidemic, neuropathologic investigations focused on leukoencephalopathy as a cause of neurologic deterioration; more recent studies emphasize neocortical abnormalities of dendrites and synapses. There continues to be ongoing debate as to whether AIDS/HIV encephalopathy/dementia is a function of viral burden within the brain as opposed to a deleterious "amplification effect" resulting from a circumscribed population of infected cells (i.e., microglia/macrophages) secreting cytokines, neurotoxins, etc. Infants and children with AIDS show HIV infection of the CNS as a cause of neurologic deterioration or (more accurately) progressive encephalopathy much more commonly than OIs and lymphoma as a proportion of all infected patients than in the comparable adult population.

In adults, HIV infection of the CNS may also lead to spinal cord lesions, specifically *vacuolar myelopathy* of AIDS. This presents clinically with spastic paraparesis, incontinence, and ataxia and shows neuropathologic features essentially identical to those found in subacute combined degeneration of the spinal cord noted in individuals with vitamin B_{12} deficiency—i.e., vacuolar change in the dorsal columns (especially of the thoracic region) and lateral corticospinal tracts (Fig. 20).

Neuropathologic features of AIDS/HIV encephalopathy include variable (from minimal to severe) abnormalities on gross inspection: the brain may appear normal or show diffuse atrophy with ventriculomegaly together with an impression of pallor or gray discoloration of the central white matter. Microscopic features include widespread low-grade inflammation with microglial nodules and perivascular lymphocytic cuffing (Fig. 21), and leukoencephalopathy manifest as patchy demyelination and astrocytic gliosis—to be distinguished from well-defined white matter lesions of MS (which occur rarely in AIDS) and severely demyelinated, often necrotic lesions of progressive multifocal leukoencephalopathy (PML; see below). The defining feature of HIV infection of brain, however, is the presence—usually in a pericapillary distribution, and especially prominent within subcortical white matter and deep gray matter—of multinucleated cells with either scant or abundant cytoplasm

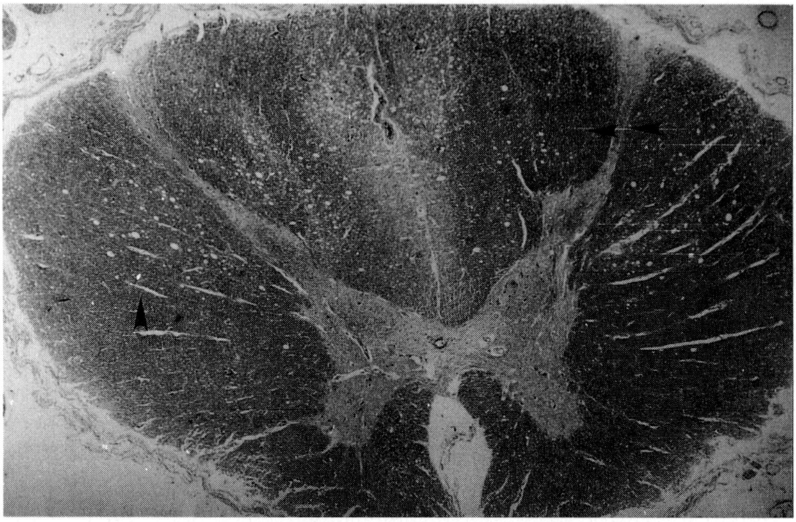

(A)

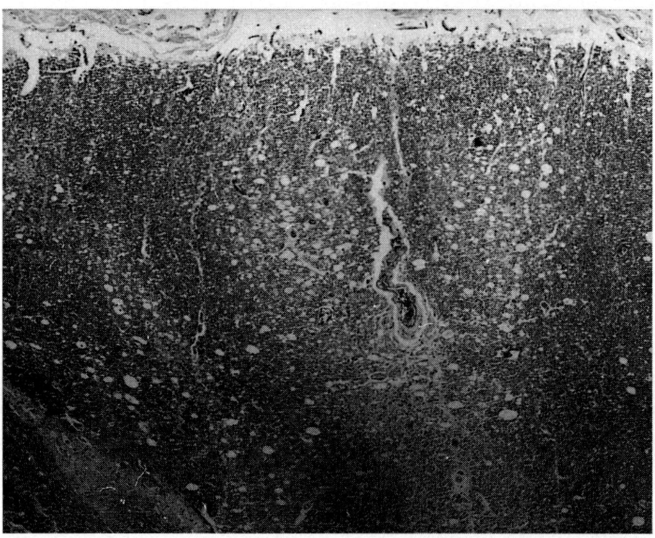

(B)

Figure 20 Vacuolar myelopathy of AIDS (VMA). (A) Thoracic spinal cord (stained with a technique to highlight myelin) shows vacuolar change most prominently within dorsal columns (especially gracile fasciculi, horizontal arrows) and less prominently within lateral corticospinal tracts (vertical arrow). (B) Detail of changes in the dorsal columns.

(Fig. 22). These cells have been further characterized as macrophages and often show immunoreactivity with antibodies to HIV gp41 or p24 antigens. However, even without immunohistochemical supporting evidence, the presence of these cells (sometimes referred to as HIV-type giant cells or HIV-GC) in the appropriate context, and assuming other causes of granulomatous inflammation/giant cell formation have been ruled out, can be used as firm evidence for HIV in the brain. Dendritic and synaptic loss from the neocortex of patients with HIV infection of the CNS have also been demonstrated.

In children with HIV progressive encephalopathy, the degree of cerebral atrophy and inflammation may be more severe than in the adult, and dystrophic calcification is usually a more prominent neuropathologic finding. Rare adults with HIV encephalopathy show predominant involvement of the cortex and deep gray matter, which manifest spongy change, marked astrocytic gliosis, and typical HIV-GC (Fig. 23).

B. Opportunistic Infections (OIs) and Neoplasms

Some of these are considered elsewhere in this chapter (see Sect. IX) and thus will only briefly be discussed here. The profound deficiency in cell-mediated immunity that characterizes AIDS may lead to opportunistic infection by fungi, viruses, atypical bacteria (especially of the acid-fast variety), and parasites. Many of the pathogens are microorganisms which immunocompetent people encounter daily without resultant disease. Primary CNS lymphoma (PCNSL) is by far the commonest neoplasm to occur in HIV-infected patients. For obscure reasons, Kaposi sarcoma (KS) is almost never found in the brain. The differential diagnosis of a mass or space-occupying lesion in the brain of an AIDS patient is an important consideration for the surgical pathologist who is asked to interpret a diagnostic biopsy from such an individual; frequently such biopsies are stereotactic, thus very small. Though mixed lesions may be found, the main considerations in such an instance are toxoplasmosis, PCNSL, fungal infection (especially aspergillosis), tuberculoma, PML, CMV, and KS (in roughly decreasing order of frequency). The possibility of a non-HIV-related lesion (glioma, metastatic cancer) must always be kept in mind. The various groups of OIs and PCNSL will be briefly considered.

1. Fungal Infection

By far the most common opportunistic fungal pathogen to infect the CNS of AIDS patients is *Cryptococcus neoformans*; as many as 5% to 10% of AIDS patients examined at necropsy show evidence of this OI, usually presenting as a meningitis, though solid masses of fungal organisms may be present within brain parenchyma as a "cryptococcoma." This microorganism is an oval or spherical fungus with a thick mucopolysaccharide capsule, of variable diameter (in the range of 2 to 15 μm). Meningitis secondary to cryptococcus often pres-

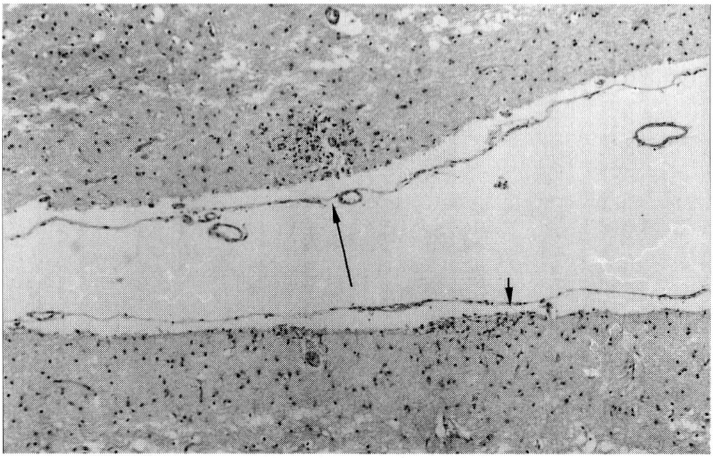

(A)

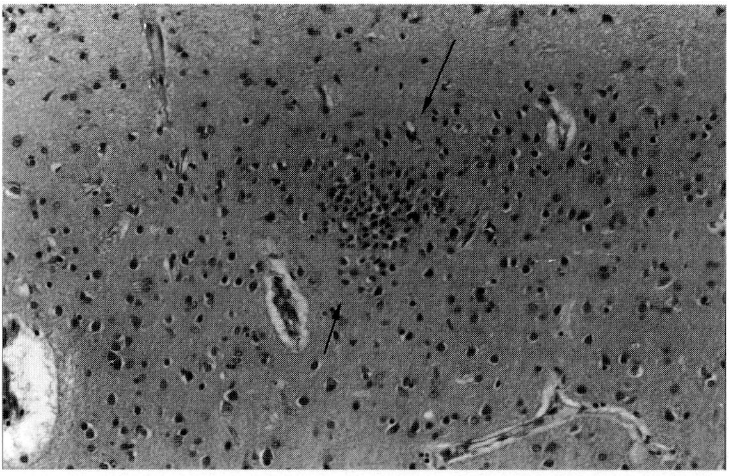

(B)

Figure 21 HIV encephalopathy; microglial nodules. The microglial nodules (MGNs) seen in CNS of a patient with AIDS are morphologically identical to those encountered in the brains of patients with other forms of viral encephalitis. (A) Note two subpial accumulations of microglia, the upper one (arrow) with features of a typical MGN, the lower one (arrowhead) manifest as a barely perceptible increase in cellularity immediately adjacent to the pia. (One of the first strains of HIV to show neurotropism, HIV-JR, was isolated from brain of this patient at autopsy.) (B) MGN (arrows) in otherwise unremarkable neocortex. (C) Magnified view of an MGN in substantia nigra shows uniform appearance of round to oval cells with slight spongy change in the affected neuropil. (D) An extraordinary event is dystrophic calcification of a MGN, as shown in this panel.

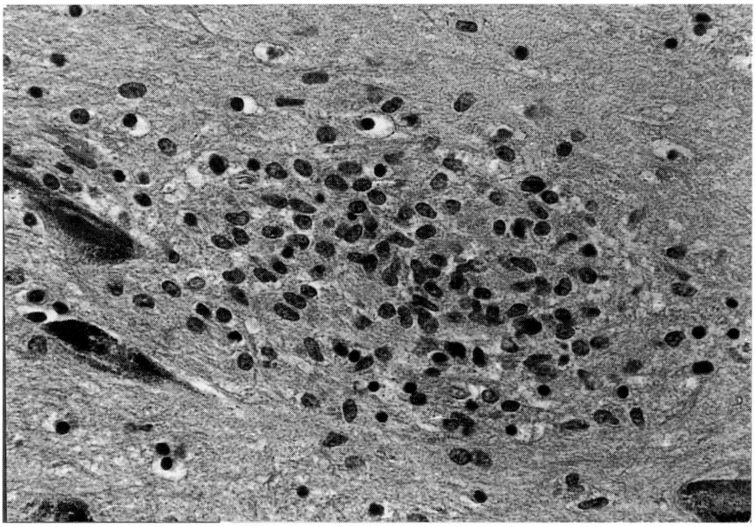

(C)

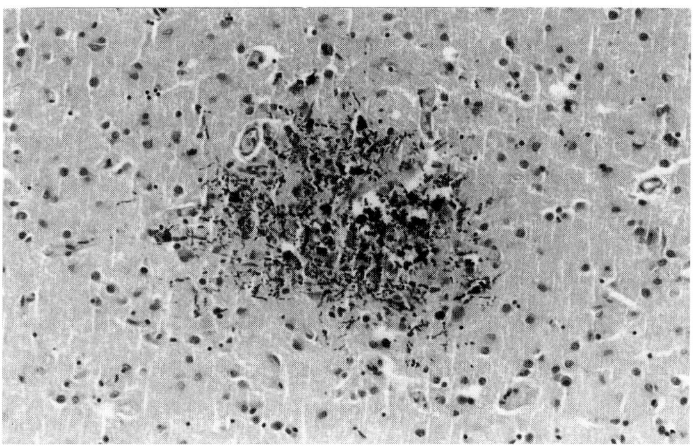

(D)

ents insidiously and is usually associated with a negligible inflammatory response in the meninges (in immunosuppressed patients or those with an intact immune system); hence a lumbar puncture may yield minimal abnormalities apart from presence of the fungal organisms (most easily demonstrated on an India ink preparation) or cryptococcal antigen. Often the CNS is the only organ system affected, though dissemination from pulmonary cryptococcosis may oc-

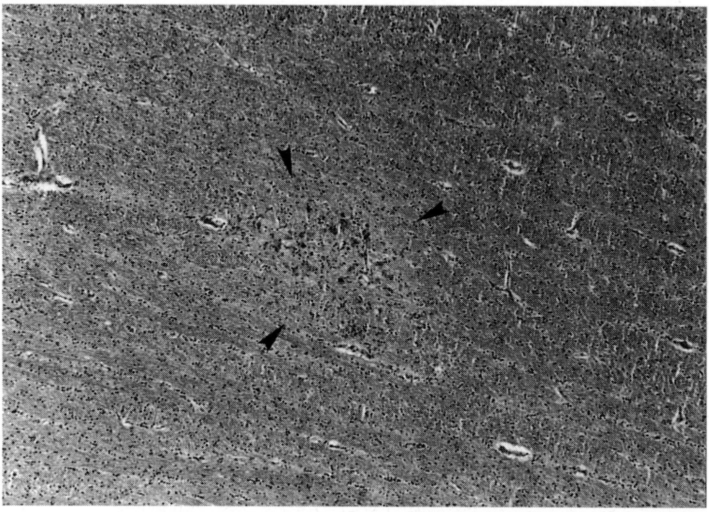

(A)

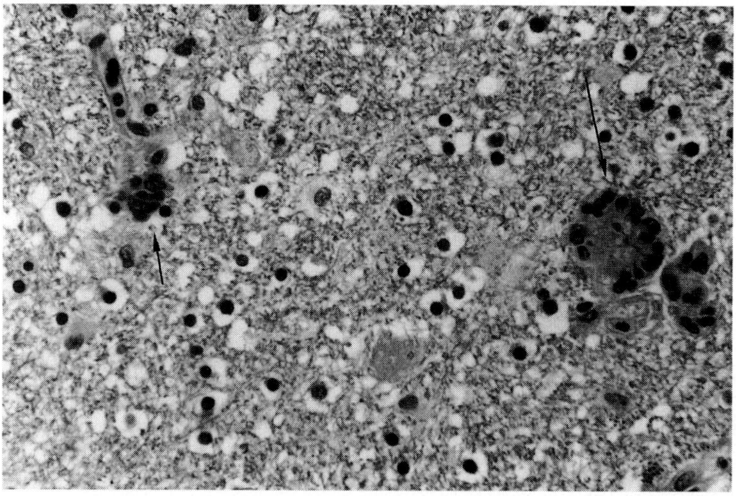

(B)

Figure 22 The varied appearances of HIV-type multinucleated (sometimes giant) cells, HIV-GC, a marker for HIV in the CNS. (A) At low magnification, clusters of HIV-GC may be seen (arrows) in regions of slight rarefaction of the white matter. (B) Two multinucleated cells, one with little cytoplasm (arrow at left), the other with abundant cytoplasm (arrow at right). HIV-GC at left shows proximity to a capillary. Surrounding neuropil shows astrocytic gliosis. (C) HIV-GC (e.g., indicated by arrows). Atypical lymphocytes nearby represent the edge of a cerebral lymphoma. (D) Immunocytochemistry using primary antibodies to HIV-1 proteins p24 or gp41 can be used to confirm presence of HIV antigens (arrow) in brain tissue.

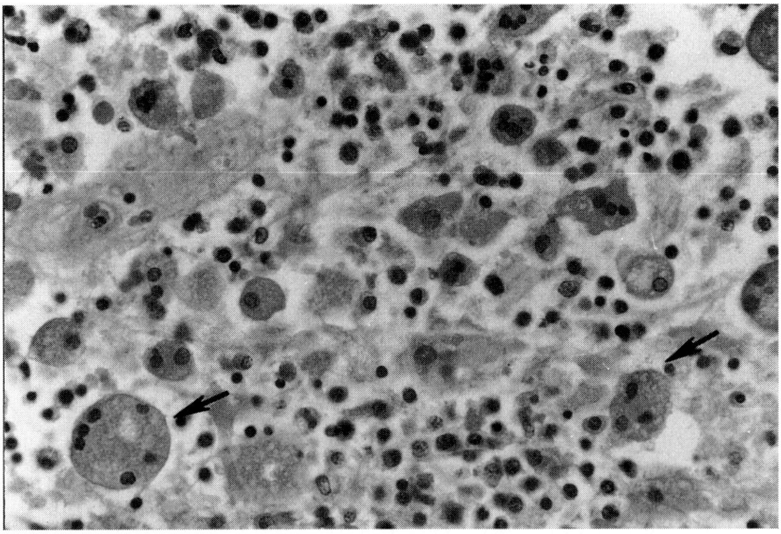

(C)

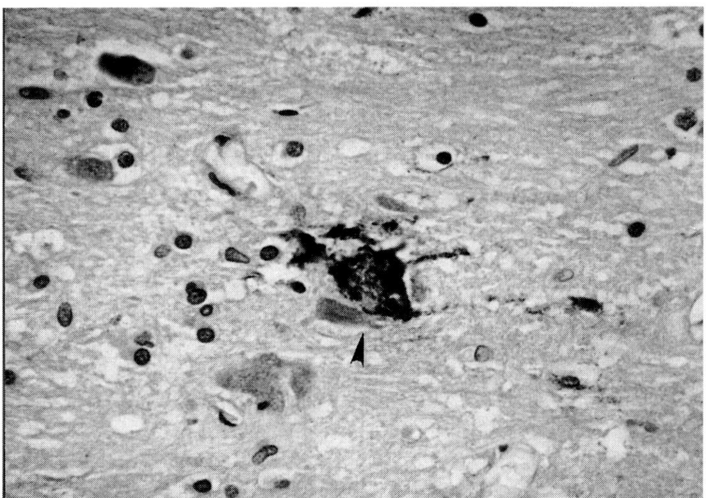

(D)

Figure 23 A very rare manifestation of HIV infection of the brain is a destructive polioencephalopathy, as in this illustration (meninges are at top). Note almost total loss of neurons, with spongiform change. Cellular appearance of the cortex is the result of microglial and astrocyte proliferation. (Case material studied by courtesy of Dr. John Deck, Toronto, Canada).

cur. Rarely AIDS patients show evidence of disseminated cryptococcosis with multiple-organ involvement.

Neuropathologic features of cryptococcal meningitis are strikingly characteristic. Externally, the brain may have a slippery feel and appear glistening, presumably related to the organism's polysaccharide coat; with minimal inflammation, the meninges are generally not opacified. On cut section, gray matter may show a cribriform appearance (Fig. 24) which is the result of a prolifer-

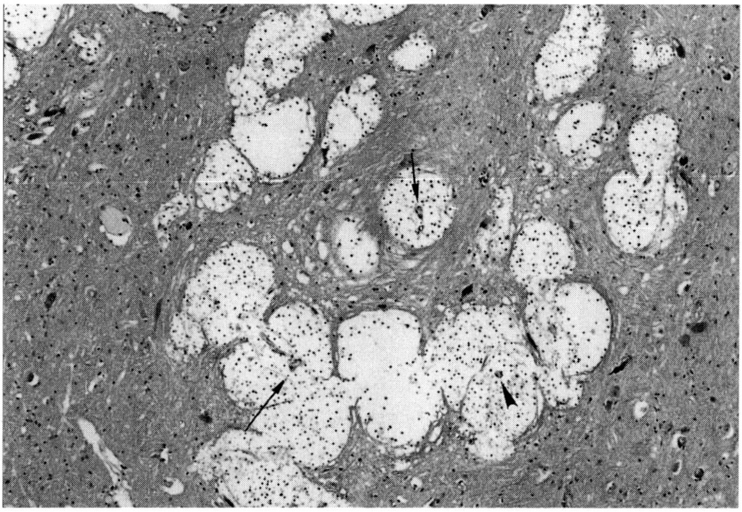

Figure 24 CNS cryptococcosis in AIDS. A cribriform appearance of gray matter often results from distended (perivascular/Virchow-Robin) spaces within which the fungal organisms proliferate. Microvessels can still be recognized at the centers of some of these clusters of microorganisms (e.g., arrows). Inflammatory response in this case is negligible.

ation of fungi in the perivascular/Virchow-Robin spaces with their resultant expansion; gray matter rather than white matter is rendered "cribriform" because of its higher microvascular density. Histologic sections confirm the presence of cryptococci in the subarachnoid and perivascular spaces; though they can be seen on routine stains, fungal organisms are most effectively illustrated using periodic acid-Schiff (PAS) or mucicarmine techniques (Fig. 25). Inflammation may be minimal, in some cases even negligible. A small minority of patients (with AIDS, other forms of immunosuppression, or a normal immune system) develop a brisk granulomatous meningoencephalitis (Fig. 8). Necrotic cryptococcomas occur rarely, in the brain substance.

Virtually any fungal organism may cause cerebral abscess or meningoencephalitis in patients with HIV-1 infection—e.g., (most commonly in the authors' experience) *Candida albicans, Aspergillus* spp. and *Coccidioides immitis* (Fig. 8). CNS involvement in aspergillosis usually occurs with disseminated infection, and because the fungus is angioinvasive and may cause thrombi or the formation of true "mycotic" aneurysms, resultant abscesses are usually markedly necrotic and prominently hemorrhagic (see below).

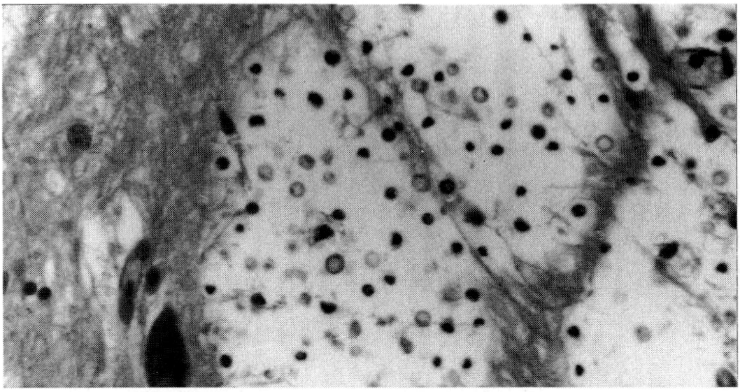

Figure 25 CNS cryptococcosis in AIDS, magnified view. The variably sized fungal organisms are most easily identified using the PAS or mucicarmine technique, which stains their polysaccharide coat. Again, note an abundance of microorganisms but virtual absence of acute/chronic inflammatory cells.

2. *Viral Infection*

While HIV-1 itself shows an affinity for the CNS (though it usually infects microglia/macrophages rather than neuroectodermal cells), immunosuppression—especially the severe compromise of cell-mediated immunity encountered with AIDS—renders the patient susceptible to OI by other viral agents, including both RNA and DNA viruses. The most commonly encountered are the following.

a. Herpesviruses. Of this group, cytomegalovirus (CMV) is the commonest viral OI in AIDS—it is found in the CNS of 15% to 20% of AIDS patients at autopsy. Within brain, spinal cord, retina (Fig. 26), and even the peripheral nervous system, CMV produces extremely heterogeneous neuropathologic manifestations, that include:

1. Low-grade (microglial nodule, MGN) encephalitis which may be indistinguishable from that associated with HIVE unless typical cytomegalic cells with nuclear and cytoplasmic inclusions are present.
2. Severe necrotizing encephalitis, with large regions of cystic encephalomalacia resembling infarcts; very rarely, CMV encephalitis can present as a mass lesion in the CNS.
3. Ventriculoencephalitis, visible grossly as a "line" of hemorrhagic necrosis of brain tissue beneath and immediately adjacent to the ventricular lining, usually of the lateral ventricles; this reflects the propensity of CMV to infect ependymal cells from the CSF and thence to move into brain parenchyma in a "ventriculofugal" fashion.

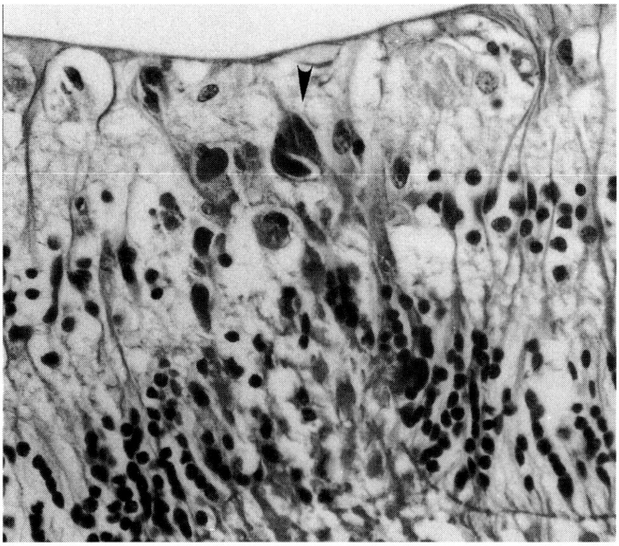

Figure 26 CMV retinitis, one of the most common complications of AIDS. Note typical cytomegalic cell (arrow) with negligible surrounding inflammatory infiltrate.

4. Myelitis and meningoradiculitis with clinical presentation as an ascending polyradiculoneuropathy (Guillain-Barré syndrome), often secondary to CMV-associated vasculopathy with microvascular thrombi in and around spinal cord nerve roots.
5. Rarely, as widespread infection of CNS microvascular endothelial cells or as foci of demyelination; predominantly vascular endothelial infection by CMV is also noted in peripheral nerve and muscle of some patients.

Figures 27 and 28 show various neuropathologic features of CMV infection in AIDS. The defining feature of all neuropathologic conditions associated with CMV infection is the characteristic cytomegalic cell with typical "owl's eye" nuclear and basophilic cytoplasmic inclusions; necrosis and inflammation surrounding these "marker" cells may vary tremendously from case to case.

Herpes/varicella zoster is a much less common OI than CMV in AIDS, and also tends to produce variable neuropathologic manifestations, among which are 1. a leukoencephalitis/leukoencephalopathy that resembles the type of demyelination noted in plaques of MS (see Chap. 5) or the more poorly delineated, sometimes necrotic foci of progressive multifocal leukoencephalopathy (PML; see below); 2. myeloradiculitis extending into peripheral nerves;

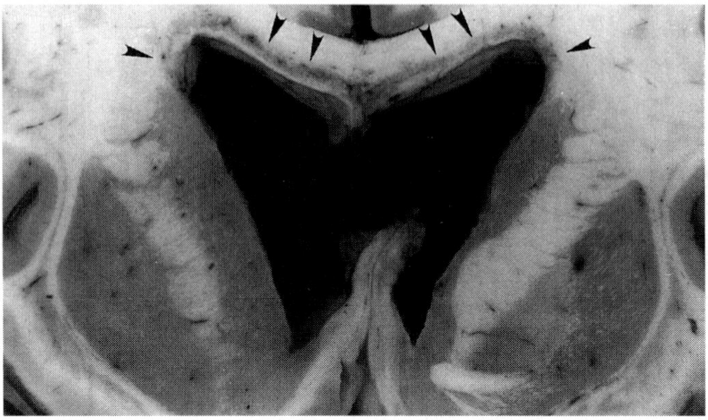

(A)

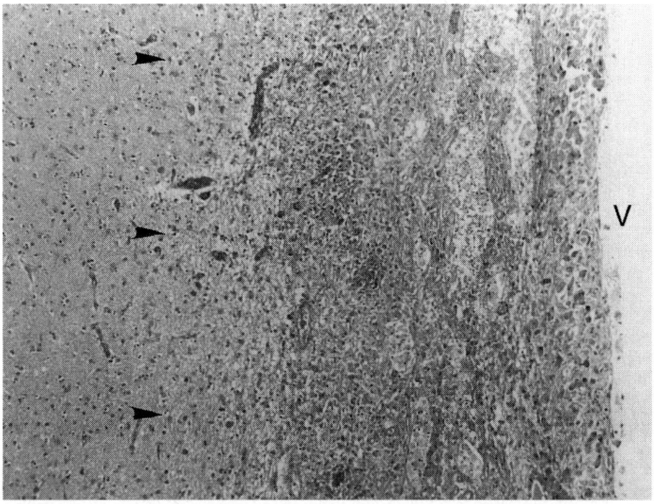

(B)

Figure 27 CMV encephalitis in AIDS. (A) Affinity of CMV for ependyma and subependymal regions (with ventriculofugal spread of virus) is sometimes suggested by gross appearance of the cut brain. In this case, note hemorrhagic necrosis in ependyma and periventricular regions lining the lateral ventricles (arrows). (B) CMV ventriculoencephalitis, low-power view. (Lateral) ventricular cavity is designated by "V" at right of the micrograph. Region bounded approximately by arrowheads and the ventricular cavity represents region of intense inflammation and necrosis largely caused by CMV infection. (C) Magnified view of another region shows numerous cytomegalic cells with typical Cowdry type A intranuclear inclusions. (D) A more subtle example of CMV ependymitis and "subependymitis" showing cytomegalic cells among ependymal lining

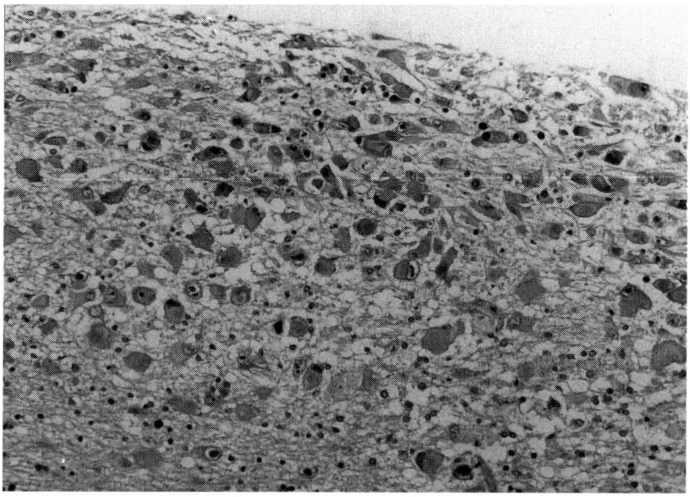

(C)

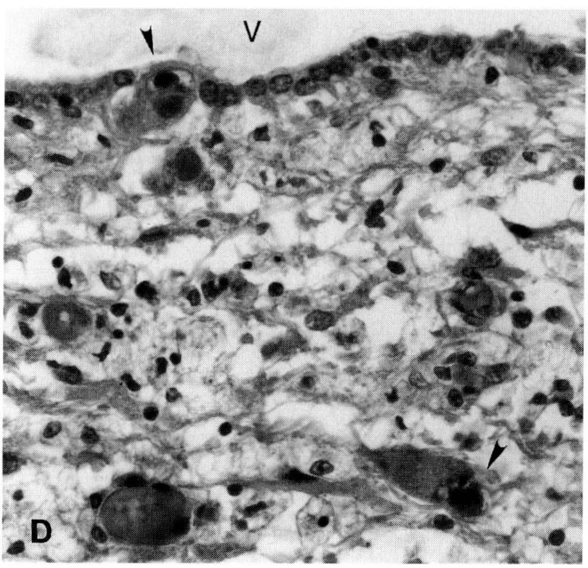

(D)

cells and in the subjacent brain parenchyma (arrows), which manifests edema but relatively little inflammation (ventricular cavity is indicated by "V"). (E) CMV encephalitis is characterized by variable associated tissue damage and inflammation. In this panel, moderate acute and chronic inflammation is noted adjacent to cytomegalic cells,

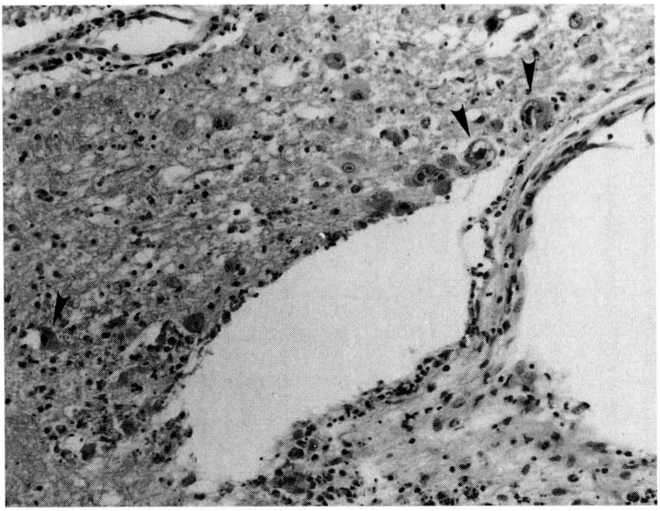

(E)

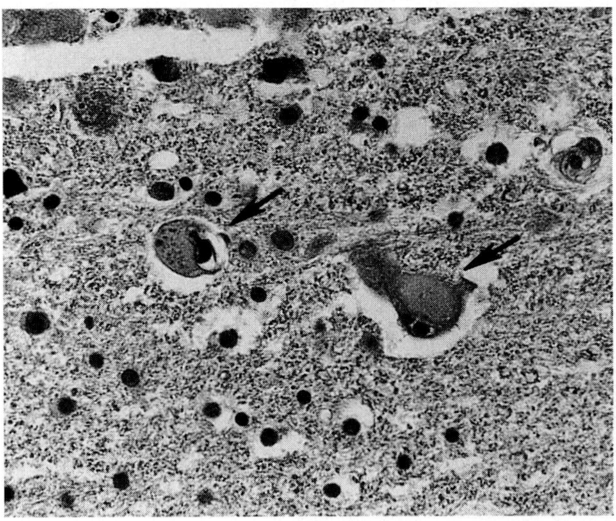

(F)

Figure 27 Continued

(arrows). (F) Frequently, in the brains of AIDS patients, scattered cytomegalic cells are seen in the neuropil (arrows) with negligible surrounding inflammatory reaction or evidence of tissue injury.

3. ventriculitis (Fig. 29); and 4. vasculitis or a noninflammatory vasculopathy.

Herpes simplex may present as a necrotizing viral encephalitis in AIDS. Epstein-Barr virus (EBV) infection has been implicated in the pathogenesis of primary CNS lymphomas, which are very common in AIDS patients (see below). The potential neuropathogenic roles of human herpesvirus 6 (HHV-6) and newly discovered KS-associated herpesviruses remain to be elucidated.

b. Progressive Multifocal Leukoencephalopathy (PML). First described in the late 1950s as a complication of immunosuppression caused by hematologic and lymphoid malignancies and their treatment, this is now most commonly seen in AIDS patients (present in 1% to 4% of brains from individuals with AIDS examined at autopsy) and thus is appropriately considered at this point. PML is a subacute demyelinating disease that affects the CNS of patients who have deficiencies in cell-mediated immunity. Clinical manifestations depend on the focus/foci of white matter lesions, and the disease is usually inexorably progressive though remissions and clinical stabilization are reported, especially among patients (including those with AIDS) who show improvement in their immune status. Coma is common in terminal stages of the illness. MRI and CT scans show typical white matter lesions; PML should be considered in the differential diagnosis of any HIV-infected patient with increased white matter signal intensity on T2-weighted MRI images of the brain. Survival is usually measured in months, especially considering that affected patients are usually critically ill even prior to the development of PML. The causal virus is a double-stranded DNA-containing papovavirus, specifically JC virus (JCV) of the polyoma subgroup. Latent JCV persistence may occur in renal tissues of many immunocompetent individuals, with reactivation of virus occurring during immunosuppression. JCV is then disseminated through the blood, and CNS lesions of PML are frequently (though by no means exclusively) encountered in an angiocentric pattern. It should be considered primarily as a lytic infection of oligodendroglia, though astrocytes are also infected by the causal agent. JCV is known to have interactions with HIV *in vitro*, and it is possible that the destructive lesions of PML cause movement into the brain of HIV-infected monocytes, which may then lead to CNS coinfection by the two agents. The fact that both PML and HIV infection of the CNS can cause white matter abnormalities and a dementia often leads to clinical confusion in attempting to decide which type of brain lesion(s) a given patient has.

Neuropathologic features of PML are characteristic on both cut sections of the fixed brain and histologic specimens. The cut surface of the white matter shows poorly demarcated ("moth-eaten") regions in an asymmetric distribution within the cerebral hemispheres (Fig. 30), brainstem, and cerebellum, a distinguishing feature that sets these lesions apart from the demyelinating plaques of MS (see also Chap. 5). Though PML is primarily a leukoencephalopathy, neo-

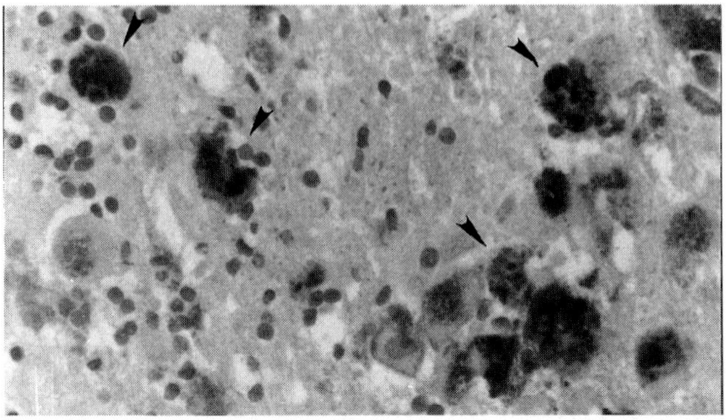

(A)

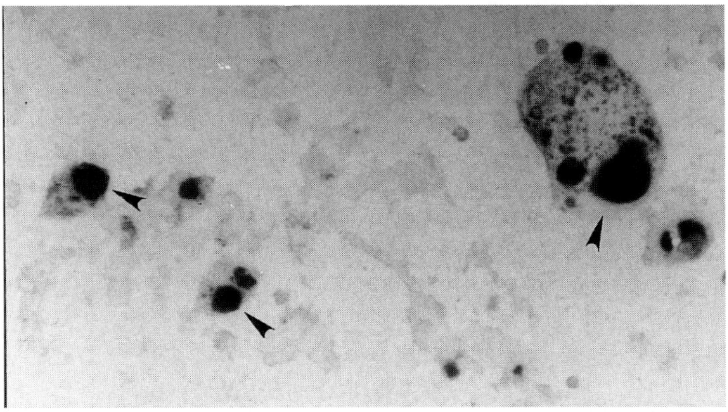

(B)

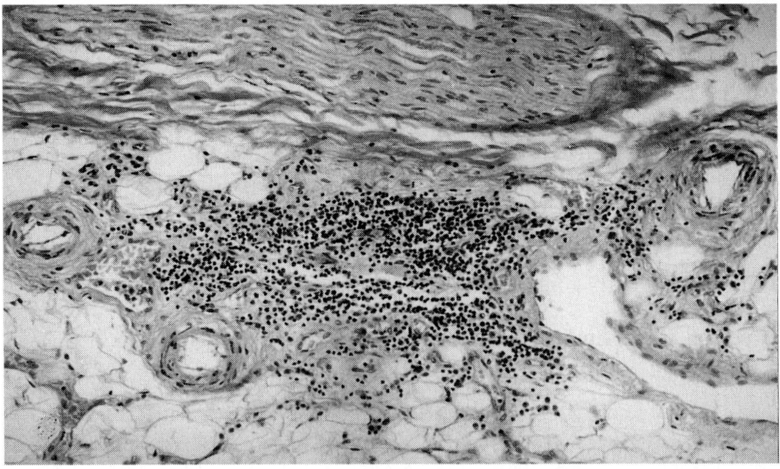

(C)

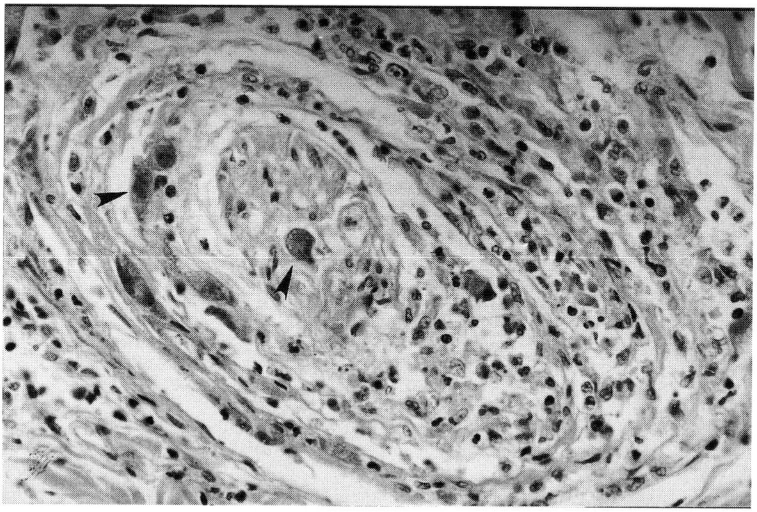

(D)

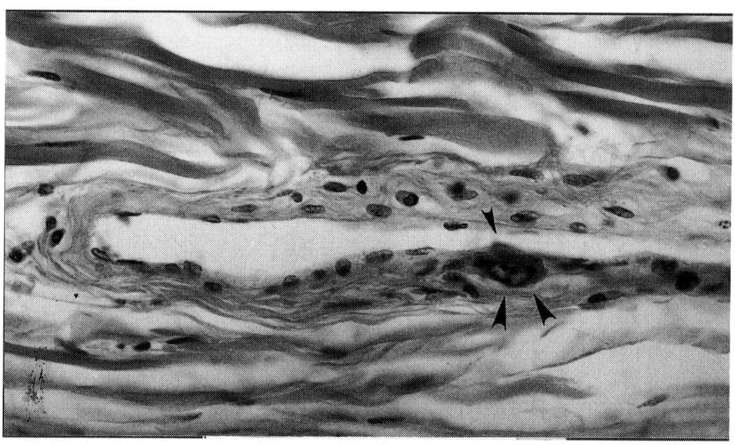

(E)

Figure 28 The presence of CMV within brain can be confirmed using immunohiostochemistry (A) incorporating anti-CMV antibodies and/or in situ hybridization (B) with CMV-specific DNA probes. Immunoreactive and probe-positive cells are indicated in both panels by arrowheads. PCR is a more sensitive technique that can confirm the presence of CMV DNA in tissue but does not localize genes to specific cell types unless the newer method of in situ PCR is utilized. CMV can also involve the peripheral nervous system, as shows in panels C to E. Note patchy peri/epineurial inflammation (C,D) and the presence of scattered cytomegalic cells and CMV inclusions, including some within microvascular endothelial cells (arrows).

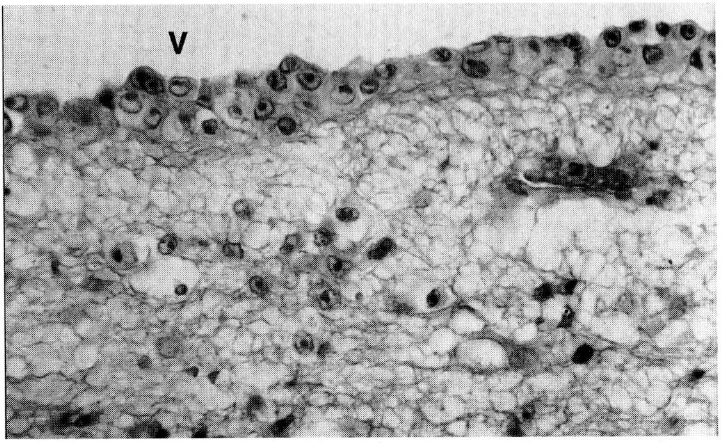

Figure 29 VZV ventriculoencephalitis in AIDS. Like CMV, VZV has an apparent affinity for ependyma. In this micrograph, note prominent Cowdry type A intranuclear inclusions within ependymal and subependymal cells, though the affected cells are *not* cytomegalic. As with CMV infection of neural parenchyma, inflammatory response can be variable and is virtually absent in this case. Tissue shows spongiosis indicative of edema, which may in part have resulted from transudation of CSF secondary to ependymal injury caused by VZV ependymitis. V = ventricular cavity.

cortex may be involved. Unlike with MS plaques, the periventricular and subpial regions are not especially prominently involved.

Histologic sections of PML foci demonstrate demyelination that is (as the gross specimen usually suggests) poorly demarcated. Though it is classified as a central "myelinopathy," PML can often cause (again, unlike MS) tissue necrosis—abundant macrophages may be encountered in regions of PML. The other histopathologic hallmarks are atypical bizarre astrocytes, often with lobulated nuclei and abundant GFAP immunoreactive cytoplasm; and oligodendroglial inclusions that present as amphophilic slightly enlarged glassy nuclei (Fig. 31) with (usually) negligible surrounding cytoplasm; i.e., they are distinctly different than the nuclear inclusions encountered with herpesvirus infections. Viral particles may be shown within oligodendrocyte nuclei or (less commonly) central myelin sheaths by electron microscopy (Fig. 32), and viral genes can be demonstrated by *in situ* hybridization immunohistochemistry (using JCV-specific probes) within the nuclei of both oligodendroglia and astrocytes (Fig. 33). *In situ* studies usually reveal more extensive and abundant viral presence than does routine light microscopy; regions that appear entirely normal by light microscopy may show abundant JCV genes.

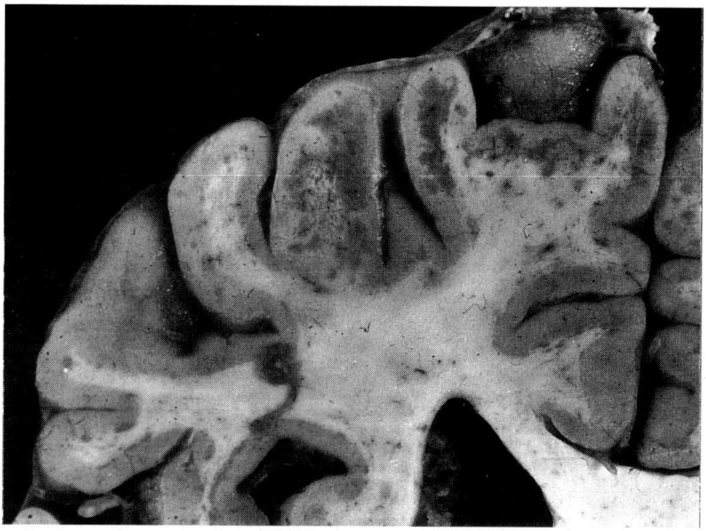

(A)

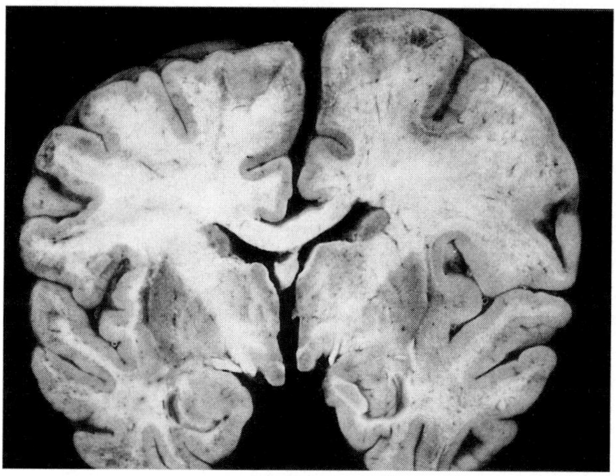

(B)

Figure 30 Progressive multifocal leukoencephalopathy (PML) in AIDS, gross appearance of cut brain. Both panels show multiple foci of grey discoloration of subcortical white matter, better demarcated from intact white matter in panel A than B. In severe PML, white matter may show patchy necrosis. In (A), lesions are present at cortex-white matter junction and extend into overlying cortex.

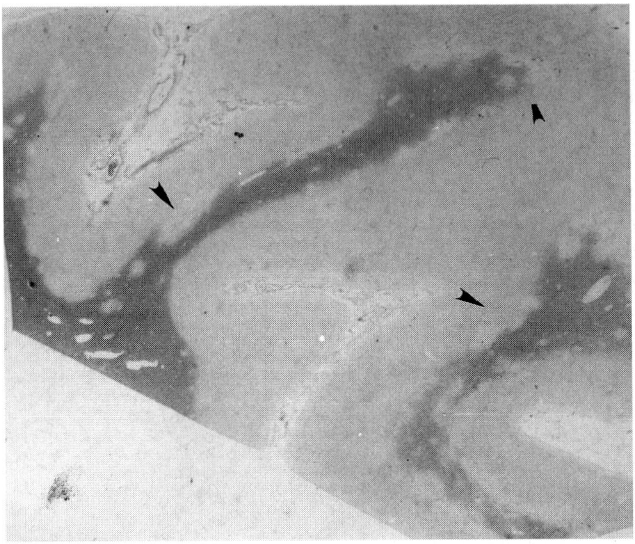

(A)

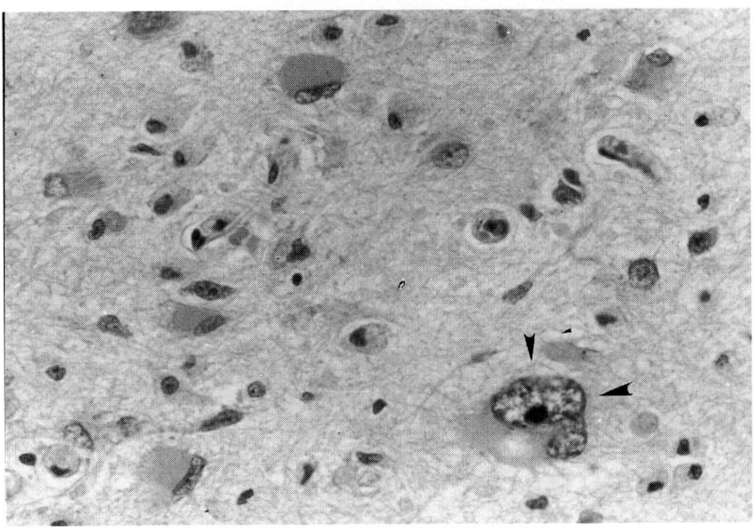

(B)

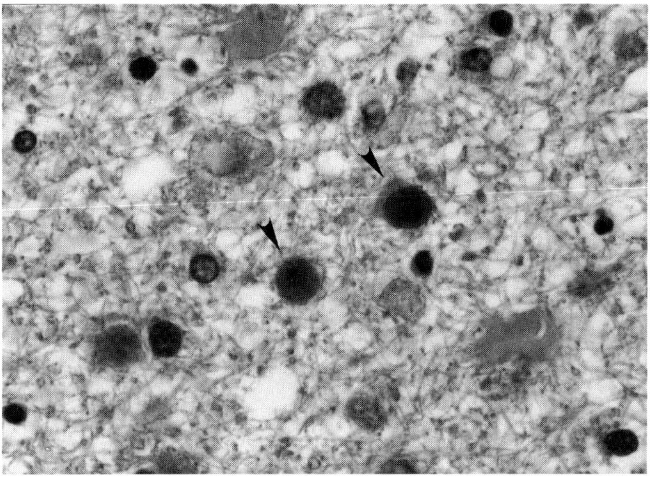

(C)

Figure 31 PML, microscopic features. (A) PML is often best appreciated on a whole mount section, as in this section of cortex and white matter stained with a technique to demonstrate myelin. Note patchy "moth-eaten" appearance to the white matter (e.g., designated by arrowheads), especially at the cortex–white matter junction. Typical microscopic appearances include the presence of atypical, bizarre astrocytes, often with lobulated nuclei (arrows, panel B), and oligodendrogial inclusions (arrows, panel C) characteristic of papovavirus infection. These inclusions differ from Cowdry type A nuclear inclusions typical of herpesvirus infections and SSPE, in that they replace the entire nucleus with amphophilic glassy material. Inclusions tend to be most abundant at the "advancing" edge of a focus of obvious PML.

Other viruses that infrequently cause OI of the brain/spinal cord of AIDS patients include adenovirus and measles virus.

3. Parasitic Infection

By far the commonest parasite to cause OI infection in AIDS, abscesses caused by *Toxoplasma gondii* also represent one of the two major differential diagnoses of a space-occupying lesion of the brain in an HIV-infected individual (the other is primary CNS lymphoma; PCNSL). The causal parasite has a worldwide distribution, with a relatively higher incidence of infection in warmer climates.

T. gondii is an obligate intracellular parasite, the definitive host for which is the cat. The organism is ingested with contaminated food, enters the bloodstream through the gastrointestinal tract, and disseminates to several organs (especially brain, heart, and skeletal muscle), where it establishes persistent latent infection.

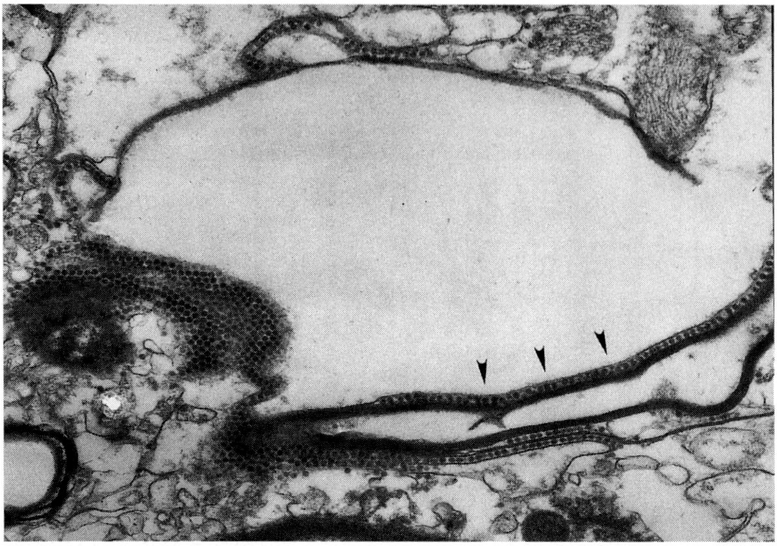

(A)

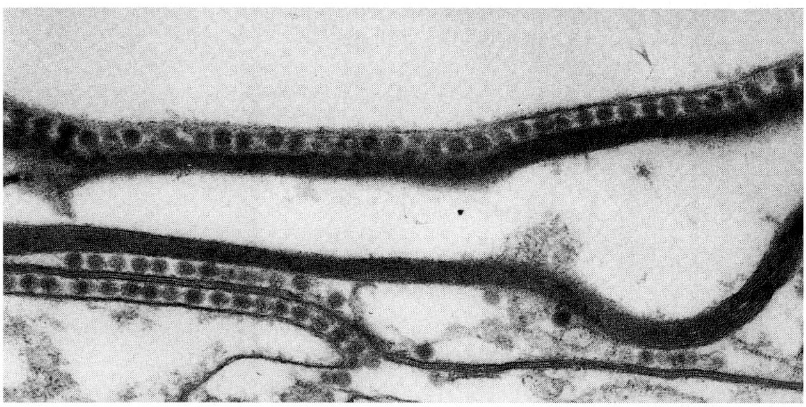

(B)

Figure 32 PML, ultrastructural features. Spherical papovavirus virions are usually detected in oligodendroglial nuclei. Exceptionally, as in this case, they are identified between myelin lamellae, suggesting a direct mechanism for myelin injury in this patient. Region designated by arrowheads in panel A is shown at higher magnification in (B).

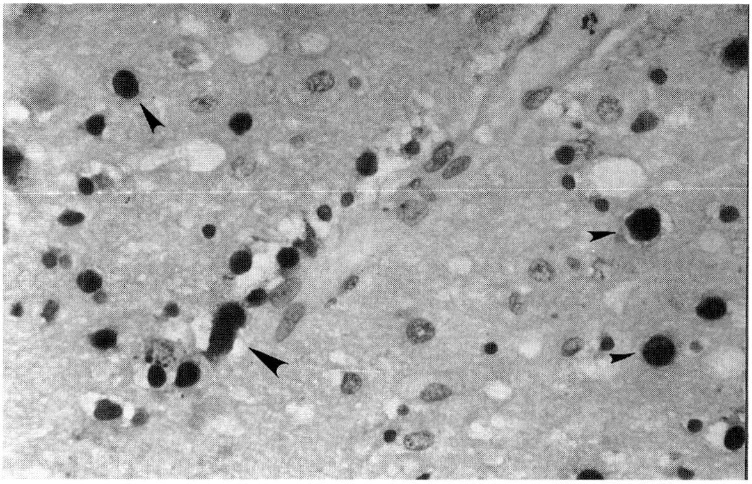

Figure 33 PML—in situ hybridization. DNA probes specific for papovavirus (in this case JC virus) can be linked to a marker (e.g., biotin) that in turn may be used to detect the presence of viral genes in affected tissue sections. Arrowheads indicate some of the many immunoreactive oligodendroglial nuclei.

Normal cell-mediated immunity serves to maintain the parasite in a quiescent or latent state. Toxoplasmosis as an OI in AIDS patients appears to have variable frequency among AIDS patients in different geographic zones; i.e. it is most common among AIDS patients in the southeastern U.S. (e.g., among Haitian and other Caribbean immigrants to Miami) and less common in San Francisco and Los Angeles. CNS toxoplasmosis is encountered in approx. 8% to 15% of AIDS patients examined at necropsy. Among AIDS patients who undergo stereotactic or open brain biopsy to establish definitive diagnosis of a mass lesion, toxoplasmosis has been seen (in our experience) in almost 25% of such patients.

As with many other OIs, the clinical presentation of CNS toxoplasmosis may be extremely variable and relatively nonspecific, though signs and symptoms are usually of subacute onset and rapid progression. Clinical manifestations reflect localization of the abscess(es). Seropositivity for *T. gondii* is not specific in allowing for the diagnosis, and neuroimaging studies of mass lesions show few specific features; i.e., they are usually round/spherical and show ring enhancement with surrounding edema on CT scans, though they can be irregular or hypodense. Neuroimaging studies also tend to underestimate the numbers of lesions eventually discovered at autopsy, though in this regard MRI scans are more sensitive than CT scans. CNS toxoplasmosis in AIDS is a fatal infection unless treated early and aggressively with appropriate antibiotics.

Neuropathologic features include (on cut sections of fixed brain) the presence of large poorly delineated soft pale or hemorrhagic mass lesions with surrounding edema (Fig. 34) usually situated at the cortex–white matter junction or in the deep central gray matter; brainstem and cerebellum may also be involved. Latent CNS toxoplasmosis may produce no gross abnormalities of the brain. Microscopic sections show different features depending on whether infection is inactive/latent or active/acute. In the former situation, intact cysts or bradyzoites are encountered throughout the parenchyma. With active infection, lesions resemble bacterial or fungal abscesses (see above), with a central necrotic zone containing abundant histiocytes and PMNs; an intermediate zone of congestion, vascular proliferation, and a characteristic myofibroblastic hyperplasia affecting the walls (media and adventitia) of medium-size or small blood vessels; and an outer zone of slight inflammation, vascular changes, and scattered microglial nodules. Tachyzoites of *T. gondii* (approx. 2 μm in diameter) are difficult to detect in the central zone of such an abscess and are more easily found (together with encysted organisms) in the intermediate zone. The outer zone is more likely to show encysted parasites (Fig. 35). The clinicopathologic evolution of CNS toxoplasmosis can also be subdivided into necrotizing, organizing, and chronic phases, lasting (respectively) less than a few weeks, weeks to months, and many months.

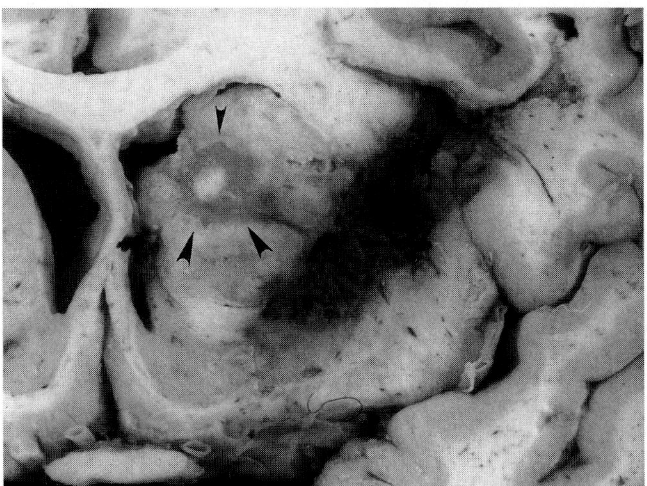

Figure 34 CNS toxoplasmosis in AIDS. Necrotic foci were present throughout the brain, e.g., in the basal ganglia (as indicated by arrowheads). The elongated hemorrhagic region represents a biopsy needle track into which secondary hemorrhage had occurred.

In a brain biopsy from an AIDS patient with suspected toxoplasmosis, the number of encysted organisms or bradyzoites may be small in comparison to the degree of tissue necrosis and inflammation. Great care must be taken to examine multiple sections/levels of the biopsy to find the organisms; this can be facilitated by use of *T. gondii*-specific antibodies in an immunohistochemical procedure.

Other parasites that are much less common as OIs in the CNS of AIDS patients include acanthamoeba, achloric algae (*Prototheca*), trypanosomiasis, and cysticercosis.

4. Bacterial Infection

Symptomatic bacterial meningoencephalitis is a relatively rare complication of HIV infection and AIDS. Infection of the CNS by mycobacteria is, however, infrequently observed, though as a cause of morbidity and mortality it is much less common than the previously described viral, fungal, and parasitic OIs. *Mycobacterium avium-intracellulare* (MAI) infection is most often encountered (on routine H&E-stained sections) as a collection of perivascular foamy histiocytes; the bacteria are, however, easily demonstrated on acid-fast stains of the tissue. The "granulomas" are thus poorly formed collections of histiocytes, lacking multinucleated giant cells and other inflammatory components. Most often, MAI infection of the brain is encountered as an incidental finding at autopsy; rarely, it can produce meningoencephalitis or focal necrosis.

Mycobacterium tuberculosis (MTB) infection, while encountered infrequently in European and North American AIDS patients, is more common among Africans and Haitians with HIV infection. The increasing presence of MTB infection in North America appears to parallel the increasing incidence of AIDS, and drug-resistant strains of MTB have emerged. Neuropathologic manifestations are similar to those of MTB meningoencephalitis seen in non-AIDS patients (see above). In the acute phase, the meningeal exudate may include large numbers of PMNs, thus resembling a purulent/suppurative meningitis, while in the chronic phase typical epithelioid granulomas and Langhans'-type giant cells are seen. Tuberculomas have rarely been seen in AIDS, but of course must be included in the differential diagnosis of mass lesion in an HIV-infected individual.

Neurosyphilis can result from the deficient cell-mediated immunity characteristic of AIDS-indeed, a more virulent and aggressive form of spirochetal infection may result. Presentation has usually been in the secondary or tertiary stages, with myelopathy or meningoencephalitis. Rare examples of gumma, and "quaternary" syphilis with meningovascular disease and treponemal involvement of brain, have been described in HIV-infected patients.

Other bacteria that have occasionally been encountered as etiologic agents responsible for meningoencephalitis or brain abscess in AIDS include

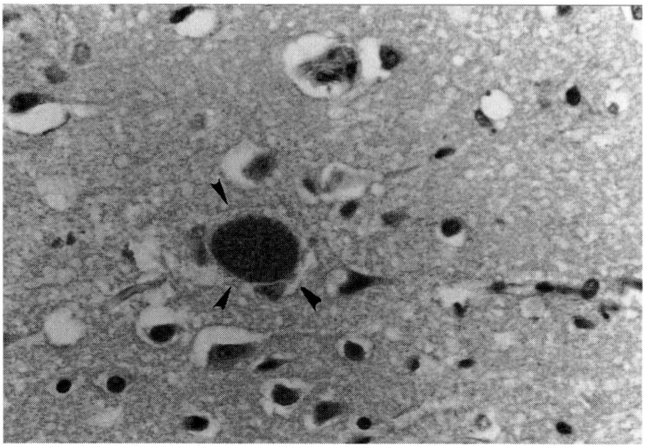

(A)

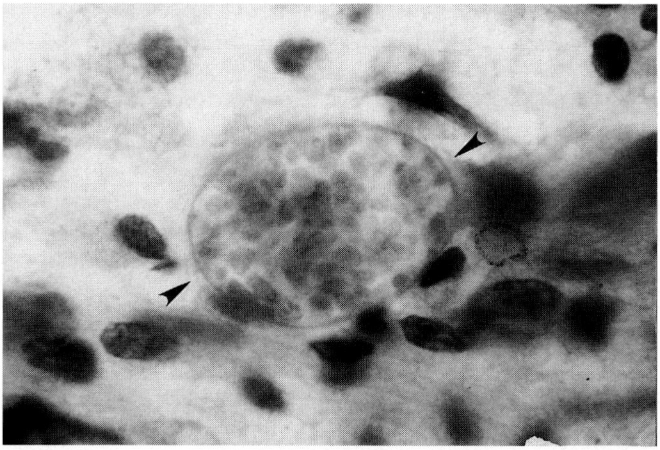

(B)

Figure 35 CNS toxoplasmosis, microscopic and ultrastructural features. (A) Encysted organisms (arrows) are present in otherwise unremarkable cerebral cortex. (B) Magnified view of a *Toxoplasma* cyst (arrows) in an abscess. (C) Edge of an abscess showing extensive necrosis, acute and chronic inflammation. Two vessels (arrows) show a typical adventitial thickening secondary to myofibroblast proliferation, shown at higher magnification in (D). When this vascular change is noted in the brain biopsy of an immunosuppressed patient (especially with AIDS), which also demonstrates necrosis and inflammation, toxoplasmosis must be considered the likely causal agent—even though relatively few bradyzoites may be detectable by routine light microscopy. (E) Typical ultrastructural appearance of encysted bradyzoites. (Electron micrograph courtesy of Dr. Richard Mertens, Cedars Sinai Medical Center, Los Angeles.)

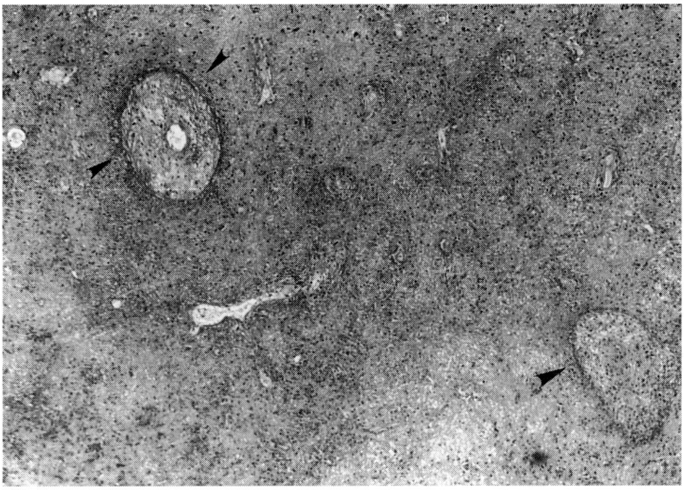

(C)

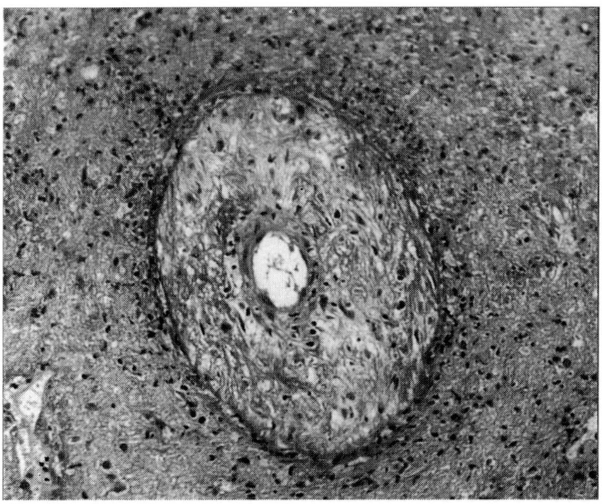

(D)

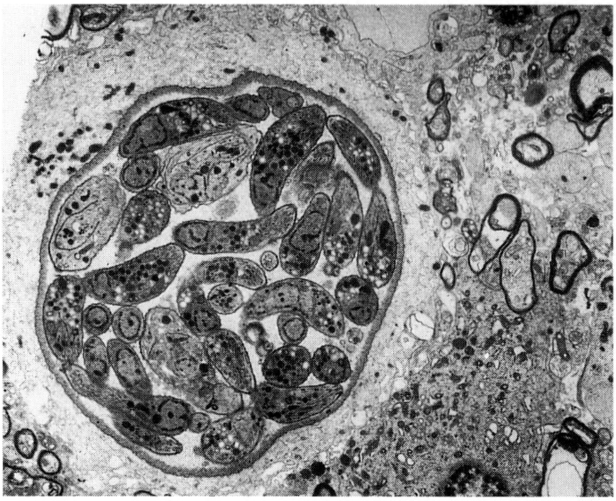

(E)

Figure 35 Continued

Listeria monocytogenes, *Nocardia asteroides*, *Streptococcus pneumoniae*, and *Streptococcus milleri*.

5. *Neoplasms*

Lymphoma is by far the commonest "opportunistic" neoplasm to involve the CNS, either as meningeal spread of systemic or disseminated (usually non-Hodgkin's) lymphoma or as primary CNS lymphoma (PCNSL)—also discussed and illustrated in Chapter 6. Non-Hodgkin's lymphomas (NHLs) in general (i.e., *not* just those involving the brain) are 50 to 60 times more common in AIDS than in the general population. PCNSL is usually of non-Hodgkin's type. Molecular studies incorporating PCR technology and *in situ* hybridization have implicated Epstein-Barr virus in the etiopathogenesis of PCNSL in AIDS and non-AIDS patients. While convincing evidence for the presence of EBV genes and antigen in PCNSL cells has been presented, the precise role of this herpes-virus in the origin and evolution of the neoplasm remains to be determined. Clinically, PCNSL in AIDS presents as a single or multiple space-occupying lesions; patients with this diagnosis usually have a very poor prognosis despite aggressive therapy; death is often due to a combination of the PCNSL and OIs. Most PCNSLs are of B-cell type, cytologically aggressive and show extensive (usually central) necrosis, which renders their definitive diagnosis problematic at the time of frozen or permanent section; i.e., they can be difficult to distinguish from some of the necrotizing OIs already described. Neuropathologic features of these tumors are further discussed in Chapter 6, and a representative example is illustrated in Figure 36.

Kaposi sarcoma (KS), a common systemic malignancy seen in HIV-infected individuals, *rarely* involves the dura or brain parenchyma; when it does, gross appearances are of a well-demarcated mass lesion and histologic features are as for visceral KS. Because HIV infection is common and both primary and metastatic neoplasms of brain parenchyma are relatively common lesions, gliomas and metastatic brain tumors will on occasion be found in the CNS of HIV-infected individuals. There is no good epidemiologic evidence for an increased incidence of either in association with HIV infection.

6. Cerebrovascular and Miscellaneous Lesions

"Stroke" as a complication of HIV infection has been briefly described in Chapter 2. Cerebral hemorrhage and infarcts occur infrequently as a complication of AIDS, more often in the pediatric population than adults. They may have one or more of multiple etiologies, including: endocarditis (bacterial, fungal, or nonbacterial/marantic); thrombocytopenia or coagulopathy; extensive bleeding into a necrotic focus associated with CNS infection (e.g., due to fungus, toxoplasmosis) or neoplasm (especially PCNSL); and HIV-associated vasculopathy.

Abnormalities secondary to nutritional and/or metabolic abnormalities are often noted in AIDS patients, including:

1. Anoxic-ischemic/hypoxic encephalopathy, not an unexpected finding in patients who experience a variety of cardiorespiratory disturbances, many due to overwhelming pulmonary infection by OIs.
2. Alzheimer's type II astrocytosis, usually associated with hepatic encephalopathy but frequently seen in the CNS of AIDS patients with apparently normal liver function.
3. Wernicke's encephalopathy.
4. Central pontine myelinolysis and (more commonly) multifocal necrotizing leukoencephalopathy (MNL), the latter a necrotizing change most commonly found in the basis pontis, clearly associated with immunosuppression and seen in patients with AIDS and other causes of immunodeficiency (see Chap. 5).

Complications of AIDS treatment may involve the CNS or PNS. Perhaps the best documented of these is a mitochondrial myopathy associated with the administration of zidovudine, which appears to result from depletion of mitochondrial DNA (mtDNA) from affected muscle fibers.

C. Other Retroviruses

Although HIV-1 infection overshadows other retroviral infections of the CNS/PNS, it is by no means the only agent in this group to be associated with neurologic disease. HIV-2, endemic to West Africa and rarely encountered in

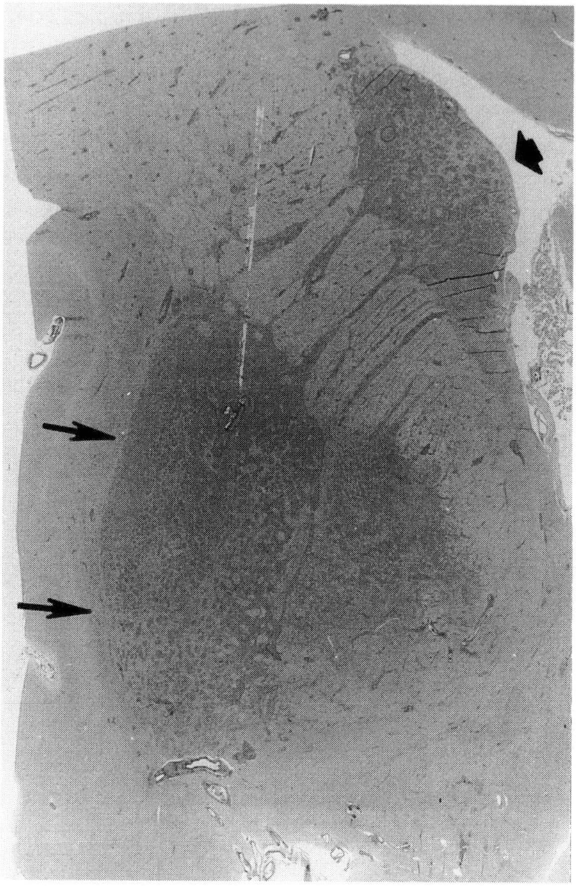

(A)

Figure 36 Primary CNS lymphoma (PCNSL) in AIDS (see also Chap. 5). (A) Whole-mount section of basal ganglia from a patient with AIDS shows the lentiform (arrows) and caudate (arrowhead) nuclei extensively infiltrated by lymphoma. This micrograph dramatically illustrates why this tumor is usually unresectable. (B) Junction between viable (at right) and necrotic (at left) brain tissues shows one vessel with pronounced fibrinoid necrosis (arrow) whereas intact vessels (arrowheads) show angiocentric proliferation of relatively uniform lymphoid cells.

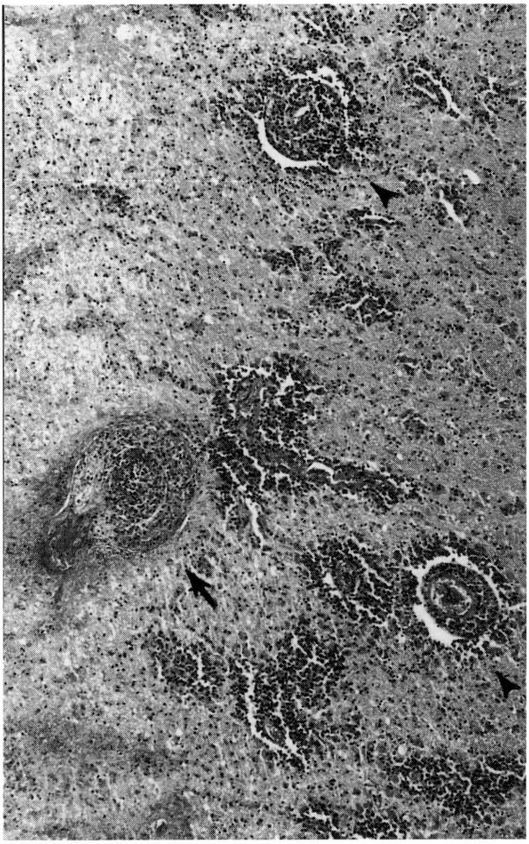

(B)

Europe or North America, can also cause AIDS. CNS infection by the virus has been described; the resultant microscopic lesions are very similar to those encountered in HIV-1 encephalitis (i.e., microglial nodules with HIV-GC).

Human T-cell leukemia virus type I (HTLV-1) was the first retrovirus associated with human disease and produces disease in the tropics and Japan, especially the island of Kyushu. The virus can be transmitted by passage of virus-infected CD4+ lymphocytes in body fluids, including blood, milk, and semen. After integration of proviral DNA into the host cell genome, a long incubation period (lasting up to 30 years) may be followed by the development of T-cell leukemia in a significant proportion of infected patients. CNS infection by HTLV-1 may also ensue. Neuropathologic features have been assessed in a small number of necropsy cases, mainly studied in Japanese patients. Disease affects primarily the spinal cord, resulting in a progressive syndrome of HTLV-1-associated myelopathy (HAM) or tropical spastic paraparesis (TSP). Histopathologic examination of affected cord shows the presence within both white and gray matter parenchyma of infiltrates of CD4+ cells in the context of chronic inflammation. White matter degeneration follows the inflammation, and longstanding lesions (with 9+ years' clinical duration) may appear more degenerative than inflammatory.

Myelopathic changes are most commonly and "reproducibly" encountered within lower thoracic cord segments, the lateral white matter—especially corticospinal tracts—being most severely affected; neurons are relatively spared. An autoimmune mechanism of disease pathogenesis has been suggested and is being investigated in a rat model. HTLV-1 genes have been demonstrated within affected spinal cord segments using PCR.

IX. NEUROPATHOLOGIC COMPLICATIONS OF (NON-AIDS-RELATED) IMMUNOSUPPRESSION

Though AIDS is the commonest naturally occurring form of immunosuppression, with an especially profound abnormality of T-cell-mediated immunity, iatrogenic immunosuppression is commonly encountered among patients who are undergoing chemotherapy/radiation therapy for hematologic, lymphoid, and solid malignancies, and patients who have received bone marrow, heart, lung, heart-lung, liver, or kidney transplants. Familiarity with the spectrum of neurologic/neuropathologic abnormalities likely to be encountered in such critically ill individuals—among whom infections figure prominently—is mandatory for both neurologists and pathologists. In most large clinical and autopsy series that have examined various "populations" of transplant patients, cerebrovascular lesions (including anoxic/ischemic change that in its extreme form manifests as cortical laminar necrosis, hemorrhage, and infarcts) emerge as the commonest complications, though "infections" generally run a close second.

Among heart and heart-lung transplant recipients, encephalitis/abscess is most commonly caused by *Aspergillus fumigatus*, *Candida albicans*, *T. gondii*, and *Nocardia*, whereas meningitis results from *Listeria monocytogenes* and cryptococcosis. Among liver and bone marrow transplant patients, fungal abscesses are most commonly the result of infection by *Aspergillus* and *Candida*, while cryptococcal and coccidioides meningoencephalitis are less commonly seen—the latter almost exclusively in the southwestern U.S., a region in which *Coccidioides immitis* is endemic (e.g., in the San Joaquin Valley of California). Whereas CNS candidiasis may produce disseminated microabscesses throughout the brain, coccidioidomycosis generally results in a severe granulomatous meningoencephalitis with vasculopathic complications (see above). *Aspergillus* abscesses usually occur in the setting of disseminated fungal infection and, because of the angioinvasive nature of this microorganism, tend to be (at least in late stages) extraordinarily hemorrhagic (Fig. 37). Although disseminated viral infections (e.g., by CMV) are a serious complication of organ transplantation, symptomatic CMV encephalomyelitis appears to be extremely rare. Evidence of a low-grade "microglial nodule"-type encephalitis in brain tissue from liver transplant patients suggests the presence of CNS viral infection, though in many instances this cannot be attributed to a specific agent. Occasional patients have developed PML after organ transplantation, and bone marrow transplantation may infrequently be complicated by adenovirus or mumps virus encephalitis (Fig. 38). Rarely, immunosuppressed patients may develop localized mass lesions resulting from infection with MAI, as illustrated in Fig. 39.

X. SLOW/ATYPICAL VIRAL AND PRION INFECTIONS

Two groups of diseases will be considered: subacute sclerosing panencephalitis (SSPE), and "prion diseases," the best-understood examples of which are spongiform encephalopathy (Creutzfeldt-Jakob disease, CJD) and Gerstmann-Sträussler-Scheinker disease (GSSD). A third entity, progressive rubella panencephalitis, is, partly due to its extreme rarity, rather poorly characterized as a nosologic entity and is thus mentioned only in passing.

A. Subacute Sclerosing Panencephalitis

SSPE is a rare (four or five cases per year observed in the U.S.; an estimated one case per million cases of measles) cause of dementia in children and adolescents associated with measles virus infection or vaccination. In North America, disease onset is characteristically in the early teen years, though cases have been observed as early as infancy; the latent interval after vaccination is approx. 8 years; after antecedent measles virus infection, 11 or 12 years. A small minority of SSPE patients give no history of previous measles virus infection or vaccination. Parainfluenza virus (type 3) has also been implicated in the etiology of some cases of SSPE. The disease presents with personality changes followed by rapidly progressive dementia which culminates in death within a few weeks to many years; i.e., survival is highly variable. Characteristic EEG abnormalities occur. Infection of the CNS by a defective measles virus has been implicated as a cause of the illness, and measles virus RNA and antigen are found in the brains and CSF of affected individuals. In patients with an intact immune system, CSF synthesis of antimeasles virus antibodies is virtually diagnostic of SSPE.

Neuropathologic features of SSPE include widespread chronic inflammation (featuring lymphocytes and plasma cells) and astrogliosis throughout the

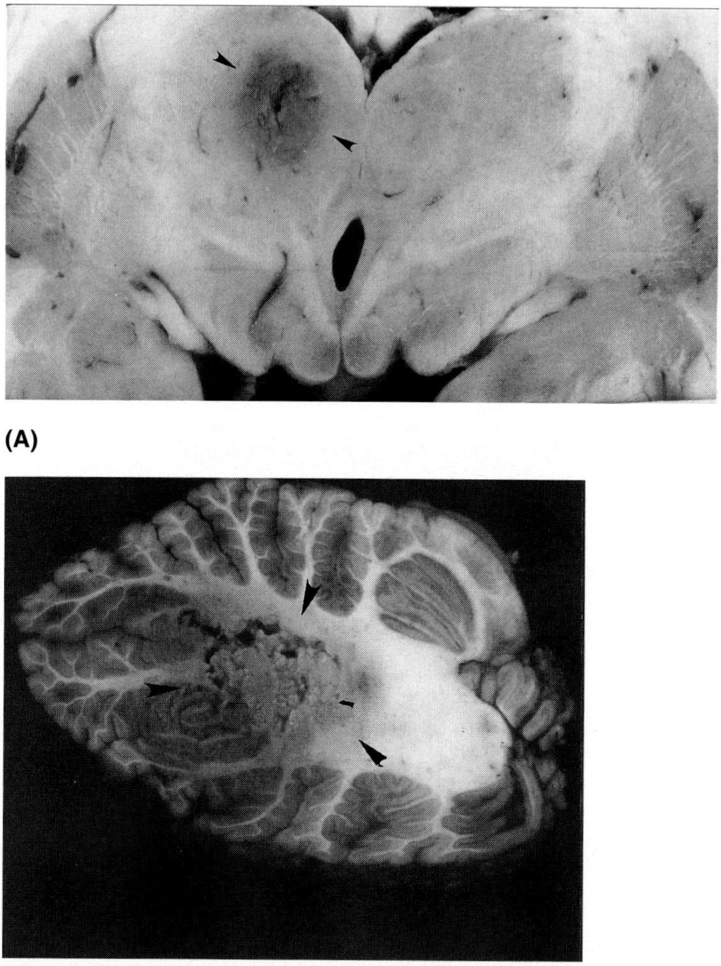

(A)

(B)

Figure 37 *Aspergillus* abscesses in brains of immunosuppressed patients. Panels A,B show poorly defined regions of necrosis in (A) diencephalon of a patient with AIDS, and (B) cerebellum of a patient with aplastic anemia. By contrast, panel C demonstrates extensively hemorrhagic abscesses (larger in the right cerebral hemisphere, indicated by arrowheads) in a child with complex immunodeficiency and lymphoma, who died with disseminated aspergillosis following a bone marrow transplant. (D) Angioinvasive nature of this fungus is highlighted in this section (stained with a methenamine silver technique to show the microorganisms). Arrowheads indicate only portion of the vessel wall that remains intact.

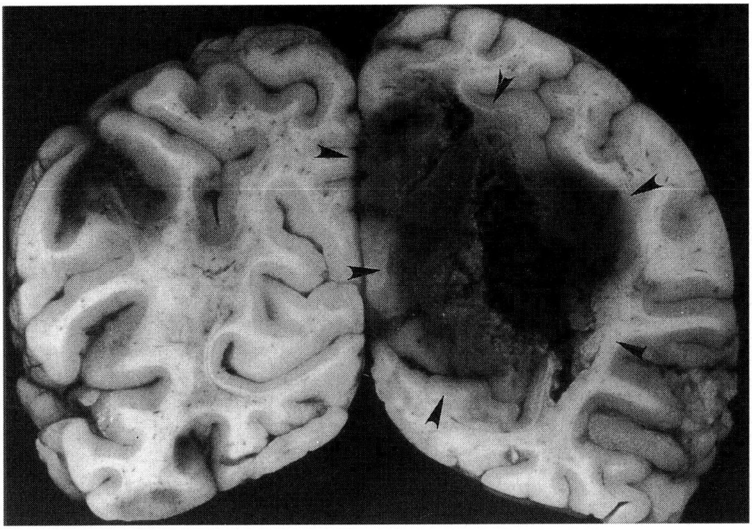

(C)

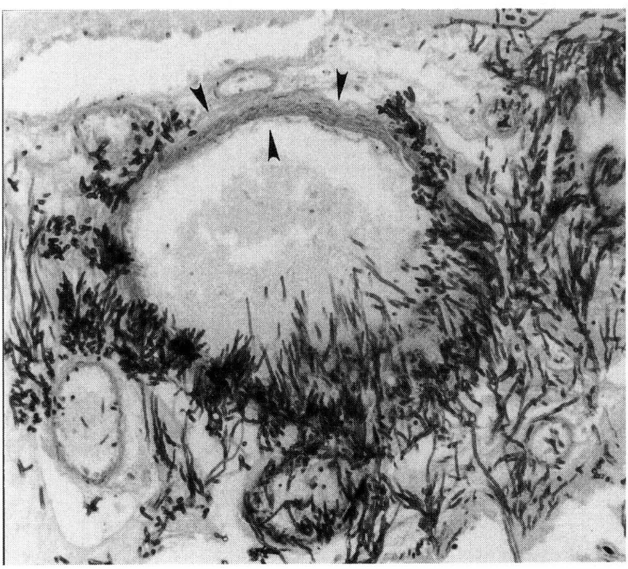

(D)

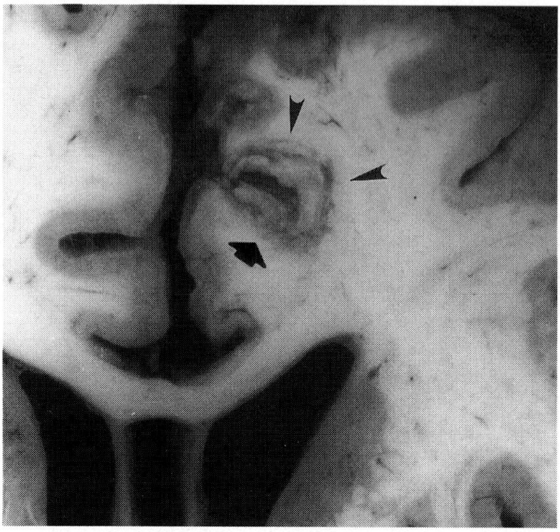

Figure 38 Mumps encephalitis in a profoundly immunosuppressed child. At autopsy, multifocal encephalomalacia was noted throughout the brain—e.g., in this focus adjacent to the right cingulate gyrus, designated by arrowheads. Widespread inflammation was noted throughout the brain, and viral particles were demonstrated by electron microscopy.

CNS, with typical Cowdry type A intranuclear inclusions in various cell types (including neurons). As well, many oligodendroglia show PML-like inclusions, i.e., presenting as effacement of the nucleus with amphophilic staining properties (Fig. 40). Molecular studies (including *in situ* hybridization and PCR) show the presence of measles virus genes in affected brain; as well, mutations of the measles virus gene from wild type are characteristically observed. If the encephalitis is particularly destructive, gitter cells/foamy histiocytes may be abundant. Ultrastructural study usually reveals the presence of characteristic intranuclear viral particles.

Immunocytochemical studies have implicated enhanced expression of various cytokines (by both resident CNS and infiltrating cells) in SSPE pathogenesis and progression. Immunosuppressed individuals may develop a form of progressive measles encephalitis.

B. "Prion" Diseases

The term prion, coined in the early 1980s by S. Prusiner to describe an agent or group of agents with novel biological properties that produce rapidly pro-

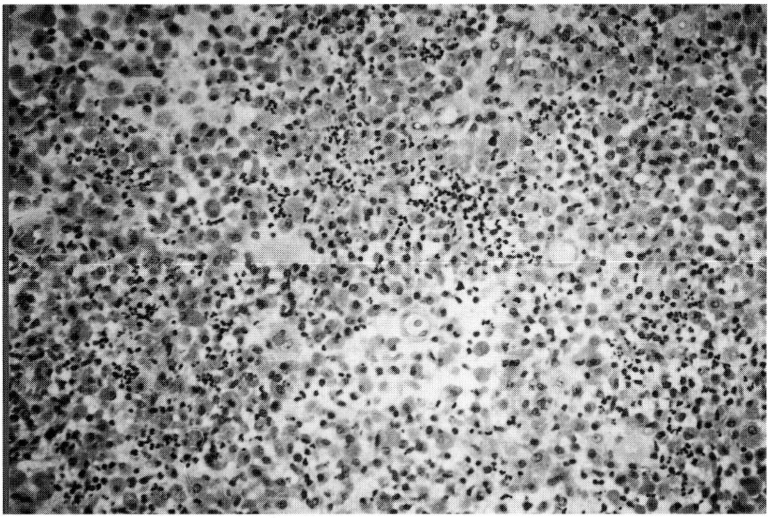

(A)

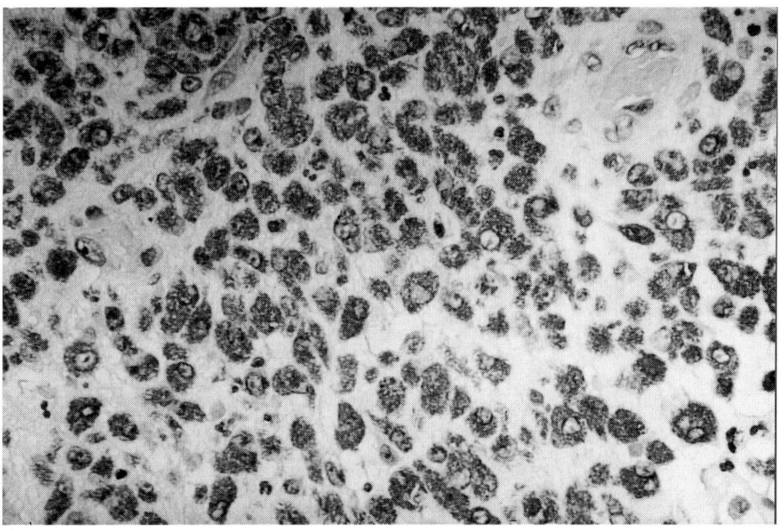

(B)

Figure 39 Dural-based lesion in a patient with systemic lupus erythematosus (SLE), thought (on neuroimaging studies) to represent a meningioma. At surgical resection, fields of histiocytes, some with a distinctly oval or spindle-shaped cell morphology, were seen (A); rare foci of PMNs suggestive of acute inflammation (as in this field) were noted. Staining for acid-fast bacteria (B) showed the presence of numerous intracellular, rod-like microorganisms, confirmed on culture to be *Mycobacterium avium-intracellulare* (MAI). This is a distinctly unusual presentation for MAI infection, which is most commonly found in perivascular macrophages in the CNS of patients with AIDS.

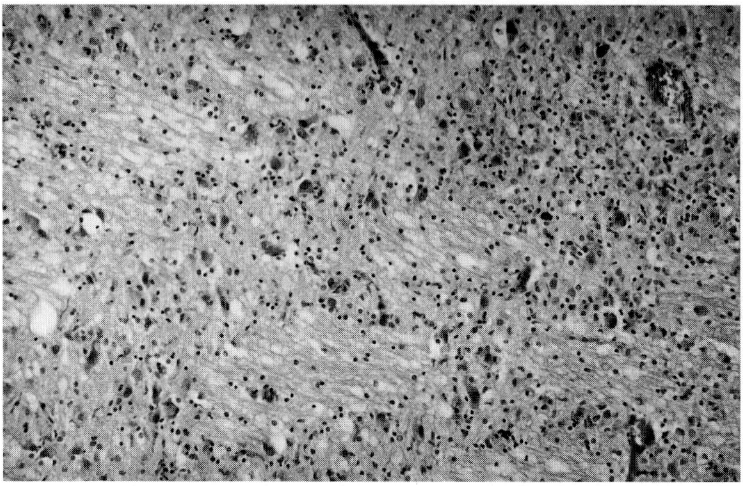

(A)

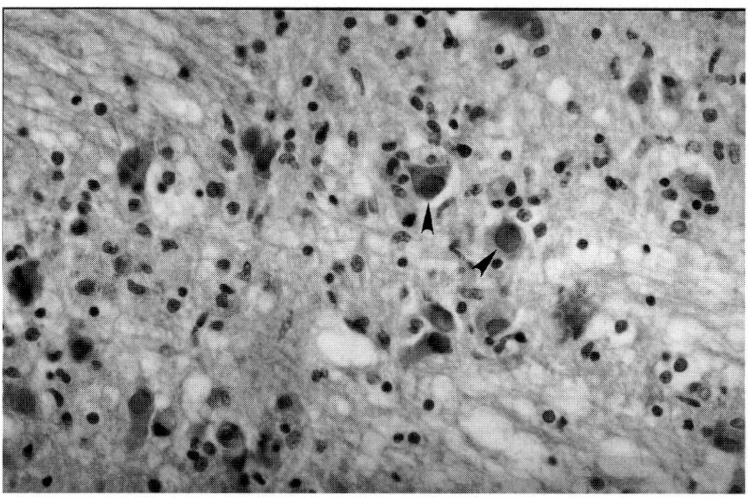

(B)

Figure 40 Subacute sclerosing panencephalitis (SSPE). This patient showed especially severe involvement of the brainstem, sections of which are illustrated. (A) Multifocal chronic inflammation including microglial nodules and perivascular cuffing by mononuclear inflammatory cells are characteristically present. (B) Nuclear inclusions may be of the Cowdry type A form, or (as in this panel) glassy nuclei which show effacement of the normal chromatin pattern (arrows)—i.e., an appearance similar to the papovavirus inclusions of PML. The presence of virus can be confirmed by electron microscopy or in situ hybridization.

gressive dementia with spongiform change in cerebral gray matter, has come to symbolize a field of research that (at the very least) has revolutionized our understanding of both infectious and degenerative diseases. For instance, prion diseases have sporadic, transmissible, and inherited variants, yet "transmission" of the disease from human to experimental animal or from one human to another (by direct inoculation of infected CNS tissue) can apparently occur without an obvious nucleic acid component to the transmissible agent. Cross-species transmission of prion diseases clearly occurs, and within the mid-1990s a bovine form of spongiform encephalopathy (BSE) has been implicated in the causation of a rare human variant of spongiform encephalopathy.

The best-understood examples of human spongiform encephalopathy (also referred to as transmissible spongiform encephalopathy; TSE) will be described briefly prior to a brief consideration of pathogenetic mechanisms.

1. Kuru

This progressive ataxia caused by a degenerative disease of the cerebellum (with profound Purkinje and granule cell loss and "plaques" in the cerebellar cortex observed at necropsy), though now largely extinct as the result of the discontinuation of cannibalistic rituals, was first observed among Fore peoples of Papua New Guinea. Apparent transmission of the disease during the practice of handling and consuming brain tissue from the deceased suggested to investigators that similar subacute neurodegenerative conditions may be transmissible.

2. Creutzfeldt-Jakob Disease (CJD)

Also known as subacute spongiform encephalopathy, this is a rare (one or two cases per million per year in the U.S.) cause of rapidly progressive dementia, usually setting in in elderly or middle-aged individuals, who rarely survive longer than 1 or 2 years. EEG changes associated with clinical evidence of myoclonus are characteristic. Brain tissue examined at biopsy or autopsy shows characteristic spongiosis of the neuropil, many of the vacuoles apparently originating in neuronal cell bodies. With time, there are cortical neuron loss and astrocytic gliosis (Fig. 41). Cerebellar degeneration (similar to that seen in Kuru, though usually lacking Kuru plaques) is often encountered and accounts for the ataxia observed in many affected individuals. CJD has been inadvertently transmitted from one human to another by contaminated dural grafts, deep EEG electrodes, corneal transplants, and administration of growth hormone apparently extracted from infected pituitary glands.

3. Gerstmann-Sträussler-Scheinker Disease (GSSD)

This rare condition, estimated to be only one-tenth as common as CJD, is an inherited, slowly progressive syndrome of cerebellar degeneration in which dementia occurs as a late manifestation. Spongiform change similar to that seen

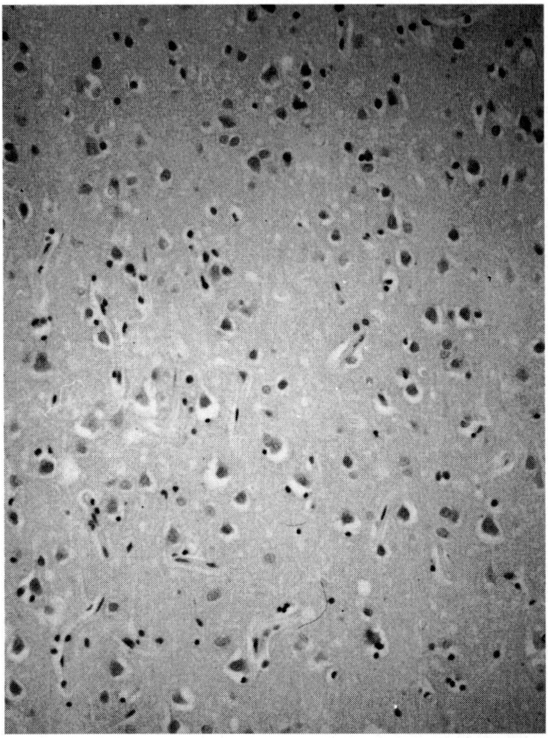

(A)

Figure 41 Spongiform encephalopathy (CJD), microscopic features. (A) A subtle degree of spongiosis is noted in otherwise intact cortex. (B) Severe CJD, symptomatic for many months, in another patient. Note large vacuoles that impart a cribriform appearance to the entire cortex. Extensive proliferation of reactive astrocytes is also present. (C) Ultrastructural features of CJD in a brain biopsy. Note large vacules (arrows) that appear to arise from splitting of membranes. Intact cell processes (including myelinated fibers) are present elsewhere in the field.

in typical CJD is observed in both neocortex and cerebellum, and large amyloid plaques are encountered, especially in the cerebellar molecular layer (Fig. 42). More widespread neuron loss and gliosis may occur throughout the CNS. The amyloid plaques (in contradistinction to those observed in AD/SDAT) show absence of a significant neuritic component and are composed of the pathogenic protease resistant (prion) protein (PrP) encoded by the PRNP gene (see below).

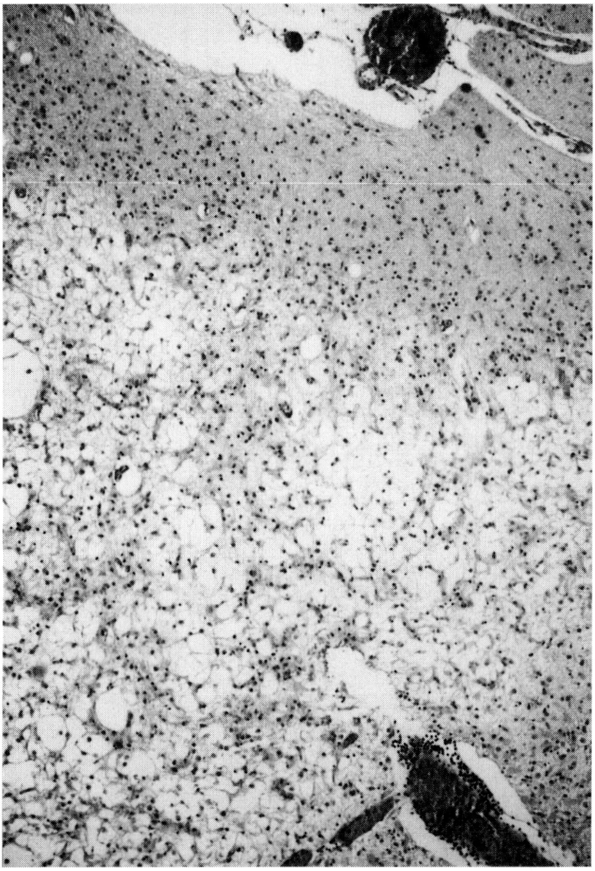

(B)

4. Familial Fatal Insomnia (FFI)

This extremely rare degenerative condition presents with a sleep disorder, dysautonomia, myoclonus, ataxia, and pyramidal and extrapyramidal signs. Neuropathologic features include thalamic atrophy and variable spongiform change throughout the brain.

Spongiform encephalopathies observed in animals include BSE, transmissible mink encephalopathy, and scrapie in sheep; the last has been especially valuable as a model for studying human transmissible spongiform encephalopathies.

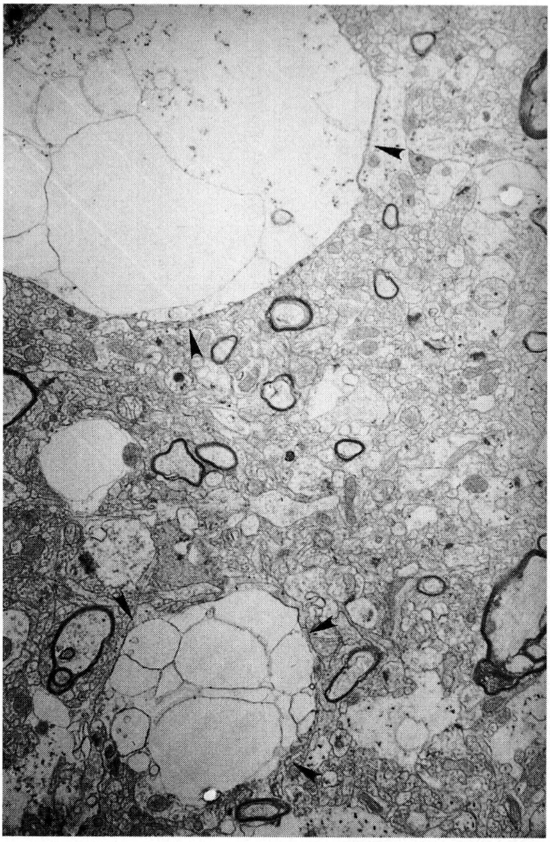

(C)

Figure 41 Continued

The prion protein (PrP) encoded by the *PRNP* gene on chromosome 20—and mutations in the PRNP gene—appear to play key roles in the pathogenesis of transmissible spongiform encephalopathies and their genetically determined variants. Two isoforms of the PrP have been found: PrP^{c}, with a molecular weight (MW) of 33 to 34 kDa, appears to be a normal cellular (plasma membrane) glycoprotein highly expressed in neurons. The "prion hypothesis" states that pathogenic prions, however, consist of the abnormal isoform PrP^{Sc}, and that the c form of the protein can "evolve" into the pathogenic Sc isoform by a change in its conformation.

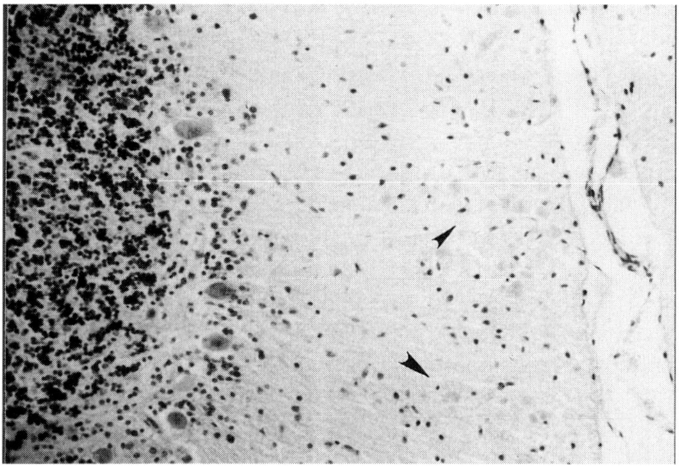

(A)

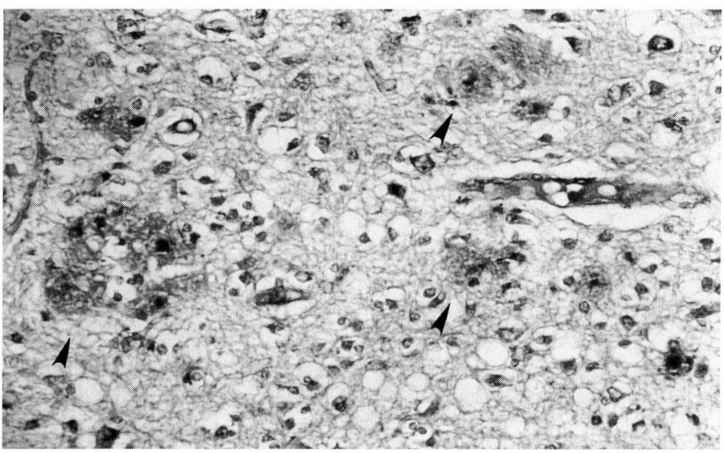

(B)

Figure 42 Gerstmann-Sträussler-Scheinker disease (GSSD), considered a familial "prion disease" closely linked to (and much less common than) CJD. Spongiform change, gliosis, and amyloid deposits are prominent throughout the central neuraxis. Cerebellum and cortex are sites of prominent amyloid plaques (lacking a neuritic component), which are relatively inconspicuous on routine (H&E) stains (arrows, A) but more readily apparent on PAS-stained sections (arrows, B).

This conformational alteration in PrP is a defining feature in the (hypothesized) pathogenesis of all the previously described prion diseases. It appears to be a random event in sporadic spongiform encephalopathies, an occurrence induced by exogenous PrP^{Sc} in transmitted forms of disease, and the result of instability of mutant PrP^{c} in familial forms (especially GSSD and FFI)—virtually all of which result from mutations in the PRNP gene. Once it has formed, the PrP^{Sc} appears to act as a template by "imposing" an abnormal/pathogenic conformation on newly synthesized PrP^{c}. This, in turn, results in replication and accumulation of sufficient PrP^{Sc} to produce neurologic disease. The massive juggernaut of research effort aimed at understanding the "prionopathies," utilizing cutting-edge technology of molecular neurobiology, is likely to solve the riddle of this mysterious group of rare conditions within the next few years and may well provide insights into the neuropathogenesis of nonprion types of dementia.

XI. PARASITIC INFESTATIONS

While relatively rare in neuropathologic practice in developed countries, these diseases represent a major factor in neurologic morbidity and mortality in third-world nations. Cerebral toxoplasmosis as a complication of AIDS has been considered elsewhere, and several other examples are briefly discussed below. For detailed discussion of these entities, the reader is referred to standard reference texts.

A. Protozoal Infections

Cerebral amebic abscess results from infection by *Entameba histolytica,* an intestinal parasite native to tropical and subtropical climates. Cerebral disease usually follows upon lung, GI tract, or liver involvement. A single necrotic or hemorrhagic cerebral abscess is usually identified; on microscopic section, typical trophozoites (15 to 25 μm in diameter and resembling foamy histiocytes) are identified. Primary amebic meningoencephalitis results from infection by *Naegleria fowleri,* a widely distributed organism especially common in fresh water. This rare CNS infection manifests as a highly necrotizing hemorrhagic meningoencephalitis; characteristic amoebae (Fig. 43) are found in the inflammatory infiltrates. Granulomatous amoebic encephalitis results from CNS infection (usually) by *acanthamoeba,* an organism with a worldwide distribution.

Clinically significant infection usually occurs in chronically ill and/or immunosuppressed patients. The characteristic granulomatous inflammation is centered on arteries and veins.

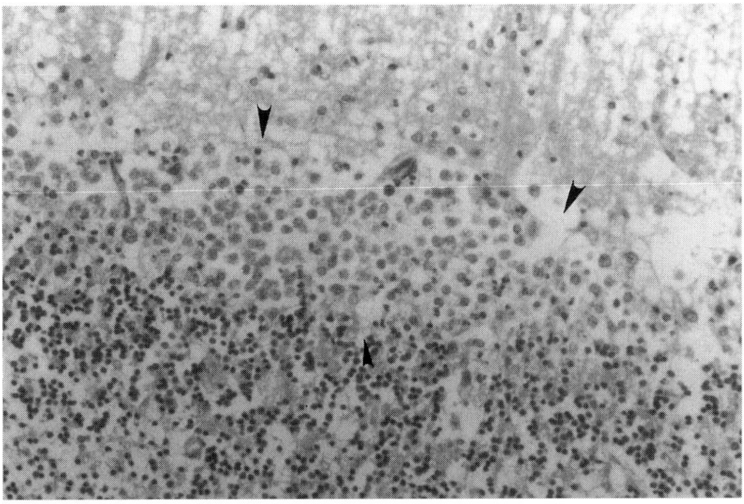

(A)

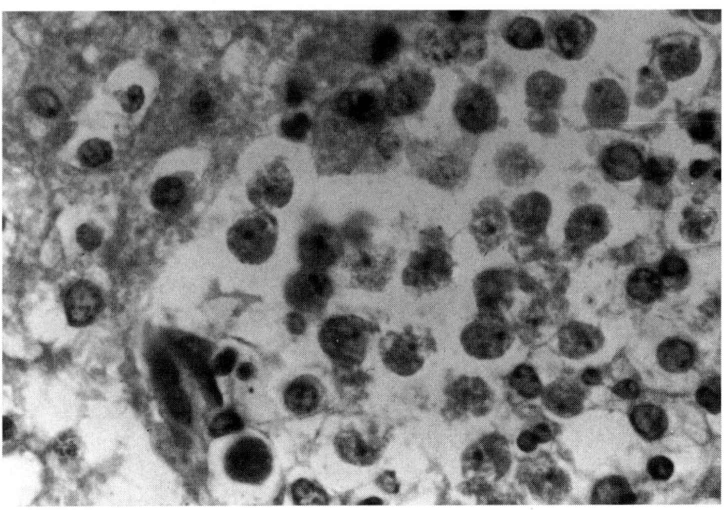

(B)

Figure 43 *Naegleria fowleri* meningoencephalitis. Pale amoebic organisms are seen at low (arrowheads, A) and high (B) magnification. As these micrographs indicate, the trophozoites can be difficult to distinguish from normal constituent cells of the brain or associated inflammatory elements. *Naegleria* meningoencephalitis is usually very necrotizing.

B. Toxoplasmosis

This has been considered as one of the most common OIs observed in the CNS of patients with AIDS. Congenital toxoplasmosis results from transplacental spread of protozoans, usually the result of primary infection of a pregnant mother. The brain in such cases shows multiple zones of necrosis, especially in the periventricular regions, with widespread cerebral calcification. Cerebral destruction may be so severe as to resemble that seen with hydranencephaly.

C. Malaria

CNS complications usually result from infection by one of four species of plasmodium endemic to subtropical/tropical climates. Cerebral disease is most common in young children and visitors to an endemic region since neither group has immunity to this parasite. Occlusion of cerebral capillaries is a pivotal event in the evolution of neurologic complications caused by malaria; capillary necrosis, perivascular hemorrhages, and cerebral edema commonly result.

D. Trypanosomiasis

This is usually subdivided into a consideration of the African and American forms of disease, the latter found commonly in South and Central (rather than North) America. Infection results from the organism *Trypanosoma cruzi.* Neuropathologic features include cerebral edema with widespread petechial hemorrhages, and parasites are visible within glial cells or at the centers of microglial nodules throughout the CNS.

E. Helminthic Infections

This group of conditions is the result of infestation by tapeworms (cestodes), flukes (trematodes, e.g., schistosomiasis), or roundworms (nematodes, e.g., trichinosis, strongyloidiasis)—of which selected examples will be discussed.

Cysticercosis is one of the most common parasitic infestations of the CNS worldwide and possibly the one most likely to be encountered in the U.S., especially in hospitals and clinics in states that border Mexico. The responsible agent is the larval form of the pork tapeworm *Taenia solium,* which produces disease after ingestion of foodstuffs contaminated by ova. Clinical manifestations often include seizures, signs of raised intracranial pressure, and dementia; sudden death may result from acute hydrocephalus. Neuropathologic features include the presence of one to many cysts within the CNS, usually in the brain substance, leptomeninges, or ventricular cavities. The cyst wall shows a characteristic three-layered appearance (Fig. 44). The cysts typically induce minimal

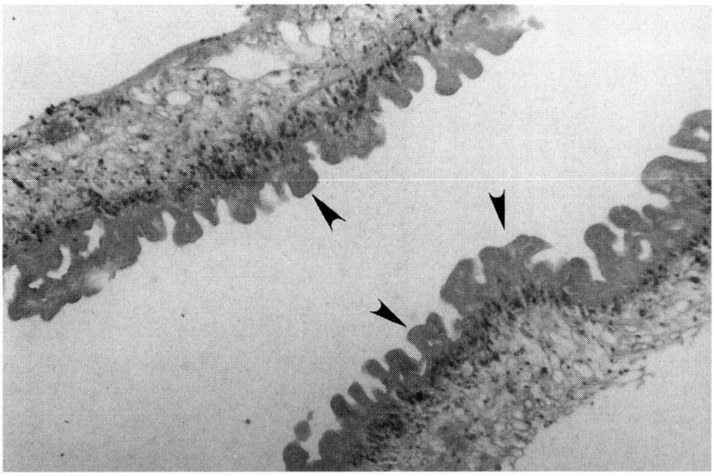

Figure 44 Cyst wall of cerebral cysticercosis showing typical trilaminar appearance. The cyst lining (arrows) is eosinophilic; nuclei are much smaller than those of any normal human diploid cell, and are arranged in a characteristic pseudostratified "palisade." Neither hooklets nor scolex are seen in this micrograph.

reaction within surrounding brain until they die, at which time a marked purulent and granulomatous reaction may develop to the dead cysticerci. Sometimes, the scolex and hooklets of the parasite can be identified, but often—e.g., at the time of presentation of a "cystic intraventricular structure" for evaluation at the time of frozen section—only the characteristic cyst wall will be identified.

Echinococcosis (hydatid disease) usually results from infestation by larvae of *Echinococcus granulosus*, for which canines are the definitive host. Human cysts usually localize to the lungs and liver (rarely involving the CNS) after accidental ingestion of ova.

XII. RICKETTSIAL INFECTIONS

Rickettsial infections represent a rare cause of neurologic disease. Rickettsiae are obligate intracellular bacteria (pleomorphic coccobacilli) that usually infect animals, and only infrequently cause human disease that may involve the CNS. Their definitive hosts are usually rodents or other mammals. Pathologic features of infection include multiorgan microvascular injury that produces extremely heterogeneous CNS manifestations. Human disease is subclassified into four main categories, viz.: spotted fever, e.g., Rocky mountain spotted fever

(RMSF); typhus fever; scrub fever; and miscellaneous (e.g., Q fever, ehrlichiosis).

Rickettsial disease appears to be mediated by infection of microvascular endothelium, with its subsequent injury and death. Increased vascular permeability may result, microthrombi may develop and perivascular inflammation by mononuclear inflammatory cells is common. Fibrinoid necrosis and a PMN infiltrate in and around the vessel wall are uncommon features. Cerebral microinfarcts and meningoencephalitis sometimes occur, and microglial nodule-like lesions are sometimes present. As expected, an affected brain at necropsy shows (relatively nonspecific) edema and petechial hemorrhages at the cortex–white matter junction. Microorganisms can be detected in tissue sections using the Brown and Hopps stain.

XIII. LYME DISEASE

Though a "fashionable" diagnosis in the last decade of the 20th century, Lyme disease has poorly defined neuropathologic features, primarily because only rare patients have undergone brain biopsy or autopsy. It is seldom fatal. Lyme disease is caused by a tickborne spirochete, *Borrelia burgdorferi* (Bb), a loosely coiled spirochete 9 to 30 μm in length. Its main vector is the deer tick *Ixodes scapularis*, the bite of which can transmit the causal agent to man. Human disease that results from infection with the spirochete manifests as a multisystem disorder with variable CNS and PNS involvement; the condition is described as "Lyme-borreliosis." The host immune response to the organism may have a major pathogenetic role; autoimmune phenomena may also be of importance in causing symptoms.

Neuropathologic features include CNS and PNS abnormalities. Within brain, meningoencephalitis is often seen, typical microglial nodules having been identified within brain. Chronic illness may result in demyelination. The PNS shows some similarities to Guillain-Barré syndrome, and (rarely) mononeuritis multiplex may occur. Multifocal inflammatory infiltrates composed of lymphocytes, histiocytes, and plasma cells are often centered on vasa nervorum. Microvascular thrombosis and recanalization are sometimes seen. In chronic examples of Lyme-borreliosis, axonal degeneration may be found.

XIV. DISORDERS OF "POSSIBLE" INFECTIOUS ETIOLOGY

"Paraneoplastic" CNS/PNS abnormalities with a significant inflammatory component are discussed in Chapter 8. In these and similar conditions, chronic, usually multifocal CNS inflammation develops for mysterious reasons. Because the pattern of inflammatory change is similar to that encountered with "conventional" viral infections, a viral etiology is usually invoked to explain the neuropathologic change. At least some of these entities may turn out to have nonviral (e.g., autoimmune) etiologies.

One of the most intriguing diseases in this group is Rasmussen encephalitis (RE), first recognized as an important cause of epilepsy in the 1950s. RE is characterized by epilepsia partialis continua, slowly progressive neurologic deterioration (evolving over months to years), lateralized cerebral atrophy, and neuropathologic features suggestive of chronic encephalitis. Overall, it is a relatively rare cause of seizures. Disease onset is almost always before the age of 15 years but rarely within the first 2 years of life. Various herpesviruses have been implicated as causal pathogens for RE, but PCR and *in situ* hybridization studies—though they frequently show herpesvirus genes as "footprints" of infection in RE-affected tissue—have not been conclusively linked to the disease. Recent evidence suggests an autoimmune component to RE, based on animal experiments showing an RE-*like* picture in rabbits immunized with the GluR3 glutamate receptor. Neither "viral" nor "autoimmune" theories of pathogenesis adequately explain the striking unilaterality of the cerebral lesions.

Neuropathologic features (most commonly assessed in cortical resection specimens derived from surgical treatment/hemispherectomy) include variable atrophy. Histologic sections show widespread involvement of cortex and white matter (though more commonly the former) by multifocal patchy inflammation, astrocytic gliosis, and variable degrees of chronic inflammation (Fig. 45) including microglial nodules and perivascular cuffing by mononuclear inflammatory cells, especially T-lymphocytes. Microglial activation is highlighted by immunohistochemical markers for these cells.

Cystic encephalomalacia may be present, but large regions of the cortex show an entirely normal appearance—the transition from normal to affected areas is often very sharply demarcated. Capillary proliferation is sometimes seen in and adjacent to foci of injury.

Will RE be proven to have a viral cause? Might it represent the result of infection by an as yet unknown or uncharacterized virus, or one that is ubiquitous but induces an inflammatory/degenerative disease only in susceptible individuals? If so, what are the determinants of that "susceptibility"? The molecular tools that have allowed for a profound understanding of many types of CNS/PNS infection can now be brought to bear on RE and other puzzling inflammatory disorders that injure neural tissue.

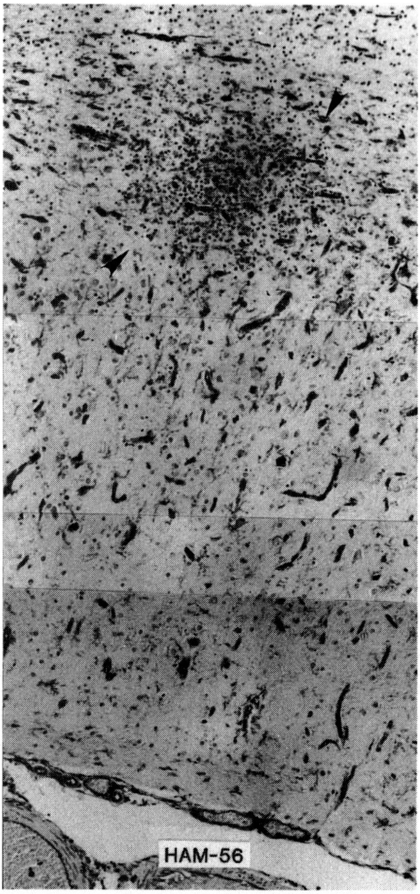

(A)

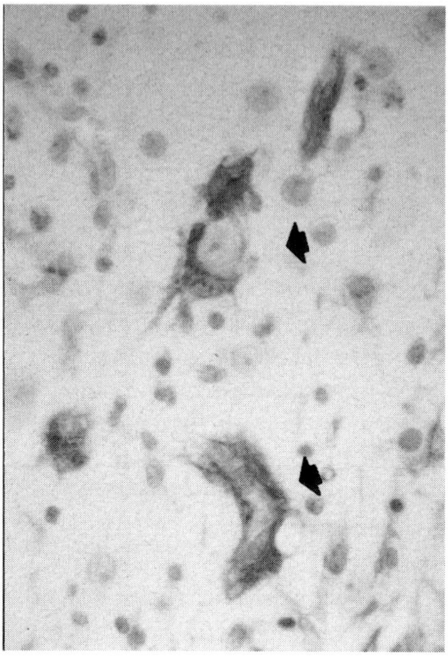

(B)

Figure 45 Chronic (pathogen-free) Rasmussen-type encephalitis. Commonly, widespread multifocal chronic inflammation is present, manifest as microglial nodules and perivascular cuffing by mononuclear inflammatory cells (usually T-cells). (A) Section of affected brain immunostained with a macrophage/microglial marker, HAM-56. Note prominent rodlike microglia throughout the cortex, and a large microglial nodule (arrows) near the cortex–white matter junction. (B) Section immunostained with an antibody to HLA-DR, an MHC class II marker. Note prominently immunoreactive cells around neurons (upper arrow) and a microvessel (lower arrow). (C) Anti-GFAP immunohistochemistry highlights the laminar nature of reactive astrogliosis; also note prominent subpial (Chaslin-type gliosis, small arrowheads) and a single subpial microglial nodule (large arrowhead). (D) Section stained with primary antibody to β-2-microglobulin (an MCH class I marker) shows prominently immunoreactive perivascular cells adjacent to a positively stained microglial nodule.

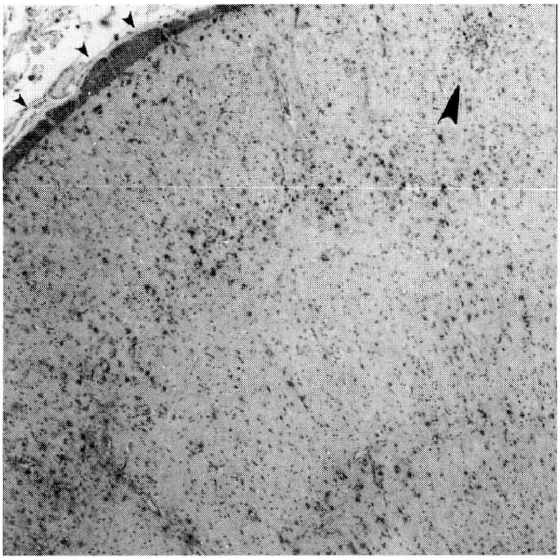

(C)

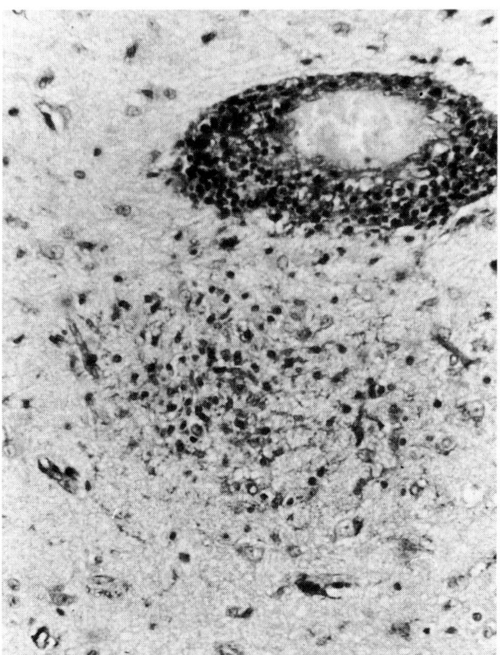

(D)

REFERENCES

1. Achim CL, Wang R, Miners DK, Wiley CA. Brain viral burden in HIV infection. J Neuropathol Exp Neurol 1994; 53:284–294.
2. Adams H. The neuropathology of viral infections of the nervous system. Br J Hosp Med 1973; 10:394–401.
3. Anderson NE, Willoughby EW, Synek BJL, Croxson MC, Glasgow GL. Brain biopsy in the management of focal encephalitis. J Neurol Neurosurg Psychiatry 1991; 54:1001–1003.
4. Basit AS, Ravi B, Banerji AK, Tandon PN. Multiple pyogenic brain abscesses: an analysis of 21 patients. J Neurol Neurosurg Psychiatry 1989; 52:591–594.
5. Brew BJ, Rosenblum M, Cronin K, Price RW. AIDS dementia complex and HIV-1 brain infection: clinical-virological correlations. Ann Neurol 1995; 38:563–570.
6. Calisher CH. Medically important arboviruses of the United States and Canada. Clin Microbiol Rev 1994; 7:89–116.
7. Chrétien F, Gray F, Lescs MC, et al. Acute varicella-zoster virus ventriculitis and meningomyeloradiculitis in acquired immunodeficiency syndrome. Acta Neuropathol 1993; 86:659–665.
8. Court L, Dodet B, eds. Transmissible Subacute Spongiform Encephalopathies: Prion Diseases. Amsterdam: Elsevier, 1996.
9. Darnell RB. The polymerase chain reaction: application to nervous system disease. Ann Neurol 1993; 34:513–523.
10. Dickson DW, Lee SC, Mattiace LA, Yen S-H C, Brosnan C. Microglia and cytokines in neurological disease, with special reference to AIDS and Alzheimer's disease. Glia 1993; 7:75–83.
11. Dill SR, Cobbs CG, McDonald CK. Subdural empyema: analysis of 32 cases and review. Clin Infect Dis 1995; 20:372–386.
12. Dubois-Dalcq M, Altmeyer R, Chiron M, Wilt S. HIV interactions with cells of the nervous system. Curr Opin Neurobiol 1995; 5:647–655.
13. Esiri MM. Herpes simplex encephalitis. An immunohistological study of the distribution of viral antigen within the brain. J Neurol Sci 1982; 54:209–226.
14. Farrar WE. Atlas of Infections of the Nervous System. London: Mosby Year Book, 1993.
15. Farrell MA, Droogan O, Secor DL, Poukens V, Quinn B, Vinters HV. Chronic encephalitis associated with epilepsy: immunohistochemical and ultrastructural studies. Acta Neuropathol 1995; 89:313–321.
16. Ferreirò JA, Robert MA, Townsend J, Vinters HV. Neuropathologic findings after liver transplantation. Acta Neuropathol 1992; 84:1–14.
17. Gyure KA, Prayson RA, Estes ML, Hall GS. Symptomatic *Mycobacterium avium* complex infection of the central nervous system. Arch Pathol Lab Med 1995; 119:836–839.
18. Iwasaki Y. Human T cell leukemia virus type I infection and chronic myelopathy. Brain Pathol 1993; 3:1–10.
19. Jackson AC. Acute viral infections. Curr Opin Neurol 1995; 8:170–174.
20. Kaplan K. Brain abscess. Medical Clin North Am 1985; 69:345–369.

21. Manz HJ. Pathology and pathogenesis of viral infections of the central nervous system. Hum Pathol 1977; 8:3–26.
22. Mischel PS, Vinters HV. Coccidioidomycosis of the central nervous system: neuropathological and vasculopathic manifestations and clinical correlates. Clin Infect Dis 1995; 20:400–405.
23. Mohrmann RL, Mah V, Vinters HV. Neuropathologic findings after bone marrow transplantation: An autopsy study. Hum Pathol 1990; 21:630–639.
24. Mrak RE, Young L. Rabies encephalitis in humans: pathology, pathogenesis and pathophysiology. J Neuropathol Exp Neurol 1994; 53:1–10.
25. Nagano I, Nakamura S, Yoshioka M, Onodera J, Kogure K, Itoyama Y. Expression of cytokines in brain lesions in subacute sclerosing panenecepahlitis. Neurology 1994; 44:710–715.
26. Prusiner SB. Biology and genetics of prior diseases. Annu Rev Microbiol 1994; 48:655–686.
27. Scheld WM, Whitley RJ, Durack DT, eds. Infections of the Central Nervous System. New York: Raven Press, 1991.
28. Swartz MN, Dodge PR. Bacterial meningitis—a review of selected aspects. N Engl J Med 1965; 272:898–902, 954–960, 1003–1010.
29. Singhi PD, Singhi SC. Central nervous system infections in children (bacterial, tubercular). Curr Opin Neurol 1995; 8:150–155.
30. Tompkins LS. The use of molecular methods in infectious diseases. N Engl J Med 1992; 327:1290–1297.
31. Vinters HV, Anders KH. Neuropathology of AIDS. Boca Raton: CRC Press, 1990.
32. von Einsiedel RW, Fife TD, Aksamit AJ, et al. Progressive multifocal leukoencephalopathy in AIDS: a clinicopathologic study and review of the literature. J Neurol 1993; 240:391–406.
33. Whitley RJ, Cobbs CG, Alford CA Jr, et al. Diseases that mimic herpes simplex encephalitis. Diagnosis, presentation, and outcome. JAMA 1989; 262:234–239.

5

Diseases of White Matter

I. INTRODUCTION

Diseases of white matter (*leukoencephalopathies*, as opposed to those that primarily affect the gray matter, *polioencephalopathies*) are pathologic abnormalities that involve CNS myelinated tracts. Though they are generally considered to be diseases that affect myelin and oligodendrocytes/oligodendroglia—the cells that produce CNS myelin (see Chap. 1)—the discussion below will highlight the observation that most leukoencephalopathies are not purely diseases of the myelin sheath. They can, however, generally be considered in several nosologic categories, as follows:

1. Idiopathic demyelinating conditions (mainly multiple sclerosis and its variants; usually referred to in the United Kingdom as disseminated sclerosis DS)
2. Dysmyelinating conditions, primarily the leukodystrophies (see also Chap. 9)
3. Demyelinating conditions associated with systemic (often metabolic/electrolyte) abnormalities
4. Infectious/post- or parainfectious/inflammatory conditions
5. Miscellaneous "toxic" leukoencephalopathies

II. MULTIPLE SCLEROSIS (MS) AND VARIANTS

First described by Charcot in the 1870s, MS is a commonly encountered chronic, idiopathic, inflammatory, demyelinating disease of the CNS. Though much is known about its epidemiology, the etiopathogenesis of MS remains obscure. The neuropathologic lesions observed in affected patients suggest chronic inflammation and eventual scar formation as playing a key role. The lesions of MS have a distinctive appearance grossly and microscopically, which distinguish them from other demyelinating conditions considered in this chapter.

A. Etiologic and Epidemiologic Considerations

Few diseases of the CNS have intrigued and challenged both clinical and basic neuroscientists to the extent that MS has. Attempts to discover its cause(s) have also involved major contributions from the fields of neurovirology, immunology, and neuroepidemiology. Yet its etiology remains enigmatic and elusive, as does its definitive treatment. The key feature of MS is selective destruction of oligodendrocytes and myelin, with relative preservation of axons, in foci that are usually widely distributed throughout the CNS but are confined to the CNS. The disease has a much higher prevalence in temperate zones than in the tropics and subtropical climates. There is evidence from rigorous epidemiologic studies of well-defined and stable populations, suggesting that the prevalence of MS has increased significantly throughout this century, from a rate of approximately 46/100,000 in 1915 to over 100/100,000 in the late 1970s, though at least part of this increase may be apparent, a reflection of the increasing sophistication of diagnostic and ascertainment methods, etc., that allow for the definitive diagnosis of a greater number of cases. A careful study in Olmsted County and Rochester, Minnesota (home of the Mayo Clinic), has shown age- and sex-adjusted prevalence rates of approx. 175/100,000. The annual incidence of MS is about twice as high in women as men—7 vs. 3/100,000, with a possibly rising incidence of the illness. Median age of onset is 34 years for males, 32 years for females.

Studies of changes in MS incidence as a function of migration at different ages and to/from populations with varying incidence of MS at different ages have produced fascinating data. The overall aim of this work has been to ascertain the relative roles of environmental vs. genetic risk factors for the development of MS. When individuals migrate after adolescence, they retain a risk of developing MS which coincides with their nation of origin, whereas when they migrate at a younger age they "take on" the risk associated with the environment to which they have relocated. Among groups migrating to Israel, the prevalence of MS was five to 10 times higher among northern European immigrants than among those from Africa or Asia or, indeed, among natives of Israel. Comparable investigations have been carried out in Japanese populations (in Japan and the U.S.) and among South Africans (immigrants vs. natives). Studies of this sort continue in an attempt to characterize true disease incidence among genetically well-characterized groups. In general, living in tropical/subtropical zones appears to be protective against the development of MS, whereas undefined "risk factors" are more common in the environment of temperate climates.

Theories of the etiology of MS could easily fill a book in themselves—and would make for fascinating reading! At various times, CNS trauma, exposure to heavy metals (including zinc, lead), diet (especially one high in fat), and autoimmune theories of pathogenesis have had data produced in their support. Genetic factors appear to be significant; i.e., monozygotic twins have greater than 25% concordance for MS, whereas dizygotic twins and control (nontwin) subjects show around 2% concordance for the disease. Furthermore, certain major histocompatibility complex (MHC) haplotypes are associated with MS, including A3, B7 (of MHC class I alleles), DR2, and Dw2 (of MHC class II). The neuropathologic features of MS, however, tend to favor an autoimmune/infectious/postinfectious etiology. Genetic and environmental studies support the general view that MS results from an environmental influence acting upon genetically susceptible individuals.

Over past decades, virtually every virus known to infect humans and several viruses that are thought to be restricted to subhuman primates have been implicated in the pathogenesis of MS, though at this time none has been conclusively proven to be its cause. A viral etiology for MS seems biologically attractive; a persistent infectious agent might be expected to produce multifocal death of oligodendrocytes with associated demyelination and chronic inflammation. Leading viral etiologic candidates over the years have included RNA- and DNA-containing agents, including herpesviruses (most recently human herpesvirus type 6; HHV-6), measles, and retroviruses (e.g., HTLV-1, which is known to produce a chronic inflammatory neurologic condition that involves brain and spinal cord and has some similarities to MS; see Chapter 4). Polymerase chain reaction (PCR) and in situ hybridization methodologies have been extensively utilized to look for an agent that might be *uniquely* associated with demyelinating plaques of MS; none has been proven to be of etiologic significance, though many viruses or their genes have been localized to MS plaques by various methodologies. Despite this, viruses that infect the CNS of various animals are known to produce (in these species) conditions that usually have a component of acute or chronic demyelination and thus show similarities to MS. This group of agents includes canine distemper virus (a paramyxovirus), visna virus (a nononcogenic retrovirus) in sheep, JHM virus (a coronavirus) in rats and mice, and Theiler's virus (a picornavirus) in mice.

An autoimmune pathogenesis for MS also has attractive features. An antigen on myelin might be mistaken as foreign, with the result that lymphocytes and macrophages "attack" the myelin sheath and cause it to be stripped from CNS axons. The inflammatory cells that invade the brain/spinal cord in MS have variable immunophenotypes; i.e., some are macrophages/histiocytes, others T-lymphocytes (including $CD8^+$ [cytotoxic/suppressor] and $CD4^+$ [helper/inducer]), and are found in the CNS in variable proportions, dependent on what stage of the disease is examined by the neuropathologist. Though in MS there is probably a movement of monocytes back and forth between the blood and the brain, the macrophage is regarded as a key "effector" cell in disease causation. The final common pathway of disease, demyelination, is mediated at least in part by lymphokines/cytokines secreted by infiltrating inflammatory cells—both are commonly present at various stages of MS (for an excellent review, see Navikas and Link; Ref. 22). Though no completely faithful animal model for MS exists, the best fit is a variant of an autoimmune condition, experimental allergic encephalomyelitis (EAE), in the course of which animals develop chronic inflammatory and demyelinating lesions—sometimes with a relapsing and remitting course—in the CNS after "immunization" with brain/spinal cord extracts.

Other immunologic theories for the etiology of MS include the "bystander" hypothesis, by which CNS myelin is an innocent bystander that is injured/destroyed because of an immune response occurring within the CNS; such theories might explain how more than one infectious agent could lead to a chronic demyelinating condition; i.e., various agents might induce CNS inflammation, a consequence of which would be the release of lymphocytes and macrophages that are toxic to the myelin sheat. Another scenario involves immune destruction of persistently infected oligodendrocytes; such a theory incorporates components of both the infectious and autoimmune theories described briefly above. This would result in a "dying-back" gliopathy affecting the distal (myelin-producing) components of oligodendrocytes. Attractive as this disease mechanism might appear, no agent causing persistent oligodendroglial infection that might trigger an immune response has yet been identified. Abnormal cell-mediated immune responses almost certainly have a role in the pathogenesis of MS, including its less common variants. Anomalous immune responses to myelin component proteins, especially myelin basic protein (MBP), myelin-associated glycoprotein, and proteolipid protein (PLP; or apoprotein), have also been implicated.

B. Clinical Features

MS has extremely variable clinical manifestations, depending on what part(s) of the CNS it affects. It is a disease for which clinical history and neurologic examination are still essentially diagnostic: for the diagnosis to be sustained, there must be evidence for CNS lesions disseminated in space and time. "Clinically definite" MS is defined by the presence of two attacks and clinical evidence of two separate lesions, or two attacks with clinical evidence of one lesion and "paraclinical" evidence of another, separate lesion. The disease may present with virtually any symptom (the most common are paresthesias, gait difficulty, weakness or incoordination of one or both lower extremities, or visual loss secondary to retrobulbar neuritis) or neurologic sign (common ones encountered include absent abdominal reflexes, hyperactive deep tendon reflexes, lower-limb ataxia, and bilateral Babinski signs or upgoing toes reflecting corticospinal tract demyelination).

The clinical diagnosis can be supported by several laboratory investigations. Helpful laboratory tests include:

1. Presence within CSF of IgG oligoclonal bands or evidence for increased CNS synthesis of IgG; the former correlates with the existence of plasma cells within demyelinating MS plaques.
2. Abnormalities of (electrophysiologically determined) evoked potentials (e.g., brainstem auditory and somatosensory evoked potentials).
3. Neuroimaging studies, especially magnetic resonance imaging (MRI), which is particularly sensitive to white matter/myelinated tract abnormalities; this technique shows abnormal results in as many as 95% of patients with clinically definite MS.

Unfortunately, none of these ancillary tests is fully specific on its own—all must be interpreted in the light of clinical history and the patient's neurologic examination. For instance, CSF abnormalities of IgG may be detected in a variety of inflammatory/infectious neurologic disorders. However, they are helpful aids in arriving at a diagnosis that was, as recently as 30 years ago, one made on purely clinical criteria.

MS may run an extremely variable course. Indeed, classic demyelinating plaques of MS are not infrequently encountered at autopsy in asymptomatic patients who die of other causes. At least one-fifth of MS patients have a relatively benign course for 15 years or longer. A minority have a fulminant course, progressing to death within a few weeks or months. A fortunate few experience only two or three disease "exacerbations" throughout their lifetime, during which they become symptomatic for a few days or weeks, only to make a complete recovery. Remission (or significant diminution in relapse rate) during pregnancy has been well documented in several clinical investigations but there is an increased risk of relapse in the 6-month postpartum period. Though no definitive treatment for MS currently exists, immunosuppressive therapy is of benefit to some patients (particularly during exacerbations), and encouraging clinical trials utilizing various immunomodulators (e.g., β-interferon) are currently under way.

C. Neuropathologic Features

1. Gross Abnormalities

The lesions of classic (Charcot type) MS may be apparent at the time of examination of brain and spinal cord during the necropsy. They appear as well-defined and clearly demarcated regions of myelin less on the surface of the brain and spinal cord, since these are structures (unlike the cerebral hemispheres) where myelinated tracts extend to the pial surface (Fig. 1). The prosector will be guided in his or her search for plaques by the patient's clinical history: one who experienced primarily paraparesis/quadriparesis will be expected to show mainly spinal cord abnormalities, whereas one whose major complaint during life was ataxia and vertigo would more likely have brainstem and/or cerebellar plaques. However, "clinically silent" plaques are found in the brains of almost all MS patients who come to autopsy.

At the time of brain cutting, MS plaques present much as they do on the brain/spinal cord surface—i.e., as well-demarcated regions of myelin loss—with preservation of the underlying "scaffolding" of the white matter tracts—i.e., their axonal component (Figs. 2, 3). In this way they differ from cerebral infarcts, which also show loss of brain substance but manifest absence of the axons in addition to the myelin, usually with associated cystic cavitation (see Chap. 2). MS plaques often have a gray gelatinous appearance when the brain is cut (Fig. 4). Furthermore, MS plaques are more likely to be found adjacent to a CSF interface (i.e., lining a ventricle or a pial surface), though they may occur deep within the white matter of the centrum semiovale or even adjacent to and extending into the cortex (Fig. 5), and may be relatively symmetrical between the cerebral hemispheres in both size and location (e.g., surrounding the lateral ventricles).

2. *Microscopic Features*

Most cases of MS seen at autopsy are examples of "burnt-out" disease; i.e., the patient has had the illness for years or even decades. In these individuals, the plaques of demyelination have a fairly stereotypical appearance, viz. as predicted by the gross appearance of the brain/spinal cord they demonstrate well-demarcated zones of myelin loss with relative preservation of axons (Fig. 6); these changes can be highlighted with the appropriate stains for myelin (e.g., Luxol fast blue) and axons (Bielschowsky) (Fig. 7). In fact, longstanding plaques can show significant axon loss as well, even leading to Wallerian degeneration distally, e.g., in the spinal cord (Fig. 8). Intense astrocytic gliosis is common in the plaque itself (Fig. 9), a region where oligodendrocytes are scarce or absent. The optic chiasm and nerves, frequently involved in MS, can show extremely patchy/focal demyelination (Fig. 10). Inflammation, when present, takes the form of perivascular lymphocyte cuffing, but at autopsy this is seen with variable frequency and may be absent even in severe cases of longstanding MS.

Rarely, lesions of acute/subacute MS that present with unusual neuroimaging features, sometimes even as a mass leseion, will undergo diagnostic biopsy. The neuropathologist must always be aware of this possibility when

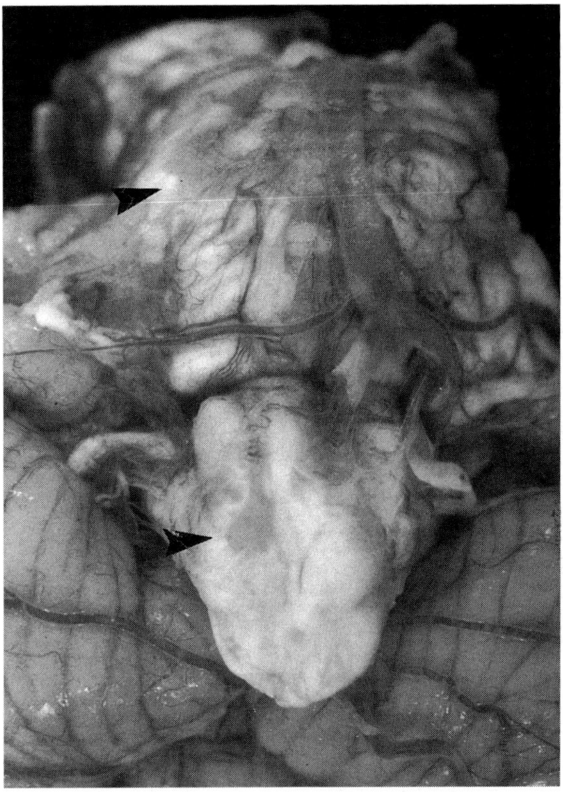

Figure 1 External view of pons and cerebellum from a patient with longstanding MS. Note well-demarcated regions/plaques of demyelination visible on both the external aspect of the pons (upper arrowhead) and at the cut section of the medulla (lower arrowhead).

reviewing surgically derived material. A lesion at this stage is more likely to show evidence of acute/subacute myelin breakdown with the presence of foamy histiocytes/gitter cells. By electron microscopy, such biopsies show perivascular inflammatory cells closely apposed to myelin sheaths, astrocytic proliferation even at some distance from demyelinating plaques, and unusual intracytoplasmic macrophage inclusions.

Some MS plaques show partial preservation of myelin. Such partly demyelinated plaques are often seen adjacent to regions of complete demyelination; these are sometimes referred to as "shadow plaques." In a given lesion, it is

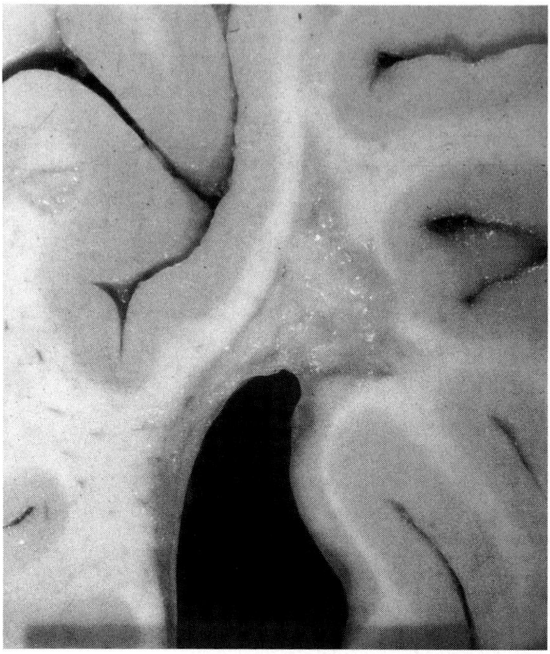

(A)

Figure 2 Demyelinating plaques of severe longstanding MS. (A) shows a single well-demarcated plaque, whereas (B) illustrates two periventricular plaques, both apparently showing more complete demyelination than that illustrated in (A).

impossible to ascertain whether such a plaque represents a focus of "partial demyelination" or "remyelination," both of which almost certainly occur in the disease (hence its relapsing and remitting nature). For an excellent review of the molecular pathophysiology of signs and symptoms in MS, see the review by Waxman, ref. 34.

3. MS "Variants"

The Charcot type of MS is by far the most common variant encountered in daily practice. Several rare entities probably linked etiologically to MS are described, as follows.

a. Acute MS (Marburg variant). A fulminant form of MS which occurs primarily in younger patients, and is usually associated with a rapidly progressive downhill course. The neuropathologic features show more prominent tissue de-

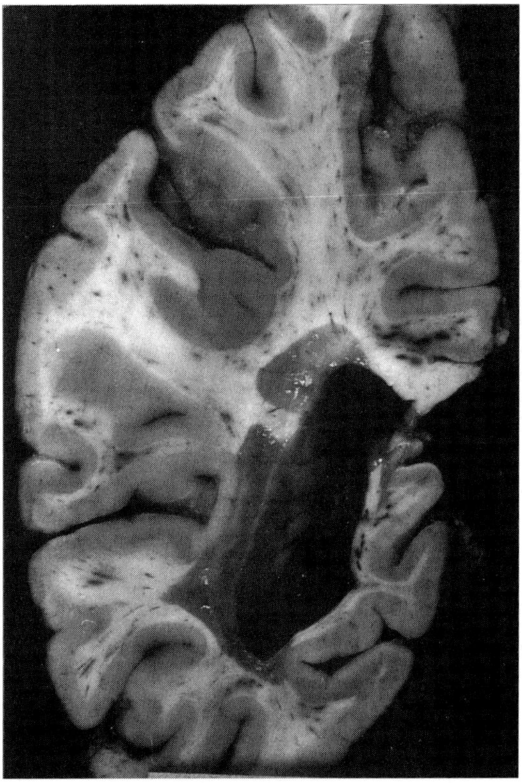

(B)

struction (i.e., not simply demyelination) with (in the acute phase) abundant tissue macrophages which sometimes show a mild to moderate degree of nuclear atypia. In the modern era, when destructive lesions (particularly if puzzling on CT or MRI) are likely to undergo diagnostic biopsy, this lesion is more commonly encountered in surgical (not just autopsy) material, as for the example illustrated in Figure 11.

b. Neuromyelitis Optica (*Devic's disease*). In this condition, demyelinating lesions typical of Charcot-type MS are encountered only in the optic nerve(s) and spinal cord, hence the descriptive name. Optic neuritis usually causes visual impairment/blindness in both eyes, though not necessarily simultaneously; myelopathy may precede or postdate visual abnormalities by months or years. Males and females are equally affected among reported examples, and onset is

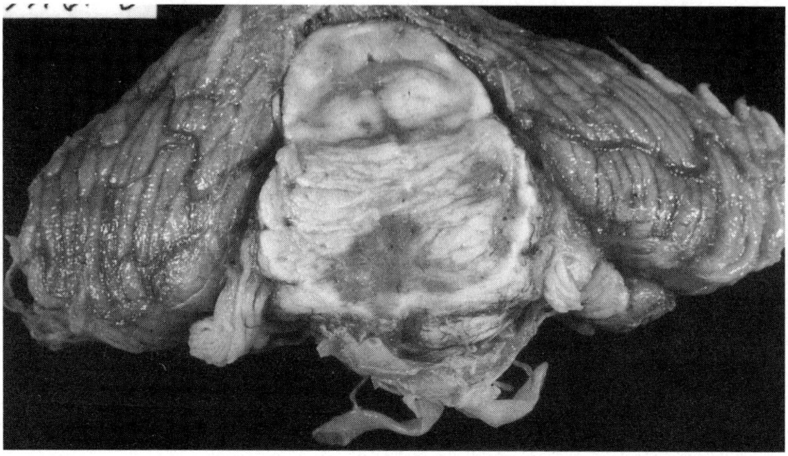

Figure 3 Multiple demyelinating plaques of MS in both the basis pontis (in some places abutting the pial surface) and pontine tegmentum.

somewhat later than for Charcot-type MS, usually between ages 30 and 50 years. The disease tends to have acute onset and to be rapidly progressive in approximately half of affected patients. A typical example is illustrated in Figure 12.

c. *Balo's Concentric Sclerosis.* First described in 1928 as "encephalitis periaxialis concentrica," this rare disease presents in young patients with acute onset, strokelike symptoms, and absence of remissions and exacerbations—i.e., a monophasic course. The morphologic appearance of affected tissue yields a spectacular onionskin-like appearance of "layers" of demyelinated and (more normally) myelinated white matter, the latter possibly representing demyelinated white matter that has become remyelinated. Intermediate forms between Charcot-type MS and Balo's concentric sclerosis have been described, especially among Japanese patients.

d. *Schilder's Disease* (*diffuse sclerosis*). This condition shows some similarities to both classical MS and leukodystrophy (see below and Chap. 9). In some ways, this may be regarded as an extreme form of MS, with bihemispheric widespread demyelination, though with scattered, otherwise typical MS plaques. Axonal injury, cavitation, and even Wallerian degeneration may occur, though there is usually sparing of the subcortical "U fibers." In such a brain encountered at autopsy, leukodystrophy must be excluded as a diagnostic consideration. Often diagnosed in adolescents (in the second decade of life), it must be in the clinical differential diagnosis of "mental deterioration" in this age group.

III. DYSMYELINATING DISEASES/LEUKODYSTROPHIES

The metabolic basis of these conditions, which result in variably severe and rapid degradation of CNS myelin in (depending on the specific disorder) children or adults, will be discussed in detail in Chapter 9. From a diagnostic viewpoint in considering the differential of abnormalities that affect white matter, these disorders usually begin earlier in life (some in infancy) though they may present during adult life, have a progressive downhill course (unlike the "waxing and waning" course of Charcot-type MS), and show diffuse white

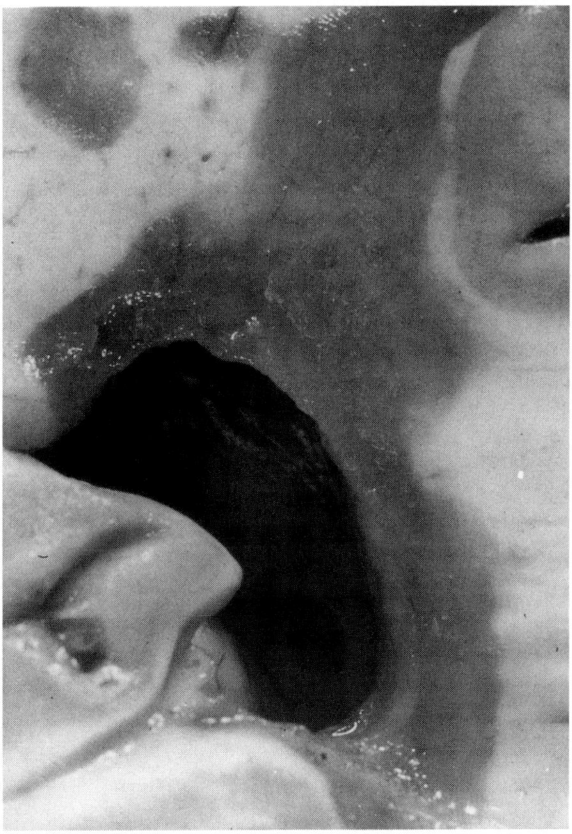

Figure 4 Magnified view of a periventricular MS plaque shows its gelatinous, glistening appearance; however, unlike in a cystic infarct, the axonal "scaffolding" of the white matter is preserved.

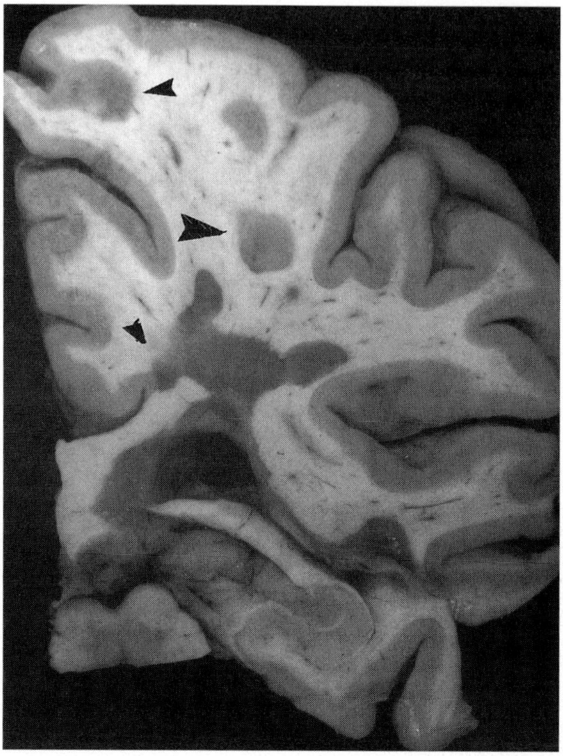

Figure 5 Though MS plaques favor proximity to CSF pathways (e.g., the ependymal lining of the ventricular system or a pial surface), they may occur in the centrum semiovale or in a subcortical location (arrowheads), sometimes even extending into the cortex.

matter abnormalities, not the multifocal, well-delineated demyelinating lesions of MS.

IV. DEMYELINATING CONDITIONS ASSOCIATED WITH SYSTEMIC/METABOLIC ABNORMALITIES

A. Central Pontine Myelinolysis (CPM)

This condition, first recognized in the late 1950s, is identified pathologically as a variably sized region of demyelination most prominent within the basis pontis. Within the pons, affected regions of demyelination may range from very tiny to very large (Fig. 13), the latter being most easily recognized in cut sections of the pons at the time of brain cutting.

1. Etiologic and Epidemiologic Considerations

The condition was initially described in alcoholic and malnourished patients, so its etiology was at first felt to be tied to these clinical states, especially alcoholism. It soon became clear, however, that in many cases metabolic abnormalities frequently found in alcoholics, rather than alcoholism *per se*, were causally associated with CPM. Specifically, CPM was associated with a rapid, sustained (usually iatrogenic) increase in serum sodium levels from a hyponatremic baseline; hyponatremia is defined in most studies as serum Na^+ below 130 mEq/L or mmol/L, and very often it is below 115 to 120 mEq/L. Indeed, CPM-like lesions can easily be induced in various experimental animals (rabbits, dogs, rats) after rapid correction of vasopressin-induced hyponatremia, though of interest, regions of demyelination are often found in white matter structures other than the pons (e.g., hemispheric white matter, hippocampal fimbria, anterior commissure, and cerebellum) which is, however, also frequently affected. Animals in which hyponatremia only was induced failed to show similar lesions. Rates of change in serum sodium levels necessary to induce CPM have been estimated (in one study) to be on the order of 8 mEq/L per day, sustained for at least 5 days. Patients with chronic hepatic disease—particularly alcohol-induced—are especially likely to show CPM (one study estimates CPM to occur in as many as 9% to 10% of such individuals) so that the initial apparent association of CPM with alcohol abuse may simply have reflected this fact. In general autopsy populations, the incidence of "incidental CPM" has been estimated to be as high as 0.5% to 1.0%.

Not all patients who are found to have CPM at necropsy have a clear-cut history of corrected hyponatremia—as many as 40% to 50% may not. Orthotopic liver transplantation is also associated with a high incidence of subsequent CPM, in as many as 10% to 15% of patients who come to autopsy. Specific etiologic factors in these individuals are extremely difficult to ascertain, since their perioperative course is almost invariably associated with wide swings not only in serum Na^+ but in serum glucose, osmolality, and plasma levels of various drugs that might contribute to myelinolysis.

2. Clinical Features

These are poorly understood. CPM is still, despite modern imaging advances, largely a postmortem diagnosis. Some studies using MRI suggest that CPM is a reversible disorder. Clinical signs and symptoms that might be expected in a patient with a (primarily) demyelinative lesion of the basis pontis would include corticospinal tract signs (hyperreactive deep tendon reflexes, spasticity, upgoing toes); however, CPM (surprisingly) often spares these descending fiber tracts. In rare patients in whom particularly detailed clinicopathologic correlation has been carried out, other features observed have included decerebrate posturing, small reactive pupils and bilateral paresis of the sixth cranial nerve. CPM al-

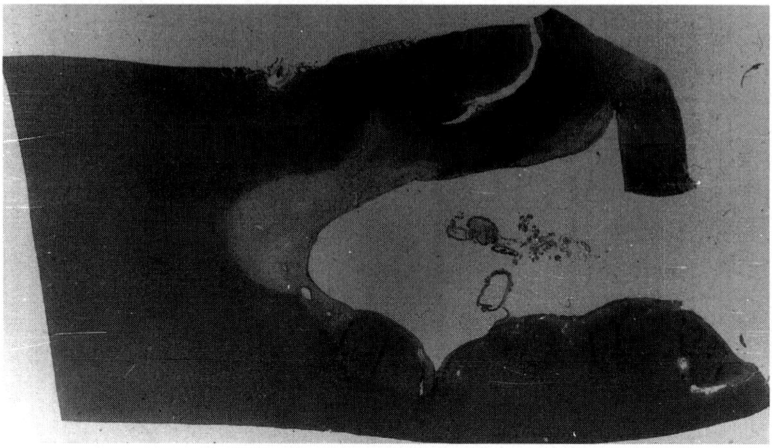

(A)

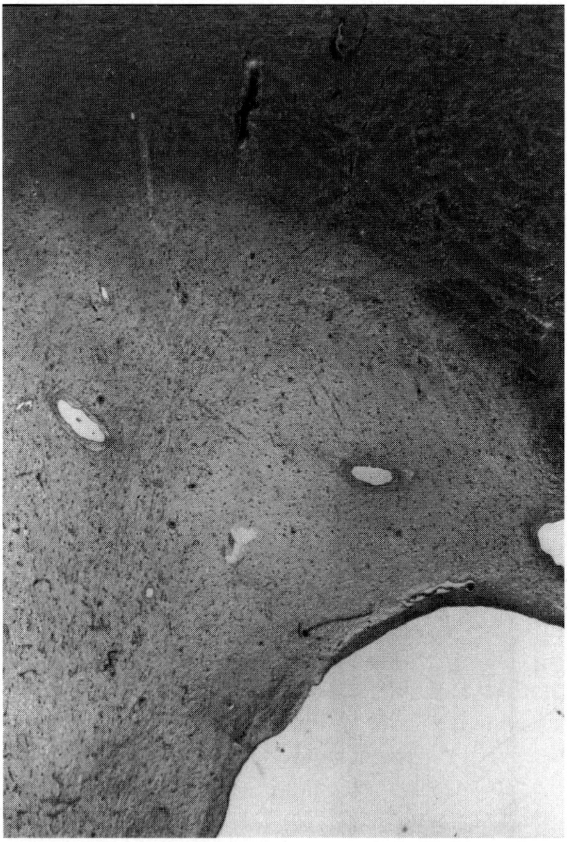

(B)

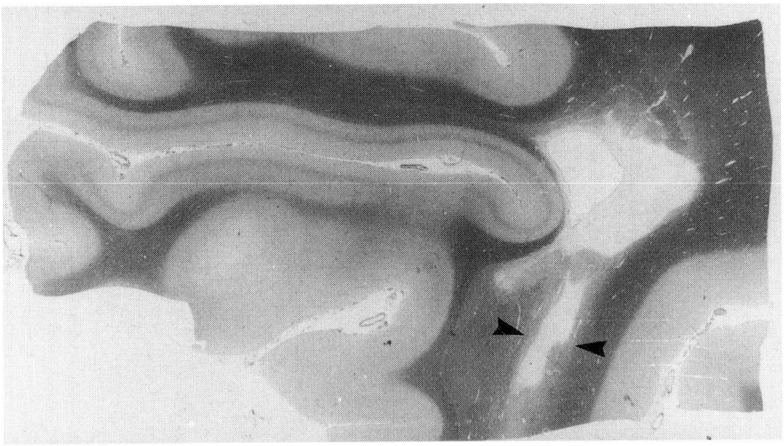

(C)

Figure 6 Well-demarcated demyelinating plaques of MS are easily seen on H&E-stained sections of affected brain, even without the benefit of microscopic examination. (A) Periventricular region from same specimen, shown at higher magnification in (B). They are particularly dramatic in sections stained specifically for myelin (C). Panel C shows a periventricular plaque and a smaller, slitlike plaque in the deeper white matter (arrowheads).

most exclusively occurs in adults though rare pediatric—including infantile—cases have been reported.

Within the past 5 to 10 years, the disease spectrum of CPM and extrapontine myelinolysis has been expanded to include a broader group of neurologic disorders, many of them reversible, that occur in patients with severe hyponatremia—usually below levels of 116 mmol/L and sometimes as low as 100 to 105. Clinical studies clearly indicate that patients in whom serum Na^+ is raised at a rate more rapid than 12 mmol/L/day worsen neurologically, whereas those in whom serum Na^+ is raised more slowly had uneventful neurologic recoveries. The terms *osmotic demyelination syndrome* and *osmotic myelinolysis* have been coined for this constellation of neurologic disorders associated with electrolyte abnormalities. Furthermore, it has been suggested that increased serum osmolality (rather than altered sodium levels *per se*) may play a role in their etiology.

3. *Neuropathologic Features*

Depending on the extent and duration of the lesion, CPM can, though infrequently, be recognized at the time of brain cutting as a region of softening

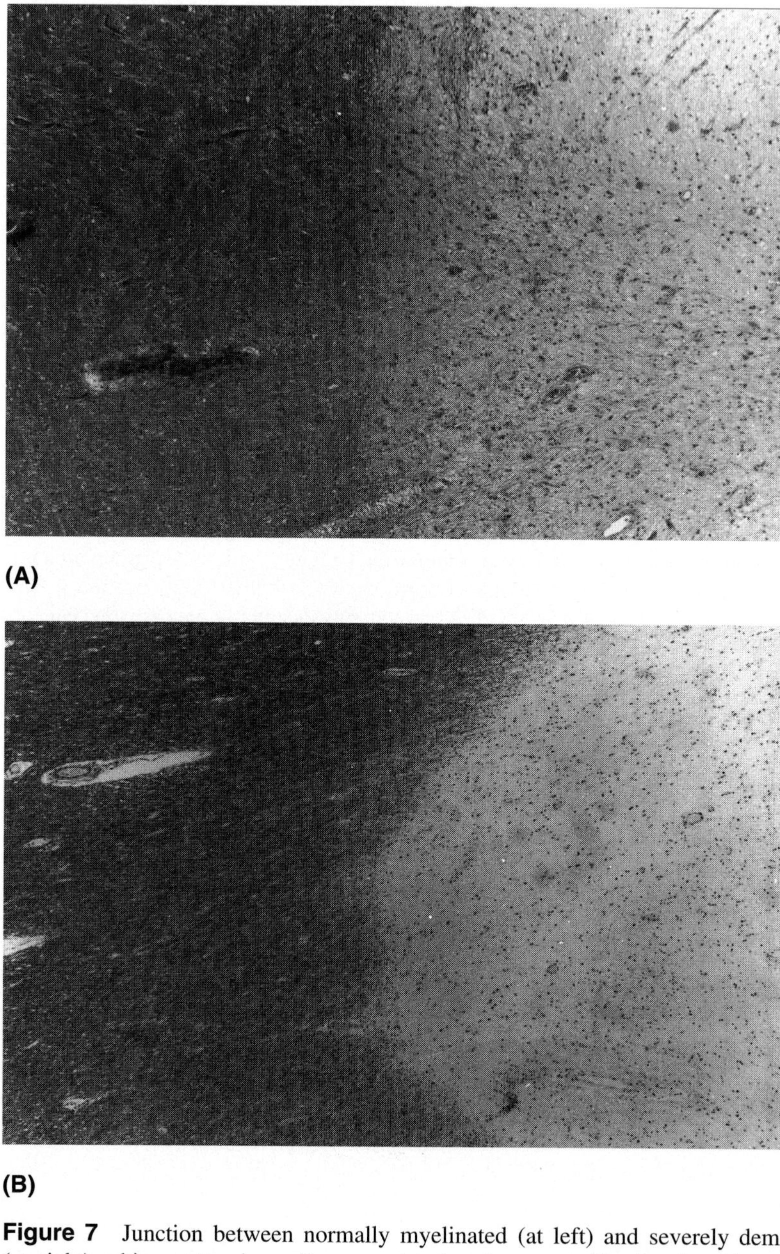

(A)

(B)

Figure 7 Junction between normally myelinated (at left) and severely demyelinated (at right) white matter is easily appreciated at low magnification in either an H&E-stained (A) or myelin-stained (B) section. The high cellularity of the demyelinated white matter is due to astrocytic gliosis, better seen in panel (A) (see also Fig. 9).

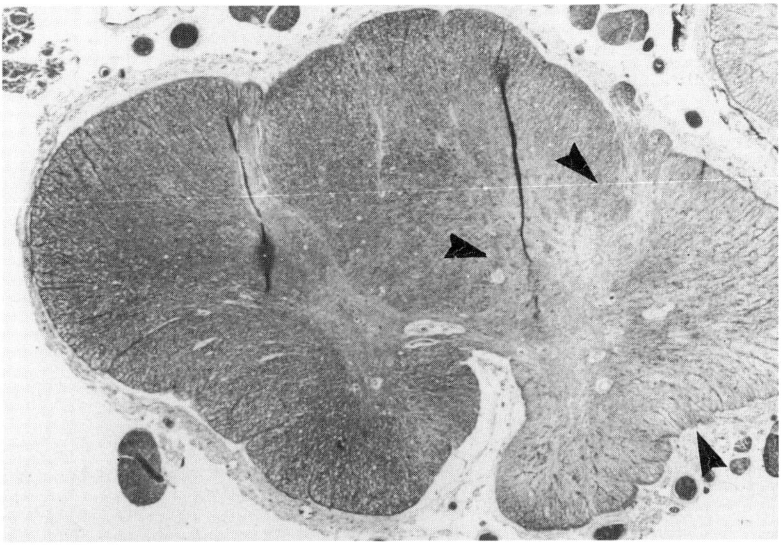

Figure 8 Demyelinating plaque (MS) in thoracic spinal cord affects almost half of its cross-sectional area (delineated by arrowheads). Typical of MS plaques, it does *not* respect tract boundaries.

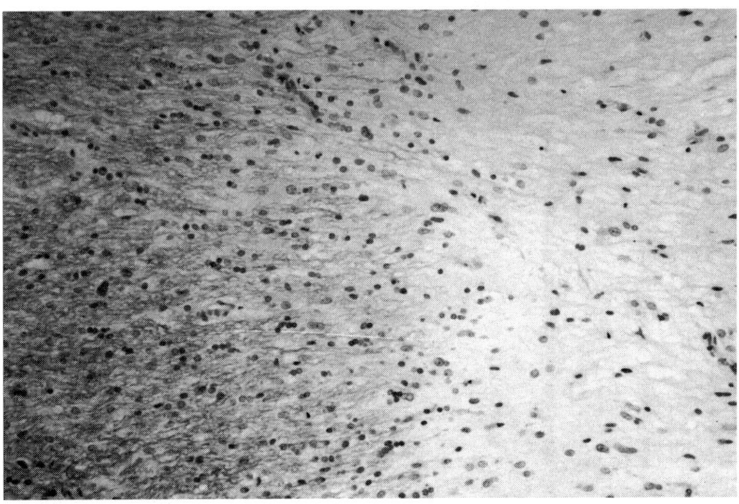

Figure 9 The relatively high cellularity of an MS plaque (right half of figure) is due to astrocytic proliferation/scarring. By contrast, left half of panel shows relatively preserved myelin, with residual oligodendrocytes.

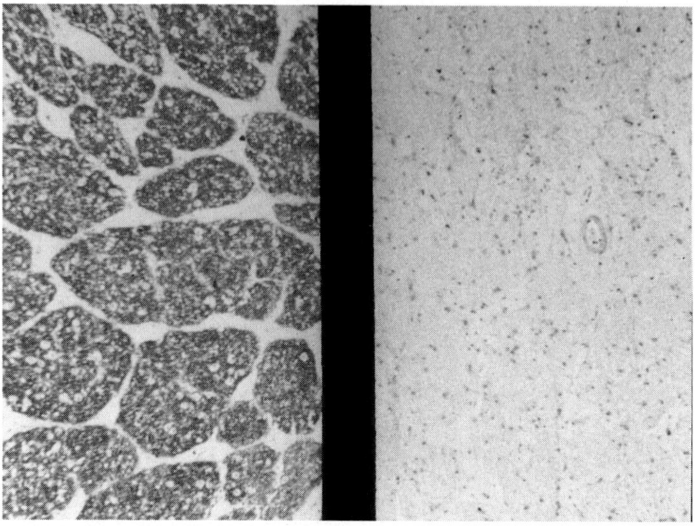

Figure 10 Optic nerves (ONs) from an MS patient stained for myelin. Whereas one ON (left panel) shows entirely normal myelination, the other (right panel) shows almost total demyelination. The two panels are from sections photographed at comparable magnifications, after identical staining conditions.

(sometimes closely resembling an ischemic infarct) in the basis pontis. However, the diagnosis is more often made at the time histologic sections are examined. Myelin-stained sections, and even H&E-stained sections, show a well-demarcated region of demyelination, *usually* with preservation of axons and neuronal cell bodies, i.e., of the pontine nuclei, in the basis pontis (Figs. 14, 15). When small, a focus of CPM is usually diamond-shaped, with only demyelination of crossing pontocerebellar tracts; when large, lesions are often cruciate, or "bat wing," in shape (Fig. 14), with frequently preservation of the descending corticospinal and corticobulbar tracts.

Microscopically, CPM is almost identical to the typical demyelinative plaques of Charcot-type MS; myelin and oligodendrocytes are absent, whereas axons *tend* to be preserved. Regions of CPM are very well demarcated from normally myelinated pontine fibers (Fig. 15). Lesions can be crudely classified as *acute*, with demyelination only; *active or subacute*, with abundant macrophages (Fig. 16); or *chronic*, with myelin loss and astrocytic gliosis left as "footprints" of the pathologic process. Cavitation does not usually occur, though in severe subacute cases abundant macrophages and neuroaxonal spheroids (indicative of axonal injury) are seen, the latter especially prominent at the edges of foci of CPM. The anatomic location and symmetry of the lesion together with the (usual) absence of cavitation distinguish a CPM lesion from a

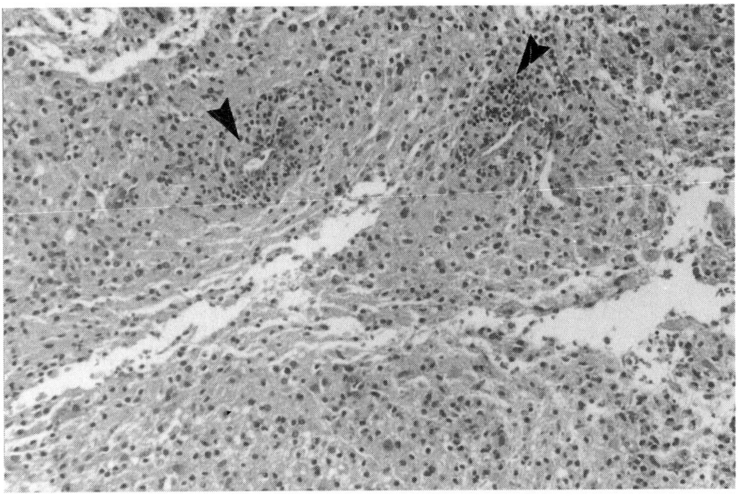

(A)

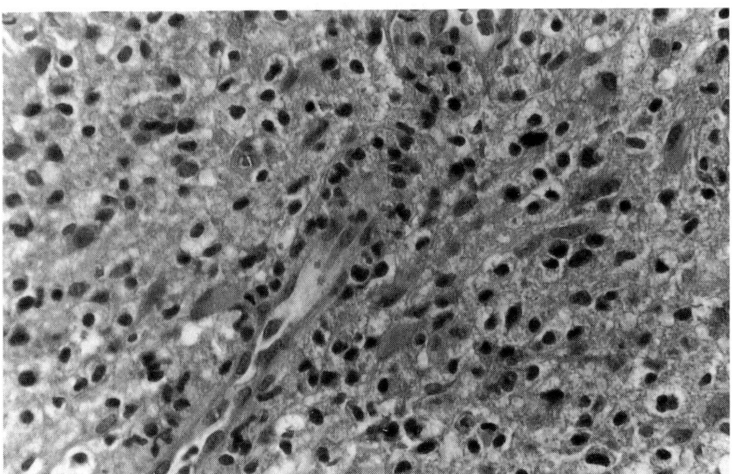

(B)

Figure 11 Acute fulminant (Marburg type) MS in a 22-year-old female with a 2-week history of numbness and paresis of the right arm and leg. Imaging studies showed multifocal brain lesions, one of which was biopsied. Sections showed a cellular but relatively monomorphous lesion with some scattered atypical astrocytes (not illustrated). Scattered perivascular cuffs of mononuclear lymphocytes were seen (arrows, panel A). At higher magnification (B), most of the cells were seen to be typical macrophages/histiocytes. The patient made a remarkably good initial recovery on steroids (subsequent clinical details not available).

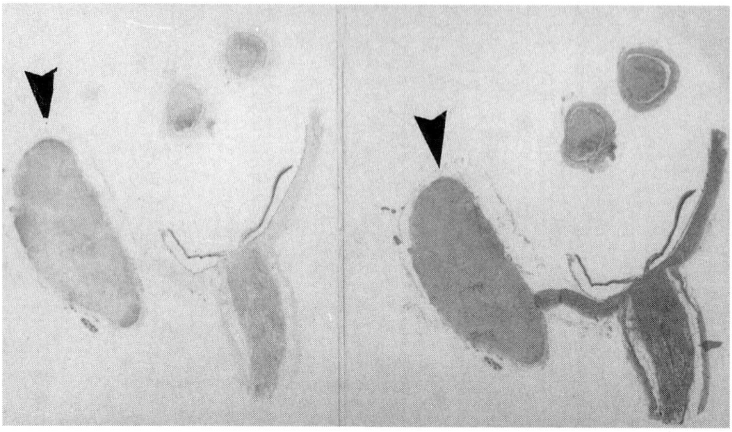

Figure 12 Neuromyelitis optica/Devic's disease. Sections are of spinal cord (arrowheads), optic nerves (two levels in transverse section), and posterior portion of eye together with ON cut in longitudinal section. Right half of photograph from sections stained with H&E; left half from parallel sections stained for myelin. Note almost complete demyelination of both ON and spinal cord; only thin subpial rims of preserved myelin are seen in both structures.

pontine infarct; only its location and "clinical context" distinguish a focus of CPM from a demyelinating plaque of chronic MS!

Extrapontine foci of CPM can occur almost anywhere where myelinated fiber tracts are present in the CNS; in our experience, foci are particularly prominent in cerebellar white matter, but they may be seen in subcortical white matter of the centrum semiovale; the thalami (where they may be quite symmetrical); internal, external, and extreme capsules; and even the lateral geniculate nuclei. At least one report describes exclusively extrapontine regions of CPM *without* involvement of the pons itself.

B. Multifocal Necrotizing Leukoencephalopathy (MNL)

This puzzling lesion is best considered here, as it also tends to favor pontine tracts, in particular the (crossing) pontocerebellar fibers; indeed, some have argued that it represents a variant of CPM, though regions of MNL are more consistently necrotic than are foci of CPM, and there are important differences in the clinical context for the two lesions.

1. Etiologic and Clinical Considerations

MNL differs from CPM in terms of the patient population in which it occurs: MNL is observed almost exclusively in the CNS of patients who are immuno-

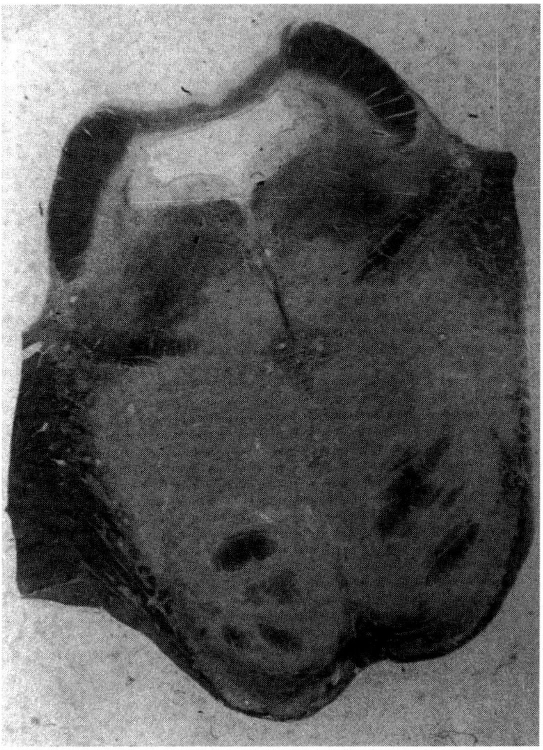

Figure 13 Severe central pontine myelinolysis (CPM) in an adult (myelin-stained section). Note almost complete (bilaterally symmetrical) demyelination of the basis pontis, with extension of demyelinated zone into the pontine tegmentum. There is, despite the extent of the lesion, *relative* sparing of the corticospinal tracts.

suppressed, whether as a function of infectious or naturally occurring disease (e.g., AIDS, leukemia, lymphoma, severe combined immunodeficiency [SCID]), or iatrogenic immunosuppression following bone marrow or organ transplantation. Lesions identical to MNL were initially described in patients with CNS or extra-CNS malignancies who had received cranial radiotherapy and/or intrathecal chemotherapy. MNL may be quite common, depending on how thoroughly the pons is examined; the lesions are tiny and almost never predictable from any grossly apparent feature of the pons (or any other region of the brain) at the time of brain cutting.

Precise etiologic factors have been difficult to pinpoint. Metabolic abnormalities of the type usually noted in the histories of patients with CPM are conspicuously absent. The strong association of these lesions with the immuno-

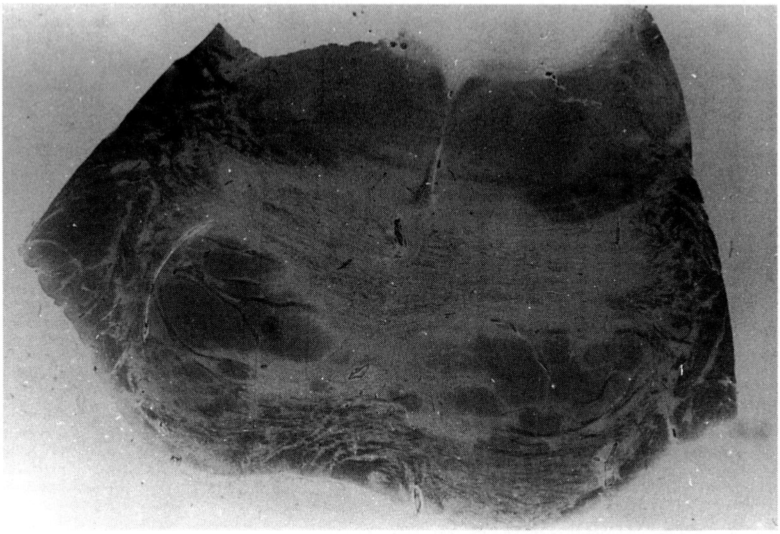

Figure 14 CPM in a 6-year-old child. This example is slightly less severe than the one illustrated in Figure 13. Note "bat wing"-type area of demyelination in basis pontis, with preservation of descending corticospinal tracts. (For case details, see Steinsapir and Vinters, 1985; Ref. 29).

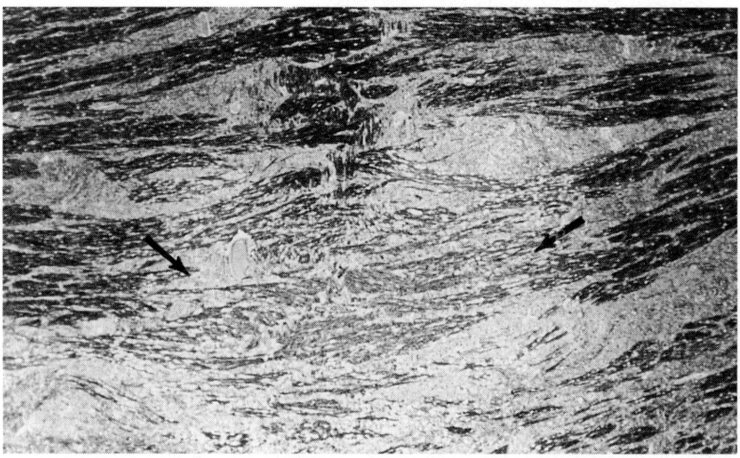

Figure 15 Low-power view of a (relatively) small region of CPM in a patient with AIDS. In this section stained for myelin, arrows indicate a region in which myelin is lost (from pontocerebellar fibers) but axons appear preserved.

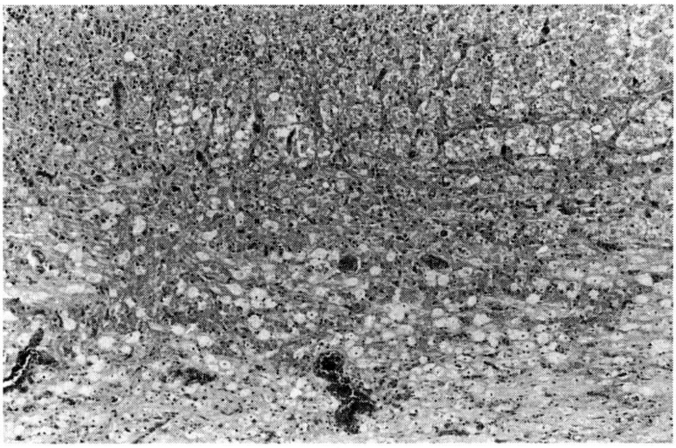

Figure 16 Microscopic appearance of severe CPM (section is from lesion illustrated in Fig. 14). Most of the cells shown are histiocytes, indicative of subacute demyelination.

suppressed state suggests that an opportunistic pathogen (e.g., an as yet unrecognized virus) may be of etiologic significance, though none has thus far been characterized. Lesions of MNL may represent unusual manifestations of cerebral anoxia/ischemia or infarct, but if so, it is puzzling that they are in general *not* associated with microvascular thrombi or any other form of microangiopathy and tend to occur almost exclusively in white matter tracts, which are widely perceived as being more resistant to anoxic/ischemic insults than are neurons. They may also result in part from medications that are frequently administered to immunosuppressed patients either prophylactically or therapeutically.

2. *Neuropathologic Features*

In one extraordinary case we have encountered and published, foci of MNL were so widespread and prominent in the basis pontis that they had caused a grossly visible expansile enlargement of this structure, suggestive of a primary brainstem neoplasm. Most often, the lesions are noted as small regions of necrosis, usually with prominent calcification and abundant neuroaxonal spheroids, predominantly in the pontocerebellar fibers (Fig. 17) with less frequent involvement of the descending corticospinal tracts. They may be single or numerous in a given case and can be found at multiple levels of the pons. Though they "favor" the basis pontis, MNL lesions can be found in extrapontine locations.

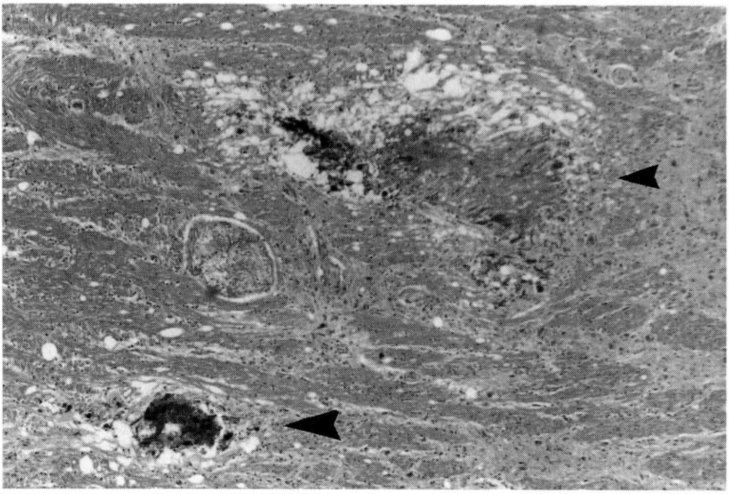

Figure 17 Multifocal necrotizing leukoencephalopathy (MNL). Two lesions (arrows) are noted in the basis pontis, an area of predilection for this lesion, usually found in immunosuppressed patients. Though of different size and configuration, both show peripheral vacuolization, central necrosis with calcification; neuroaxonal spheroids (not shown) are a prominent feature at higher magnification.

C. Marchiafava-Bignami Disease

1. Etiologic and Clinical Considerations

This is a very rare condition—a complication of ethanol abuse—characterized by degeneration of the corpus callosum and anterior commissure. Initially described in 1903, it was at first felt to be restricted to Italian patients who ingested large quantities of wine, but the condition has been reported in individuals around the world. Most cases occur in malnourished alcoholic males in the age range 45 to 60 years. Some patients are noted to have hepatic cirrhosis. Clinical manifestations are extremely variable, ranging from a frontal lobe disorder to slowly progressive dementia to hemiparesis. Systematic studies of clinicopathologic correlation are complicated by the extreme rarity of the condition and the plethora of clinical signs and pathologic features that are often to be found in long-term alcoholics who come to necropsy. Cessation of ethanol intake and improved nutritional status can lead to some amelioration of signs and symptoms, though patients who have progressed to the point of dementia persist, often for years, in a demented state. Clinical diagnosis is made with a high index of suspicion, and confirmation of callosal lesions by MRI scanning.

Indeed, the progression of neuropathologic change in the corpus callosum can be studied using serial MRI scans; these demonstrate initial diffuse swelling of this structure, taken to represent edema and demyelination, followed by (in the chronic stages) features suggestive of focal necrosis. Focal ischemic necrosis may be an explanation—or part of the explanation—for why the disorder occurs. For example, we have examined the brain of an elderly patient who developed extensive necrotic lesions of the central corpus callosum (Fig. 18) as an apparent intraoperative complication of vascular surgery (see Chap. 2).

2. Neuropathologic Features

Typically, there is destruction of the myelinated fibers in the corpus callosum, especially the central lamina of the genu, and the anterior commissure; rarely, extracallosal lesions are noted in the white matter of the centrum semiovale and middle cerebellar peduncles. Though the condition is described as a "leukoencephalopathy," cortical neuronal injury with astrocytic gliosis ("cortical laminar sclerosis") is found in layer III of the frontal and temporal cortex; presumably, this results from loss/injury of the (interhemispheric) callosal fibers. The astute reader will recognize the similarity of Marchiafava-Bignami lesions to those described as "extrapontine" CPM and MNL above, though the clinical substrates and predisposing factors for the three conditions vary sig-

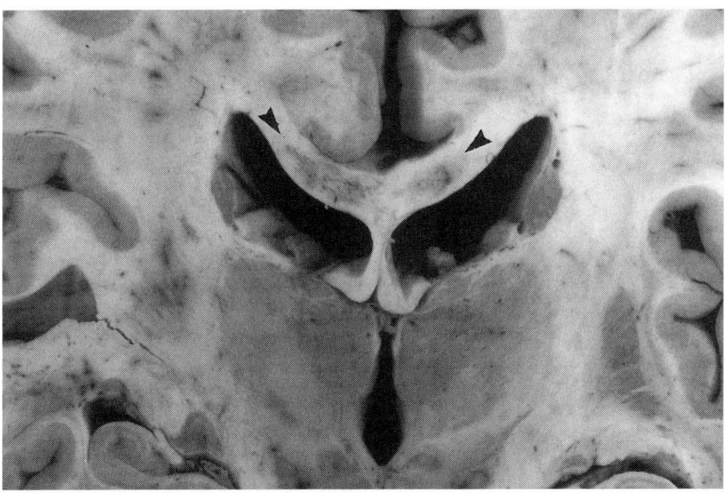

Figure 18 Marchiafava-Bignami-*like* lesion in an elderly individual who became "encephalopathic" after aortic surgeries. Note central regions of necrosis (arrowheads) in the middle of the corpus callosum. Sections showed features of subacute necrosis with large collections of macrophages; comparable lesions were found elsewhere in the brain, primarily within white matter. Etiology of the lesions was attributed to an unusual manifestation of anoxic/ischemic change with resultant necrosis.

nificantly. Nevertheless, certain common themes of etiopathogenesis may emerge over time as these disorders come to be understood more completely.

V. DEMYELINATION WITH INFECTIOUS POST- OR PARAINFECTIOUS/INFLAMMATORY CONDITIONS

Two diseases of white matter with well-defined (if incompletely understood) infectious etiologies have already been considered in Chapter 4; these are progressive multifocal leukoencephalopathy (PML) (an example of which is illustrated in Figure 19 solely for purposes of comparison with MS), and HIV encephalitis or AIDS-related leukoencephalopathy. Figure 20 highlights an approach to assessing the likely etiologic category of white matter disease, given certain gross characteristics of the lesions in cut sections of the brain.

A. Acute/Hyperacute Hemorrhagic Leukoencephalitis (AHL)

This disease, also known as Weston-Hurst syndrome, is an extremely rare idiopathic disorder of young adults characterized by a clinically fulminant course,

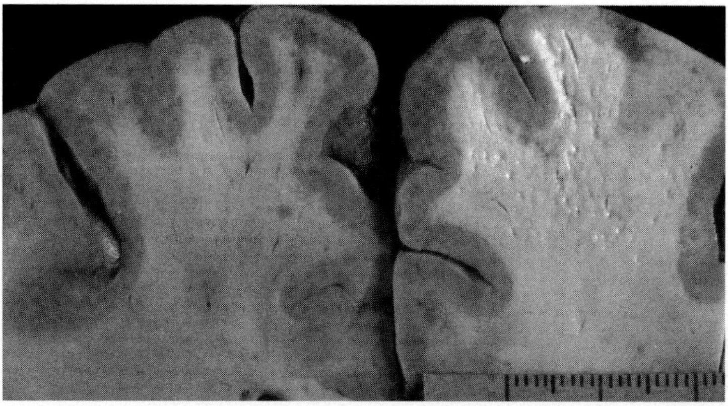

Figure 19 Progressive multifocal leukoencephalopathy in a patient with systemic lymphoma. Unlike the situation with demyelinating plaques of MS, white matter of the centrum semiovale shows ill-defined regions of "pitting," imparting a moth-eaten appearance to it. Cortex is relatively spared (grossly) though often involved on histologic sections. In this example, the abnormality is pronounced in the right cerebral hemisphere (right side of photograph), whereas that in the left is relatively spared. As is often the case, extent and severity of PML changes were asymmetrical between the two sides (see also Fig. 20).

with (usually, though not invariably) rapid progression to coma and death within 1 to 2 weeks. The brain at necropsy shows petechial hemorrhages throughout the white matter, caused by extensive microvascular injury with fibrinoid necrosis of (primarily) white matter microvessels; gross appearances of fixed brain slices are not unlike those of patients who have experienced cerebral fat emboli. Perivascular edema and hemorrhage are associated with demyelination and (sometimes) axonal injury. An allergic/autoimmune reaction to brain components (especially myelin) may represent its biologic basis; the lesions resemble those seen in hyperacute experimental allergic encephalomyelitis (EAE). It may be related to another relatively unusual entity, as follows.

B. Acute Disseminated Perivenous Encephalomyelitis (ADPVE)

In this condition, associated with a variety of viral diseases of childhood (e.g., measles, mumps, rubella) and less clearly with a history of recent vaccination, the patient becomes severely ill with a neurologic syndrome that follows shortly (usually within 1 to 2 weeks) upon the viral infection. It usually occurs in patients less than 35 years of age. Despite the fulminant onset, recovery from this illness may occur. Neuropathologic features include striking perivenous chronic (or acute) inflammation, with associated demyelination and preservation of axons throughout (especially) white matter, but also affecting gray matter. The similarities to monophasic MS are obvious. Subacute, late, and recurrent variants of the disease have been described; it is similar to the experimentally produced condition EAE. As vaccination programs in infancy render many of the putative viral pathogens thought to be responsible for cases of ADPVE rare infections of infancy and childhood, this condition may—hopefully will!—become a historical curiosity.

As Kepes (Ref. 18) has shown, large demyelinating regions in the CNS with histopathologic features intermediate between those of MS and ADPVE may rarely present as mass lesions—something for which the surgical neuropathologist must constantly be vigilant, especially at the time of frozen section of a brain biopsy from an "unusual mass lesion" in a young patient.

VI. "TOXIC" LEUKOENCEPHALOPATHIES

This is a heterogeneous group of disorders, none of them well-defined disease entities, that may result from the effects of various "insults" to the white matter (see also Chap. 9). Resultant neuropathologic lesions are also variably well characterized. White matter abnormalities that may result from exogenous, often iatrogenic, agents include the following.

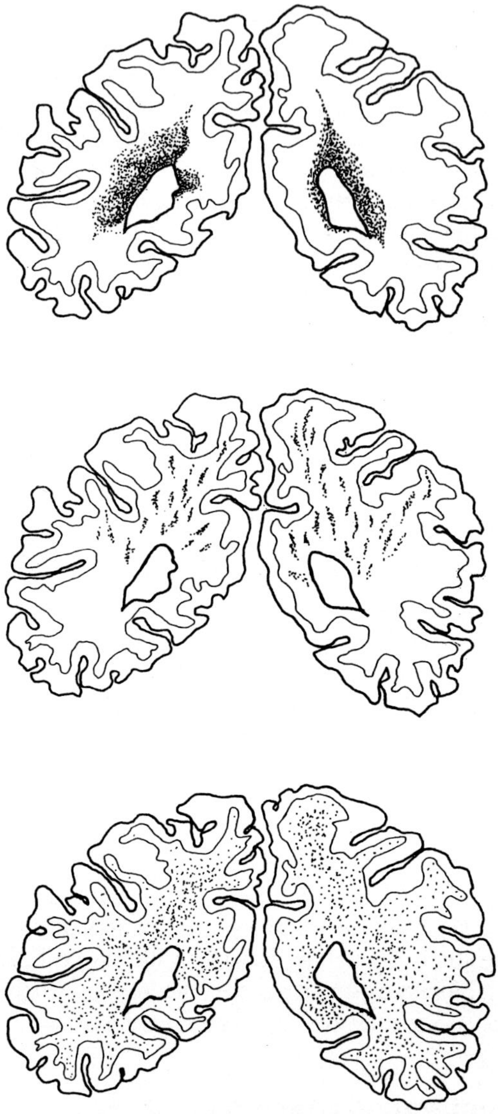

Figure 20 Schematic diagram summarizing essential differences among MS, PML, and leukodystrophy (for details, see text). (A) MS plaques: Usually well-demarcated, often periventricular and symmetrical. (B) PML: Multifocal, poorly demarcated areas of "moth-eaten" white matter, usually asymmetrical. (C) Leukodystrophy: Diffuse white matter abnormality.

A. Radiation- or Chemotherapy-Induced Leukoencephalopathy

Radiation therapy (RT), commonly administered to the CNS for the treatment of primary/metastatic brain neoplasms and hematologic/solid tumors that disseminate in the subarachnoid space, may induce MS-like plaques of demyelination in the "early" delayed phase, and white matter necrosis is usually a feature of the "late" delayed phase of RT-related injury. This is more appropriately characterized as a vasculopathy—cerebral microvessels in the radiation field often undergo fibrinoid necrosis, and/or "leak fibrin" into the surrounding neural tissue, which further undergoes coagulative necrosis. In the spinal cord, discrete foci of leukoencephalopathy may be seen in the white matter (Fig. 21) after RT or chemotherapeutic agents are administered into the CSF.

B. Cyclosporine

This drug, commonly administered in patients who receive bone marrow or solid organ transplants, has clinically documented neurotoxicity that is

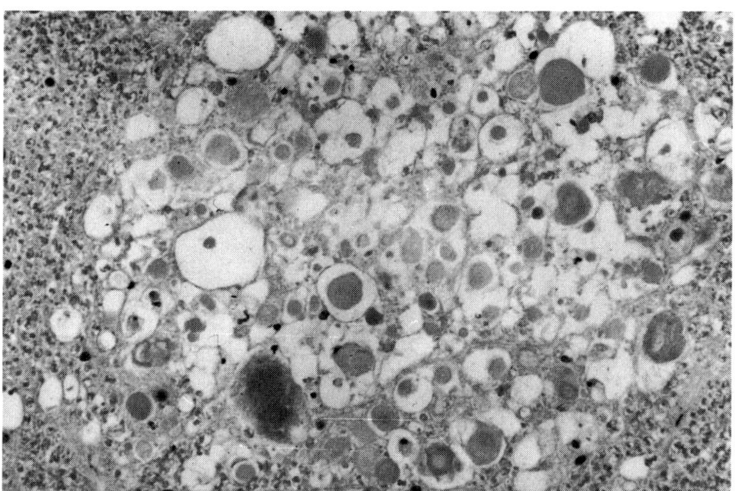

Figure 21 Patient with acute leukemia was given systemic and intrathecal chemotherapy. At autopsy, multiple small necrotic lesions (as illustrated here) were found throughout spinal cord white matter. Characteristic appearance shows vacuolated white matter containing large globular swollen axons. Focus of leukoencephalopathy is well demarcated from surrounding normal white matter (e.g., at upper left of figure).

probably largely reversible after cessation of the drug. Various clinical syndromes (including cortical blindness, seizures, quadriplegia, and even coma) may result from its administration. Neuroimaging studies in affected patients show a "diffuse disorder of white matter." White matter toxicity may explain the relatively high frequency of some specific leukoencephalopathies (e.g., CPM) in liver transplant patients, though this scenario is not currently supported by hard evidence. Autopsy studies that attempt to explain cyclosporine neurotoxicity are almost always complicated by the fact that the drug is given only to very ill patients, so that any unique effects it may have on the CNS (including the white matter) are almost impossible to assess in such a clinical milieu.

Other commonly administered drugs (e.g., amphotericin) may cause various forms of leukoencephalopathy that are not well characterized, again for the simple reason that the drugs are given to critically ill patients with a variety of systemic "lesions," both structural and metabolic. Abnormalities of the blood-brain barrier are often invoked as a mechanism of drug-induced leukoencephalopathy, though experimental evidence for same is usually lacking. Carbon monoxide (CO) poisoning may also lead to various forms of white matter damage ranging from perivascular foci of myelinolysis to large confluent zones of white matter destruction (see also Chap. 2).

Figure 22 illustrates an example of a particularly severe type of focal

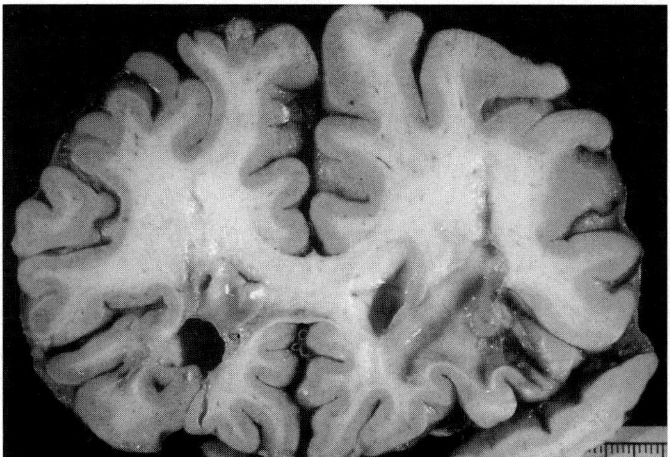

Figure 22 An abnormality of the white matter that may mimic demyelinating disease. Patient had undergone prefrontal leukotomy (now performed rarely if at all) several decades prior to death. Note asymmetric, well-demarcated, pitted, partly linear white matter cavities in centrum semiovale of both cerebral hemispheres.

leukoencephalopathy, now a historical curiosity, that has resulted from the ultimate iatrogenic intervention—prefrontal leukotomy.

REFERENCES

1. Anders KH, Becker PS, Holden JK, et al. Multifocal necrotizing leukoencephalopathy with pontine predilection in immunosuppressed patients. Hum Pathol 1993; 24:897–904.
2. Antel JP, Ruijs TCG. Oligodendrocytes and the immune system. In: Fedoroff S et al, eds. Biology and Pathology of Astrocyte-Neuron Interactions. New York: Plenum Press, 1993:271–281.
3. Burger PC, Boyko OB. The pathology of central nervous system radiation injury. In: Gutin PH, Leibel SA, Sheline GE, eds. Radiation Injury to the Nervous System. New York: Raven Press, 1991:191–208.
4. Cancilla PA, Andrews JM, Rose AS. Subacute demyelinating disease in an adult (diffuse-disseminated sclerosis). Neurology 1971; 21:825–832.
5. Chang KH, Cha SH, Han MH, Park SH, Nah DL, Hong JH. Marchiafava-Bignami disease: serial changes in corpus callosum on MRI. Neuroradiology 1992; 34:480–482.
6. Coxe WS, Luse SA. Acute hemorrhagic leukoencephalitis. A clinical and electron-microscopic report of 2 patients treated with surgical decompression. J Neurosurg 1963; 20:584–596.
7. de Groen PC, Aksamit AJ, Rakela J, Forbes GS, Krom RAF. Central nervous system toxicity after liver transplantation. The role of cyclosporine and cholesterol. N Engl J Med 1987; 317:861–866.
8. Elias SB. Oligodendrocyte development and the natural history of multiple sclerosis. A new hypothesis for the pathogenesis of the disease. Arch Neurol 1987; 44:1294–1299.
9. Ellison GW. Multiple sclerosis: why? Biomed Pharmacother 1989; 43:327–333.
10. Farrell MA, Kaufmann JCE, Gilbert JJ, Noseworthy JH, Armstrong HA, Ebers GC. Oligoclonal bands in multiple sclerosis: clinical-pathological correlation. Neurology 1985; 35:212–218.
11. Ferreiro JA, Robert MA, Vinters HV. Neuropathologic findings after liver transplantation. Acta Neuropathol 1992; 84:1–14.
12. Gilbert JJ, Sadler M. Unsuspected multiple sclerosis. Arch Neurol 1983; 40:533–536.
13. Hart MN, Earle KM. Haemorrhagic and perivenous encephalitis: a clinical-pathological review of 38 cases. J Neurol Neurosurg Psychiatry 1975; 38:585–591.
14. Hogancamp WE, Rodriguez M, Weinshenker BG. The epidemiology of multiple sclerosis. Mayo Clin Proc 1997; 72:871–878.
15. Hogancamp WE, Rodriguez M, Weinshenker BG. Identification of multiple sclerosis-associated genes. Mayo Clin Proc 1997; 72:965–976.
16. Illowsky BP, Laureno R. Encephalopathy and myelinolysis after rapid correction of hyponatremia. Brain 1987; 110:855–867.

17. Itoyama Y, Tateishi J, Kuroiwa Y. Atypical multiple sclerosis with concentric or lamellar demyelinated lesions: Two Japanese patients studied post mortem. Ann Neurol 1985; 17:481–487.
18. Kepes JJ. Large focal tumor-like demyelinating lesions of the brain: intermediate entity between multiple sclerosis and acute disseminated encephalomyelitis? A study of 31 patients. Ann Neurol 1993; 33:18–27.
19. Kleinschmidt-DeMasters BK, Norenberg MD. Rapid correction of hyponatremia causes demyelination: relation to central pontine myelinolysis. Science 1981; 211:1068–1070.
20. Lefkowitz D, Angelo JN. Neuromyelitis optica with unusual vascular changes. Arch Neurol 1984; 41:1103–1105.
21. Ludwin SK, Johnson ES. Evidence for a "dying-back" gliopathy in demyelinating disease. Ann Neurol 1981; 9:301–305.
22. Navikas V, Link H. Review: cytokines and the pathogenesis of multiple sclerosis. J Neurosci Res 1996; 45:322–333.
23. Okeda R, Kitano M, Sawabe M, Yamada I, Yamada M. Distribution of demyelinating lesions in pontine and extrapontine myelinolysis—three autopsy cases including one case devoid of central pontine myelinolysis. Acta Neuropathol 1986; 69:259–266.
24. Opelz G, Terasaki P, Myers L, et al. The association of HLA antigens A3, B7, and DW2 with 330 multiple sclerosis patients in the United States. Tissue Antigens 1977; 9:54–58.
25. Riggs JE, Schochet SS Jr. Osmotic stress, osmotic myelinolysis, and oligodendrocyte topography. Arch Pathol Lab Med 1989; 113:1386–1388.
26. Rodriguez M. Multiple sclerosis: basic concepts and hypothesis. Mayo Clin Proc 1989; 64:570–576.
27. Rodriguez M, Scheithauer B. Ultrastructure of multiple sclerosis. Ultrastruct Pathol 1994; 18:3–13.
28. Slager UT. Central pontine myelinolysis and abnormalities in serum sodium. Clin Neuropathol 1986; 5:252–256.
29. Steinsapir KD, Vinters HV. Central pontine myelinolysis in a child with the Shwachman-Diamond syndrome. Human Pathol 1985; 16:741–743.
30. Sterns RH, Riggs JE, Schochet SS Jr. Osmotic demyelination syndrome following correction of hyponatremia. N Engl J Med 1986; 314:1535–1542.
31. Swanson JW. Multiple sclerosis: update in diagnosis and review of prognostic factors. Mayo Clin Proc 1989; 64:577–586.
32. Tourtellotte WW, Pick PW. Current concepts about multiple sclerosis. Mayo Clin Proc 1989; 64:592–596.
33. Victor M. Alcoholic dementia. Can J Neurol Sci 1994; 21:88–99.
34. Waxman SG. Pathophysiology of demyelinated and remyelinated axons. In: Cook SD, ed. Handbook of Multiple Sclerosis. 2nd ed. New York: Marcel Dekker, 1996:257–293.
35. Wiley CA, Johnson RT, Reingold SC. Neurological consequences of immune dysfunction: Lessons from HIV infection and multiple sclerosis. J Neuroimmunol 1992; 40:115–120.

36. Wright DG, Laureno R, Victor M. Pontine and extrapontine myelinolysis. Brain 1979; 102:361–385.
37. Wynn DR, Rodriguez M, O'Fallon WM, Kurland LT. Update on the epidemiology of multiple sclerosis. Mayo Clin Proc 1989; 64:808–817.
38. Zweiman B, Lisak RP. Cell-mediated immunity in neurologic disease. Hum Pathol 1986; 17:234–245.

6

Neoplasms

I. INTRODUCTION

Neoplasms of the nervous system and its adjacent structures are a diverse group of lesions, in both their clinical manifestations and pathologic features. This chapter will discuss the common tumors of the brain, spinal cord, pineal and pituitary glands, leptomeninges, skull, and spine. For sake of convenience, some hamartomas and nonneoplastic mass lesions (e.g., cysts) are discussed in conjunction with neoplasms.

Tumors of the brain and spinal cord are relatively uncommon, especially when compared with the frequency of neoplasms in other organ systems, such as lung, breast, and gastrointestinal tract. The incidence of primary CNS neoplasia is only about 4 to 5/100,000 people annually. As such, except in a specialized tertiary care setting, the experience of a pathologist is limited by the rarity of these tumors. Some of these lesions are quite distinctive and readily recognized by even novice residents; others are exceedingly rare and difficult to classify definitively even by the most experienced neuropathologist.

It is our aim to provide only an overview of CNS neoplasia, focusing on the important clinical, gross, and histopathologic features of the more common and important lesions. While these tumors are sometimes seen at autopsy, our intention is to emphasize those that comprise neurosurgical biopsy specimens. When appropriate, ancillary diagnostic aids will be mentioned. For a thorough, detailed discussion of CNS neoplasms, the reader is referred to the excellent text written by Drs. Burger, Scheithauer, and Vogel, and the key references listed in the bibliography.

II. BIOPSY INTERPRETATION

Among the most stressful events many general pathologists encounter are intraoperative consultations on brain biopsy specimens. In a matter of a few minutes the pathologist is expected to accurately render a critical diagnosis, often on a tiny specimen. The primary purpose of frozen section is not to cause a marked elevation in the pathologist's blood pressure, but to lead to an accurate and correct diagnosis and to aid the neurosurgeon in determining the extent of the surgical procedure. For example, meningiomas, solitary metastases, ependymomas, hemangioblastomas, cerebellar astrocytomas, and cystic lesions are usually completely resected if they can be accurately recognized intraoperatively. There are several steps which can help a pathologist render a correct diagnosis.

It is imperative that the pathologist be aware of the patient's age and sex and the precise anatomic location of the lesion, preferably with prior review of pertinent neuroradiographic images. A clear channel of communication with the neurosurgeon should be available such that any questions and concerns may be addressed.

In addition to the usual H&E-stained frozen tissue section, we recommend the preparation and evaluation of an air-dried or alcohol-fixed touch imprint or squash preparation, especially for minuscule stereotactic biopsies. Air-dried cytologic preparations are rapidly stained by a Romanowsky technique (e.g., Diff-Quik) and alcohol-fixed smears with hematoxylin and eosin. The nuclear and cytoplasmic features and background of these cytologic preparations are often extremely helpful in defining the nature of the lesion. Smear preparations are thoroughly discussed and well illustrated by Chandrasoma and Apuzzo, as well as by Burger et al.

Often it is not imperative to render a precise diagnosis at the time of frozen section. It may suffice for the pathologist to inform the surgeon that he has biopsied and adequately sampled a viable lesion which appears neoplastic, inflammatory, or infectious. If an infectious etiology is suspected, tissues should be submitted for appropriate cultures or ultrastructural examination. If a diagnosis of lymphoma is suspected, tissues should be snap-frozen for appropriate marker studies; we also fix some of the tissue in B-5 (or similar fixative) for the superb nuclear morphology such sections provide. Glutaraldehyde fixation for all unusual neoplasms is recommended in the event ultrastructural analysis is needed for accurate diagnosis. In academic centers, tissues may be saved for research or other studies (e.g., oncogene analysis) if available and useful in a given patient.

In approaching a surgical biopsy or resection specimen, we recommend using the algorithm outlined in Table 1. Obviously, some knowledge of the normal microscopic anatomy of the brain is required before attempting to interpret CNS biopsy specimens. Unfortunately there is no magical way to become familiar with the many types of CNS neoplasia other than through hard work and experience. Generally, an accurate diagnosis can be rendered on examination of routinely stained histologic sections, without ancillary techniques needed. At times immunohistochemical stains may be helpful in characterizing some neoplasms, especially poorly differentiated ones (Table 2). Patients with infectious and vascular lesions, demyelinating diseases, and dementias may intentionally or otherwise undergo brain biopsy; these conditions are discussed elsewhere in this book.

III. PEDIATRIC VERSUS ADULT NEOPLASMS

While there is a striking overlap in the morphologic features of CNS neoplasms in adult and pediatric patients, significant age-dependent differences in the relative frequency of different types of tumors exist. These are outlined in Table 3. In adults, about two-thirds of brain tumors are supratentorial; in children about two-thirds are infratentorial. CNS tumors are the second most common form of cancer in children under 15 years of age, second only to acute leukemia. Children also have a higher incidence of embryonal neoplasms. Adults are much more likely to have high-grade astrocytomas and metastases.

IV. GLIOMAS

Glioma is a broad term that encompasses low- and high-grade astrocytomas (including glioblastoma multiforme), oligodendrogliomas, ependymomas, and the fairly frequent occurrence of mixtures of these elements (*mixed gliomas*). These tumors usually show *glial fibrillary acidic protein* (GFAP) immunopositivity and lack collagen or reticulin. A diagnosis of glioma, while somewhat vague, is often as specific a diagnosis as can be determined at the time of frozen section; a more definitive and specific diagnosis is then rendered after study of the permanent sections. The etiology of most gliomas is unknown, although anaplastic astrocytomas and glioblastomas have been described arising many years after CNS radiation therapy. Recent studies have focused on genetic abnormalities as a pathogenetic mechanism—e.g., loss of tumor suppressor genes.

A. Astrocytomas

Astrocytomas are the most common primary tumors of the CNS. They are composed of neoplastic astrocytes in a *fibrillary*, GFAP-positive background. Astrocytomas vary in their degree of differentiation and, hence, in their resemblance

Table 1 Examination of Brain Tissue Sections

I. Look for normal tissues

-Brain or spinal cord
-Leptomeninges
-Pituitary or pineal gland
-Nerve & ganglion

II. Architectural characteristics of a lesion (if one is present)

1) Circumscription
   - Discrete and well-demarcated (favors benign)
   - Irregular and infiltrative (favors malignant)

2) Background
   - Fibrillary (suggests glial)
   - Other (e.g., cystic, mucinous)

3) Cellularity
   - Hypocellular (does not exclude tumor)
   - Normocellular
   - Hypercellular
     - Uneven and more extensive (favors neoplasm)
     - Mixed infiltrate (favors inflammatory)
     - Gliosis, Rosenthal fibers (favors reactive)

4) Cellular pattern
   - Sheets
   - Microcystic
   - Rosettes
   - Fascicles
   - Alternating fascicles and loose areas
   - Papillary
   - Whorls
   - Perivascular pseudorosettes

5) Vascular pattern
   - Prominent vessels
   - Tangled abnormal vessels (vascular malformation)
   - Vascular endothelial hyperplasia (GBM)
   - Vascular hyalinization (meningioma/neurilemoma)
   - Thrombosed vessels
   - Multiple delicate, thin-walled vessels (oligodendroglioma)

6) Cytology
   - Nucleus
     - Atypia/pleomorphism
     - Nucleoli
     - Inclusions
     - Pseudoinclusions
     - Mitotic figures (including atypical mitoses)
   - Cytoplasm
     - Fibrillary
     - Indistinct
     - Scant
     - Spindloid
     - Epithelioid

7) Specific findings
   - Necrosis
   - Psammoma bodies (meningioma)
   - Verocay bodies (neurilemoma)
   - Calcification (craniopharyngioma, pituitary adenoma, oligodendroglioma, etc.)
   - Infectious agents (fungi, toxoplasma, etc.)
   - Other

III. Re-evaluate and summarize

1) Summarize the architecture, cytology, and specific features—in correlation with the precise anatomic location and clinical history.
2) Compare to differential.
3) Make diagnosis.

Table 2 Pattern of Usual Immunohistochemical Positivity in CNS Neoplasms

Primary antibody	Tumors showing positivity
Glial fibrillary acidic protein (GFAP)	Astrocytic: low grade astrocytoma, anaplastic astrocytoma, glioblastoma multiforme, astroblastoma Ependymoma Subependymoma Anaplastic ependymoma Gliosarcoma Ganglioglioma Mixed glioma
Synaptophysin & neurofilament	Ganglion cell neoplasms Central neurocytoma Pineocytoma Medulloblastoma / neuroblastoma
Epithelial membrane antigen (EMA)	Meningioma Metastatic carcinoma
S-100 protein	Neurilemoma Neurofibroma Oligodendroglioma Anaplastic oligodendroglioma Anaplastic ependymoma Astrocytoma Melanoma Chordoma
HMB-45	Melanoma
Factor VIII / CD-34 CD-31	Hemangioblastoma Hemangioma
Vimentin	Meningioma Sarcoma
Cytokeratin	Metastatic carcinoma Choroid plexus papilloma Choroid plexus carcinoma Craniopharyngioma Chordoma Most germ cell tumors
Leu-7	Oligodendroglioma Anaplastic oligodendroglioma
Chromogranin	Pituitary adenoma Metastatic neuroendocrine tumors
Alpha fetoprotein (AFP)	Embryonal carcinoma Endodermal sinus (Yolk sac) tumor
Placental alkaline phosphatase (PLAP)	Germinoma
Leukocyte common antigen (LCA) L-26 (B-cell marker) UCHL-1 (T-cell marker) Kappa and lambda light chains	Monoclonal staining patterns usually seen in lymphomas Polyclonal staining patterns usually seen in reactive inflammatory infiltrates and infections

Table 3 Comparison of Pediatric and Adult Brain Tumors by Anatomic Location

Location	Pediatric	Adult
Supratentorial		
1) Cerebral hemisphere and corpus callosum	Astrocytoma (mostly low-grade) Ependymoma Oligodendroglioma	Astrocytoma (mostly glioblastoma multiforme) Meningioma Metastatic carcinoma Oligodendroglioma Ependymoma
2) Region around the third ventricle	Astrocytoma (mostly pilocytic and low-grade) Oligodendroglioma	Astrocytoma (mostly glioblastoma multiforme; rarely pilocytic) Oligodendroglioma Ependymoma
3) Lateral and third ventricle	Ependymoma Choroid plexus papilloma Subependymal giant cell astrocytoma	Ependymoma Meningioma Subependymoma Choroid plexus papilloma Colloid cyst (third ventricle only)
4) Pituitary region	Craniopharyngioma Pituitary adenoma	Pituitary adenoma Craniopharyngioma Meningioma

5) Pineal region	Germ cell neoplasms	Germ cell neoplasms
6) Optic chiasm and optic nerve	Astrocytoma (mostly low-grade)	Meningioma Astrocytoma (mostly low-grade)
Infratentorial		
1) Cerebellum	Medulloblastoma Astrocytoma (mostly low-grade) Dermoid cyst	Hemangioblastoma Metastatic carcinoma Astrocytoma (often high-grade)
2) Brainstem	Astrocytoma (low-grade, anaplastic or glioblastoma multiforme)	Astrocytoma (mostly anaplastic or glioblastoma multiforme) Meningioma Neurilemoma (acoustic neuroma) Neurofibroma
3) Cerebellopontine angle	Ependymoma Choroid plexus papilloma	Acoustic neuroma Meningioma Epidermoid cyst Choroid plexus papilloma
4) Fourth ventricle	Ependymoma Choroid plexus papilloma	Ependymoma Meningioma

to normal astrocytes. Astrocytomas are graded by a variety of schemata, but we prefer that outlined in Table 4 because of its simplicity and reproducibility. There is a strong relationship between the grade of an astrocytoma and proliferative indices (e.g., S-phase in flow cytometry, PCNA, Ki-67), and an inverse relationship between grade and survival. As such, grading relates to prognosis and is used in determining therapy, including cranial radiation and chemotherapy. Most astrocytomas are solitary, although rarely are they multifocal.

It is imperative that the pathologist and neurosurgeon be aware of the cellular heterogeneity of astrocytomas. These tumors must be well sampled to ensure an accurate diagnosis. It has been clearly documented that the grade may vary significantly within different regions of an astrocytoma. As such, a diagnosis of a "high-grade astrocytoma" can never be completely excluded with a small, limited sample that shows only features of low-grade astrocytoma.

1. Low-Grade Astrocytomas (grades 1 & 2)

Low-grade astrocytomas can be found in any region of the brain. Their incidence is directly related to the quantity of white matter, and these tumors are thus usually found in the cerebral hemispheres. Most of these well-differentiated neoplasms are manifest in young people, including children; survival is measured in many years or decades, with cures sometimes achieved.

Grossly, these tumors present as expansile masses with irregular, poorly delineated margins (Figs. 1–3). Most are solid and a pale gray to yellow-tan color. Cysts of varying size may be present and are sometimes a dominant feature. The cortical–white matter junction may be obliterated by infiltrating tumor.

Microscopic examination of low-grade astrocytomas reveals neoplastic astrocytes which are crowded (Fig. 4), although in grade 1 neoplasms the increased cell density is subtle and may be difficult to recognize at the time of frozen section. Neoplastic astrocytes are irregular in distribution and have a poorly defined, infiltrative border. They exhibit slight nuclear irregularity and

Table 4 Grading of Astrocytic Tumors (Daumas-Duport criteria)

Four criteria
1) Nuclear atypia
2) Mitoses
3) Vascular endothelial hyperplasia
4) Necrosis

Grade

0 criteria	=	grade 1	(low-grade astrocytoma)
1 criterion	=	grade 2	(low-grade astrocytoma)
2 criteria	=	grade 3	(anaplastic astrocytoma)
3–4 criteria	=	grade 4	(glioblastoma multiforme)

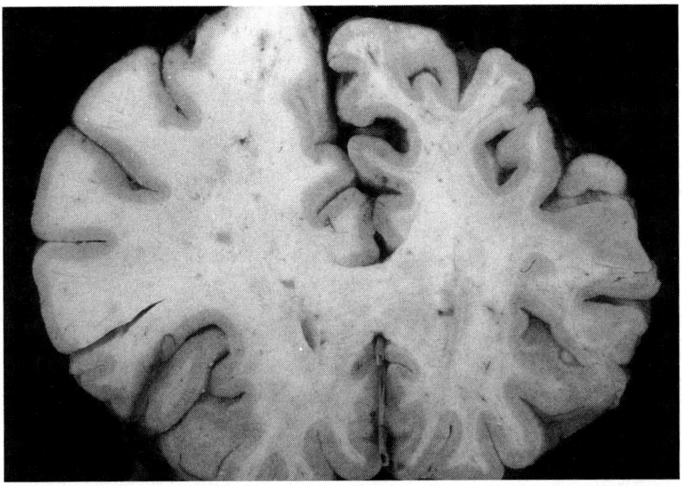

Figure 1 Astrocytoma. The white matter of the left frontal lobe is expanded by a large, infiltrative, fibrillary astrocytoma. The tumor has indistinct borders and has caused focal effacement of the cortex/white matter junction, with enlargement of the gyri.

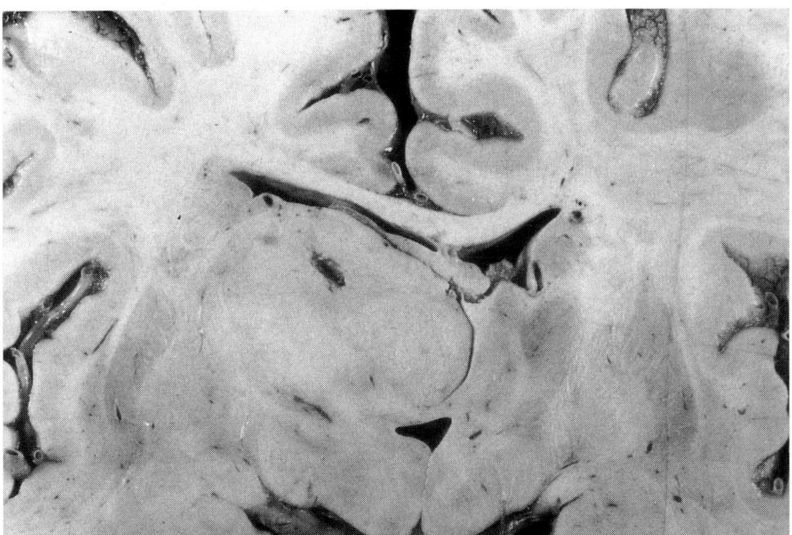

Figure 2 Astrocytoma. An indistinct neoplasm is expanding the deep gray matter of the left cerebral hemisphere, with effacement of thalamus and internal capsule, shift of midline structures, and compression of the left lateral and third ventricles.

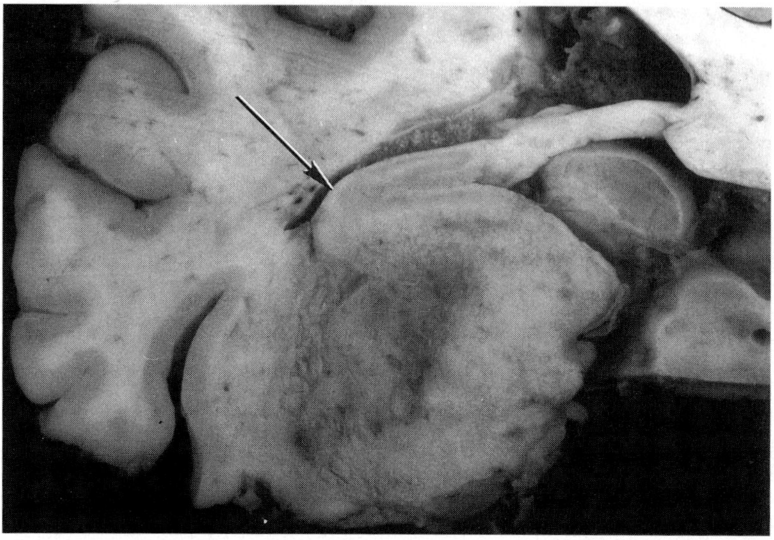

Figure 3 Astrocytoma. The medial temporal lobe inferior to the hippocampus (arrow) is extensively effaced by a poorly delineated, expansile neoplasm which shows areas of cystic change.

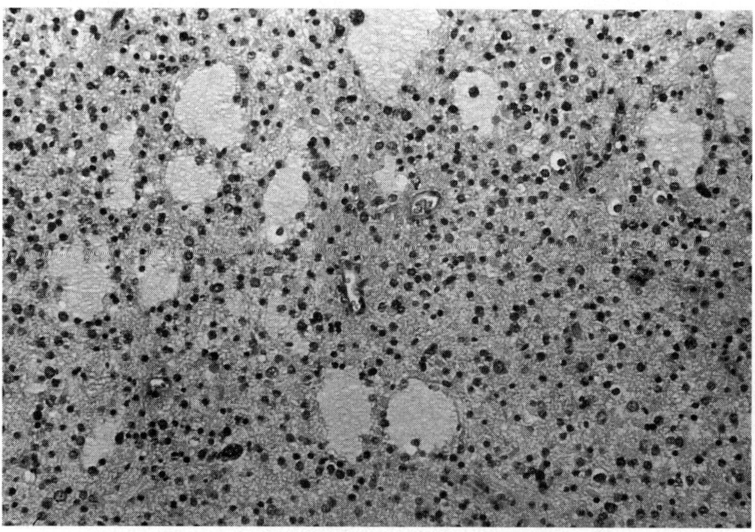

Figure 4 Low-grade astrocytoma. At scanning magnification this fibrillary astrocytoma is characterized by increased cellularity, with irregularity in cell distribution and frequent nuclear overlap. The background is finely fibrillary and microcystic, both features helpful in diagnosing astrocytoma.

atypia, hyperchromasia, extremely rare mitosis, and abundant eosinophilic fibrillary cytoplasm (Fig. 5). This fibrillary cytoplasmic background is extremely helpful in determining the nature of an astrocytoma at the time of intraoperative consultation.

Perineuronal "satellitosis"—the crowding of neoplastic astrocytes around neurons at the periphery of the tumor—is an extremely helpful clue to the diagnosis of malignancy (Fig. 6). Secondary structures of Scherer include subpial or perivascular collections of neoplastic astrocytes (Fig. 7) and usually indicate a higher grade of malignancy. Extensive necrosis (with palisading of nuclei at the periphery), vascular endothelial hyperplasia, and atypical mitosis are not identified in low-grade astrocytomas.

Specific types of low-grade astrocytomas are the following.

a. Pilocytic Astrocytomas ("spongioblastoma"). These are slowly growing, firm, often well-demarcated, lobulated tumors that arise around the third ventricle (where they may cause obstructive hydrocephalus), within the thalamus or hypothalamus. They are rare in the more peripheral portions of the cerebral hemispheres. Many pilocytic astrocytomas present with a mural nodule of tumor in the wall of a large cyst, and most occur in children or young adults. As they may be cured by surgical resection, it is important to recognize them. Microscopic characteristics include a compact fibrillary stroma containing mostly elongated cells with bipolar, fibrillary, cytoplasmic processes, alternating

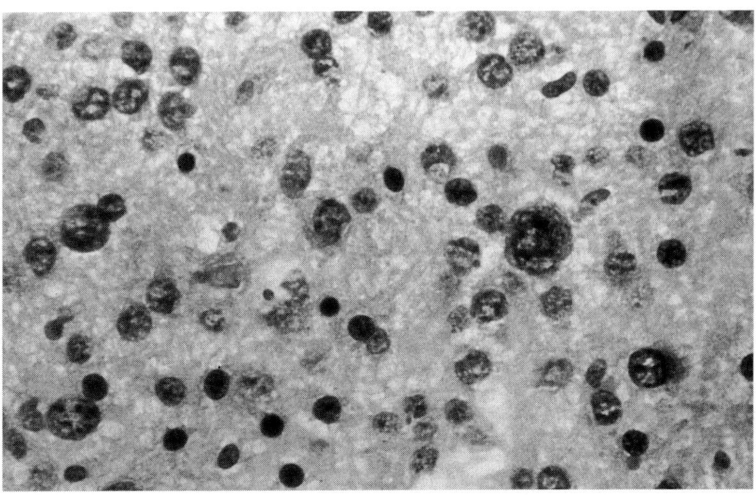

Figure 5 Low-grade astrocytoma. Higher magnification of Figure 4 shows striking variation in nuclear size, hyperchromasia, irregular spacing of nuclei, and fibrillary background.

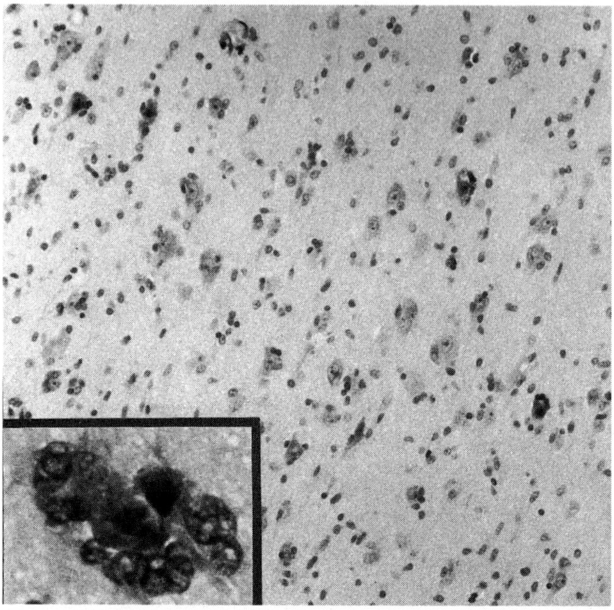

Figure 6 Astrocytoma. Neoplastic astrocytes frequently cluster around neurons when they infiltrate the outer cortex, a process known as satellitosis. This feature is often readily identified at scanning magnification (inset highlighting perinuclear clustering).

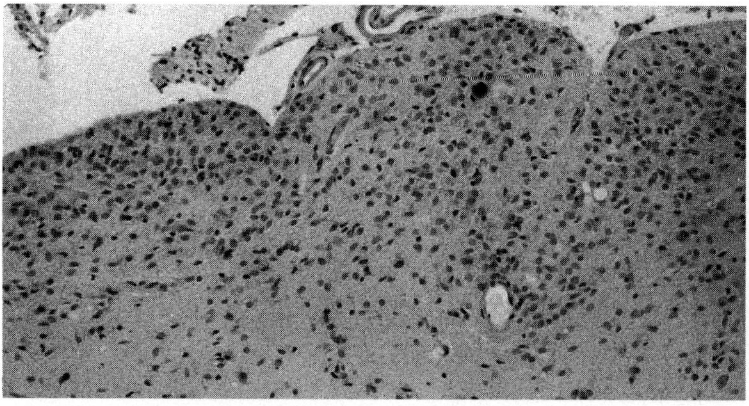

Figure 7 Astrocytoma. The subpial regions show crowded clusters of neoplastic astrocytes, a process unique to astrocytomas known as secondary structures of Scherer. These are usually indicative of high-grade malignancy.

with a loose microcystic stroma containing stellate astrocytes (Figs. 8, 9). Rosenthal fibers are highly eosinophilic, round, ovoid to beaded structures which are a helpful clue in recognizing pilocytic astrocytomas; however, as they also occur in reactive gliosis, they are not pathognomonic. Atypia is usually minimal and mitotic figures are exceedingly rare. Prominent vessels may be seen but are to be distinguished from the true endothelial hyperplasia associated with high grade astrocytic neoplasms.

b. Cystic (protoplasmic) Astrocytomas. These are soft, gelatinous, and sometimes macroscopically cystic. Histologically, these tumors contain loose, stellate cells with delicate processes forming a fine, weblike matrix, with microcystic changes (Fig. 10). Large cysts are common.

c. Cerebellar Astrocytomas. Cerebellar astrocytomas are primarily tumors of children, comprising about 25% of pediatric brain tumors. These neoplasms may be found in either the cerebellar hemispheres or the vermis. Grossly, they are solid, well-circumscribed masses which are fairly homogeneous; they may also represent a mural nodule in the wall of a cyst containing xanthochromic fluid. Microscopically, the pattern is characteristically a variable admixture of solid pilocytic components (often with Rosenthal fibers) and loose, microcystic, protoplasmic elements (Figs. 11, 12). While some atypia and multinucleation

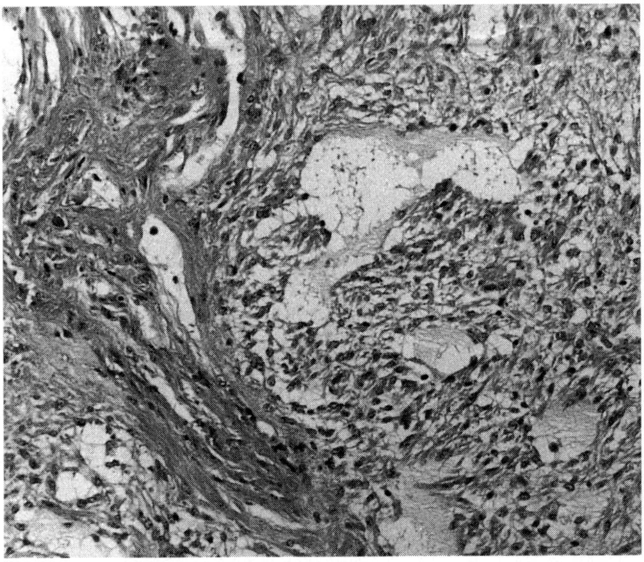

Figure 8 Pilocytic astrocytoma. These tumors are composed of cells with oval nuclei and polar cytoplasmic processes. The stroma in some areas is more compact and fibrillary, with other areas showing cystic change.

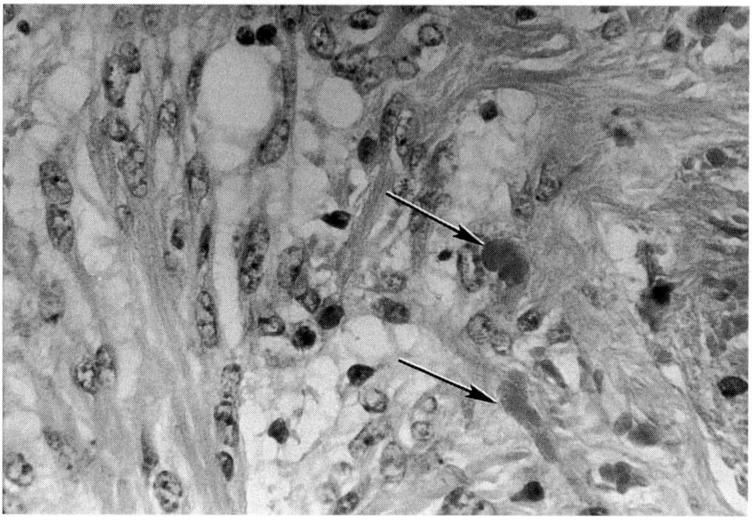

Figure 9 Pilocytic astrocytoma. High magnification of Figure 8 highlights the characteristic polar pilocytic cells. The presence of eosinophilic Rosenthal fibers (arrows) is common and a helpful diagnostic clue.

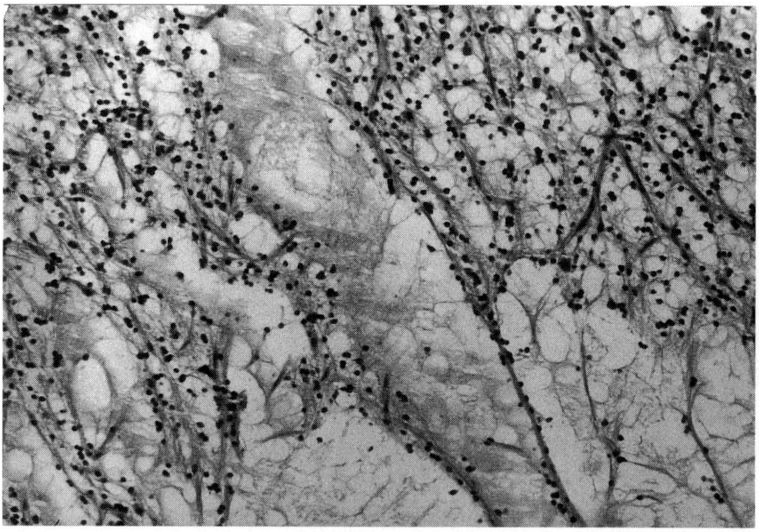

Figure 10 Cystic astrocytoma. This tumor contained scattered clusters of neoplastic astrocytes between cysts of varying size.

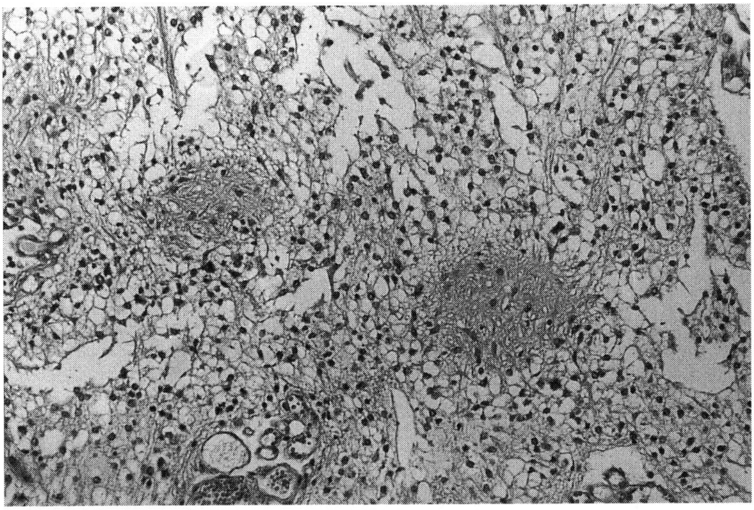

Figure 11 Cerebellar astrocytoma. Scanning magnification shows islands of compact fibrillary stroma in a loose cystic background.

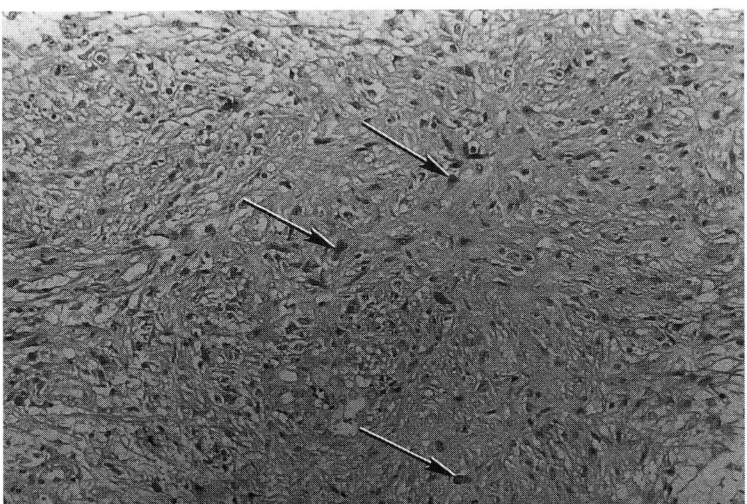

Figure 12 Cerebellar astrocytoma. Sometimes abundant Rosenthal fibers are seen in the compact areas of these neoplasms. Arrows indicate several of these.

of tumor cells and vascular proliferation may be seen; these do not alter the excellent prognosis. The presence of mitoses may, however, be indicative of dedifferentiation to a malignant neoplasm, although such transformation is exceedingly rare. Complete surgical excision of the tumor is often curative, although many recur following subtotal resection—e.g., cases with brainstem infiltration.

d. Gemistocytic Astrocytomas. These supratentorial tumors are readily recognized by their characteristic plump cells with abundant eosinophilic cytoplasm, eccentric nuclei, and short cytoplasmic processes (Fig. 13). While gemistocytic astrocytes predominate, there is also an admixture of neoplastic fibrillary astrocytes (which appear to be the proliferative cells). Mixed, polyclonal, perivascular, lymphoid infiltrates are common (Fig. 14). The prognosis of gemistocytic astrocytomas is less favorable than that of the above subtypes, and some authors believe these tumors should be automatically grouped with anaplastic (grade 3) astrocytomas.

2. Anaplastic Astrocytomas (grade 3)

These are neoplasms having an intermediate grade of malignancy and age of presentation between low-grade astrocytomas and glioblastoma multiforme. Average survival exceeds 2 years. Over time, dedifferentiation of low-grade astrocytomas into anaplastic astrocytomas commonly occurs, although some

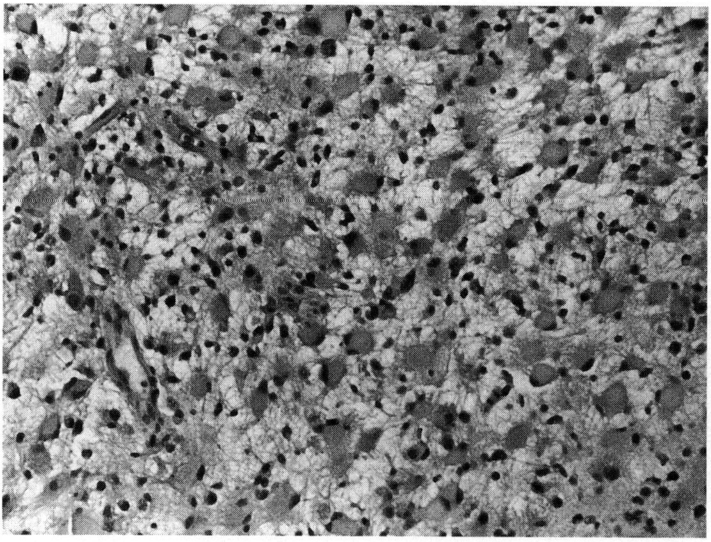

Figure 13 Gemistocytic astrocytoma. These tumors are readily recognized by their predominant cell type—the plump, eosinophilic gemistocyte.

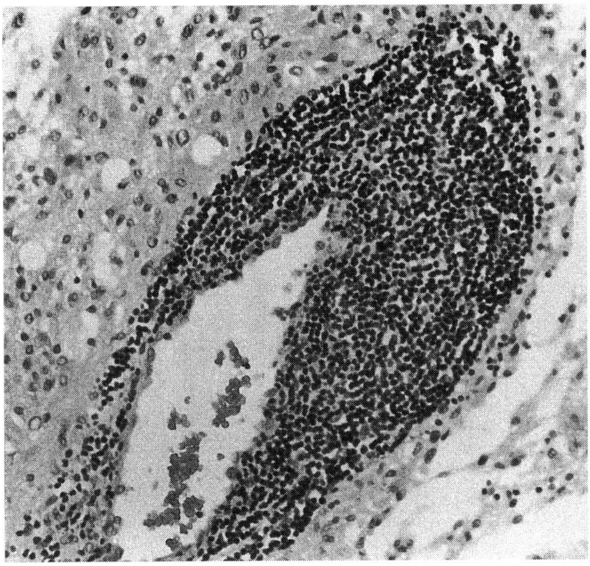

Figure 14 Astrocytoma. Perivascular lymphoid collections are common in gliomas. Such infiltrates are polyclonal in nature and should not cause one to think of the atypical glial proliferation as reactive rather than neoplastic.

anaplastic astrocytomas arise de novo. Grossly and microscopically these tumors are poorly demarcated. Histologically, they demonstrate increased cellular density and atypia, scattered mitosis, but absence of necrosis or vascular endothelial hyperplasia. Infiltration of the leptomeninges may occur, resulting in fibroplasia—a finding to be considered in the differential diagnosis of gliosarcoma.

3. *Glioblastoma Multiforme (grade 4)*

Glioblastoma multiforme (GBM) describes the most common CNS tumor type in adults. It usually arises from malignant transformation of a lower-grade astrocytoma or, less commonly, oligodendroglioma or ependymoma. These tumors may, however, arise de novo as GBM without a preexisting lower-grade phase. Rarely, GBMs are multifocal. Survival is usually less than a year.

On gross examination, GBMs may appear relatively well demarcated, with surrounding edema (Fig. 15). Most are infiltrative and poorly circumscribed. They grow rapidly and often are hemorrhagic, yellow, necrotic, and huge (Fig. 16). Most are cerebral, with a characteristic propensity to infiltrate the contralateral hemisphere across the corpus callosum, resulting in "butterfly" lesions (Figs. 17, 18). Less commonly, GBMs involve the brainstem, cerebel-

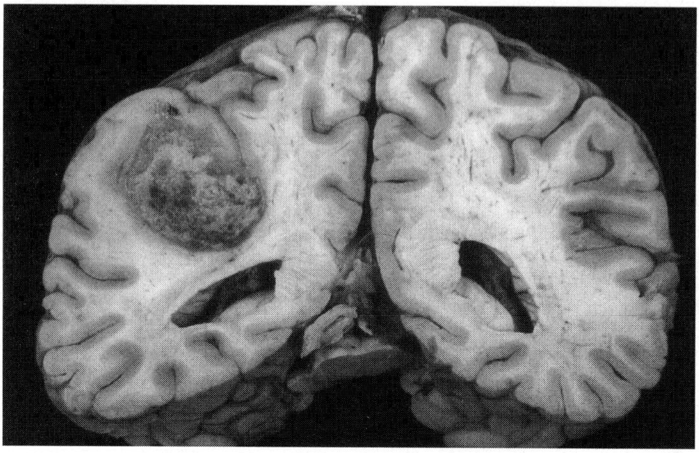

Figure 15 Glioblastoma multiforme. Some glioblastomas appear deceptively circumscribed, as did this tumor from the parieto-occipital cortex of a 63-year-old woman. Necrosis and hemorrhage are clues to the high-grade nature of this neoplasm.

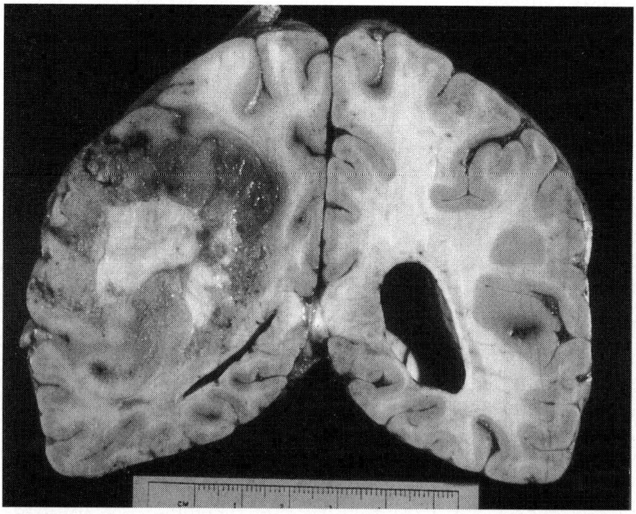

Figure 16 Glioblastoma multiforme. Many glioblastomas are large, extensively necrotic neoplasms effacing large portions of the cerebral hemispheres.

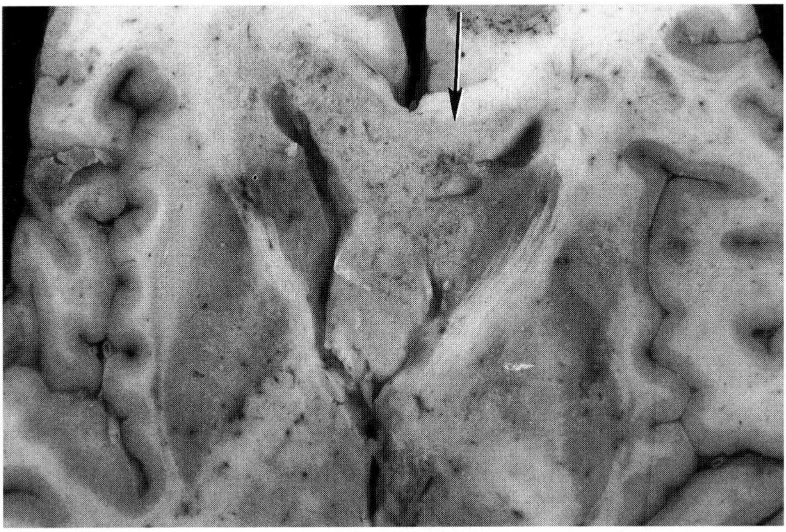

Figure 17 Glioblastoma multiforme. Growth of a neoplasm across the corpus callosum is a helpful gross and radiographic clue to the diagnosis of glioblastoma multiforme. This neoplasm effaces the genu of the corpus callosum (arrow), causes marked expansion of the septum pellucidum, and infiltrates the white matter of both cerebral hemispheres.

lum, and spinal cord. At these critical sites, their rapid growth rate is particularly devastating.

Microscopically, GBMs are highly cellular, poorly circumscribed neoplasms. Tremendous variation exists in their morphologic expression: small round cell, spindle cell, anaplastic giant, and multinucleate cell subtypes exist (Figs. 19–21). Mitosis are numerous, including atypical mitoses, and the fibrillary astrocytic background seen with lower-grade astrocytomas is preserved. Classically, GBMs have vascular endothelial hyperplasia (Figs. 22, 23), sometimes with glomeruloid tufting. Areas of confluent coagulative necrosis, surrounded by a palisaded rim of neoplastic glial cells (Figs. 24, 25), are best appreciated at low magnification. GBMs have a tendency to invade the leptomeninges (Fig. 26) and may spread along CSF pathways. During intraoperative consultation, smear preparations are often useful in assessing glioblastomas (Fig. 27).

4. *Uncommon Astrocytic Neoplasms*

Brainstem astrocytomas are most commonly found in children and usually involve the pons (Fig. 28). These tumors are diffuse, are often of low grade, and

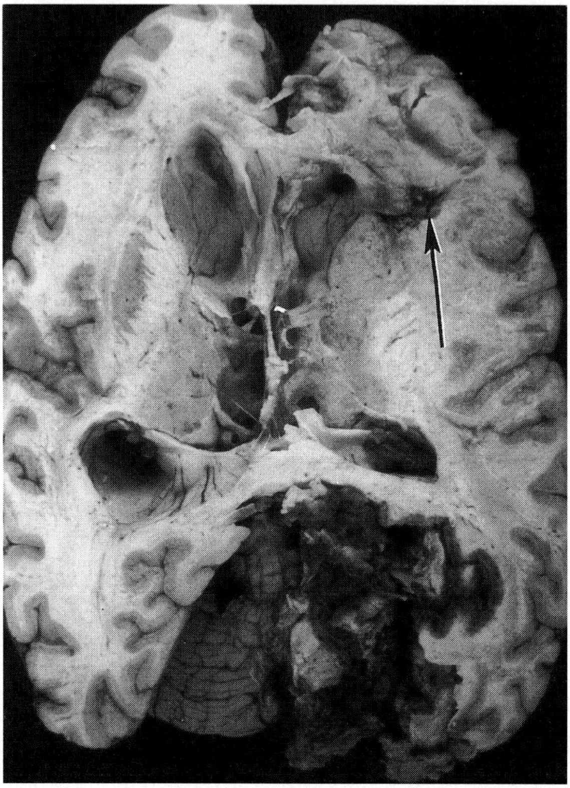

Figure 18 Glioblastoma multiforme. This tumor presented in a 61-year-old woman, who was treated with radiation and chemotherapy. There is prominent cystic degeneration of the white matter in the right frontal lobe (arrow), with edema. The right posterior cerebral artery territory infarct is due to transtentorial herniation of the uncus.

may show fibrillary or pilocytic differentiation. They frequently infiltrate the meninges or cause obstruction of the fourth ventricle. Anaplastic astrocytomas and glioblastomas are also found in this region, but are less common.

Nasal gliomas are rare tumors which probably are hamartomatous in nature. They are usually associated with a defect in the cribriform plate and may present as masses involving the palate or bridge of the nose. Histologically, nasal gliomas are composed of admixtures of fibroconnective and glial tissues (Fig. 29).

Optic nerve astrocytomas/gliomas are slow-growing tumors usually seen in children. They are associated with neurofibromatosis type 1, in which condition they may be bilateral. Clinically, they present with visual loss and propto-

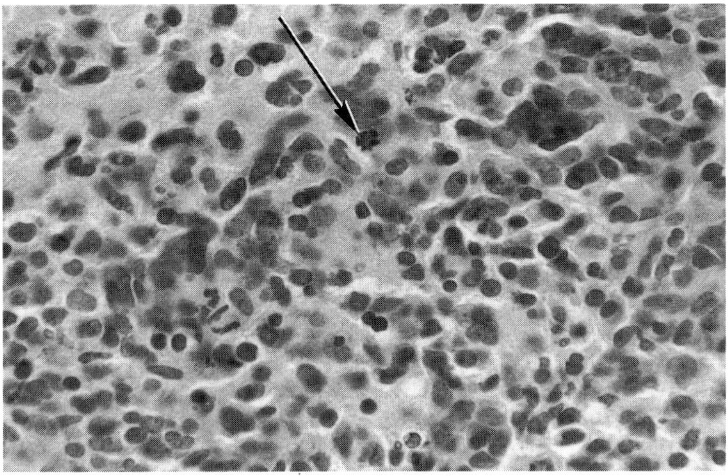

Figure 19 Glioblastoma multiforme. Tremendous variation in the histologic appearance of glioblastomas exists. This tumor is composed of many small, crowded cells with round to angulated nuclei and scanty fibrillary eosinophilic cytoplasm. A mitotic figure is highlighted by an arrow.

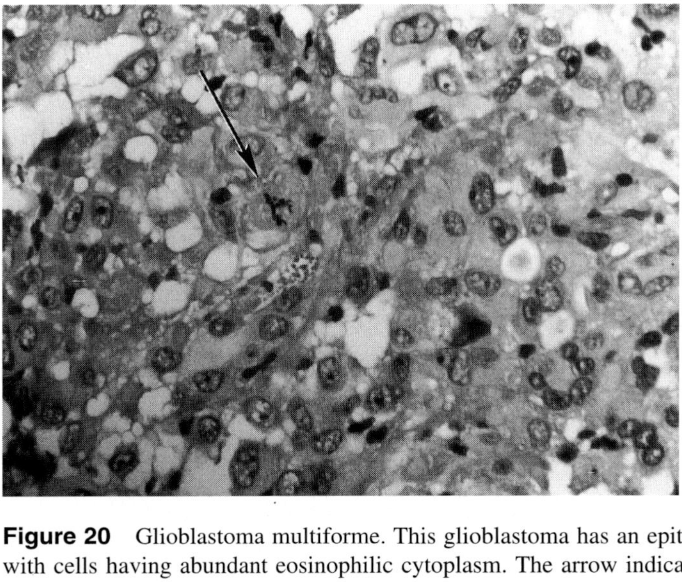

Figure 20 Glioblastoma multiforme. This glioblastoma has an epithelioid appearance, with cells having abundant eosinophilic cytoplasm. The arrow indicates an atypical (tripolar) mitotic figure.

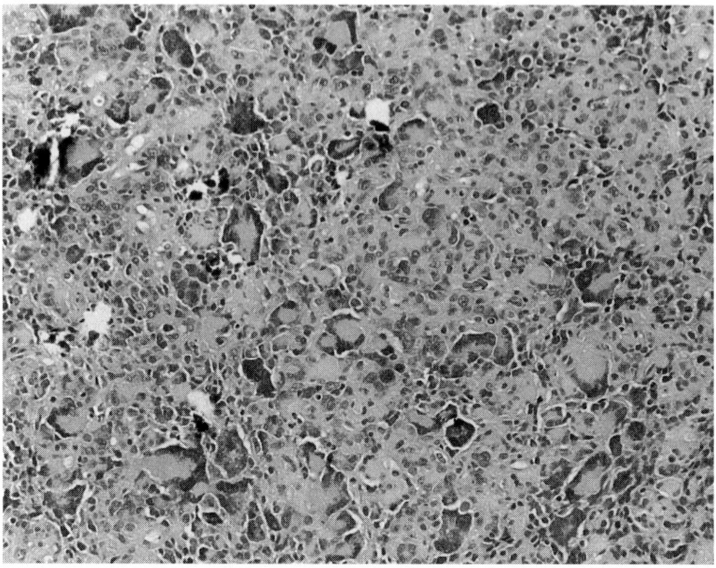

Figure 21 Glioblastoma multiforme. Marked nuclear atypia, including many bizarre tumor giant cells, is demonstrated in this glioblastoma.

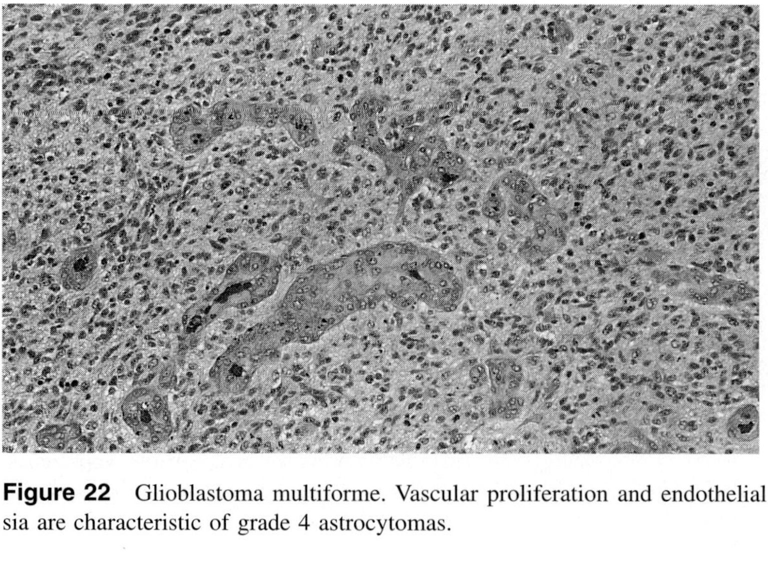

Figure 22 Glioblastoma multiforme. Vascular proliferation and endothelial hyperplasia are characteristic of grade 4 astrocytomas.

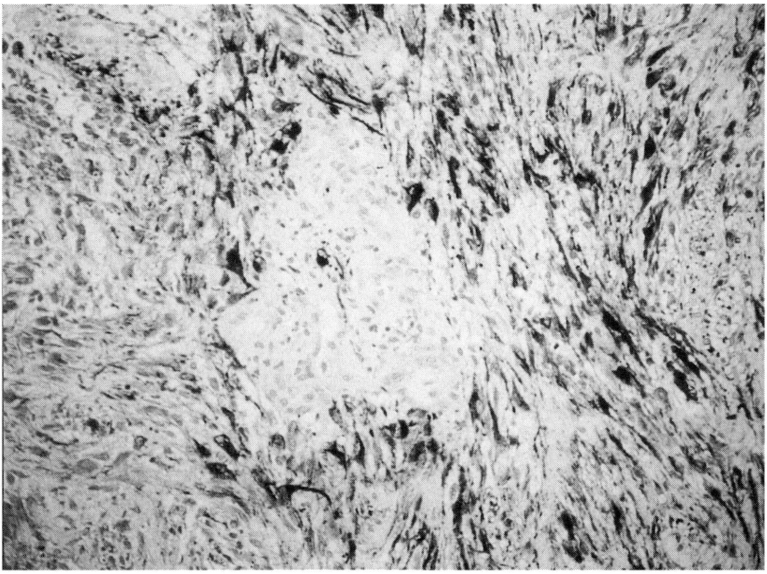

Figure 23 Glioblastoma multiforme. GFAP immunohistochemistry reveals the presence of dark cytoplasmic staining in the majority of neoplastic astrocytes, in contrast with the central, nonstaining area of glomeruloid vascular proliferation.

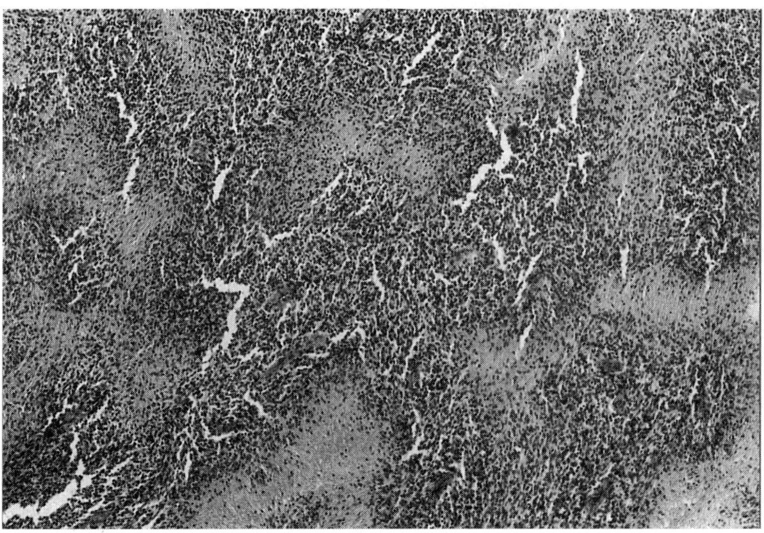

Figure 24 Glioblastoma multiforme. The presence of pale-staining areas of necrosis, surrounded by palisaded rims of tumor cells, is a helpful clue to the diagnosis of glioblastoma multiforme.

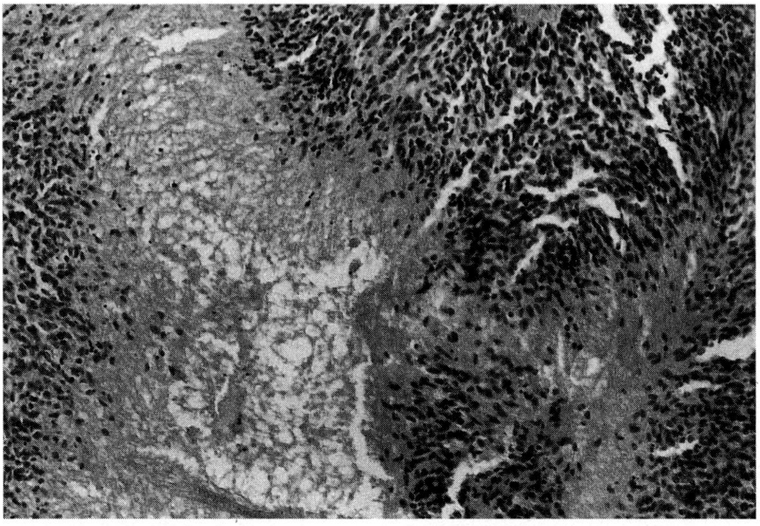

Figure 25 Glioblastoma multiforme. Higher-power view of Figure 24 highlighting the regions of necrosis and perpendicular orientation of tumor cells at their periphery.

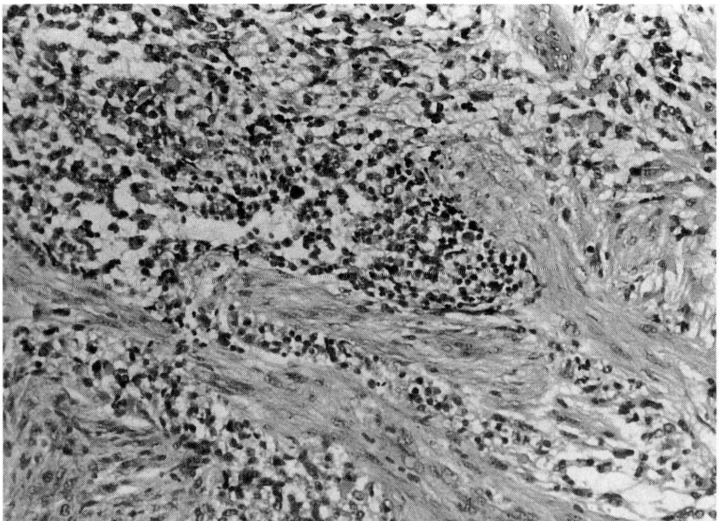

Figure 26 Glioblastoma multiforme. Many glioblastomas infiltrate the leptomeninges and produce a pronounced reactive fibroplasia, resulting in islands of malignant astrocytes separated by cords of collagen and "benign" fibroblasts. It is important to exclude malignant changes in the mesenchymal elements since this would be indicative of gliosarcoma.

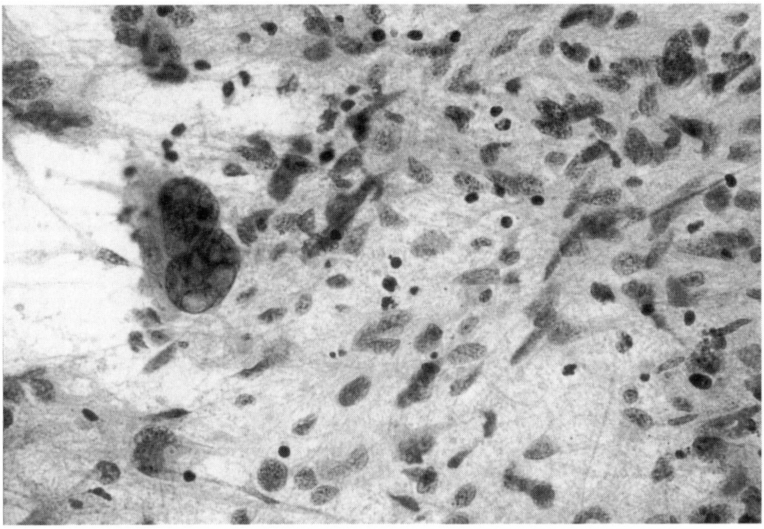

Figure 27 Glioblastoma multiforme. Cytologic smear preparation of a brain biopsy is a useful adjunct to frozen section. This preparation shows a cellular neoplasm with a fibrillary background and marked nuclear atypia. Nuclear debris is seen, indicating necrosis. A diagnosis of high-grade glioma, probably glioblastoma multiforme, can be rendered from such a preparation alone.

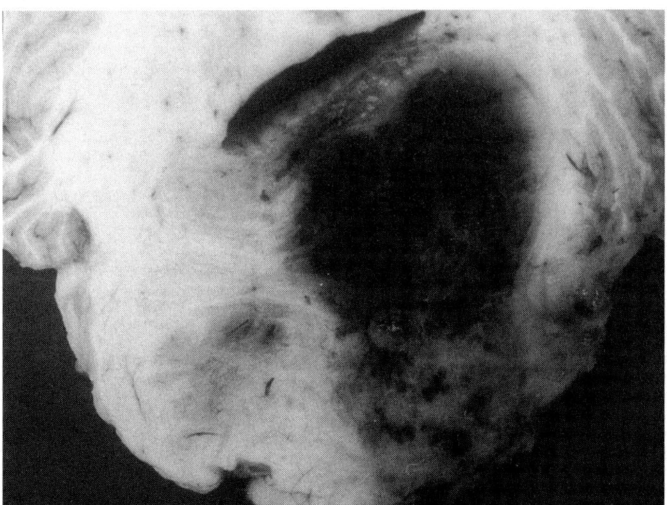

Figure 28 Brainstem astrocytoma. While most brainstem astrocytomas are of low grade, this pontine tumor is a glioblastoma multiforme. The extensive acute intratumoral hemorrhage was this 5-year-old patient's terminal event.

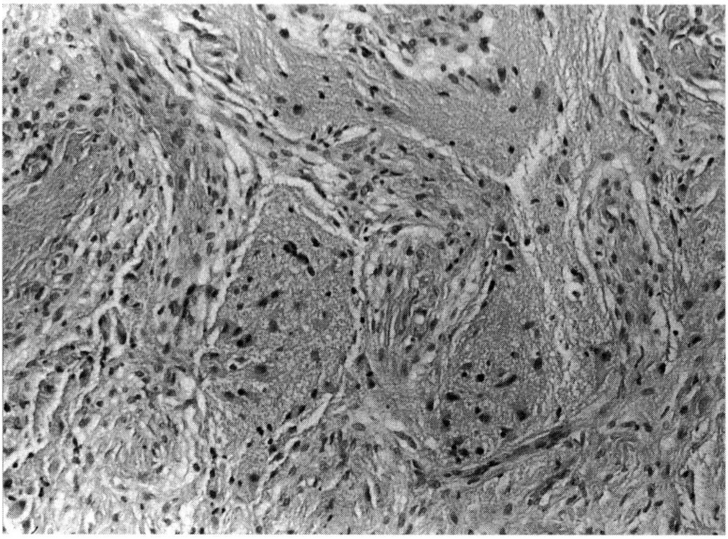

Figure 29 Nasal glioma. These rare nasal tumors are characterized by admixtures of fibroconnective septae and nests of astrocytes with abundant eosinophilic cytoplasm. Neurons may rarely be seen.

sis. Grossly, there is fusiform enlargement of the optic nerve. Microscopic sections show these tumors to have pilocytic differentiation, with expansion of the optic nerve and extension into and through the pia (Figs. 30 and 31).

Subependymal giant cell astrocytomas are mostly found in association with tuberous sclerosis complex. These nodular tumors project into the lateral ventricles and may cause obstruction of the foramen of Monro. Histologically, they consist of pleomorphic giant astrocytes with large nuclei and abundant eosinophilic cytoplasm (Fig. 32). Despite their atypical cellular composition, mitoses are uncommon, and these tumors have an excellent prognosis. GFAP stains are usually positive and neurofilament positivity may also be seen. Giant cell astrocytomas are considered by some to be hamartomatous in nature.

Pleomorphic xanthoastrocytomas are primarily tumors of children and young adults which arise in the temporal or parietal lobes. They are usually discrete, superficially situated, associated with the leptomeninges, and often partially cystic. Microscopically, pleomorphic xanthoastrocytomas are highly atypical neoplasms containing large, bizarre, multinucleated tumor cells. Numerous xanthomatous cells are usually present. Mitosis, necrosis, and vascular endothelial hyperplasia are absent. There is striking intercellular reticulin deposition. The tumors often resemble fibrous histiocytomas, but are GFAP-positive.

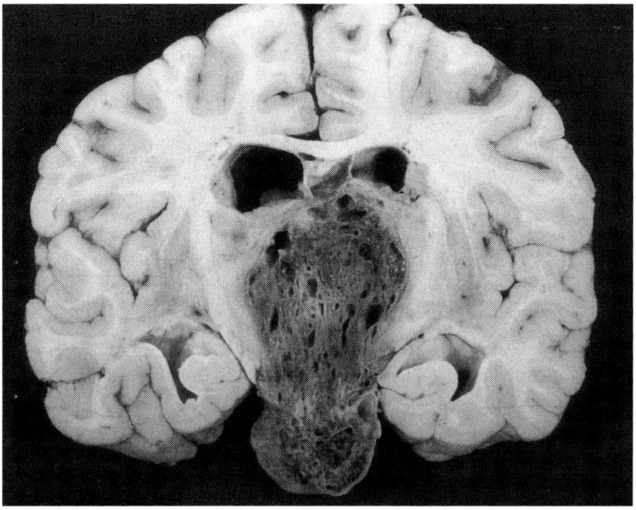

Figure 30 Optic nerve glioma. This large pilocytic astrocytoma originated from the optic chiasm of a 10-year-old boy. The tumor had been diagnosed 8 years previously, and the patient had undergone three prior resections. The glioma shows expansion and destruction of midline structures, including obstruction of the third ventricle and dilatation of the lateral ventricles. There is cystic degeneration and a brownish discoloration due to old hemorrhage.

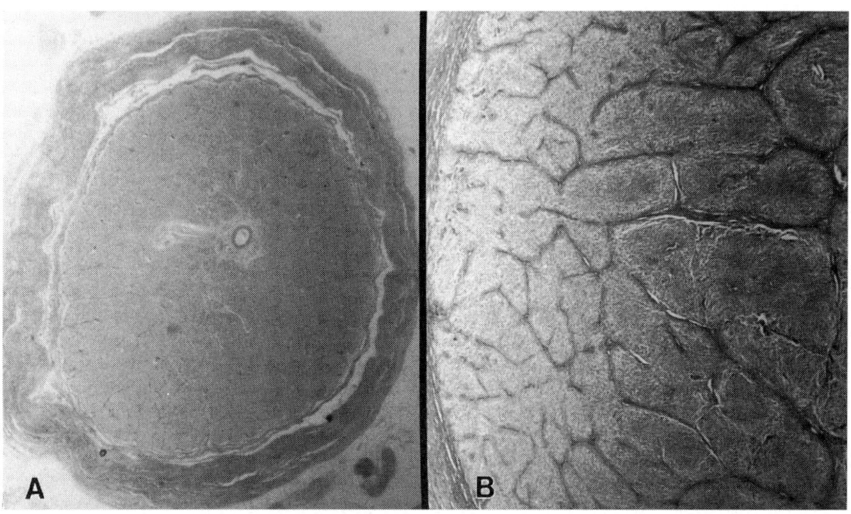

Figure 31 Optic nerve glioma. Both panels represent micrographs of optic nerve at identical magnification. Panel A shows normal optic nerve and dura. Panel B shows optic nerve with marked fusiform cross-sectional enlargement secondary to proliferation of astrocytes. Notice, however, that the normal septation of the optic nerve is retained.

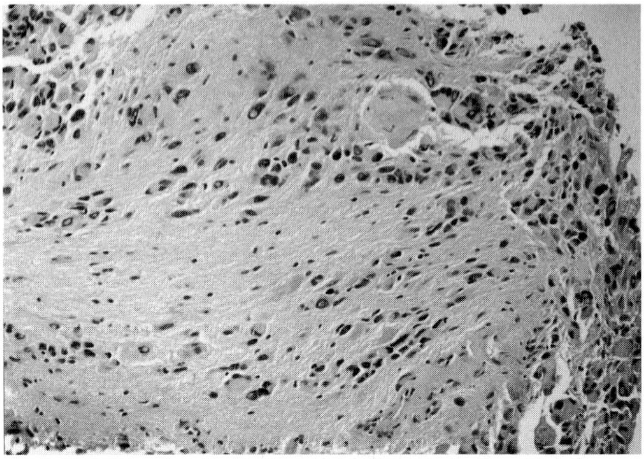

Figure 32 Subependymal giant cell astrocytoma. Such tumors are usually found in the periventricular regions of patients with tuberous sclerosis complex. They are composed of large astrocytes with abundant eosinophilic cytoplasm, which can be easily recognized at scanning magnification.

It is important to differentiate pleomorphic xanthoastrocytomas from glioblastoma multiforme, as they have a favorable prognosis.

Gliomatosis cerebri is a very rare form of astrocytic neoplasia wherein no focal mass exists. The neoplasm diffusely expands large areas of the brain, often being more extensive in some areas than others. The cerebrum is primarily affected, but the brain stem, cerebellum, and spinal cord may also be involved. Neoplastic cells are primarily pilocytic in nature, although other atypical astrocytes may be seen. The tumor is usually found in patients in their 20s and 30s; given the diffuse nature of the neoplasm, the prognosis is bleak.

Astroblastomas are circumscribed tumors composed of embryonal astrocytes ("astroblasts") usually found in the cerebral hemispheres. Histologic sections show perivascular pseudorosettelike arrangement of cells with processes radiating toward a central blood vessel, resembling the perivascular pseudorosettes of ependymomas. These tumors are very rare and usually have a favorable prognosis.

B. Differentiating Astrocytoma from Reactive Gliosis

The term "gliosis" describes a reactive astrocytic proliferation in response to injury, usually taking several weeks to become apparent in routinely stained sections. At times it may be extremely difficult to distinguish gliosis from a low-grade astrocytoma, especially at frozen section. The problem is further compounded by the fact that reactive gliosis often surrounds a glioma. Several features help to distinguish these processes:

1. Reactive astrocytes in gliosis are regularly spaced with nuclei rarely overlapping (Fig. 33). Irregularity, crowding, increased cellular density, and nuclear overlap are characteristics of gliomas.

2. Reactive astrocytes show more cellular uniformity, with lower nuclear-to-cytoplasmic ratios than neoplastic astrocytes. The cytoplasm of reactive astrocytes shows more delicate, symmetrically arranged stellate processes, best seen in GFAP-stained sections.

3. Perineuronal satellitosis by neoplastic glia (at the tumor border) is characteristic of astrocytomas and does not occur in reactive gliosis.

4. Calcification occurs in up to 15% of astrocytomas but is rare in reactive gliosis.

5. Microcysts and mitoses are important diagnostic features of gliomas which are not commonly found in gliosis.

6. Astrocytomas may infiltrate the subpial meninges, a feature not found in reactive gliosis.

7. Grossly, astrocytomas destroy the gray-white matter junction; in gliosis, this region is preserved.

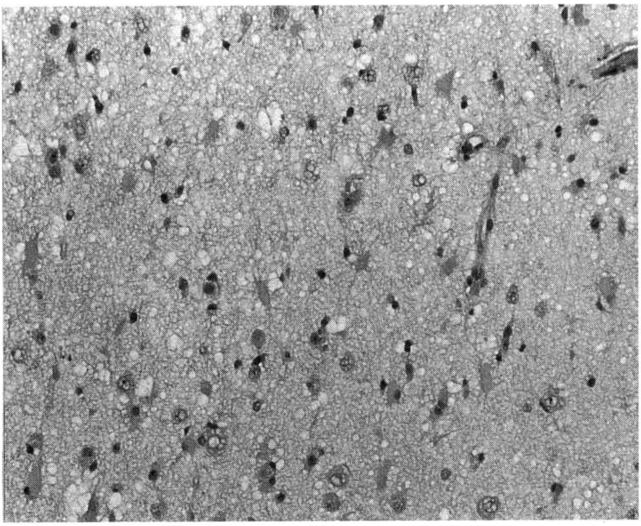

Figure 33 Reactive gliosis. Reactive astrocytes are often gemistocytic, having abundant eosinophilic cytoplasm and numerous cytoplasmic processes. Low-power view highlights their uniformity in spacing, without overlap. This specimen is from the rim of a metastatic adenocarcinoma.

C. Oligodendroglioma

Most oligodendrogliomas occur in adults, with a peak incidence in the fourth decade. They comprise about 5% of gliomas. Grossly, they are well-circumscribed, slow-growing, soft, noncystic tumors which are primarily found in the cerebral hemispheres, especially the frontal lobes (Fig. 34). Oligodendrogliomas are predominantly seen in the white matter, with extension into the cortex and leptomeninges. They frequently undergo spontaneous hemorrhage, sometimes fatal. About half of the cases are heavily calcified, a useful but nonspecific clue in neuroradiographic studies. Survival beyond 5 years is common.

In histologic sections, oligodendrogliomas are characterized by sheets of evenly distributed, uniform, epithelioid cells having a "fried-egg" appearance, characterized by clear perinuclear halos surrounding round, uniform nuclei (Fig. 35). This classic cytoplasmic clearing, while a very useful diagnostic feature, is an artifact of tissue processing and is not seen in frozen section or smear preparations (Fig. 36). Many small, delicate, "chicken wire" capillaries are interspersed, and microcalcospherites are found in over 90% of cases; mitotic figures are rare. The fibrillary background so characteristic of most gliomas is a relatively minor feature of oligodendrogliomas, and, as such, GFAP stains may be negative. While these tumors are grossly well demarcated, histologically they have an infiltrative border and often show prominent perineuronal satellitosis.

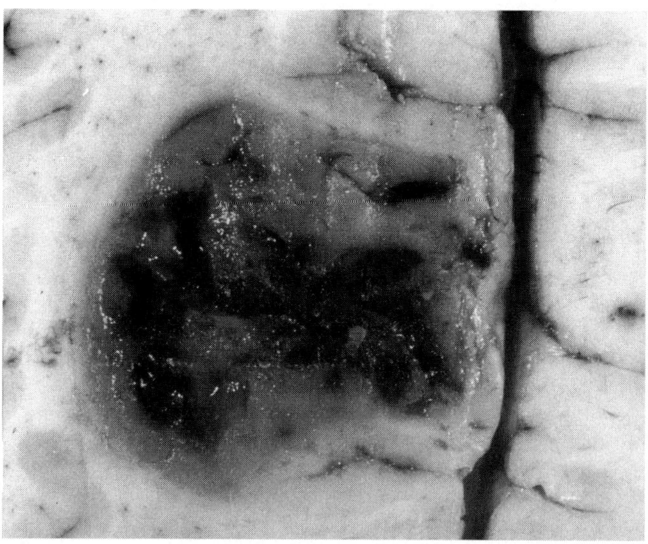

Figure 34 Oligodendroglioma. The deep cortical white matter contains a discrete light tan tumor nodule. Hemorrhage is common in oligodendrogliomas.

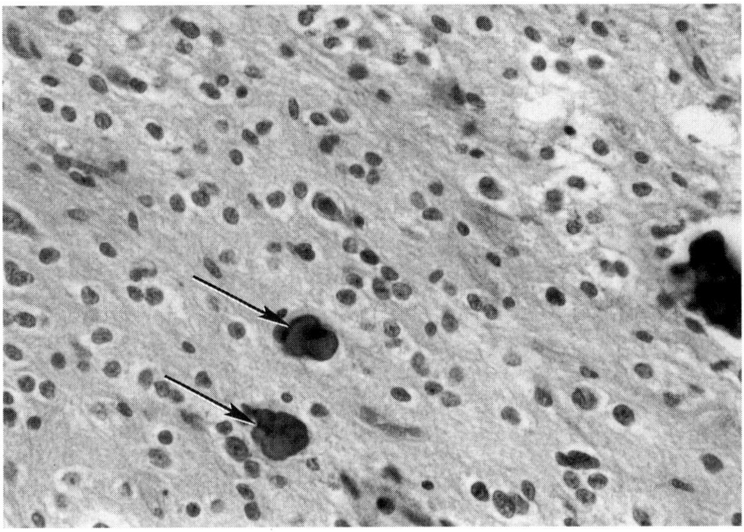

Figure 35 Oligodendroglioma. Perinuclear clearing and nuclear uniformity are characteristic of oligodendrogliomas. Stromal microcalcifications are common (arrows).

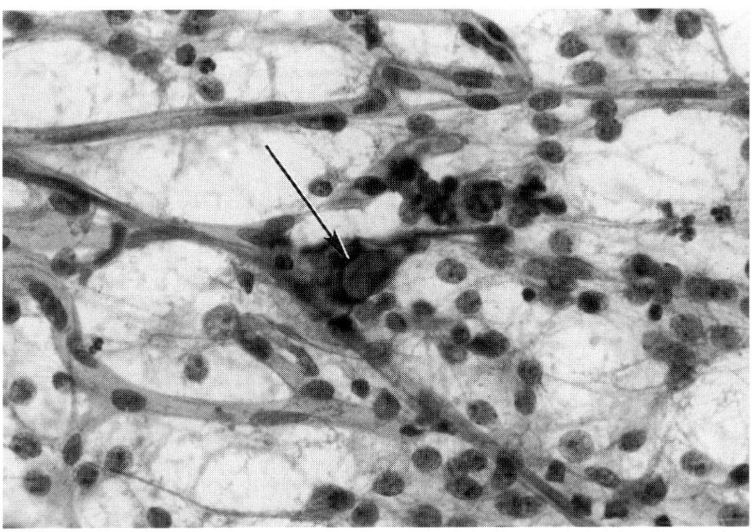

Figure 36 Oligodendroglioma. A squash preparation highlights the rich capillary content of these neoplasms. Tumor nuclei are round and uniform, with delicate chromatin and small nucleoli. The cytoplasm of tumor cells is usually striped off in smear preparation. A small calcification is seen (arrow), a helpful diagnostic clue.

Some oligodendrogliomas show areas with numerous mitosis, marked nuclear atypia, focal necrosis, and cellular crowding. Such lesions have a worse prognosis and should be considered as *anaplastic (malignant) oligodendrogliomas* rather than GBMs if the oligodendroglial elements predominate and vascular endothelial hyperplasia is absent (Figs. 37, 38).

It is not infrequent to see regions of usual astrocytoma (pilocytic, gemistocytic, protoplasmic, anaplastic) near or mixed with an otherwise typical oligodendroglioma. If such elements comprise a significant percentage of the neoplasm, the tumor should be considered a *mixed glioma (oligoastrocytoma)*. Most of these tumors behave like oligodendrogliomas.

D. Ependymomas

Ependymomas are well-demarcated, homogeneous, fleshy, slow-growing neoplasms. They may be lobulated and generally are intra- or periventricular in location (Fig. 39). Cerebral ependymomas occur in all age groups and have a tendency to expand into the surrounding brain. Infratentorial ependymomas occur primarily in children, having a predilection for the floor of the fourth ventricle, often filling it and growing through the foramina of Luschka and Magendie. Many ependymomas are calcified. They may be multiple in patients with neurofibromatosis.

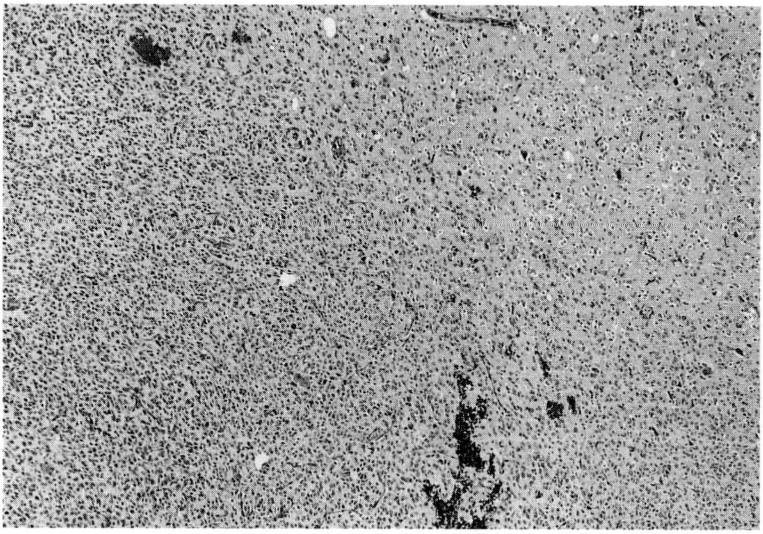

Figure 37 Oligodendroglioma. Scanning magnification shows transition between the low cellularity of a typical oligodendroglioma (top right) with the hypercellularity of an anaplastic oligodendroglioma (left).

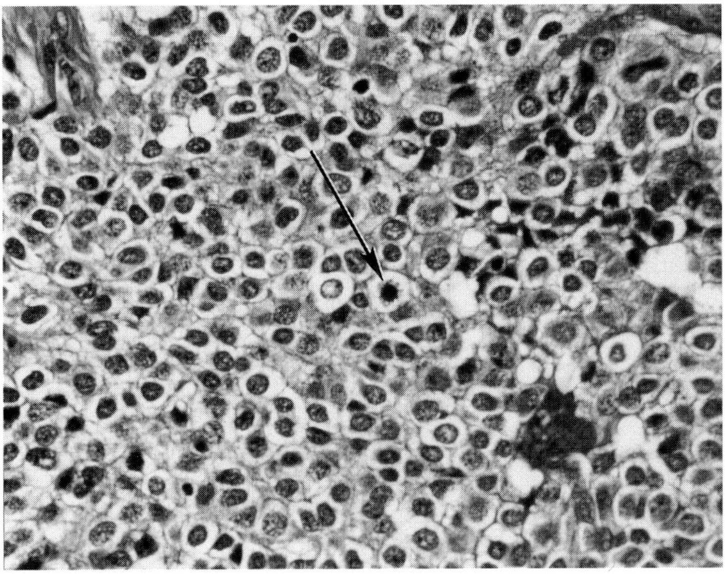

Figure 38 Anaplastic oligodendroglioma. This neoplasm reveals cellular crowding, slight nuclear irregularity, atypia, and increased numbers of mitosis (arrow).

Microscopic examination of ependymomas shows good circumscription but a highly variable cellular appearance. Some ependymomas are of low cellular density, whereas others show cellular crowding and an epithelioid appearance. Most consist of round to ovoid cells with eosinophilic cytoplasm, often with bipolar processes. Clues to the diagnosis of ependymoma are:

1. *Perivascular pseudorosettes.* These are acellular areas of fibrillary eosinophilic cytoplasm surrounding (often thickened) blood vessels, with an outer border of tumor cells (Figs. 40, 41). Perivascular pseudorosettes are frequently present even in very cellular tumors and usually are evident at scanning magnification. Sometimes they may even be appreciated in smear preparations (Fig. 42).
2. *True ependymal rosettes.* While less common than pseudorosettes, these are very helpful if present. Tumor cells are lined up around a central tubular space resembling the arrangement of cells lining the central canal of the spinal cord; cilia are often seen.
3. The presence of tubules and canals is a helpful clue.
4. Ultrastructural examination reveals ciliary bodies and blepharoplasts, specific diagnostic features of ependymomas.

Morphologic subtypes include clear cell (resembling oligodendrogliomas), tanycytic (abundant fibrillary stroma like astrocytomas), and papillary

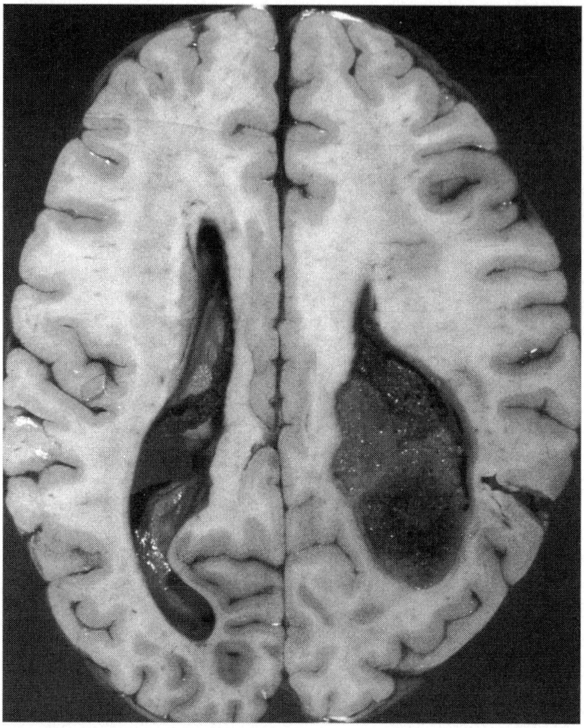

Figure 39 Ependymoma. The posterior horn of the right lateral ventricle is filled with a soft, reddish-tan neoplasm.

ependymomas. The papillary variant is characterized by singly or multilayered tumor cells covering a core of glial elements (as opposed to the connective tissue core seen in choroid plexus papillomas). Myxopapillary ependymomas are discussed with spinal cord neoplasms.

At times ependymomas may be confused with meningiomas and even metastatic carcinomas. It is useful to remember that they are immunohistochemically GFAP-positive, are EMA-negative, and have unique ultrastructural findings.

Most ependymomas are of low histologic grade. Rarely ependymomas exhibit increased cellularity, striking atypia, mitotic activity, and focal necrosis. Such lesions are associated with a poor prognosis and should be considered *anaplastic* (*malignant*) *ependymomas* rather than glioblastoma multiforme if they show predominantly ependymal differentiation.

Subependymomas are small, slow-growing, discrete, lobulated, periventricular tumors of adults. They are often found incidentally at autopsy projecting into the fourth ventricle (Fig. 43), sometimes causing obstructive hydro-

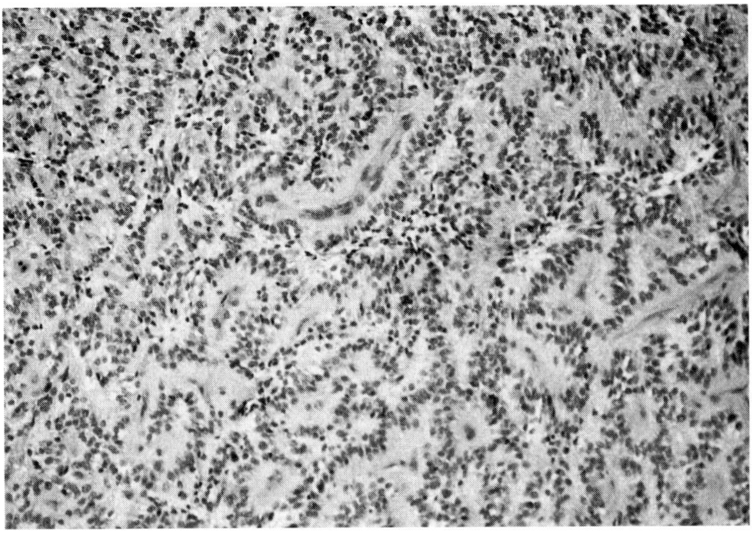

Figure 40 Ependymoma. Ependymomas demonstrate a variety of histologic patterns. Key to their diagnosis is the presence of perivascular pseudorosettes, which are acellular eosinophilic areas surrounding blood vessels. The tumor cells show a trabecular arrangement.

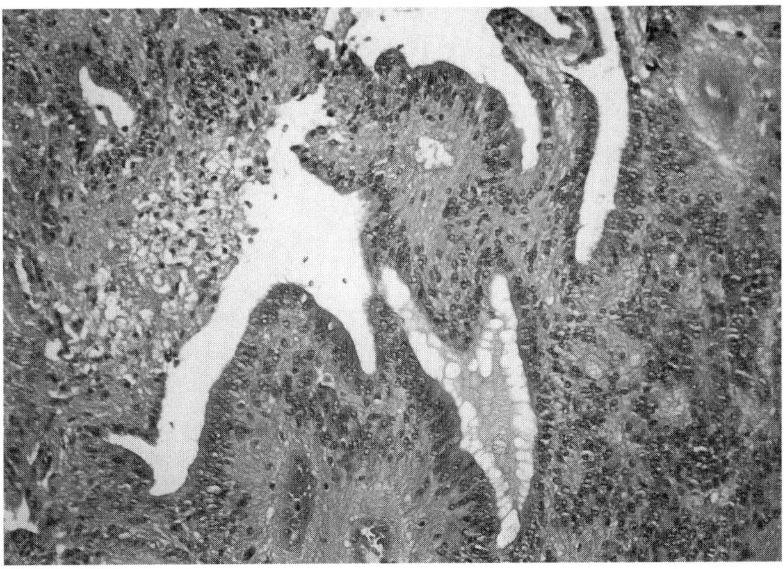

Figure 41 Ependymoma. The epithelial nature of this ependymoma is characterized by glandlike spaces and papillary structures having glial rather than fibrovascular cores. Note the presence of perivascular pseudorosettes.

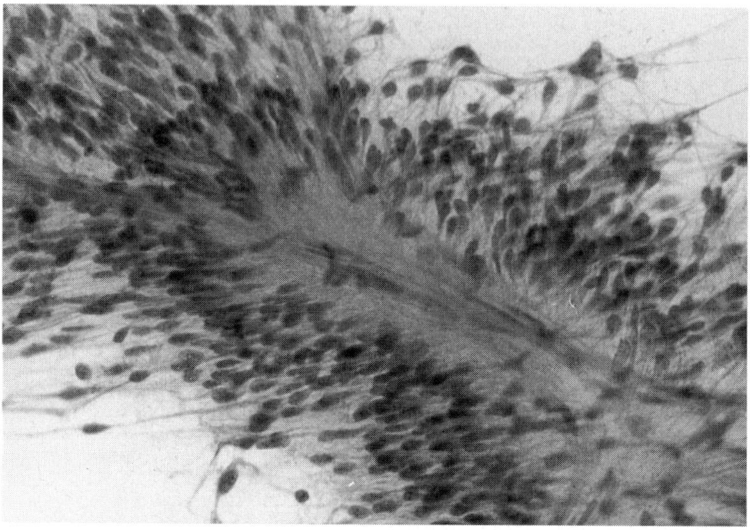

Figure 42 Ependymoma. It is important to recognize ependymomas intraoperatively since the neurosurgeon will usually attempt complete gross resection. This squash preparation shows a classic perivascular pseudorosette.

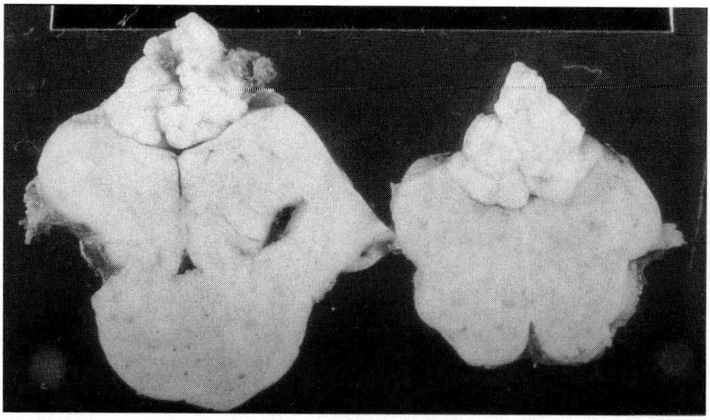

Figure 43 Subependymoma. Subependymomas commonly arise from the floor of the fourth ventricle, to which they are firmly adherent. The tumor is pale, discrete, and multilobulated, filling much of the fourth ventricle.

cephalus. Less commonly, subependymomas may present in the lateral ventricles or spinal cord and, rarely, may be multiple. They are firm, gray-tan tumors which may be partially calcified. Spontaneous hemorrhage is rare. The histologic pattern is quite distinctive. The tumors are of low grade and low cellularity, being composed of irregularly clustered nests of small uniform cells amidst a fibrillary background which often reveals microcystic changes (Fig. 44). Tumor cells exhibit both ependymal and astrocytic differentiation.

V. CHOROID PLEXUS TUMORS

Choroid plexus papillomas are rare intraventricular neoplasms most commonly found in children and young adults. About half occur in the fourth ventricle (mostly in older patients); papillomas may also arise in the lateral ventricles (in children) and, rarely, the third ventricle. Patients often present with hydrocephalus due to either obstruction or increased CSF production. Radiographically, some of these tumors show dense calcifications. Most patients are cured by surgical resection, although some papillomas recur.

Grossly, choroid plexus papillomas are red, velvety, cauliflowerlike lesions sometimes showing cystic change. They frequently "burrow" into the sur-

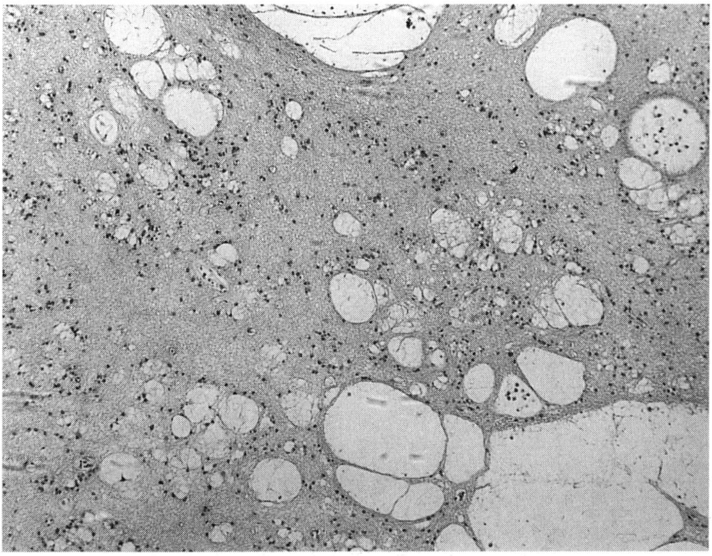

Figure 44 Subependymoma. These tumors are of low cellular density. The background is eosinophilic and fibrillary, with scattered small cysts and clusters of tumor cells.

rounding brain parenchyma, but do not infiltrate it. Histologically, papillomas very closely resemble normal choroid plexus; however, the quantity of tissue greatly exceeds that usually seen. A layer of uniform cuboidal to columnar epithelium lies on a fibrovascular core (Fig. 45). Microcalcifications are common; mitoses are rare. The differential diagnosis includes papillary ependymoma, which has a glial rather than fibrovascular core and is GFAP-positive and keratin-negative.

The presence of marked cytologic atypia, cellular stratification, necrosis, abundant mitosis, and brain invasion in a neoplasm which merges with a usual choroid plexus papilloma is diagnostic of *choroid plexus carcinoma*. These are extremely rare neoplasms, usually found in young children, which can easily be confused with metastatic adenocarcinoma.

VI. NEURONAL HAMARTOMAS/NEOPLASMS

Ganglion cell tumors generally occur in children and young adults less than 30 years of age, who usually present with seizures. They are slow-growing lesions most often found in the temporal or frontal lobes or around the third ventricle, but they may occur anywhere in the CNS. Some gangliogliomas present as partially calcified mural nodules within a cyst. Some authors believe that many

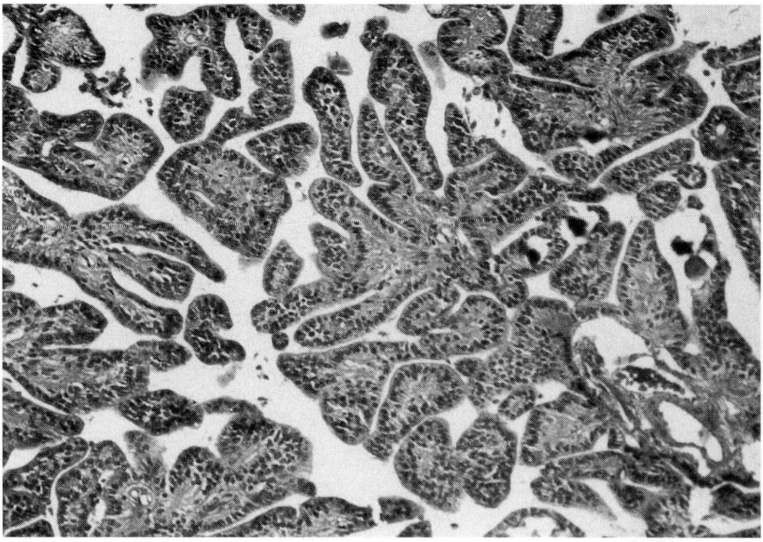

Figure 45 Choroid plexus papilloma. These intraventricular tumors resemble normal choroid plexus, but of increased abundance. The papillary fronds have a fibrovascular core and are lined by uniform cuboidal epithelium, with frequent microcalcifications.

ganglion cell tumors are hamartomas, rather than true neoplasms, although clinically most exhibit the growth characteristics of a neoplasm. They usually have a favorable prognosis, better than that of most gliomas, and only rarely behave in a malignant fashion.

Histologically, these tumors are composed of abnormal, hypercellular proliferations of neuronal (ganglion) cells, admixed with variable amounts of astrocytic and oligodendroglial elements, in a fibrillary stroma. Recognizing abnormal ganglion cells is critical to the diagnosis. These cells frequently show multinucleation, disarray, and increased cell density, and they characteristically have Nissl substance. Usually it is not difficult to distinguish them from normal or entrapped neurons. These neoplastic ganglion cells stain immunohistochemically with neurofilament and synaptophysin. Ultrastructurally, neurosecretory granules and synapses may be identified, as well as Nissl substance and neurofilaments.

Once the neoplastic ganglion cell element has been identified, the stroma must be evaluated, preferably with a GFAP stain. If astrocytic elements are minimal (e.g., at the periphery) and thought to be reactive rather than neoplastic, the lesion is classified as a *gangliocytoma.* If a significant astrocytic component is part of the neoplasm—which may be fibrillary, protoplasmic or pilocytic, but not anaplastic—the lesion is called a *ganglioglioma* (Figs. 46, 47).

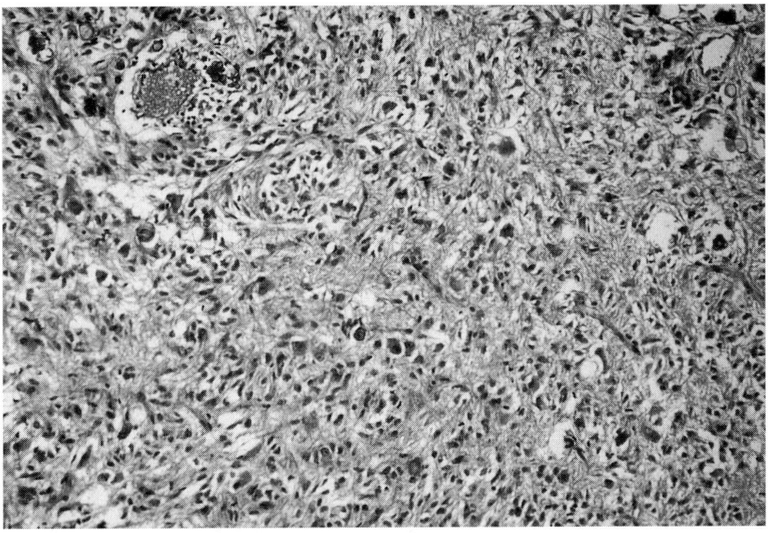

Figure 46 Ganglioglioma. Scanning view demonstrates a haphazard arrangement of neoplastic neuronal cells and astrocytes amidst a loose fibrillary background. Microcalcifications are abundant.

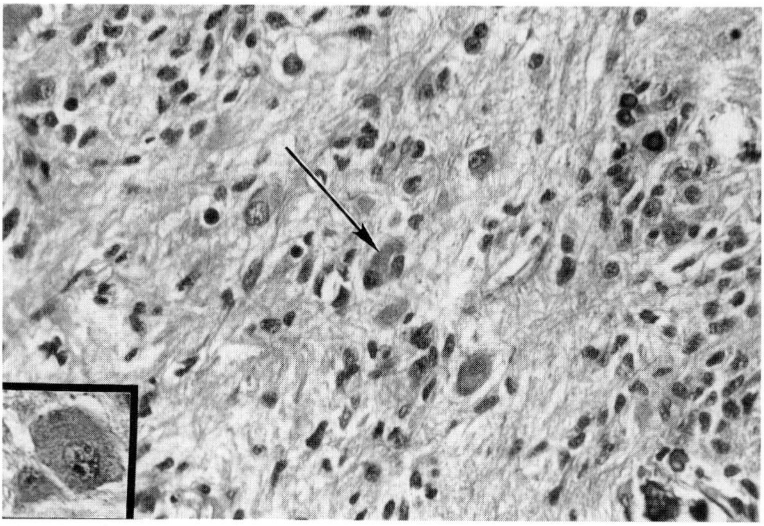

Figure 47 Ganglioglioma. Higher magnification shows atypical neuronal cells with abundant cytoplasm admixed with smaller, angulated astrocytes. Some neuronal cells are binucleate (arrow). Inset highlights closeup view of a neuronal cell.

Calcification, perivascular lymphoid infiltrates, and small cysts are commonly seen. A *desmoplastic infantile ganglioglioma* is a tumor found in patients under 18 months of age that is usually massive, firm (due to collagen deposition), and frequently cystic; it often involves the meninges.

Rarely these tumors show astrocytic atypia and numerous mitosis and should be considered *anaplastic gangliogliomas.* Such tumors have a worse prognosis. If a neoplasm has fewer mature ganglion cells than neuroblasts, without a significant astrocytic component, it is best designated a *ganglioneuroblastoma.*

Central neurocytomas are rare tumors primarily of young adults which are usually supratentorial and intraventricular in location. They represent the most common neoplasm of the septum pellucidum. These tumors are frequently calcified and generally have a favorable prognosis. They are derived from immature ganglion cells and histologically demonstrate sheets of strikingly uniform, round, clear cells resembling those of oligodendrogliomas or clear cell ependymomas (perivascular pseudorosette formation may be also be seen). Some neurocytomas may show cytologic atypia, increased mitosis, vascular endothelial hyperplasia, and necrosis, which are prognostically unfavorable.

Either immunohistochemical or electron microscopic studies are required to reach a definitive diagnosis of central neurocytoma. These neoplasms demonstrate immunopositivity for synaptophysin, neuron-specific enolase, and neurofilament, but not GFAP. Ultrastructurally, they exhibit neuronal differentiation, containing synaptic structures, microtubules, and clear or dense-core vesicles.

VII. MESENCHYMAL LESIONS

A. Hemangioblastomas

Hemangioblastomas are benign tumors primarily of middle age which may be found at a variety of locations, especially within the cerebellum and upper half of the spinal cord. The tumors are usually well-demarcated, red nodules, solid or cystic (with yellowish viscous fluid and tumor nidus), which often have a meningeal attachment. Some tumors are multiple, especially those in patients with von Hippel–Lindau syndrome (also characterized by renal, pancreatic, and hepatic cysts; renal cell carcinoma; papillary cystadenoma of epididymis or mesosalpinx; and pheochromocytoma). Hemangioblastomas may secrete erythropoietin and cause polycythemia. Surgical resection is often curative, although recurrences of subtotally resected lesions are seen.

Histologically, hemangioblastomas are composed of an admixture of thin-walled blood vessels and pale, foamy, stromal cells (Figs. 48, 49). The vascular pattern is best highlighted by a reticulin stain or immunohistochemical stain for endothelial cells (e.g., Factor VIII, CD-34, CD-31). The intervening pale cells

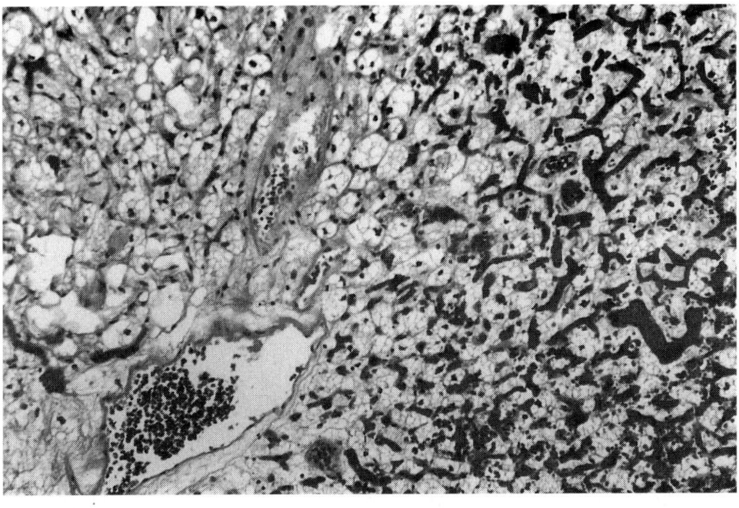

Figure 48 Hemangioblastoma. The two components, endothelial-lined blood vessels and pale stromal cells, are illustrated. The relative proportions of these elements can vary significantly.

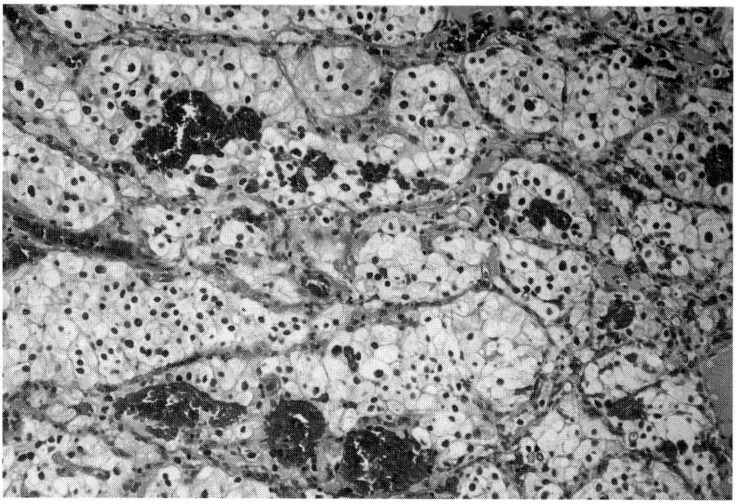

Figure 49 Hemangioblastoma. The stromal cells have pale, "bubbly" cytoplasm which is lipid-laden. In this neoplasm, they are arranged as nests and small sheets, with the vascular component being less conspicuous. Hemangioblastomas must be differentiated from metastatic renal cell carcinoma.

have abundant lipid-laden cytoplasm, the lipid being removed by routine tissue processing; Oil Red O stains can be performed on frozen sections if one wishes to confirm its presence. Enlarged, atypical, tumor nuclei are common and do not indicate malignancy. Biopsies of the wall of a cystic hemangioblastoma reveals gliosis and Rosenthal fibers, which may result in an erroneous diagnosis of pilocytic or cerebellar astrocytoma if the main portion of the neoplasm is not sampled. The pattern of hemangioblastomas mimics metastatic renal cell carcinoma (Fig. 113), which is always in the differential diagnosis.

B. Gliosarcomas

Gliosarcomas are rare neoplasms which exhibit a biphasic admixture glioblastoma multiforme and sarcoma. They are firm, fairly discrete neoplasms of older patients which favor the temporal lobes. Reticulin and collagen stains are helpful in differentiating the sarcomatous areas (reticulin-positive) from the malignant astrocytic component (reticulin-negative); an "inverted" staining pattern is observed with GFAP, which clearly delineates the malignant astrocytic elements. The sarcomatous constituent is usually fibrosarcoma, but chondrosarcoma, osteosarcoma, and rhabdomyosarcoma rarely occur. Gliosarcomas have a propensity to invade blood vessels and develop systemic metastases. Their prognosis is very poor.

C. Lymphomas

Lymphomas may arise primarily within the central nervous system (usually cerebral parenchyma) or may involve the CNS secondary to systemic disease (favoring the leptomeninges). The incidence of primary CNS lymphoma has dramatically increased in the past few decades mostly in direct association with the AIDS epidemic and increased use of immunosuppressive therapy, to the point where CNS lymphomas are among the most common neoplasms encountered in young adults. Still, overall they comprise less than 2% of intracranial neoplasms. Any age group may be affected, although primary CNS lymphomas are rare in children. Virtually all CNS lymphomas, whether primary or secondary, are high-grade non-Hodgkin's lymphomas of B-cell origin. T-cell lymphomas (including lymphomatoid granulomatosis) and Hodgkin's disease involving the CNS are rare.

Grossly, CNS lymphomas are often bulky, soft, and of gray to light tan color (Figs. 50, 51). Tumor nodules may be single or multiple, and have indiscrete borders. Air-dried, Diff-Quik-stained touch preparations (Fig. 52) are very helpful in arriving at the correct diagnosis at the time of intraoperative consultation, showing poorly cohesive cells, absence of a fibrillary background, and the presence of cytoplasmic fragments ("lymphoglandular bodies"). If the diagnosis of lymphoma is suspected and an adequate specimen is available, tissue should

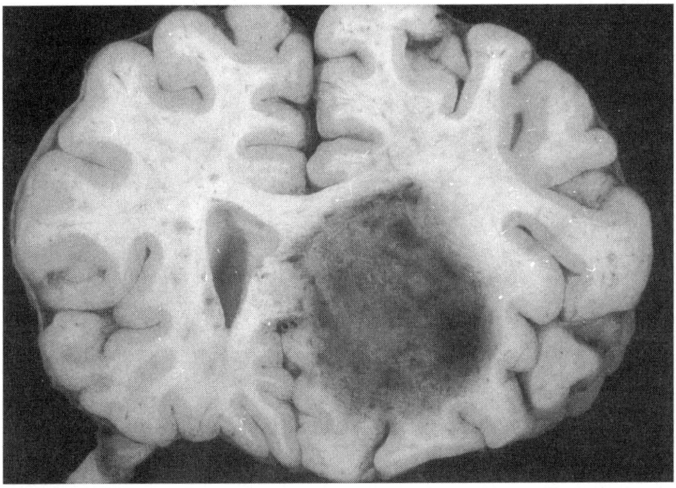

Figure 50 Lymphoma. There is a large, necrotic, focally hemorrhagic tumor mass in the deep cortical gray and white matter of this 35-year-old AIDS patient. Histologic sections revealed a primary, large-cell CNS lymphoma.

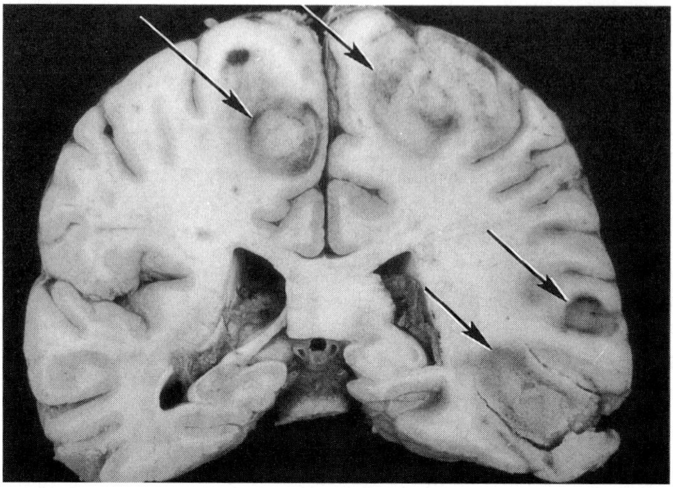

Figure 51 Lymphoma. Primary CNS lymphomas are frequently multifocal, as illustrated in this case (arrows). The patient was a 31-year-old man with AIDS. Microscopic sections showed multifocal, plasmacytoid, B-cell lymphoma.

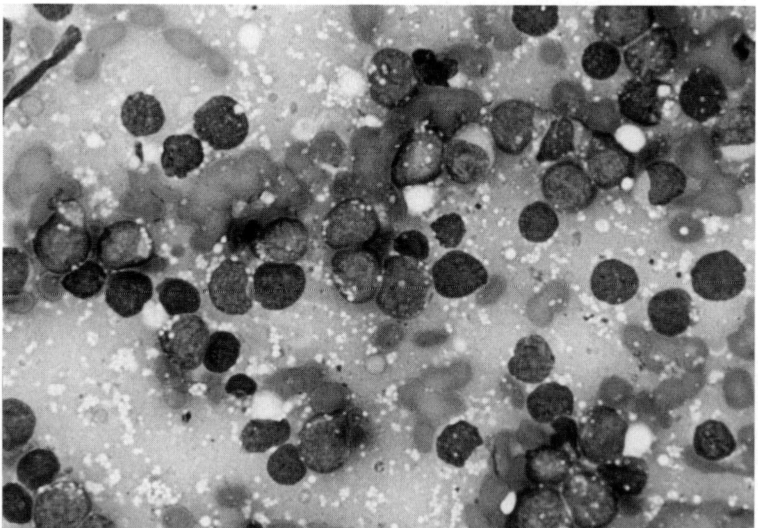

Figure 52 Lymphoma. In our experience, air-dried, Diff-Quik-stained touch preparations are the preferred method of diagnosing primary CNS lymphoma intraoperatively. The neoplastic cells in this preparation are poorly cohesive, lack fibrillary cytoplasm, and contain cytoplasmic vacuoles. Rounded cytoplasmic fragments (lymphoglandular bodies) are seen. A diagnosis of high-grade Burkitt-like lymphoma was rendered.

be snap frozen for possible marker studies and preserved in B-5 fixative for superior cytologic details. Lymphoma cells are very fragile, and biopsies should be handled with great care to avoid cell rupture and crush artifact.

Histologically, CNS lymphomas resemble their nodal counterparts and are classified in a manner analogous to peripheral lymphomas. Consultation with a hematopathologist is often helpful to ensure their precise subclassification. The cells are recognized as either mature-appearing or atypical lymphoid cells that show a striking affinity for blood vessels, the pattern of angiocentricity (highlighted by a reticulin stain) and affinity for the perivascular Virchow-Robin space being useful diagnostic clues (Figs. 53, 54). In time, a sheetlike proliferation of cells effaces the normal brain parenchyma. Fibrillary background is absent and epithelioid cells are not seen. Tumors from patients previously treated with corticosteroids are often extensively necrotic and suboptimal or inadequate for diagnosis.

Immunohistochemical studies confirming the lymphoid origin of the neoplasm, determining the monoclonality of a B- or T-cell lineage (thereby excluding a polyclonal reactive inflammatory infiltrate), and excluding other possible tumors are an integral part of the workup of lymphomas (Fig. 55). Primitive neuroectodermal tumors and metastatic small-cell carcinomas are morphologically in the differential diagnosis, but can easily be excluded immunophenotypically. Some institutions use gene rearrangement analysis to aid to the diagnosis

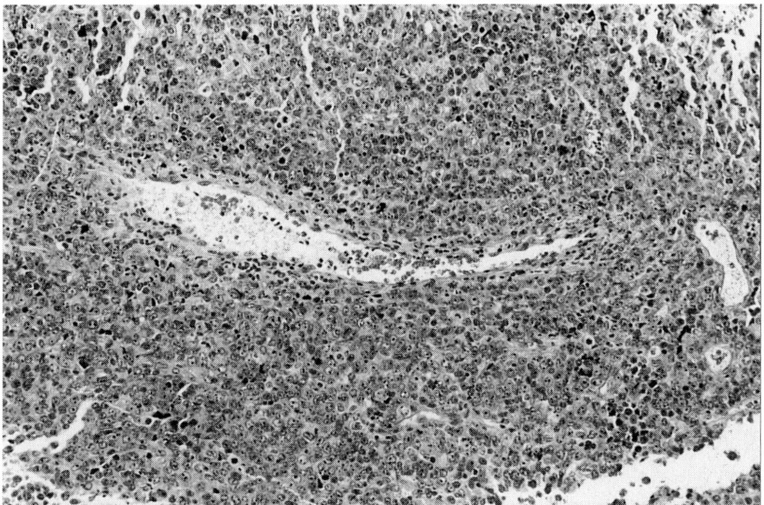

Figure 53 Lymphoma. Marked angiocentricity is a clue to the diagnosis of primary CNS lymphoma. The central, longitudinally sectioned vessel is encased by sheets of poorly differentiated tumor cells.

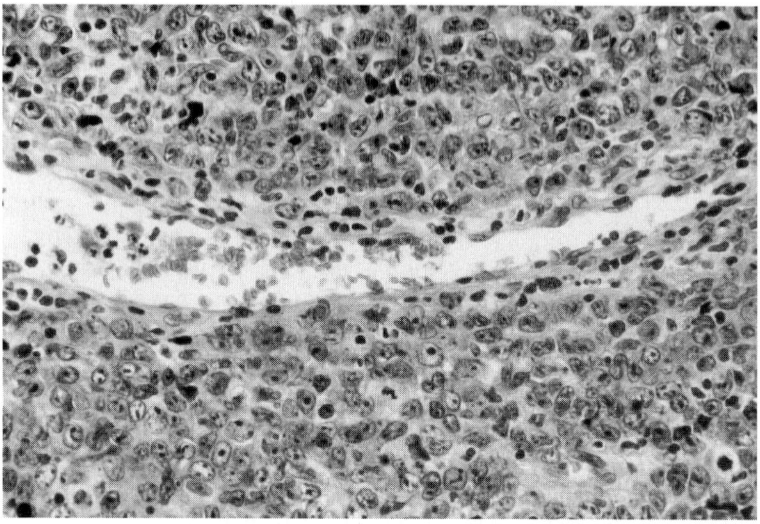

Figure 54 Lymphoma. Higher magnification of Figure 53 highlights the superb nuclear detail provided by B-5 fixation. The tumor was immunopositive for leukocyte common antigen and L-26, with lambda light-chain restriction. It is a B-cell immunoblastic lymphoma.

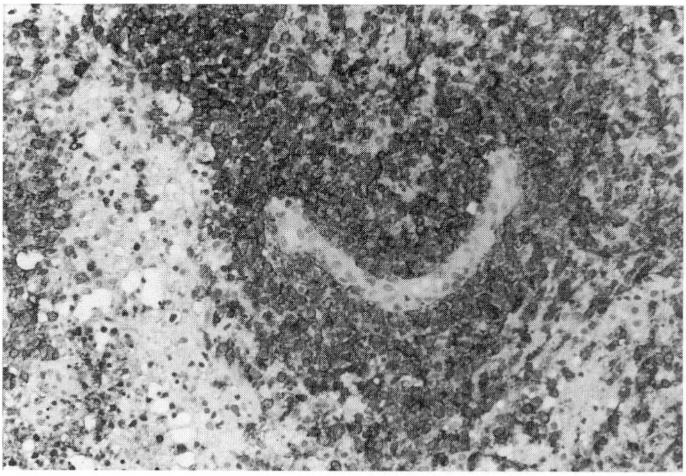

Figure 55 Lymphoma. Immunohistochemical stain for L-26 shows a proliferation of neoplastic B-lymphocytes surrounding a small (nonstaining) blood vessel.

of lymphoma, although in our experience this is not necessary except for rare problematic cases.

D. Leukemias

Leukemias usually secondarily seed the meninges and are found on CSF cytologic preparations. Rarely, patients with myelogenous leukemia may form mass lesions within the leptomeninges or brain parenchyma called chloromas (Fig. 56). These tumors grossly and histologically resemble lymphomas and are differentiated by a knowledge of the clinical history and appropriate histochemical stains (e.g., chloracetate esterase).

Clinically significant vascular neoplasms and hamartomas are common and are discussed in Chapter 2.

VIII. EMBRYONAL NEOPLASMS

A. Primitive Neuroectodermal Tumors (PNETs)

PNETs are undifferentiated neoplasms which consist of cells that resemble the primitive neuroectoderm of the fetus. PNETs presumably arise from rests of

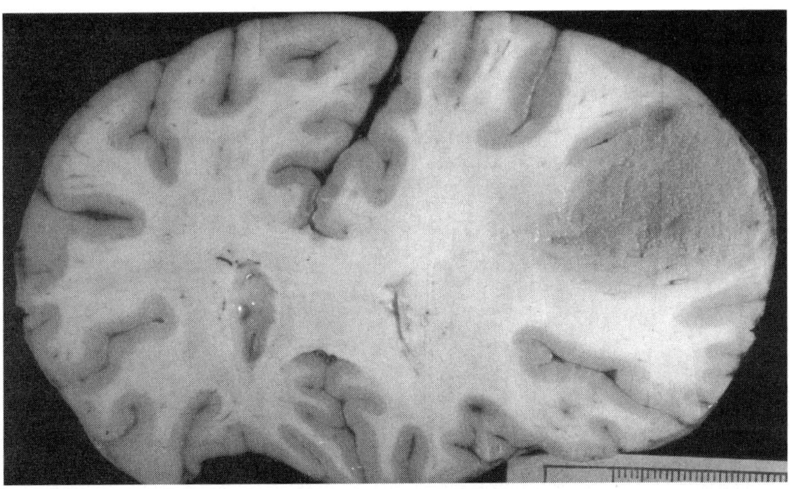

Figure 56 Leukemia. Most leukemias do not show grossly evident CNS involvement, preferentially seeding the subarachnoid space. This patient has a large friable tumor nodule in the right frontal lobe which was shown to be composed of myelogenous leukemia blast cells (i.e., chloroma). There is pronounced edema and a right-to-left shift of midline structures. Histologically, such neoplasms often bear a striking resemblance to lymphoma.

germinal cells which have the potential to differentiate into glial or neuronal elements. These rapidly growing, malignant neoplasms mostly develop in children.

Grossly, PNETs are often cystic and hemorrhagic, usually sharply demarcated, with compression of adjacent brain (Fig. 57). Histologically, they are infiltrative, small, "blue cell" neoplasms characterized by crowded darkly staining cells having scanty cytoplasm (Figs. 58, 59). Pleomorphism, mitoses, and necrosis are common. These tumors must be distinguished from other small-cell neoplasms, such as lymphoma and metastatic small cell carcinomas. PNETs have a propensity to metastasize along CSF pathways.

PNETs are subdivided primarily by their anatomic location and clinical presentation, as well as subtle histopathologic differences. There is debate as to whether these subdivisions are mostly arbitrary rather than based on true biologic differences. If specific criteria are not identified, such neoplasms may be diagnosed as *undifferentiated PNETs*.

B. Medulloblastoma

Medulloblastoma is the most common PNET, arising in the vermis or one of the cerebellar hemispheres. Medulloblastoma is primarily a tumor of childhood, with over half of the cases presenting in the first decade of life. They are the second most common CNS tumor of childhood; only astrocytomas are more prevalent. There is a slight male preponderance.

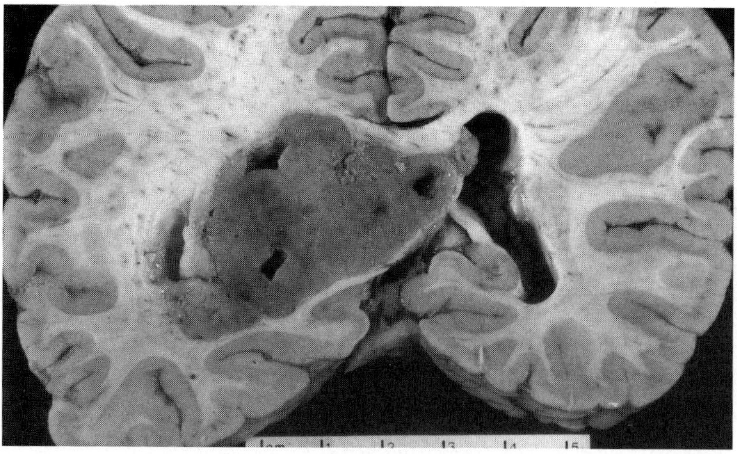

Figure 57 Primitive neuroectodermal tumor. A large, partially cystic tumor effaces the medial left cerebral hemisphere, with extension across the midline. Histologic sections showed a PNET. Such neoplasms frequently develop intracranial metastasis.

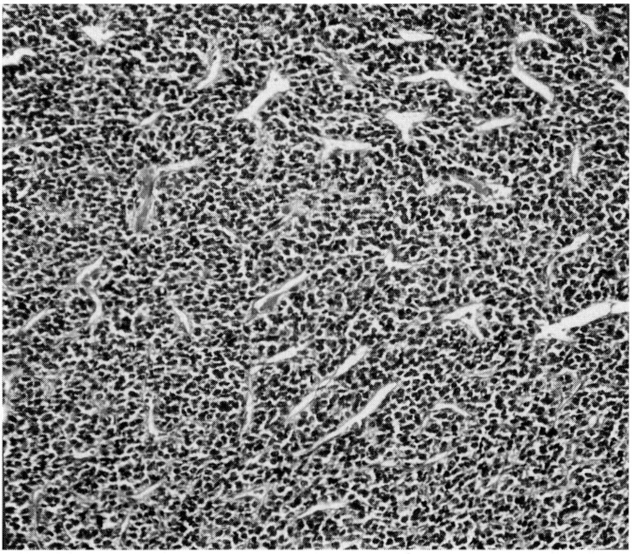

Figure 58 Primitive neuroectodermal tumor. These neoplasms are characterized by sheets of small undifferentiated cells separated by delicate fibrovascular septae.

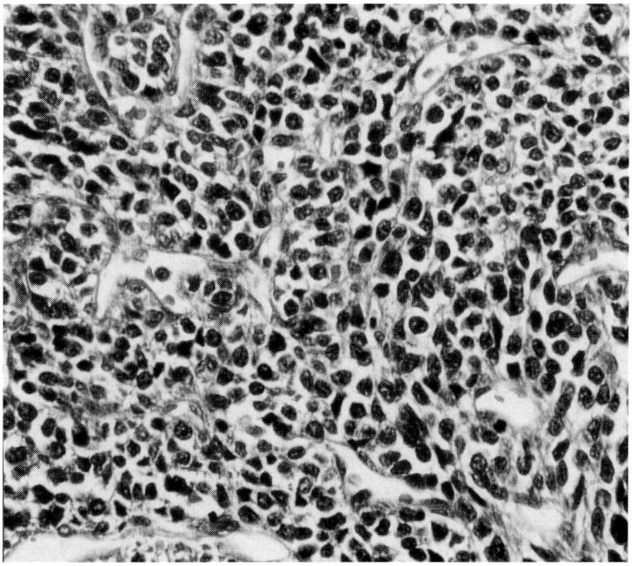

Figure 59 Primitive neuroectodermal tumor. Higher magnification of Figure 58 demonstrates the small-cell size and scanty cytoplasm. Immunohistochemical stains are usually required to exclude other small-cell neoplasms, such as metastatic oat cell carcinoma or lymphoma.

Grossly, medulloblastomas are relatively well circumscribed, uniform, pale, gray-tan tumor masses. Some are soft and friable; others are firm. CNS metastases may present as many pale plaques and nodules which "sugar-coat" the brain and spinal cord surfaces, with subsequent infiltration of the parenchyma. Extracranial metastases are rarely seen, more commonly if the child has a ventriculoperitoneal shunt through which tumor cells may "escape" the cranial cavity.

Microscopically, medulloblastomas are characterized by sheets of crowded, small, primitive cells with scanty, ill-defined, pale cytoplasm, and usually without distinct pattern or differentiation (Figs. 60, 61). Despite the gross appearance of circumscription, there is infiltration of the cerebellum or subarachnoid space. Tumor nuclei may be round or ovoid, and mitoses are usually frequent. The background is finely fibrillary. About a third of cases contain Homer-Wright rosettes, characterized by cells radially arranged around an eosinophilic, fibrillary (not tubular) center, a feature highly indicative of medulloblastoma. Virtually all medulloblastomas are immunoreactive for synaptophysin and neurofilament, indicating neuronal differentiation. Rarely, glial differentiation and GFAP positivity may be observed.

Desmoplastic medulloblastomas contain abundant connective tissue and are more common among the superficial, lateral hemispheric tumors of young adults than the midline medulloblastomas of childhood. They have a more fa-

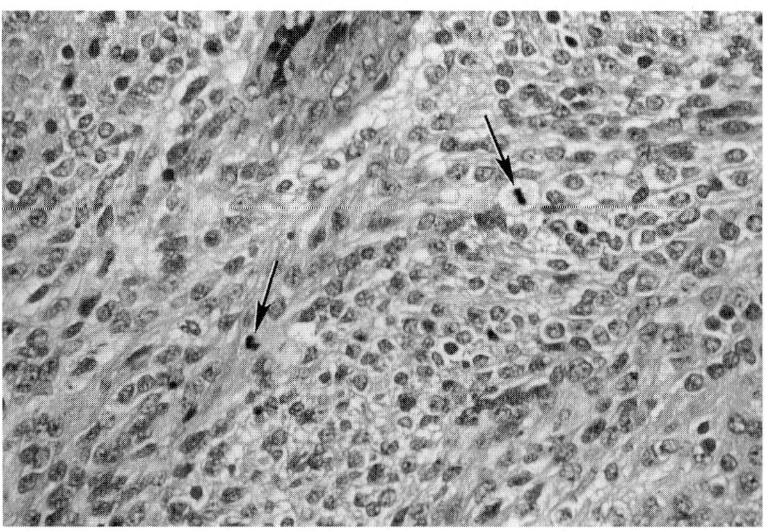

Figure 60 Medulloblastoma. Medulloblastomas are characterized by their cerebellar location. Histologically, most are composed of small primitive cells with numerous mitosis (arrows), like other PNETs.

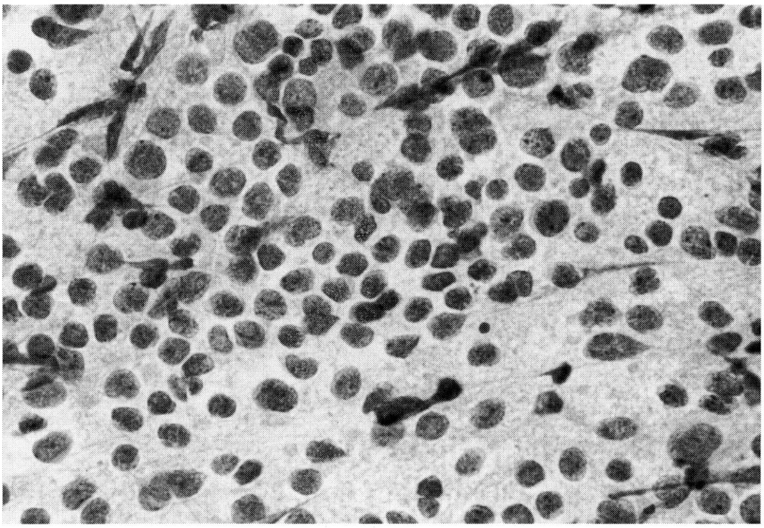

Figure 61 Medulloblastoma. Smear preparations reveal high cellularity and lack of cohesion, with the small primitive round cells frequently stripped of their cytoplasm. The fibrillary background characteristic of gliomas is absent.

vorable prognosis. The desmoplasia is thought to be a reaction caused by tumor infiltration of the leptomeninges, which may induce arrangement of small neoplastic cells as rows between strands of fibrous tissue. Follicular architecture is often seen, characterized by loosely textured, finely fibrillated islands surrounded by sheets of undifferentiated tumor (Fig. 62). These islands are reticulin-free, in contrast to the reticulin-rich tumor surrounding them. The cells within these islands often show immunophenotypic evidence of neuronal and (to a lesser degree) astroglial differentiation.

A rare variant of medulloblastoma is *medullomyoblastoma*, with smooth or striated muscle fibers amidst the PNET background. These tumors are desmin- and muscle-specific actin-positive, and may arise in the cerebellum, pineal gland, or other regions. *Pigmented papillary medulloblastoma* includes melanin-containing cuboidal epithelium showing papillary or tubular formations; some consider these neoplasms to be of "retinal anlage" differentiation.

C. Cerebral Neuroblastomas

These are rare tumors originating in the cerebral hemispheres of young children. They are well demarcated, soft, gray masses, often with hemorrhage or cystic degeneration. The tumor histologically is virtually the same as peripheral

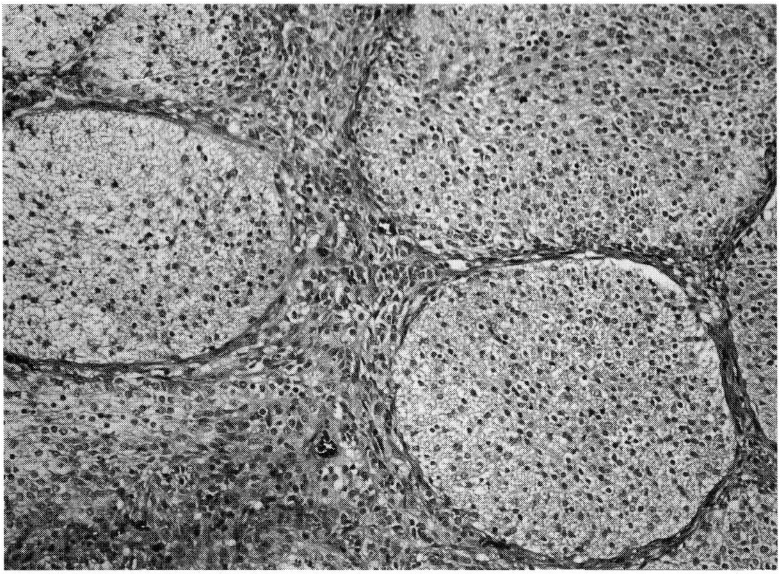

Figure 62 Desmoplastic medulloblastoma. Follicle formation, characterized by circumscribed pale islands amidst the more crowded small-cell tumor, is peculiar to this variant of medulloblastoma.

neuroblastoma or medulloblastoma, and may contain rosettes (Fig. 63). These tumors are synaptophysin- and neurofilament-positive. Rarely, maturation of the blastic cells into ganglion cells is present (*ganglioneuroblastoma*). A fibrous stroma is not uncommon.

D. Medulloepitheliomas

These are generally manifest in very young children, including neonates, and show rapid clinical growth. These tumors are considered to be the most primitive and multipotential neoplasms within the CNS. They are usually found in the cerebral hemispheres, often close to the ventricles. Grossly, they appear well demarcated, with hemorrhage and necrosis. Histologically, they are composed of papillary and tubular aggregates of stratified columnar cells resembling primitive neural tube epithelium, but they may also mimic metastatic carcinoma and choroid plexus carcinoma. Rarely, there is differentiation into ganglion cells, astroglia, or ependyma.

E. Ependymoblastomas

These are rare primitive neuroectodermal tumors with true ependymal rosette formation and perivascular pseudorosettes, usually arising around the fourth

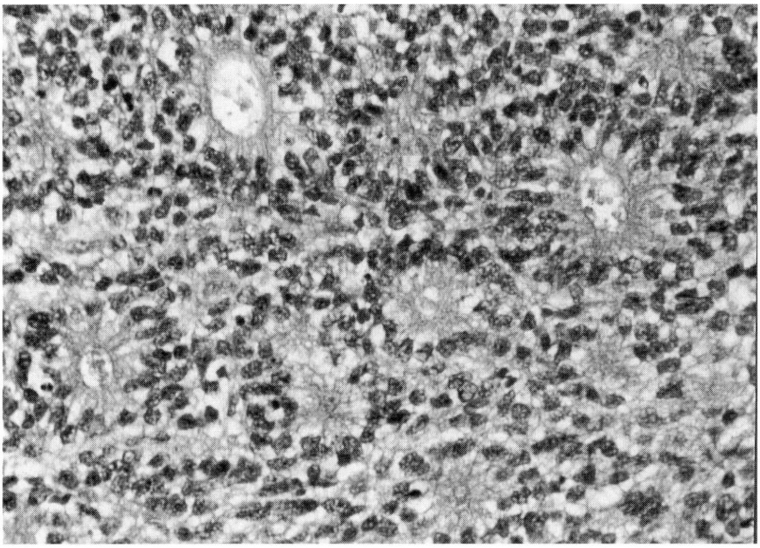

Figure 63 Neuroblastoma. The presence of rosettes is an important clue to the diagnosis of neuroblastoma. Like medulloblastomas, these tumors are usually synaptophysin- and neurofilament-positive, but are cerebral rather than cerebellar in location.

ventricle of children. Meningeal infiltration and dissemination along CSF pathways may occur. The tumor consists of small primitive cells with mitoses and necrosis. These tumors are GFAP-positive and synaptophysin-negative. Ultrastructural studies are often required for definitive diagnosis; these reveal ciliary bodies and blepharoplasts in the tumor cells.

F. Polar Spongioblastoma

This is a very rare tumor of children and adolescents arising around the fourth ventricle or in the spinal cord. It is characterized by palisaded cords of neoplastic cells separated by cords of fibrillary stroma that lack GFAP immunopositivity. Many tumor cells show evidence of astrocytic differentiation.

G. Pineoblastomas

These are PNETs that originate in the pineal gland. These tumors are found in both adults and children and have an aggressive clinical course. Rosettes may be seen.

H. Olfactory Neuroblastomas

These are tumors arising in the nasal cavity which may extend into the frontal lobes. These tumors are quite similar in appearance to cerebral neuroblastomas.

Rosette and ganglion cell differentiation may be exhibited. Olfactory neuroblastomas may demonstrate a nodular pattern of growth, the center of the nodule showing neuron-specific enolase immunopositivity and the rim showing S-100 positivity.

Germ cell tumors are discussed with tumors of the pineal region.

IX. PITUITARY TUMORS

A. Pituitary Adenomas

These are usually neoplasms of middle-aged or older patients, mostly women, which cause effacement of the normal anterior pituitary architecture and, with time, hypopituitarism, expansion of the sella turcica, and compression of the optic chiasm and hypothalamus. These tumors are soft, usually tan (Fig. 64), and microscopically characterized by sheets of fairly uniform cells with abundant cytoplasm having a variety of histologic patterns, including trabecular, sinusoidal, and papillary (Figs. 65–67). These histologic patterns have no prog-

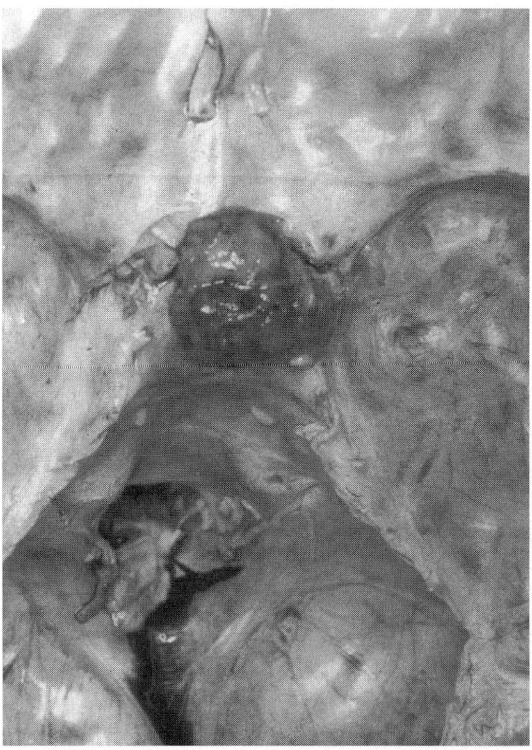

Figure 64 Pituitary adenoma. A soft, tan tumor nodule is seen bulging from the sella turcica.

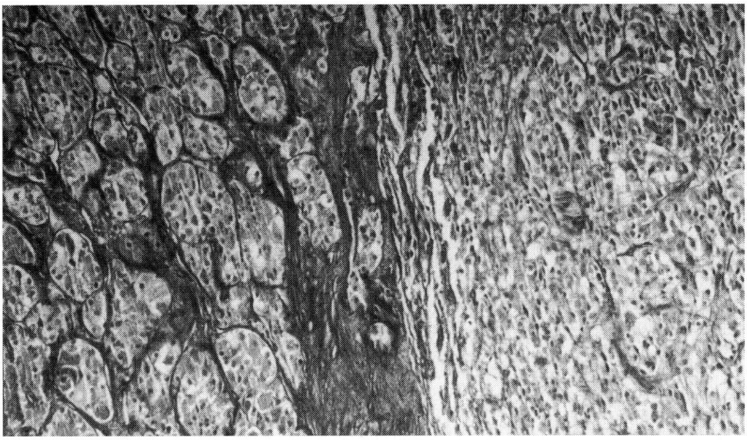

Figure 65 Pituitary adenoma. Histologic section stained with PAS-Orange G highlights the distinction between relatively normal pituitary with organoid arrangement of cells (left), and loss of organoid pattern and sheetlike arrangement of neoplastic cells (right).

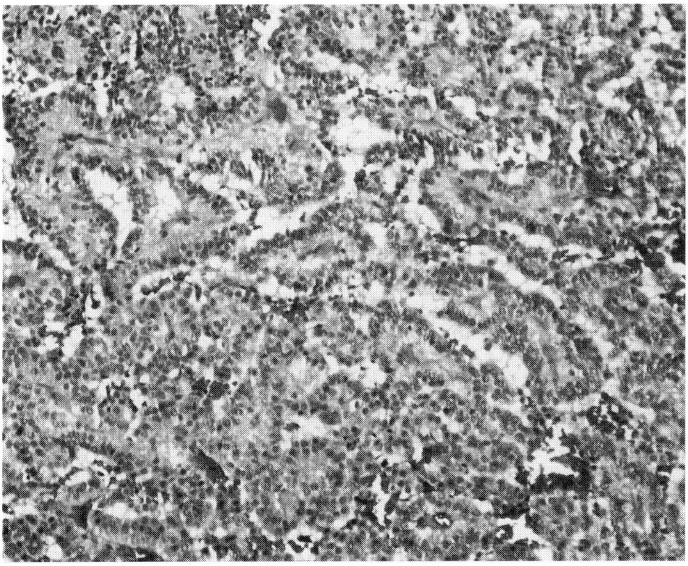

Figure 66 Pituitary adenoma. Pituitary adenomas may manifest a variety of histologic patterns. This tumor demonstrates papillary architecture.

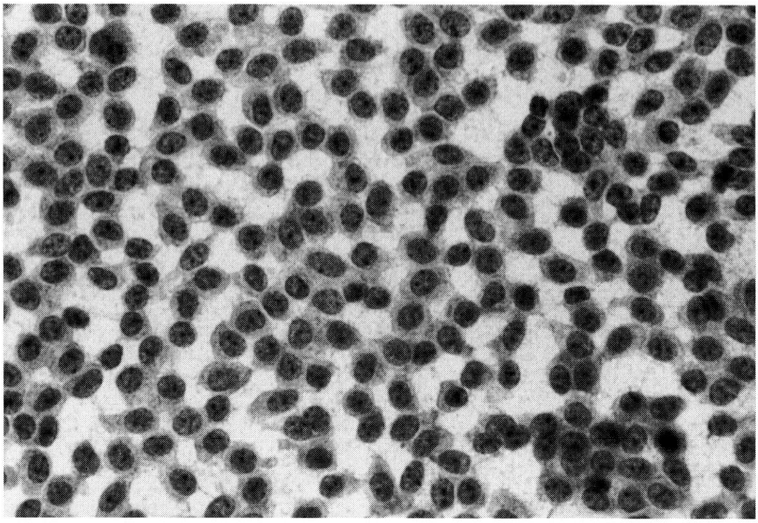

Figure 67 Pituitary adenoma. We find that the use of an intraoperative smear preparation is often more helpful than a frozen section. Smears of an adenoma show poorly cohesive sheets of cells having small, round, uniform nuclei. Cytoplasm is usually stripped by the smearing process, but in this case distinct cytoplasmic borders are seen.

nostic significance. Most adenomas are cured by surgery, but some recur and hypopituitarism may develop. Radiation and pharmaceutical agonists may also be therapeutically effective.

Traditionally, pituitary adenomas were divided into three types based on the predominant cytoplasmic staining characteristic: eosinophilic, basophilic, and chromophobic. From a practical level, it is best to consider these tumors as being either functional or nonfunctional, depending on whether serum hormone production can be measured. Nonfunctional (chromophobe) adenomas present as large tumors causing a mass effect. Functional adenomas are usually much smaller (including microadenomas) and encompass growth hormone, prolactin, and ACTH-producing neoplasms. Functional adenomas are usually manifest by syndromes of inappropriate hormone production, the hormones being demonstrable within tumor cells using immunohistochemical stains. The incidence of functional adenomas has increased over the past few decades due to advancements in radioimmunoassay and neuroimaging techniques, with functional adenomas now comprising about three-quarters of pituitary adenomas.

Pituitary adenomas may sometimes resemble oligodendrogliomas, ependymomas, and meningiomas. If confusion exists, their strong chromogranin positivity is diagnostically very helpful. Ultrastructurally, these cells contain characteristic secretory granules.

Nuclear atypia and hyperchromasia are not indicative of malignancy, nor is infiltration through the dura, bone, and into the sinuses (i.e., *invasive adenoma*; Fig. 68). Metastases are the most reliable manifestation of pituitary carcinomas, which are very uncommon. Like most malignancies, pituitary carcinomas usually demonstrate brisk mitotic activity, marked nuclear atypia, and necrosis.

B. Craniopharyngiomas

These are primarily tumors of childhood and early adult life, being the most common supratentorial tumor during the first decade. Patients may present with visual deficits, hydrocephalus, or endocrine disturbances. Craniopharyngiomas are grossly well-defined neoplasms which occur in the suprasellar region and may extend into the third ventricle, optic chiasm, or hypothalamic regions. They are partially solid, are often cystic, and contain a dark "motor oil"-like fluid which is rich in cholesterol crystals when examined by polarized light. Radiographically, calcification of craniopharyngiomas is common.

Histologically, most craniopharyngiomas are characterized by anastomosing cords and nests of loosely cohesive squamous epithelium which shows a distinct palisaded border, frequent nests of anucleate keratin (Figs. 69, 70), multinucleate giant cell reaction, cholesterol clefts, and calcification (adamant-

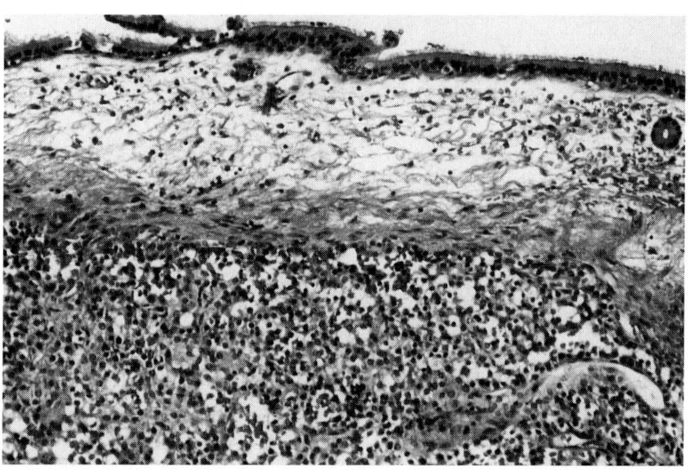

Figure 68 Invasive pituitary adenoma. Extension of a pituitary adenoma through dura and bone into the sinuses is not indicative of malignancy. Here the ciliated respiratory mucosa (top) is being undermined by sheets of cells from a large invasive pituitary adenoma.

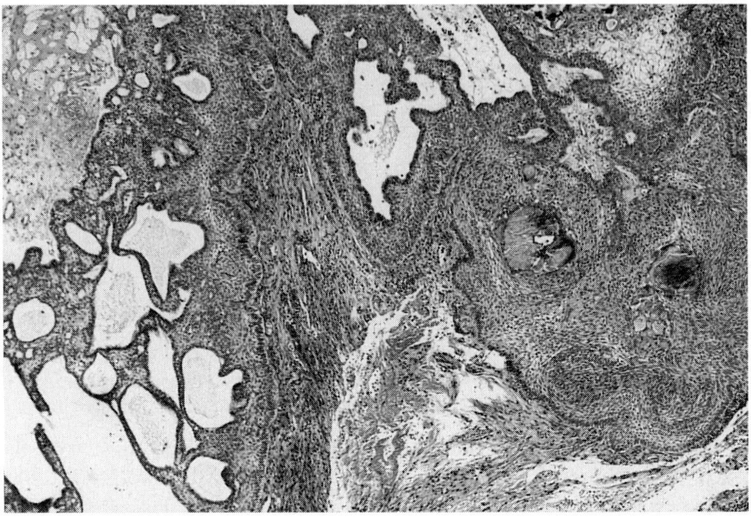

Figure 69 Craniopharyngioma. Scanning magnification is often diagnostic, revealing nests and cords of squamous epithelium in an adamantinomatous pattern separated by loose fibrous stroma. The empty cystic spaces were filled in vivo with a dark oily fluid.

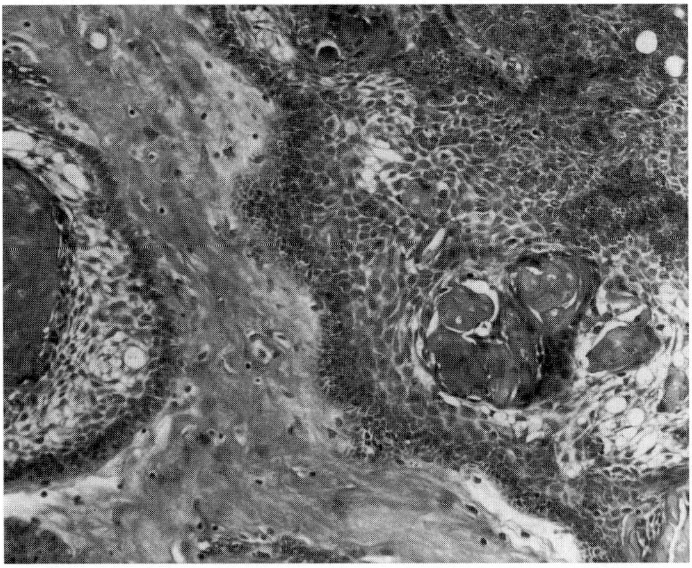

Figure 70 Craniopharyngioma. Nests of squamous epithelium whose keratinocytes show a loose arrangement. There are a distinct palisaded border and many islands of anucleate keratinization.

inomatous pattern). Craniopharyngiomas may have a more solid histologic appearance, with solid sheets of squamous cells surrounding fibrovascular cores, leading to a papillary pattern. These tumors may infiltrate the surrounding brain as solid nests, resulting in pronounced gliosis, often with Rosenthal fibers (a potential diagnostic problem if the border is biopsied for frozen section). They are difficult to completely resect, and recurrences are common.

X. TUMORS OF THE PINEAL REGION

Pineal tumors are uncommon, but are thought to derive from pineal cells or their precursors. These neoplasms usually present with signs of increased intracranial pressure, gaze paralysis (Parinaud's syndrome), or mass effect. Gliomas, meningiomas, and pineoblastomas may arise at this site and are discussed elsewhere in this chapter.

Pineocytomas (pinealomas) are well demarcated, slow-growing neoplasms which may be seen in any age group. They are histologically quite similar to the normal pineal gland and are mostly distinguished by their larger size. Calcifications may occur.

Primary *germ cell tumors* involving the CNS are uncommon but usually arise in the region of the pineal gland. These tumors are mostly manifest in children and young adults, with a male predilection. Germ cell tumors may also involve the suprasellar region (Fig. 71), third ventricle, posterior fossa, or mul-

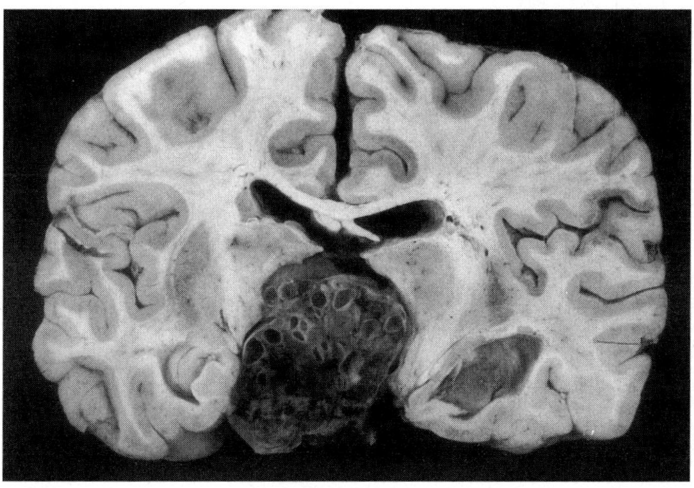

Figure 71 Suprasellar teratoma. This 14-year-old male had a large teratoma of the suprasellar region which clinically caused panhypopituitarism and compression of the second and third cranial nerves. The tumor was soft, hemorrhagic, and multicystic.

tiple sites may be simultaneously affected. These tumors are histologically analogous to their gonadal and mediastinal counterparts and are classified using the same histologic criteria as germinomas (dysgerminomas) or nongerminomatous neoplasms including: *embryonal carcinomas*, *mature and immature teratomas*, *endodermal sinus (yolk sac) tumors*, *choriocarcinomas*, and *mixed germ cell tumors*. Over half of CNS germ cell tumors are germinomas (Fig. 72).

XI. ACOUSTIC NEUROMAS

Acoustic neuromas constitute about 5% to 10% of intracranial neoplasms and typically arise from the acoustic nerve but may involve cranial nerves V, VII, or XII. These tumors are discrete, solid, and tan, but may show cystic and xanthomatous changes. They are histologically indistinguishable from neurilemomas (discussed below). Occasionally they are bilateral, especially in patients with neurofibromatosis type 2, and are found predominantly in middle-aged or older patients.

At times it may be difficult to distinguish an acoustic neuroma from a meningioma. Acoustic neuromas are more likely to be cystic and yellow, to lack a broad dural attachment and psammoma bodies and whorls, and show strong S-100 positivity and absence of EMA staining.

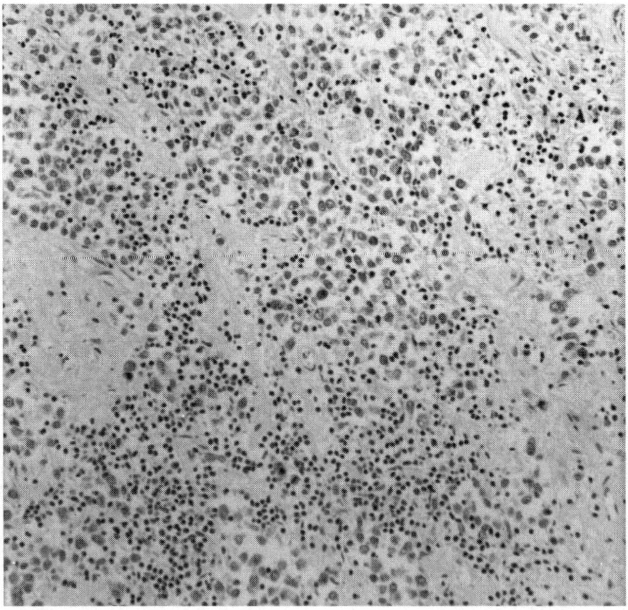

Figure 72 Germinoma. Like its gonadal counterparts, the pineal germinoma is characterized by a variable admixture of small lymphocytes and sheets of primitive cells with large nuclei.

XII. INTRACRANIAL MENINGES

A. Meningiomas

These are common neoplasms of meningeal origin which comprise about 15% of primary brain tumors. They occur primarily in adults, with a peak incidence in the fifth decade, and have a female predilection. These tumors are well circumscribed, slow-glowing, rounded or lobulated, and usually firmly attached to the dura. They may be broad-based, polypoid, or flat. Meningiomas displace and compress rather than infiltrate the brain, and usually are easily separated from it. While meningiomas may occur anywhere meninges are found, they have a predilection for the parasagittal regions, cerebral convexities (Fig. 73), olfactory groove (Fig. 74), falx cerebri, and sphenoid ridge. Less commonly, they arise in the choroid plexus. Many meningiomas are incidental autopsy

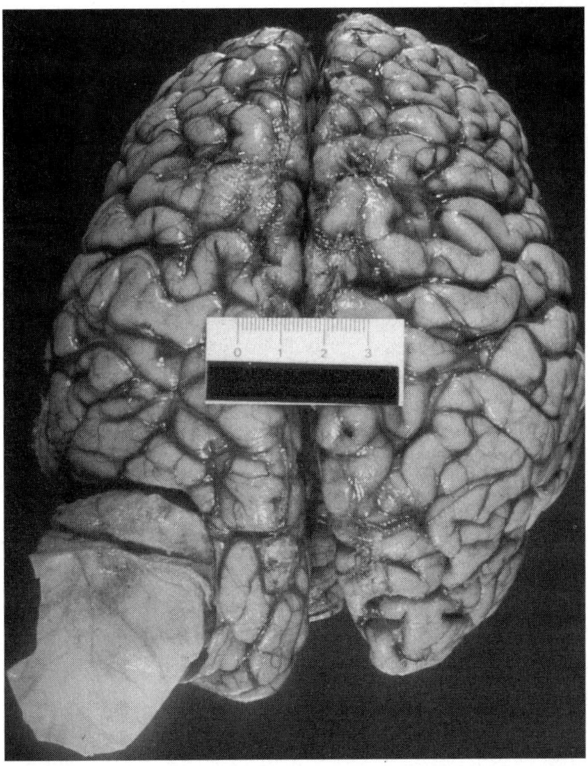

Figure 73 Meningioma. Many meningiomas are incidental autopsy findings, as was this large tumor overlying the left occipital lobe. The absence of clinical symptoms is indicative of its slow growth rate and displacement, rather than infiltration, of normal brain.

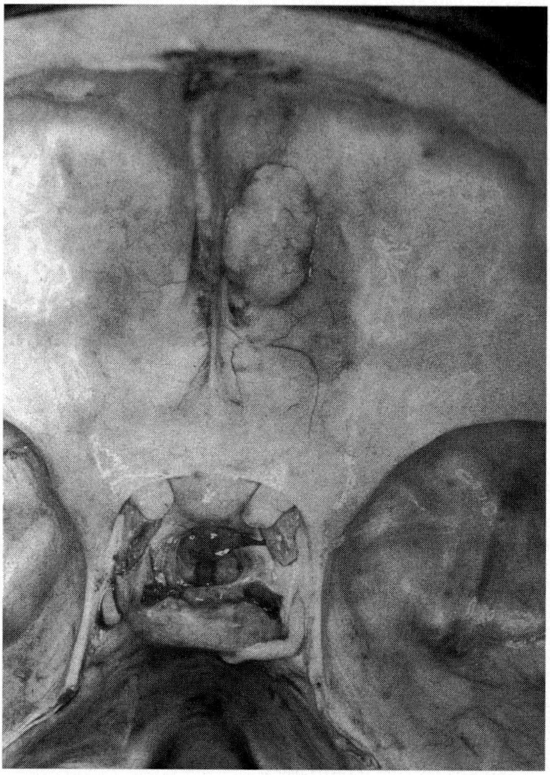

Figure 74 Meningioma. A lobulated, pale, ovoid tumor is firmly attached to the dura. The olfactory groove is a favored site of origin for meningiomas.

findings. Up to 5% may be multiple. Recurrences following surgical resection are common, especially if the lesion is incompletely removed.

Meningiomas show a uniform, firm, yellowish-white to gray cut surface (Fig. 75), and may be gritty. Sometimes they are yellow, corresponding microscopically to xanthomatous change. They are characteristically vimentin-, epithelial membrane antigen-, and reticulin-positive, and ultrastructurally contain interdigitating cellular processes and desmosomes.

Microscopically, meningiomas have a variable histologic appearance, these variations usually having no prognostic significance. They are most often characterized by sheets and nests of uniform cells with round to ovoid nuclei, separated by thin fibrous septae (meningothelial meningioma). Cells are frequently arranged in whorls (Figs. 76 and 77), the center of which may contain a calcified, laminated, *psammoma body* (Figs. 78–80). Intranuclear vacuolation and pseudoinclusions are common.

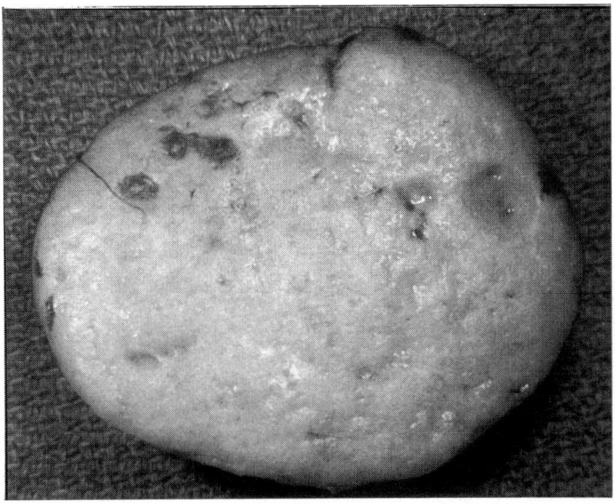

Figure 75 Meningioma. This tumor was removed from the left frontal cerebral convexity of a 68-year-old man. On cut section, it is uniform, gray-white, and contains a few small cysts.

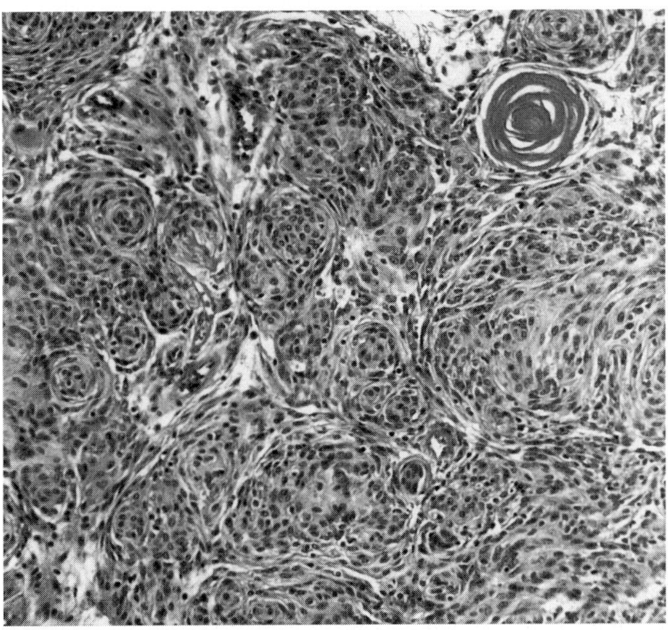

Figure 76 Meningothelial meningioma. Typical scanning view showing whorled nests of tumor cells separated by fibrovascular septae.

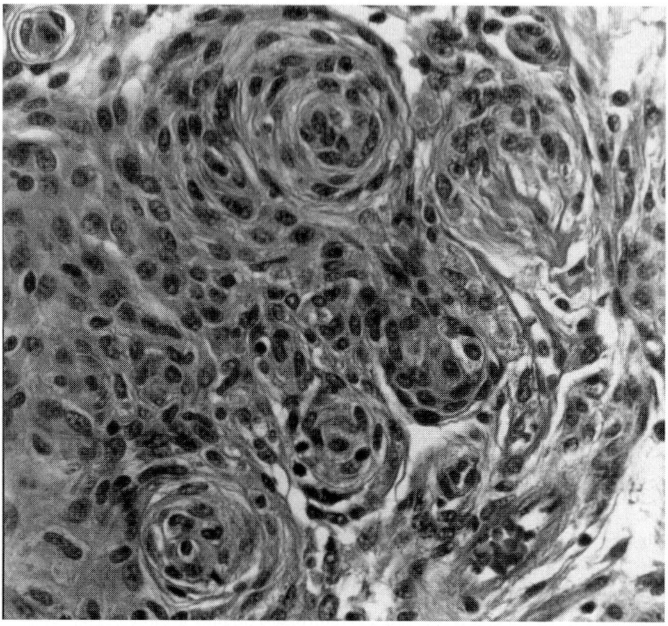

Figure 77 Meningothelial meningioma. Higher magnification showing whorling and uniform, round to ovoid cells.

A tumor may be called a *psammomatous meningioma* if psammoma bodies are a predominant feature. Some meningiomas consist of fascicles of elongated spindle cells that are separated by abundant collagenous stroma (*fibroblastic meningioma;* Fig. 81). Since fibroblastic meningiomas often lack psammoma bodies and whorls, they may be confused with acoustic neuromas if they arise at the cerebellopontine angle; an EMA and S-100 protein stain may help differentiate them. A GFAP stain may be useful in differentiating a low-grade pilocytic astrocytoma from fibroblastic meningioma. As their name implies, *transitional meningiomas* have features in common with both meningothelial and fibroblastic meningiomas.

Benign meningiomas may extend into the skull (Fig. 82) and stimulate new bone formation over a broad region (*meningioma en plaque*). They may also infiltrate the soft tissues and scalp beyond the skull (Fig. 83), without malignant connotations. Dural sinuses may also be infiltrated; however, invasion of the brain is not seen in otherwise benign meningiomas.

Secretory meningiomas are an interesting variant which show discrete, eosinophilic, cytoplasmic inclusions within tumor cells that are PAS-positive (Fig. 84). Positivity to keratin and CEA is demonstrated in cells around the

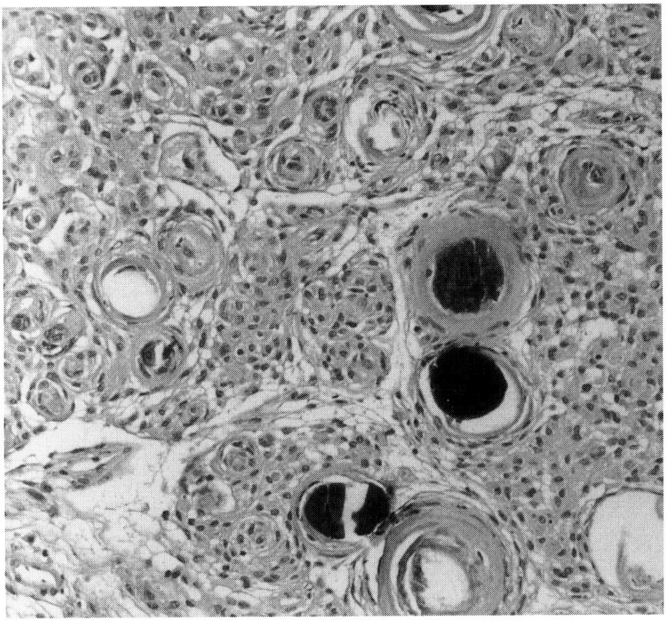

Figure 78 Meningothelial meningioma. Many meningiomas contain calcified psammoma bodies, usually found at the center of whorls of tumor cells. If psammoma bodies are present in large numbers, the tumor may be called a psammomatous meningioma.

eosinophilic inclusions. *Microcystic (angiomatous) meningiomas* contain numerous microcysts, abundant hyalinized blood vessels, foamy histiocytes, nuclear atypia, and often lack a significant compliment of the psammoma bodies and whorls so characteristic of most meningiomas (Figs. 85, 86). They may resemble hemangioblastomas, but are usually of dural origin.

Papillary meningiomas are unusual in that they are locally aggressive and may metastasize. They occur in a younger population than typical meningiomas and are characterized by a papillary architecture, the papillae being an artifact of tissue processing. These tumors are cellular, mitotically active, and often invasive. They usually lack whorls and psammoma bodies and must be differentiated from ependymomas, especially since the "papillae" may show a "pseudorosette" morphology. Choroid plexus papillomas and metastatic carcinomas are also in the differential diagnosis.

The presence of cellular atypia in a meningioma is not uncommon and, by itself, is not diagnostic of malignancy, especially in the absence of mitoses. Similarly, benign tumors may show focal areas of increased cellularity, necrosis, hemorrhage, and a sheetlike pattern of growth, without malignant connota-

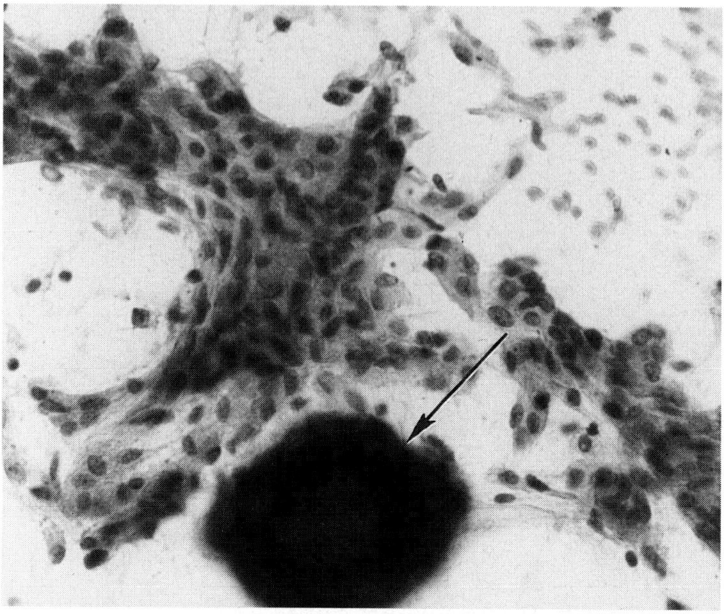

Figure 79 Meningioma. Intraoperative smear preparations often show mostly cohesive clusters of tumor cells, with scattered individual cells. Cellular whorling or the presence of a psammoma body (arrow) are helpful clues to the correct diagnosis.

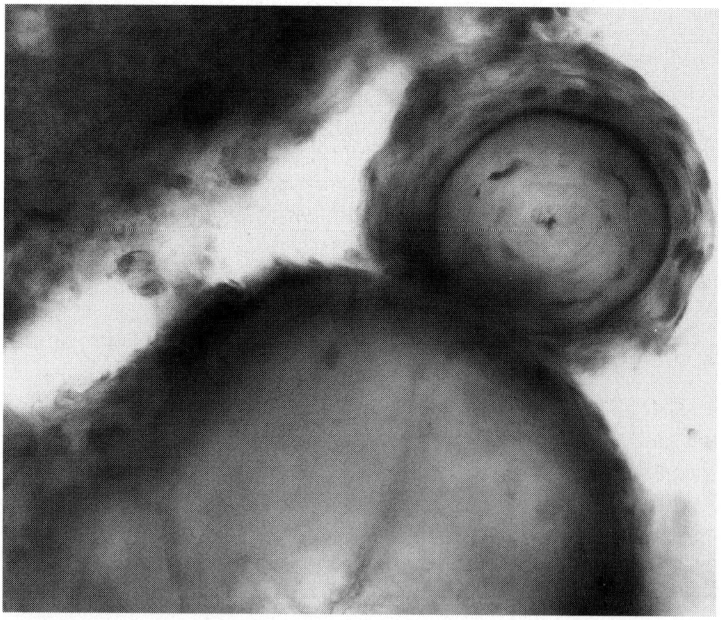

Figure 80 Meningioma. If present in sufficient numbers on an intraoperative smear preparation, psammoma bodies make the diagnosis of meningioma relatively straightforward. It is necessary to focus up and down to appreciate their three-dimensional quality.

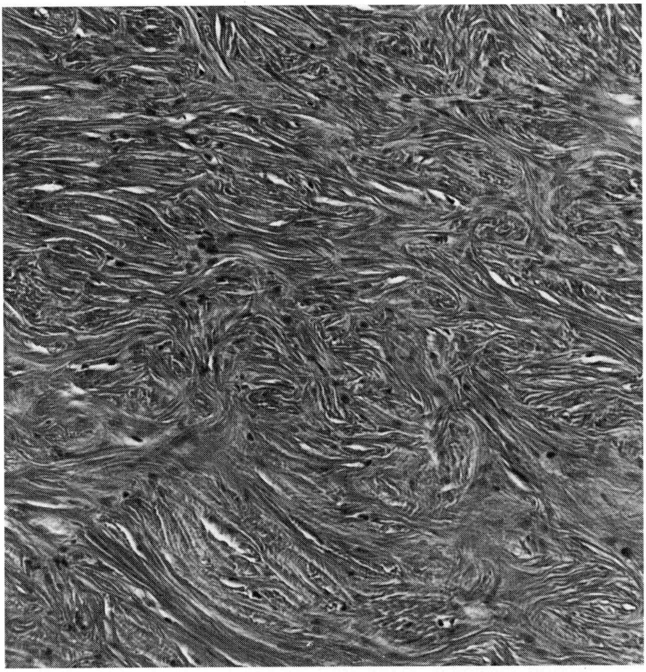

Figure 81 Fibroblastic meningioma. A fibroblastic meningioma is characterized primarily by collagenous stroma, with scattered intervening spindle cells.

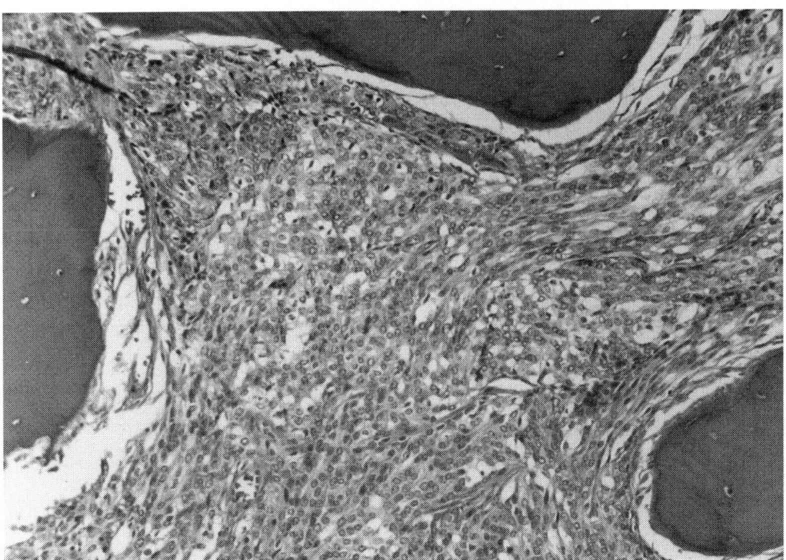

Figure 82 Meningioma. The extension of a meningioma into the skull is common. The medullary space of the calvarium is permeated by tumor, with bone spicules separated by sheets of uniform meningothelial cells. This pattern of infiltration does not imply malignancy.

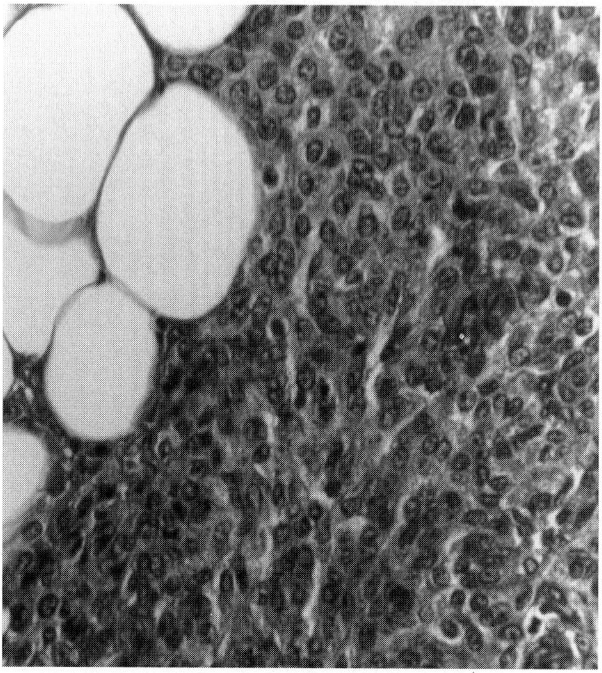

Figure 83 Meningioma. Some meningiomas present as scalp masses, having infiltrated through the skull into the subcutaneous fat. The tumor cells (right) are crowded but strikingly uniform.

tions. It is best to consider such lesions *atypical meningiomas* since they have a higher frequency of recurrence and subsequent malignant transformation.

The presence of significant atypia, with or without necrosis and hemorrhage, in a rapidly growing, cellular neoplasm with numerous mitoses and invasion of the brain, is indicative of *malignant meningioma* (Figs. 87, 88). Similarly, invasion of vascular spaces is ominous and may herald the presence of distant metastases. Although metastases are rare, they are definitively diagnostic of malignancy. It is possible in some patients to see dedifferentiation of a benign meningioma in recurrences, ultimately ending with a malignant neoplasm. The histologic pattern of some malignant meningiomas merges with sarcoma (usually fibrosarcoma).

B. Meningeal Sarcomas

These are extremely rare, frankly malignant neoplasms that arise from mesenchymal elements (Fig. 89). Sarcomas usually occur in younger patients or those

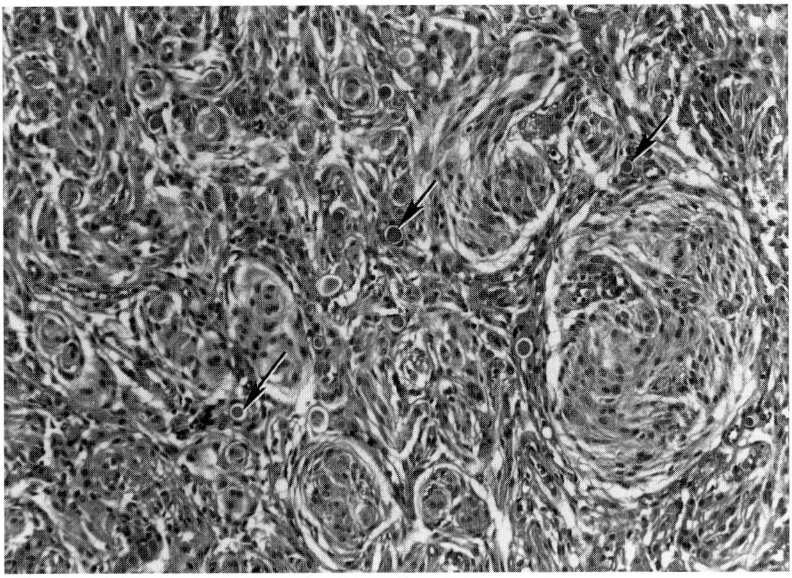

Figure 84 Secretory meningioma. Secretory meningiomas contain distinct, rounded, eosinophilic, cytoplasmic inclusions. There are many of these inclusions in this photomicrograph, two of which are highlighted by arrows.

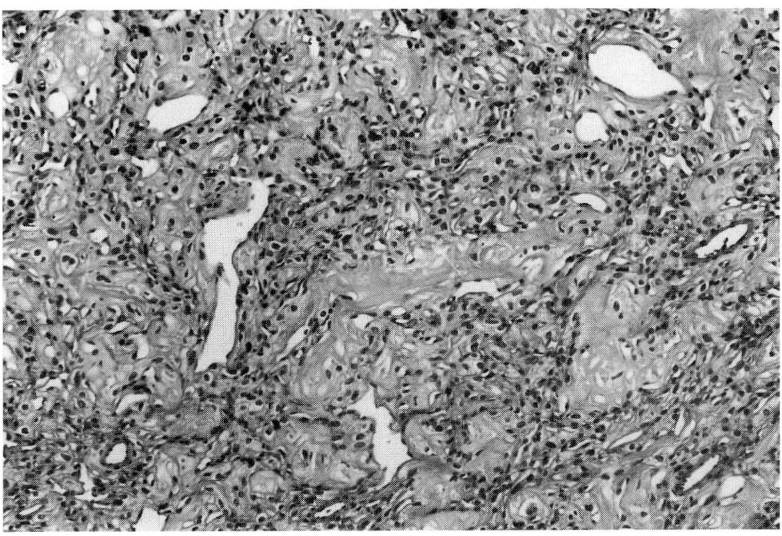

Figure 85 Angiomatous meningioma. Prominent hyalinized blood vessels, separated by scattered meningothelial cells, are the most dominant feature of this tumor. The cellular whorls and psammoma bodies usually seen in meningiomas are absent.

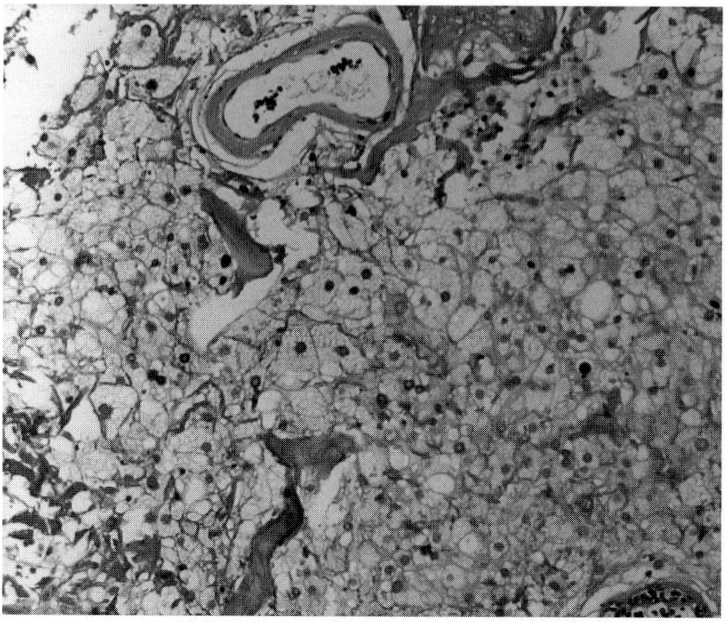

Figure 86 Angiomatous meningioma. Some meningiomas contain many foamy histiocytes, which may impart a yellow color to the neoplasm. Note the hyalinized vessel at the top of the photomicrograph.

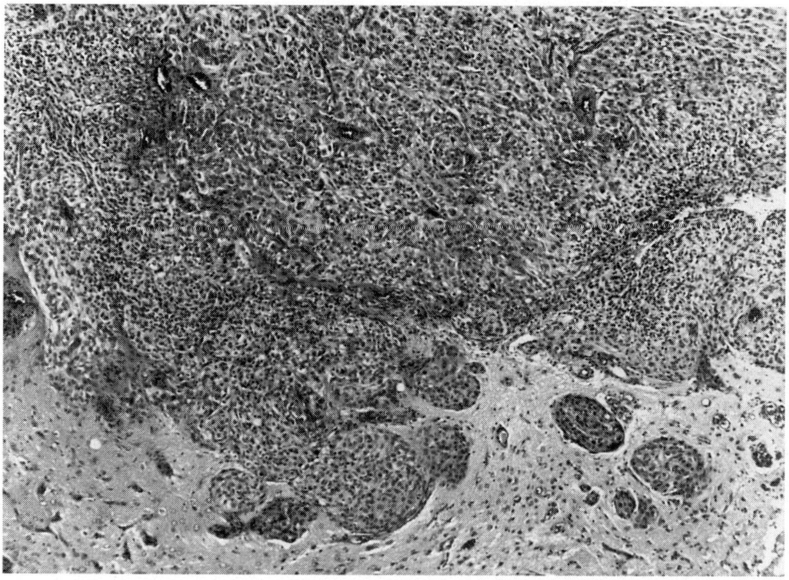

Figure 87 Malignant meningioma. Invasion of brain parenchyma by a meningioma is an ominous sign and is indicative of malignancy. The cerebral cortex (bottom) is infiltrated by small nests of tumor and is gliotic.

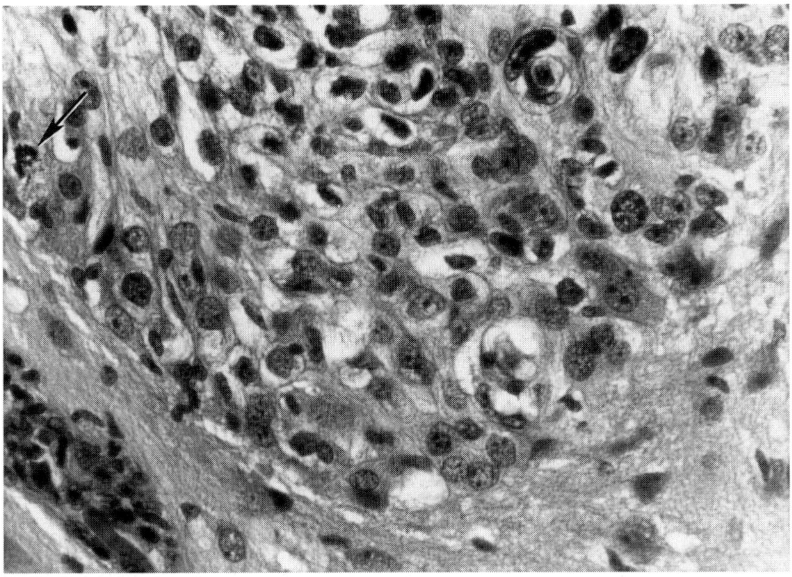

Figure 88 Malignant meningioma. Higher magnification of Figure 87 shows significant cellular atypia and an occasional mitotic figure (arrow) within an intracortical nest of invasive meningioma.

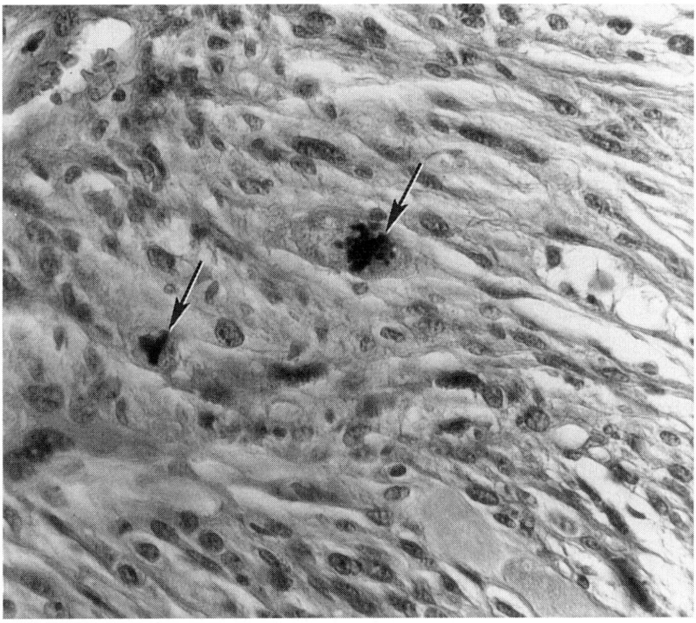

Figure 89 *Meningeal sarcoma.* The presence of atypical mitotic figures (arrows) is a clue to the malignant nature of this meningeal sarcoma.

who have had prior cranial radiation therapy. These tumors may manifest a great variety of histologic patterns and are classified based on their manner of differentiation into fibrosarcoma, leiomyosarcoma, mesenchymal chondrosarcoma, mesenchymal osteosarcoma, liposarcoma, malignant fibrous histiocytoma, or undifferentiated sarcoma. The gross and microscopic appearance of these neoplasms is analogous to their soft-tissue counterparts and will not be documented here. CNS metastasis from other sites must be considered in the differential diagnosis.

C. Hemangioblastomas

These may occur primarily in relation to the meninges and have been previously discussed in this chapter.

D. Lipomas

Lipomas are rare, usually clinically silent neoplasms unless they cause a local mass effect (e.g., spinal cord compression). They frequently arise in the midline and generally involve the corpus callosum, hypothalamus, or spinal canal. Grossly, they are bright yellow (Fig. 90). Microscopically, they consist primarily of adipocytes with admixtures of blood vessels, bone, cartilage, fibrous tissue, and neuroglial elements.

E. Hemangiopericytomas

These are low-grade malignant neoplasms thought to arise from pericytes in the meninges, rather than meningothelial cells. These tumors are analogous to

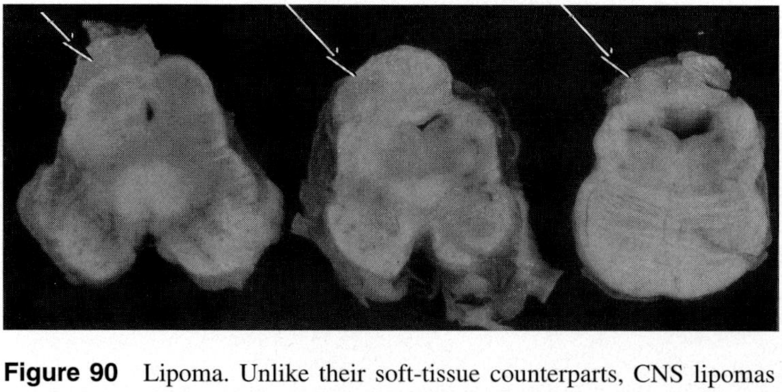

Figure 90 Lipoma. Unlike their soft-tissue counterparts, CNS lipomas are very rare, usually incidentally discovered tumors. This yellow lipomatous mass of the quadrigeminal plate (arrows) was fortuitously found in a 41-year-old woman who had olivopontocerebellar atrophy.

their soft-tissue counterparts. While grossly they often resemble meningiomas by their dural attachment, they are associated with heavy bleeding during surgery. Histologically, hemangiopericytomas consist of sheets of mostly uniform elongated cells containing numerous branching ("*staghorn pattern*") dilated blood vessels (Figs. 91, 92). The tumors are reticulin-rich and may show mitotic figures. They have a tendency to multiple recurrences and may metastasize. In the past, such lesions were often referred to as "angioblastic meningiomas," but they lack EMA positivity, whorls, and psammoma bodies.

F. Diffuse Meningeal Melanosis

Patches of meningeal hyperpigmentation are not uncommon unless extensive (*diffuse meningeal melanosis*). Such pigmented lesions may be associated with a proliferation of nevoid melanocytes within the meninges often resembling blue nevi. These patients may also have cutaneous giant (hairy) nevi. *Primary malignant melanomas* of the meninges are extremely rare, but are associated with the usual cytologic features of malignancy plus invasion and intracranial or extracranial metastases. These cases may arise in the setting of meningeal

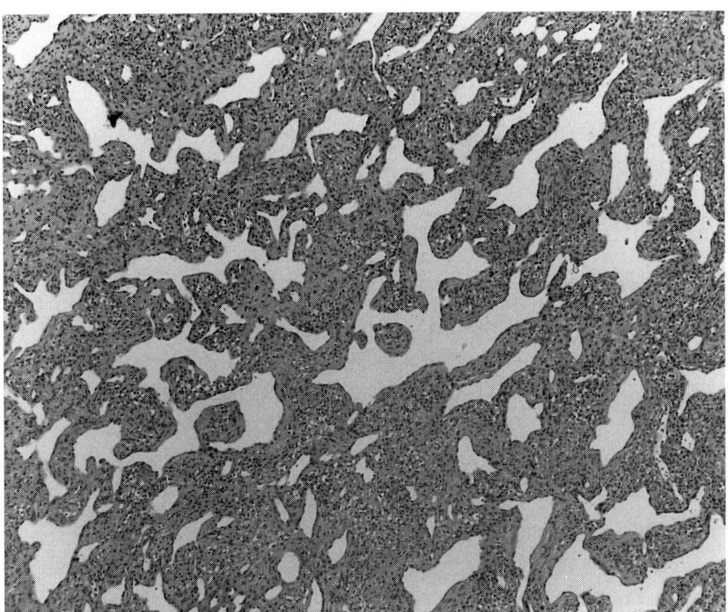

Figure 91 Hemangiopericytoma. Scanning view shows a highly vascular neoplasm with "staghorn" pattern of blood vessels.

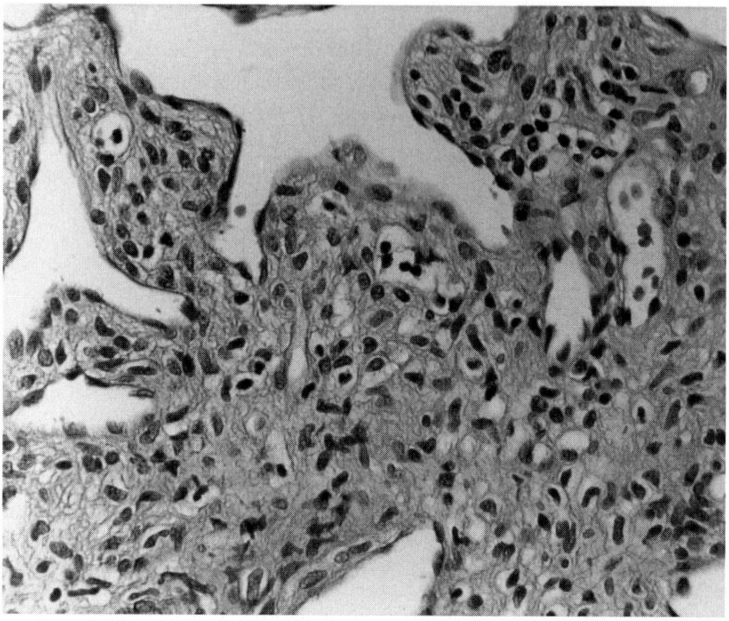

Figure 92 Hemangiopericytoma. Higher magnification shows vascular spaces that are separated by uniform, ovoid to angulated cells. These tumors are not of meningothelial origin, but rather are analogous to soft-tissue hemangiopericytomas.

melanosis, but exclusion of metastases from an occult, non-CNS primary is problematic and often impossible.

XIII. SPINAL CORD AND ITS COVERINGS

A spectrum of neoplasia occurs within the spine. Mostly these tumors are analogous to those described above; however, unique aspects of tumors in this region are discussed below.

A. Astrocytomas

These are relatively rare when compared with their counterparts in the brain, occurring perhaps only 5% as frequently. Astrocytic tumors are usually found in the cervical and upper thoracic cord of children and young adults and are fusiform, expansile neoplasms. Most spinal astrocytomas are low-grade, are often pilocytic, and may be associated with a cystic cavity. Despite a small size, their destruction of fiber tracts has devastating clinical consequences.

B. Ependymomas

These are circumscribed tumors, mostly of adult life, constituting the majority of masses arising in the region of the central canal. Ependymomas comprise over half of spinal gliomas and, unlike spinal astrocytomas, are mostly localized to the lower cord including the conus medullaris, cauda equina, sacrum, and adjacent paravertebral soft tissues. Those involving the filum terminale take the form of a well-demarcated, ovoid mass. Myxopapillary differentiation predominates, a feature unique to tumors of the filum terminale and conus medullaris. Nonetheless, the histopathology is often analogous to that of intracranial ependymomas.

Myxopapillary ependymomas are characterized by mostly uniform cuboidal cells arranged in a papillary fashion around a vascular core, with pseudorosette formation and an abundant mucicarmine-positive stroma (Figs. 93, 94). Calcification is rare. These tumors may cause erosion of the vertebral bodies and if strikingly mucinous may be confused with chordomas; their GFAP positivity is an important distinguishing feature.

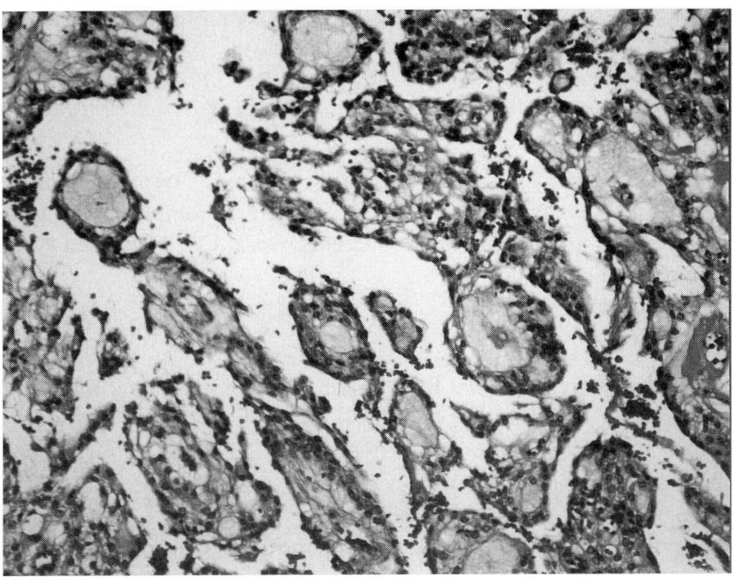

Figure 93 Myxopapillary ependymoma. These neoplasms are localized to the distal spinal cord and may exhibit prominent papillary formation, the papillae frequently containing small pools of mucin around blood vessels.

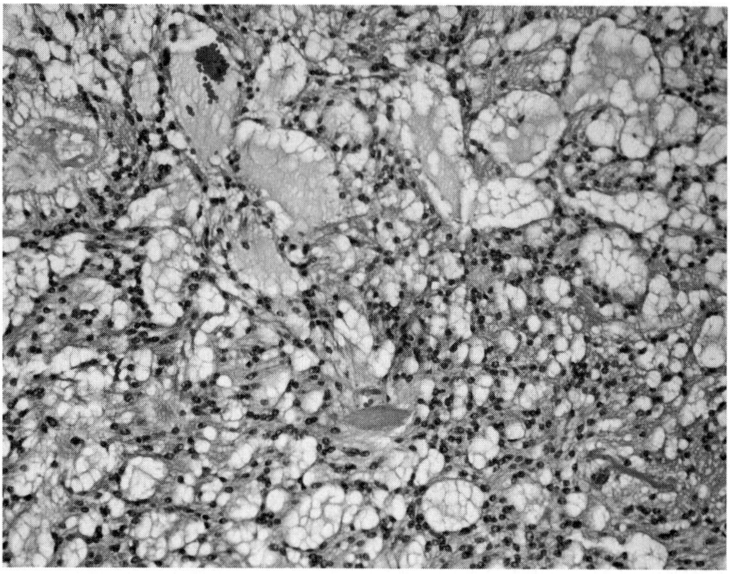

Figure 94 Myxopapillary ependymoma. Even the more solid portion of a myxopapillary ependymoma reveals abundant mucinous material separating irregular clusters of uniform tumor cells.

C. Meningiomas

Meningiomas are firmly attached to the dura and frequently form a collarlike mass around the cord. It may be difficult to distinguish fibroblastic meningiomas from neurofibromas and neurilemomas without the aid of S-100 and EMA immunohistochemical stains.

D. Neurilemomas

Two common nerve sheath tumors are found, neurofibromas and neurilemomas. Both are slow-growing.

Neurilemomas (*schwannomas*) are derived from Schwann cells and form discrete encapsulated masses which project from the nerve. Generally they are attached to a spinal nerve root, compressing it rather than infiltrating or effacing normal nerve fibers. They usually have a uniform, pale, gray-to-tan cut surface, but may show areas of cystic degeneration and hemorrhage.

Histologically, neurilemomas are composed of varying quantities of two cellular patterns. The Antoni A pattern is composed of interlacing fascicles of cells which contain fairly uniform ovoid to spindle-shaped nuclei in a hyalinized stroma (Fig. 95). These tumor nuclei may show a palisaded arrangement

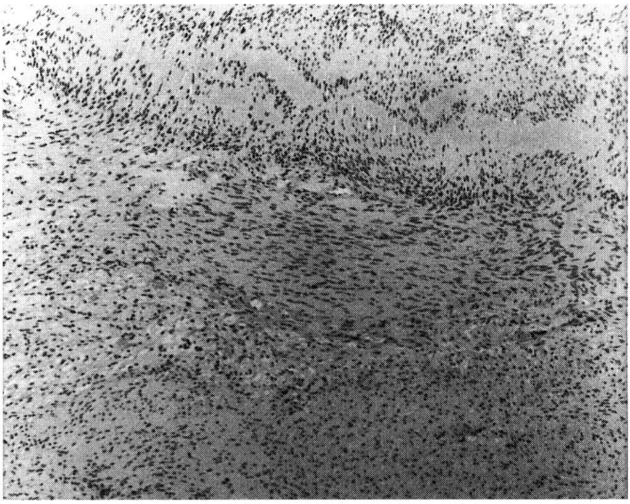

Figure 95 Neurilemoma. The cellular areas of neurilemomas (Antoni A) may show palisading of tumor nuclei, as seen at the top of this photomicrograph. These linear nuclear arrangements are known as Verocay bodies, and are a useful diagnostic clue.

(Verocay bodies). Cellular atypia, without mitosis, is thought to represent a degenerative change. Antoni B areas are hypocellular and contain widely separated stellate cells in a loose myxoid stroma which may contain hemorrhage, lipophages and hyalinized vessels (Fig. 96).

Neurilemomas of the cranial cavity are called *acoustic neuromas*, are generally attached to the eighth cranial nerve, and have been discussed previously in this chapter. Neurilemomas may resemble fibrous meningiomas, tanycytic ependymomas, subependymomas, and some astrocytomas. They can be differentiated from these neoplasms by immunohistochemical stains (Table 2), or if difficulties persist by ultrastructural examination.

E. Neurofibromas

These cause fusiform expansion of the affected nerve. Cut sections show a uniform, gelatinous, semitranslucent surface, without cystic change or hemorrhage. These tumors are characterized by proliferations of Schwann cells and fibroblasts within the nerve, causing disruption and displacement of normal axons. The stroma is myxoid, but may be fibrillary and composed of collagen. Tumor cells have spindle or wavy nuclei with pointed ends, which are haphazardly arranged (Figs. 97, 98). While some neurofibromas have regions resembling Antoni A areas of neurilemomas, Antoni B differentiation is not identified.

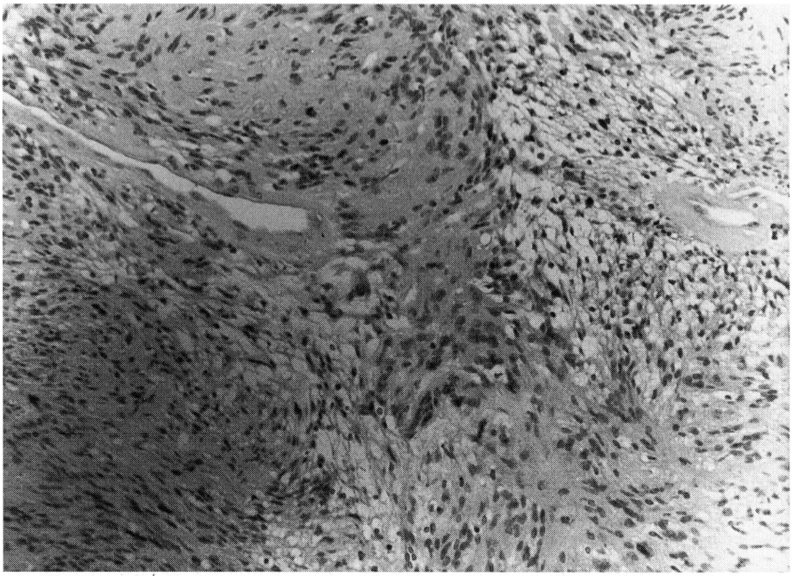

Figure 96 Neurilemoma. These tumors typically contain more compact, hyalinized Antoni A areas (bottom left) admixed with looser, less cellular Antoni B (top right).

Neurofibromas may be solitary, or multiple and part of the autosomal-dominantly inherited von Recklinghausen's neurofibromatosis. Neurofibromatosis type 1 affects about one in 5000 people and is characterized by peripheral nerve sheath tumors, including plexiform neurofibromas, cutaneous café-au-lait spots, and optic nerve/visual pathway gliomas. Neurofibromatosis type 2 is less common (about one in 50,000) and is characterized by bilateral acoustic neuromas, meningiomas, spinal cord ependymomas, and neurilemomas and neurofibromas at other sites.

F. Malignant Nerve Sheath Tumors (neurogenic sarcomas)

These are rare and usually not subclassified, although most occur in the setting of neurofibromatosis. They usually arise from peripheral nerves, and it is rare for them to be found within the cranial cavity or spinal canal. Such tumors demonstrate lack of circumscription, increased cellularity, fascicular arrangement of cells, atypia, mitotic activity, and distant metastasis. S-100 or myelin basic protein immunopositivity, if present, is helpful in differentiating these tumors from other spindle cell sarcomas.

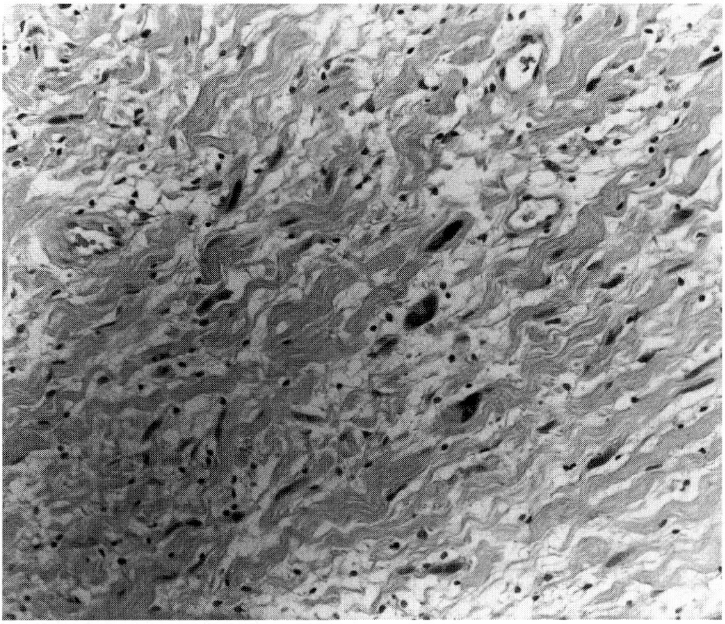

Figure 97 Neurofibroma. Plexiform neurofibromas are composed of Schwann cells in a loose mucinous matrix. The tumor nuclei may show some atypia which, in the absence of mitosis, is of no prognostic consequence.

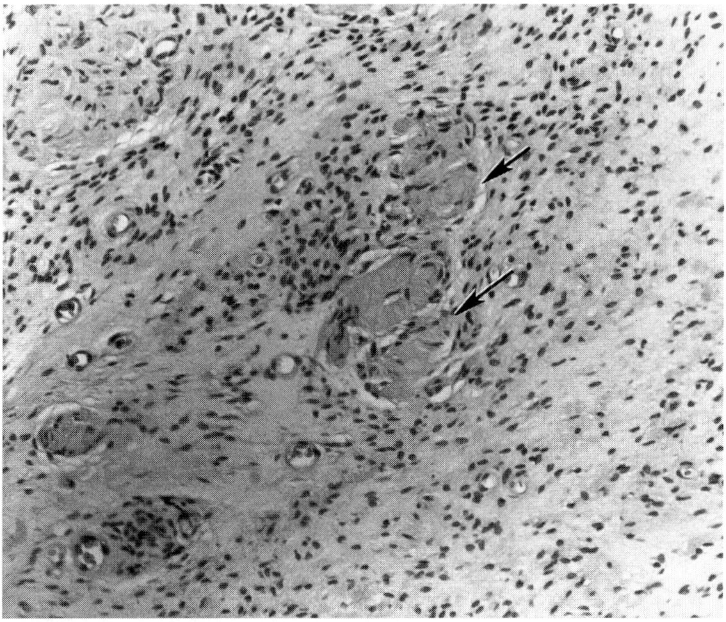

Figure 98 Neurofibroma. In a background of diffuse neurofibroma—characterized by a proliferation of uniform, often wavy spindle cells—some tactile bodies (arrows), which resemble Meissner's corpuscles of the dermis, are seen.

XIV. TUMORS OF THE SKULL AND SPINE

A large variety of benign and malignant neoplasms may arise within the spine and skull. At times these tumors may cause compression of the CNS, necessitating neurosurgical resection and submission of specimens to pathology. At such occasions, a knowledge of the x-ray and histologic appearance of osseous neoplasms is most useful.

Commonly encountered primary benign tumors of the skull and spine include aneurysmal bone cysts, fibrous dysplasia, hemangiomas, giant cell tumors of bone (Fig. 99), and sacrococcygeal teratomas. Intraosseous meningiomas have been addressed previously in this chapter. It is beyond our scope to provide a detailed discussion of these tumors; the reader is referred to a textbook of bone pathology.

A spectrum of primary malignant neoplasms of bone may be found in the spine or skull, although such tumors are rare. These include histiocytosis X (eosinophilic granuloma), osteosarcoma (Figs. 100, 101), chondrosarcoma, multiple myeloma/plasmacytoma, and lymphoma. At the time of frozen section,

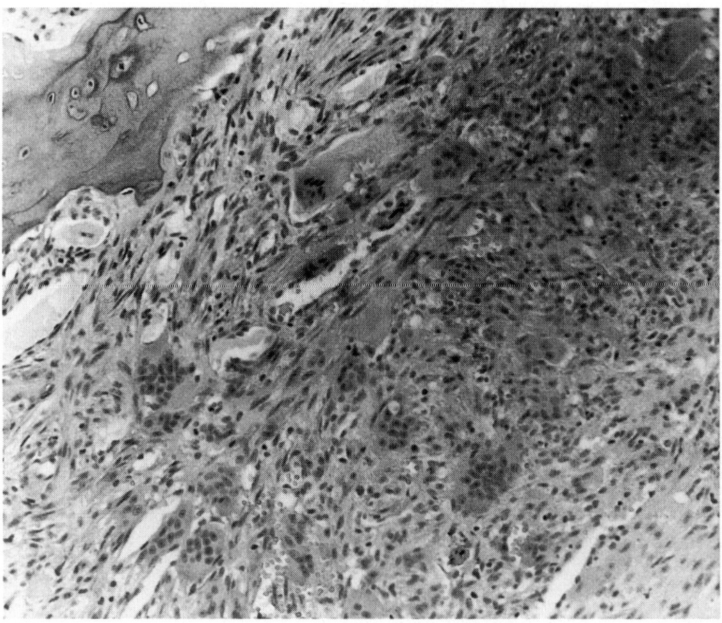

Figure 99 Giant cell tumor of bone. This neoplasm of the thoracic vertebrae caused marked bone destruction and presented with spinal cord compression. There are many multinucleate, osteoclast-like, giant cells admixed with smaller, quite uniform, mesenchymal cells.

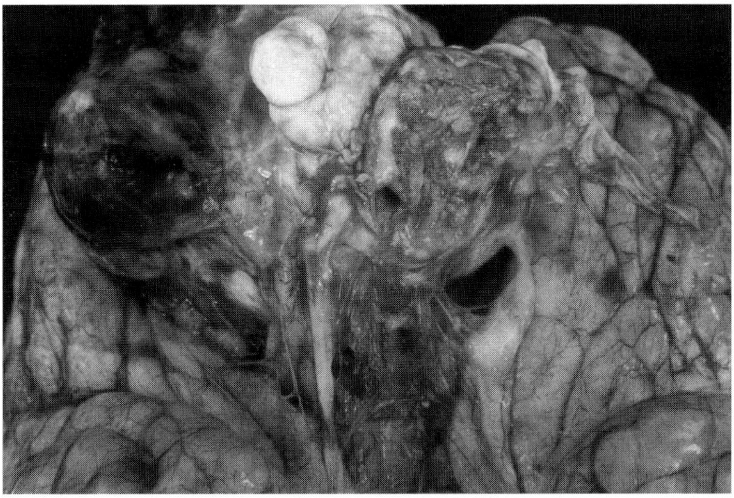

Figure 100 Osteogenic sarcoma. This tumor originated from the right orbit of a 17-year-old female who 16 years previously had had an enucleation and 6000-R localized radiation therapy for retinoblastoma. This pale, bosselated, hemorrhagic, and necrotic mass is infiltrating and compressing the frontal lobes.

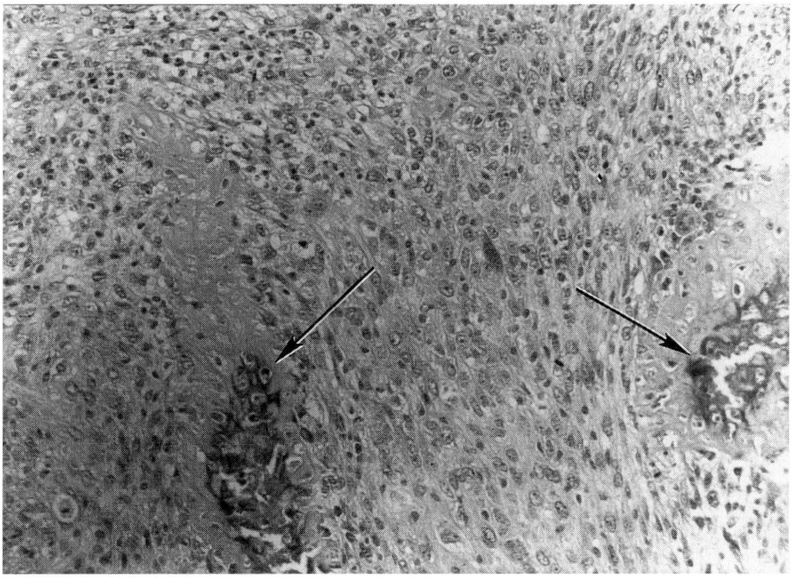

Figure 101 Osteogenic sarcoma. Tissue sections of the neoplasm illustrated in Figure 100 show a cellular spindle cell tumor containing islands of osteoid production which are centrally calcified (arrows).

touch preparations are especially helpful in diagnosing lymphomas and myelomas.

Chordomas are tumors of low malignant potential which originate from remnants of the embryonic notochord. Hence, they are limited to the skull and spine. Chordomas are midline neoplasms usually arising from the clivus or in the sacrococcygeal region, and are variably soft to firm, pale gray, and lobulated. They are usually slow-growing but may cause significant bone destruction. Metastases are rare. Histologically, they are composed of lobules of myxoid stroma containing variably arranged aggregates of atypical cells having abundant vacuolated (physaliphorous) cytoplasm (Figs. 102, 103).

Metastases to bone are common and may result in destructive lesions, with tumor extending into the epidural space, causing compressive symptoms. Metastatic breast and prostatic adenocarcinomas to the vertebral column are particularly common symptomatic lesions.

XV. METASTATIC NEOPLASMS

Metastases of malignant neoplasms to the CNS are very common in adults, comprising up to 30% of clinically significant brain tumors, but are extremely rare in children. Most metastases arise from primary sites within the lung, breast, kidney, skin (melanoma), and gastrointestinal tract (Figs. 104–109). These tumors generally maintain the histologic appearance seen in the primary

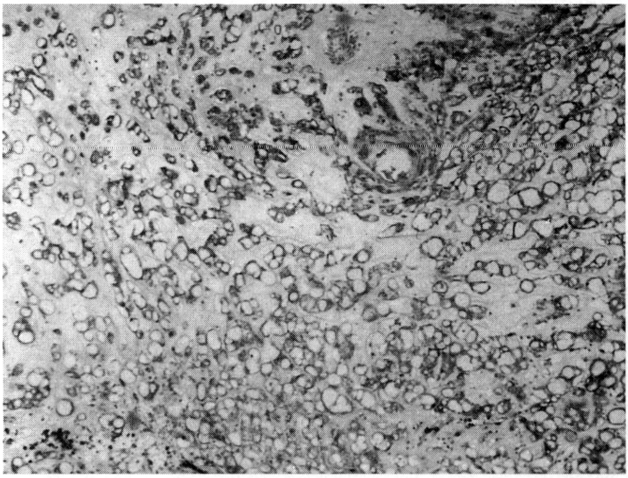

Figure 102 Chordoma. Scanning magnification shows myxoid stroma within which are many tumor cells with abundant foamy cytoplasm ("physaliphorous" cells). These cells demonstrate immunopositivity for cytokeratin and S-100 protein.

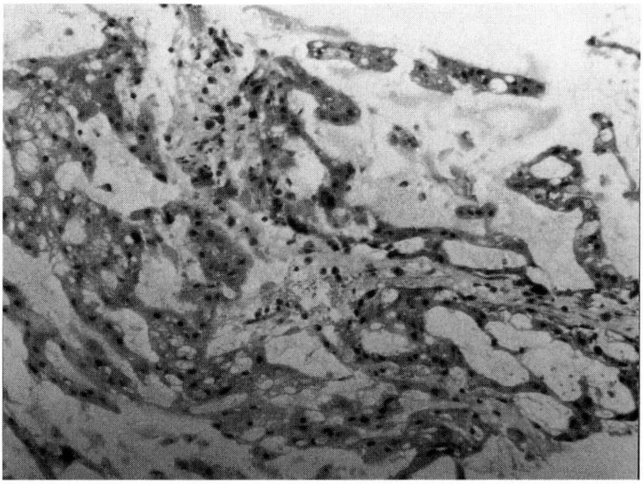

Figure 103 Chordoma. There is a chordlike arrangement of cells in a basophilic mucinous matrix. Many cells have bubbly (physaliphorous) cytoplasm.

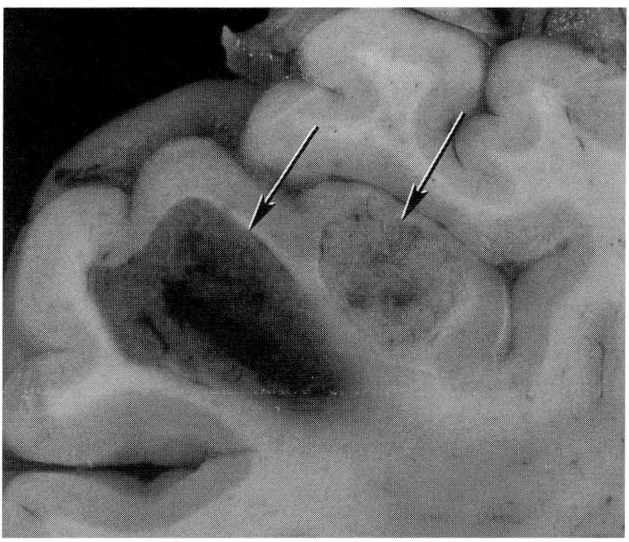

Figure 104 Metastatic carcinoma. Many metastatic tumors present with multiple lesions at or near the cortex–white matter junction. There are two discrete, necrotic, tan to hemorrhagic tumor nodules in the subcortical tissues (arrows).

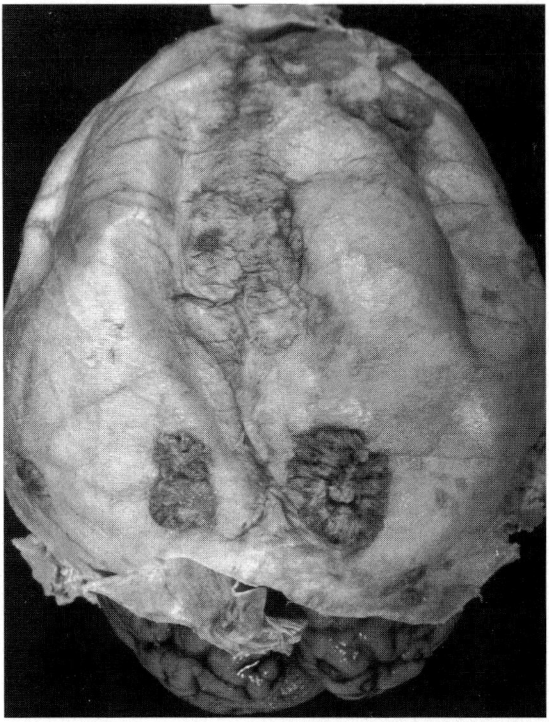

Figure 105 Metastatic carcinoma. The dura contains many nodules and plaques of tumor which were contiguous with masses in the calvarium. This 60-year-old woman had unresectable renal cell carcinoma diagnosed 3 months prior to death, with widespread systemic metastasis.

lesion (Figs. 110–116). There are frequently abundant mitotic activity, extensive necrosis, and marked nuclear pleomorphism. It is useful to remember that primary carcinomas of the CNS are uncommon, these being of choroid plexus or germ cell origin and often having distinctive histologic features.

Metastatic lesions are often multiple and widespread, a radiologic clue to the diagnosis in a patient with a known malignancy, but solitary metastases are not rare. While most of these neoplasms arise from hematogenous spread, some tumors may directly invade the brain or spine and its coverings, e.g., oropharyngeal and salivary gland tumors, may extend through the skull. Metastatic neoplasms can involve either the brain parenchyma (especially watershed regions) or leptomeninges, and grossly are often hemorrhagic and necrotic. The frequency of metastases to different sites seems mostly to be related to relative brain mass, cerebral metastases being most common.

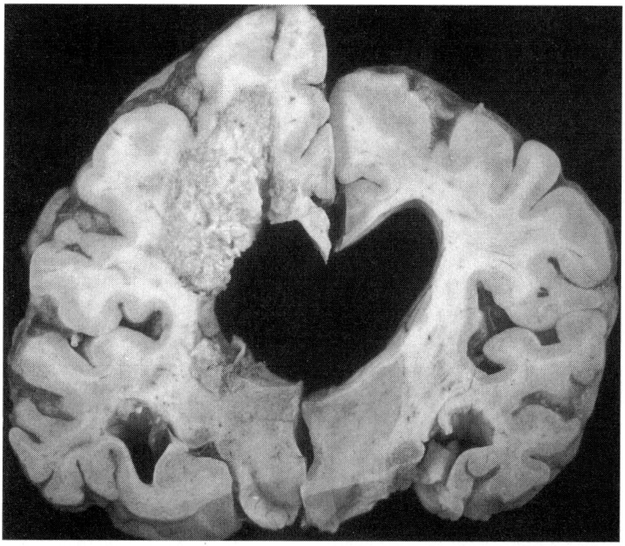

Figure 106 Metastatic carcinoma. The atrophic brain from this elderly patient with Alzheimer's disease shows a large, friable, necrotic nodule of metastatic colonic adenocarcinoma in the frontoparietal region adjacent to dilated lateral ventricles.

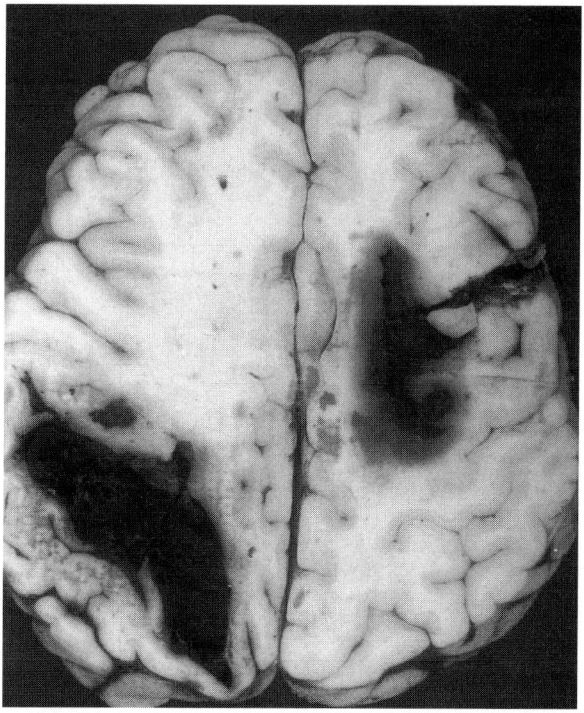

Figure 107 Metastatic carcinoma. Large hemorrhagic lesions are characteristic of metastatic choriocarcinoma. The patient was a 33-year-old female, 4 months postpartum, who developed intrauterine choriocarcinoma with multiple systemic metastasis.

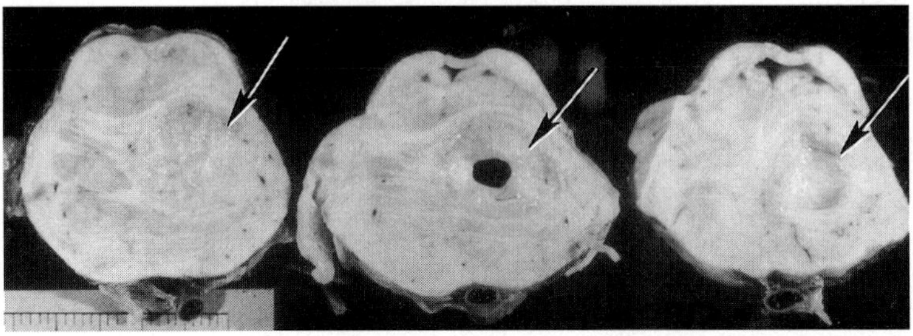

Figure 108 Metastatic carcinoma. Sections of pons show an ill-defined area of necrotic metastatic oat cell carcinoma destroying much of the right basis pontis (arrows).

Some tumors become clinically manifest with a brain metastasis before their primary site of origin is known, which may present a challenge at the time of frozen section since the pattern of a metastatic tumor is rarely specific as to site. Such tumors usually originate from the lung or gastrointestinal tract.

XVI. CYSTIC LESIONS

Cystic lesions of the brain are thought to be congenital in nature and are characterized by their epithelial lining and location. They are usually surrounded by a rim of gliotic, sometimes calcified, parenchyma.

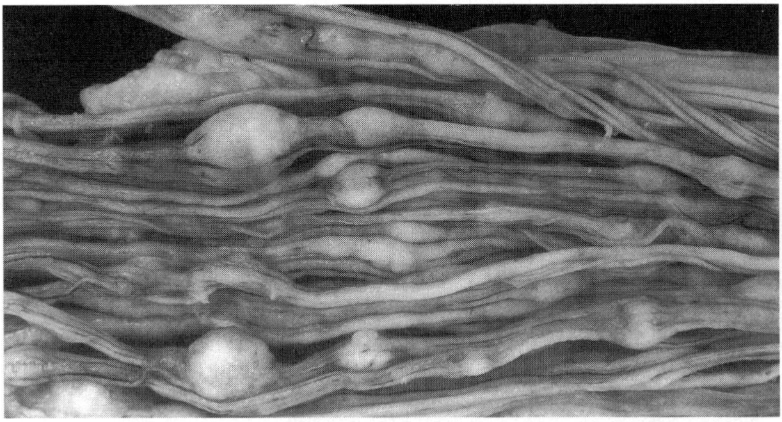

Figure 109 Metastatic carcinoma. The cauda equina contains many nodules of metastatic carcinoma.

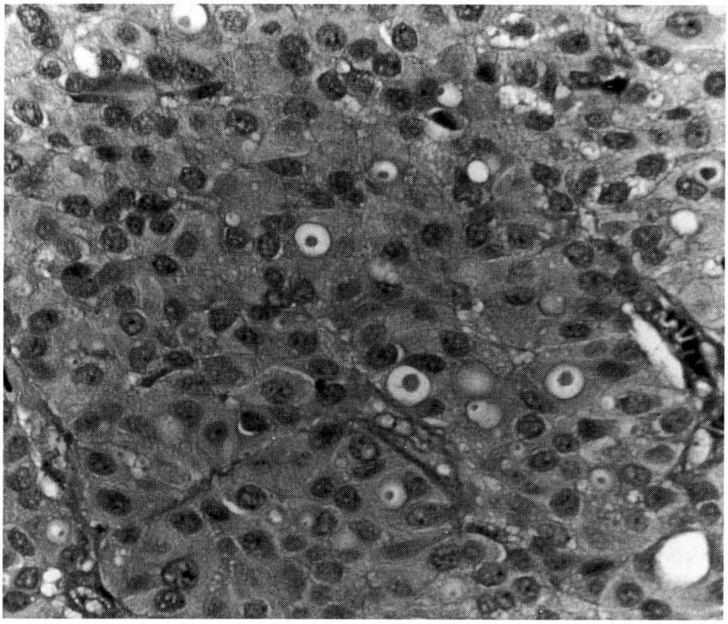

Figure 110 Metastatic carcinoma. At the time of frozen section, this dural tumor mimicked a secretory meningioma. Touch imprints, however, showed the neoplastic cells to be clearly epithelial, rather than meningeal, in nature. The patient was found to have mammary carcinoma.

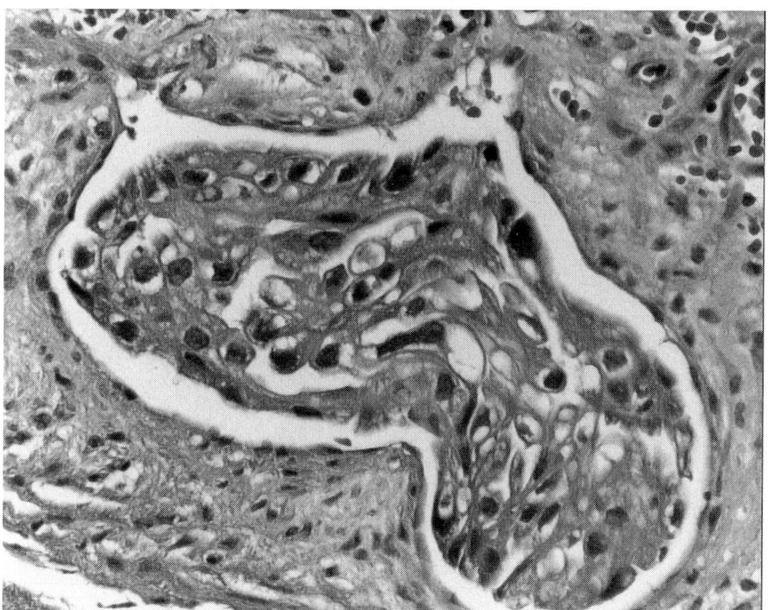

Figure 111 Metastatic carcinoma. A plug of tumor is seen within a vascular space of an organizing subdural hematoma. The patient was a young woman who had disseminated, poorly differentiated ductal adenocarcinoma of the breast.

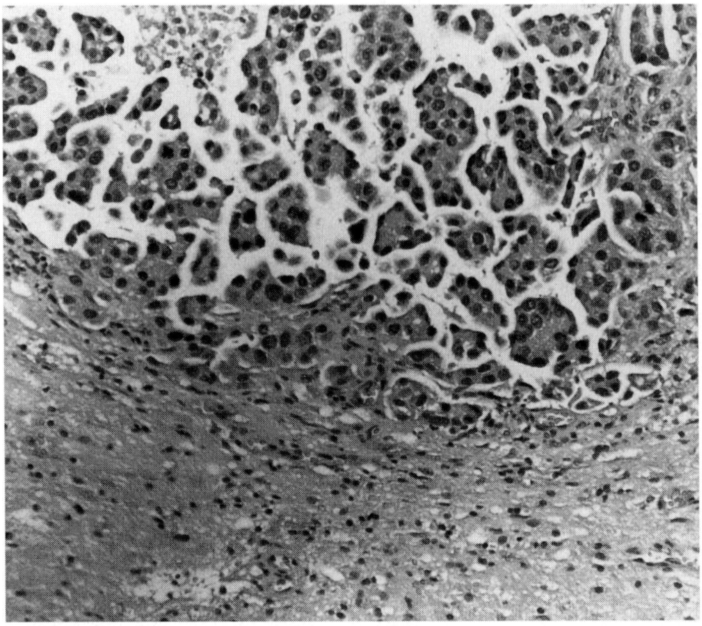

Figure 112 Metastatic carcinoma. Metastatic adenocarcinoma is seen abutting gliotic brain tissues (bottom). The patient had papillary adenocarcinoma of the breast.

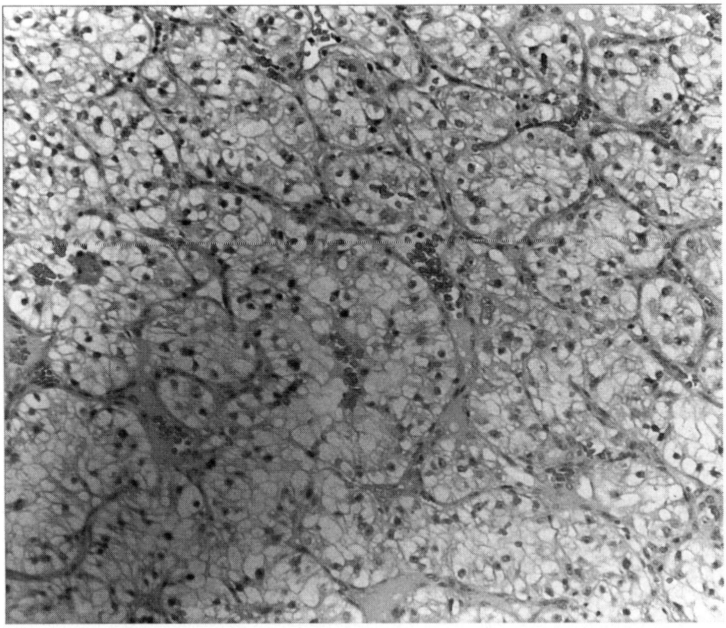

Figure 113 Metastatic carcinoma. This middle-aged man presented with a cerebellar tumor. He was subsequently found to have a large renal cell carcinoma, the primary site of this metastasis. The appearance mimics that of hemangioblastoma (see Figs. 48, 49).

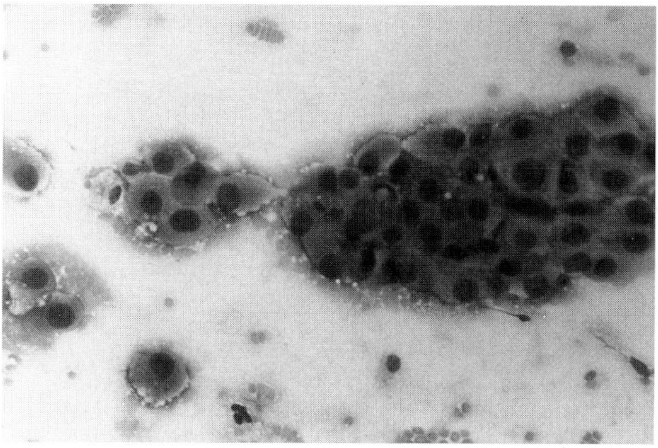

Figure 114 Metastatic carcinoma. During intraoperative consultation, touch imprints or smear preparations are helpful in determining whether a neoplasm is metastatic or primary. The cohesive nature of these epithelioid cells is that of a metastatic carcinoma, rather than a glioma.

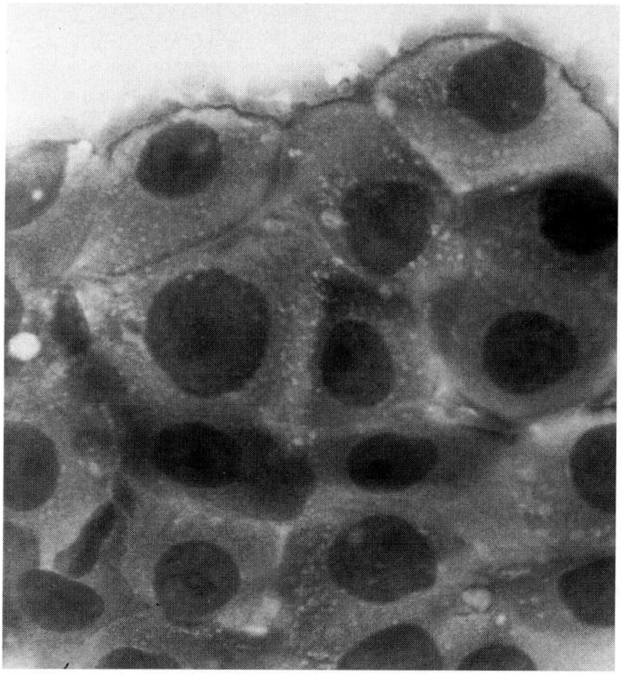

Figure 115 Metastatic carcinoma. Higher magnification of Figure 114 reveals marked nuclear atypia, prominent central nucleoli, and abundant, finely vacuolated cytoplasm. The patient was found to have a primary carcinoma in the lung.

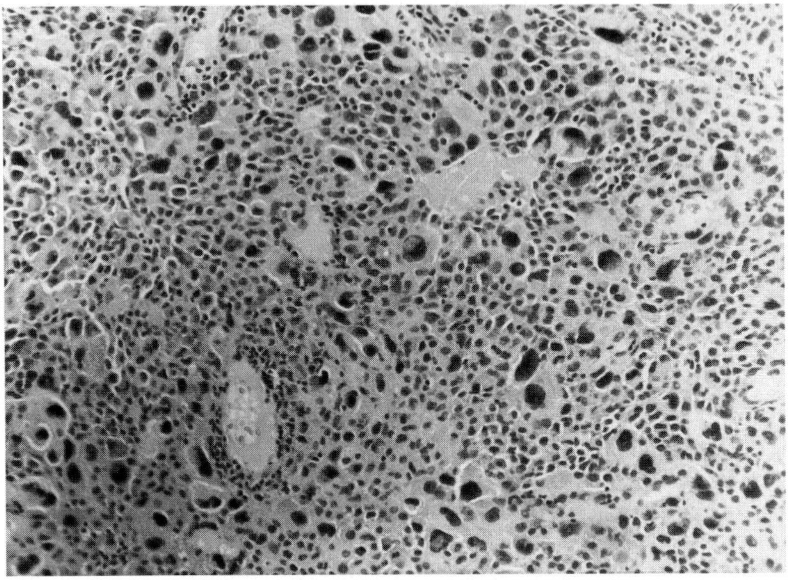

Figure 116 Metastatic melanoma. This highly pleomorphic neoplasm presented as a mass in the cerebral hemisphere of a young woman who had a cutaneous Clark level IV melanoma excised 3 years previously. The tumor is highly cellular and contains many giant cells. At first glance it resembles glioblastoma multiforme, except that vascular endothelial hyperplasia and pseudopalisaded necrosis are not seen; a fine, dusty brown pigment (melanin) was found in the cytoplasm of many cells.

Epidermoid cysts are usually manifest after the fourth decade of life and primarily involve the cerebellopontine angle and parasellar regions, but may occur almost anywhere within the CNS (Fig. 117). These well-demarcated cysts are often extensively invaginated into the parenchyma. They grossly contain flaky, pale, keratinous material with a shiny "mother-of-pearl" cyst lining. Histologically, the lining consists of a keratinizing squamous epithelium resembling the epidermis, resting on a thin layer of collagen but lacking skin appendages. Intraoperative smears of the cyst contents show sheets of keratinocytes. Ruptured cysts can cause a severe chemical meningitis.

Dermoid cysts are well-defined midline lesions of the scalp, skull, posterior fossa, or lumbosacral region, involving the CNS parenchyma or leptomeninges. Grossly, these cysts contain a thick, yellow, oily secretion and may contain fine, vellus hairs. Microscopically, in addition to a keratinizing squamous epithelial lining, dermoid cysts also contain skin appendages (hair follicles, sebaceous and eccrine sweat glands; Fig. 118); however, no other elements to suggest a teratoma are found. As with epidermoid cysts, examining smears of

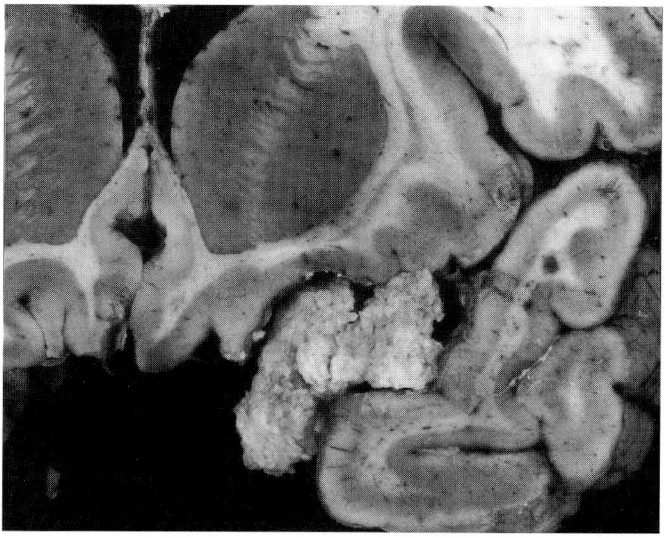

Figure 117 Epidermoid cyst. There is an epidermoid cyst at the junction of the left temporal lobe and Sylvian fissure. The cyst has pale, cheesy contents and is surrounded by a thin membrane. Histologic sections revealed a squamous epithelial lining with keratinous contents. The lesion was an incidental finding in a 27-year-old male who died of congenital heart disease.

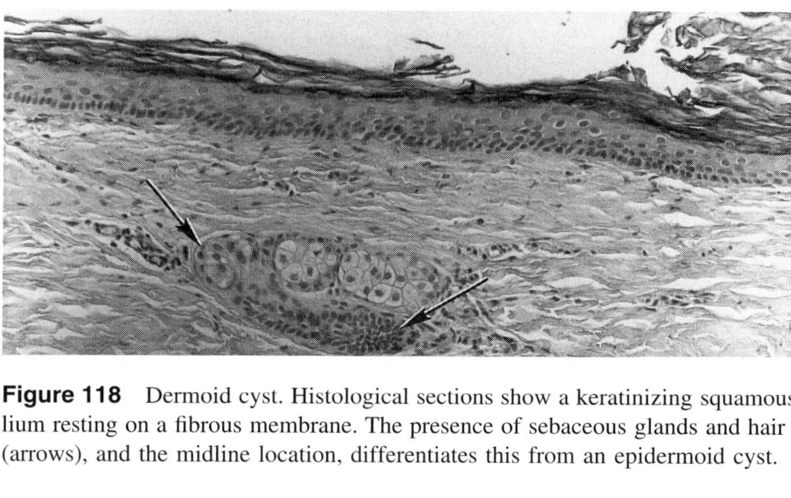

Figure 118 Dermoid cyst. Histological sections show a keratinizing squamous epithelium resting on a fibrous membrane. The presence of sebaceous glands and hair follicles (arrows), and the midline location, differentiates this from an epidermoid cyst.

the cyst contents during intraoperative consultation may be helpful in arriving at a correct diagnosis.

Colloid cysts classically arise in the roof of the third ventricle between the columns of the fornices and choroid plexus (Fig. 119). These uncommon tumors are rarely manifest before young adulthood, when they may present with intermittent obstruction of the foramen of Monro, with the potential for fatal acute hydrocephalus. They are rounded cysts, usually several centimeters in diameter, having a thin membranous wall and thick gelatinous contents. Histologically, the lining consists of uniform columnar-to-cuboidal epithelium, which is frequently ciliated and mucin-producing (Fig. 120). A thin external fibrous membrane surrounds the epithelium. The contents are mucinous and contain desquamated cells and histiocytes. The exact cell of origin is not well established.

Rathke's cleft cysts form between the pars distalis and pars intermedia of the pituitary gland, but may extend into the suprasellar regions. Larger cysts can cause pituitary compression, especially if hemorrhage has caused rapid cyst expansion. Most Rathke's cleft cysts are usually an incidental autopsy finding.

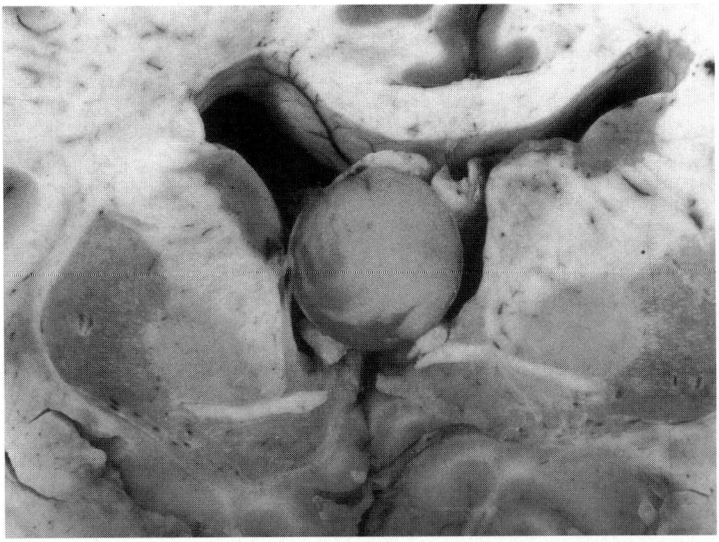

Figure 119 Colloid cyst. The classic gross appearance of a colloid cyst, with rounded mass containing thick gelatinous material arising between the columns of the fornices. The patient, a 30-year-old male, presented with severe headaches and subsequently became unresponsive.

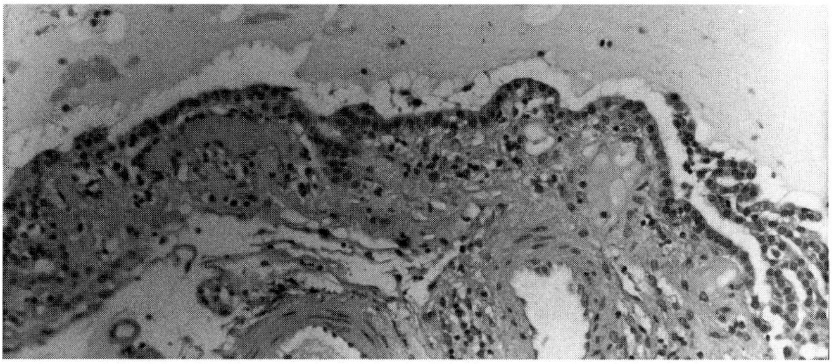

Figure 120 Colloid cyst. Histological sections show the cyst wall to be composed of fibrous tissue upon which a layer of uniform cuboidal epithelium rests.

They are filled with mucoid fluid and lined by a columnar-to-cuboidal epithelium which may be ciliated, with occasionally intermixed goblet cells and hyalinized stroma. Squamous metaplasia may be seen.

Leptomeningeal cysts are sacs of watery liquid occurring in a cleft of the arachnoid membrane. They may arise anywhere in the CNS and sometimes present as large mass lesions. *Ependymal cysts* are uncommon and lined by a ciliated columnar-to-cuboidal, nonstratified epithelium resting on glial or fibrous tissues, often occurring in the anterior cervical or upper thoracic spinal cord. As the name implies, they are thought to be of ependymal derivation and the cells are GFAP-positive. *Pineal cysts* may present as cystic masses mistaken for neoplasms; they must be differentiated from teratomas and gliomas. *Enterogenous* (*neurenteric*) *cysts* are intradural cysts of the spine and spinal cord often presenting in children or young adults. They are composed of a columnar, mucin-producing epithelium (Fig. 121), usually nonciliated and resembling that of the gut (more rarely, bronchial epithelium).

Meningoceles, meningoencephaloceles, and meningomyeloceles are due to congenital malformations of the neural tube that form during the third to fourth week of embryogenesis. They are characterized by defects in the bone, skeletal muscle, and fibroconnective tissues overlying the affected portion of the CNS. *Meningoceles* are external saccular protrusions of the meninges through dorsal defects, usually in the lumbar vertebrae. If associated with protrusions of brain, spinal cord, and nerve roots, such defects are called, respectively, *meningoencephaloceles* and *meningomyeloceles*. These latter malformations are obviously much more severe and debilitating than meningoceles.

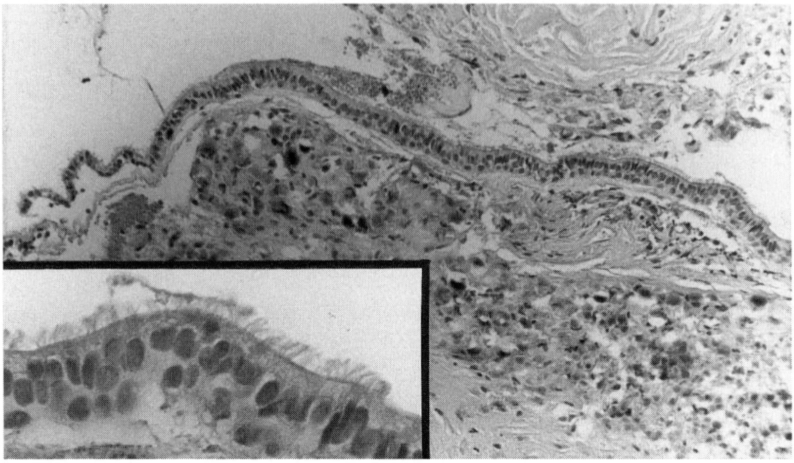

Figure 121 Enterogenous cyst. These intradural spinal cysts are lined by columnar epithelium which may be ciliated, resembling bronchial epithelium (inset). The fibrous wall exhibits extensive dystrophic calcifications.

REFERENCES

1. Bjornsson J, Scheithauer BW, Okazaki H, Leech RW. Intracranial germ cell tumors: pathobiological and immunohistochemical aspects of 70 cases. J Neuropathol Exp Neurol 1985; 44:32–46.
2. Burger PC. Use of cytological preparations in the frozen section diagnosis of central nervous system neoplasia. Am J Surg Pathol 1985; 9:344–354.
3. Burger PC. The anatomy of astrocytomas. Mayo Clin Proc 1987; 62:527–529.
4. Burger PC, Rawlings CE, Cox EB, McLendon RE, Schold SC Jr, Bullard DE. Clinicopathologic correlations in the oligodendroglioma. Cancer 1987; 59:1345–1352.
5. Burger PC, Scheithauer BW. Atlas of Tumor Pathology. Tumors of the Central Nervous System. 3rd series, fascicle 10. Washington: Armed Forces Institute of Pathology, 1994.
6. Burger PC, Scheithauer BW, Vogel FS. Surgical Pathology of the Nervous System and Its Coverings. 3rd ed. New York: Churchill Livingstone, 1991.
7. Burger PC, Vogel FS. Frozen section interpretation in surgical neuropathology. I. Intracranial lesions. Am J Surg Pathol 1977; 1:323–347.
8. Burger PC, Vogel FS. Frozen section interpretation in surgical neuropathology. II. Intraspinal lesions. Am J Surg Pathol 1978; 2:81–95.
9. Chandrasoma PT, Apuzzo MLJ. Stereotactic Brain Biopsy. 1st ed. New York: Igaku-Shoin, 1989.
10. Clark GB, Henry JM, McKeever PE. Cerebral pilocytic astrocytoma. Cancer 1985; 56:1128–1133.

11. Coffin CM, Wick MR, Braun JT, Dehner LP. Choroid plexus neoplasms. Clinicopathologic and immunohistochemical studies. Am J Surg Pathol 1986; 10:394–404.
12. Daumas-Duport C, Scheithauer BW, Kelly PJ. A histologic and cytologic method for the spatial definition of gliomas. Mayo Clin Proc 1987; 62:435–449.
13. Daumas-Duport C, Scheithauer B, O'Fallon J, Kelly PJ. Grading of astrocytomas. A simple and reproducible method. Cancer 1988; 62:2152–2165.
14. De la Monte SM, Flickinger J, Linggood RM. Histopathologic features predicting recurrence of meningiomas following subtotal resection. Am J Surg Pathol 1986; 10:836–843.
15. Dietrich DR, Toxicological and pathological applications of proliferating cell nuclear antigen (PCNA), a novel endogenous marker for cell proliferation. Crit Rev Toxicol 1993; 23:77–109.
16. Hart MN, Earle KM. Primitive neuroectodermal tumors of the brain in children. Cancer 1973; 32:890–897.
17. Ito S, Chandler KL, Prados MD, et al. Proliferative potential and prognostic evaluation of low-grade astrocytomas. J Neuro-Oncol 1994; 19:1–9.
18. Jeffreys R. Pathological and haematological aspects of posterior fossa haemangioblastomata. J Neurol Neurosurg Psychiatry 1975; 38:112–119.
19. Jennings MT, Gelman R, Hochberg F. Intracranial germ-cell tumors; natural history and pathogenesis. J Neurosurg 1985; 63:155–167.
20. Kraus JA, Koopmann J, Kaskel P, et al. Shared allelic losses on chromosomes 1p and 19q suggest a common origin of oligodendroglioma and oligoastrocytoma. J Neuropathol Exp Neurol 1995; 54:91–95.
21. Krouwer HGJ, Davis RL, Silver P, Prados M. Gemistocytic astrocytomas: a reappraisal. J Neurosurg 1991; 74:399–406.
22. Le Chevalier T, Smith FP, Caille P, Constans JP, Rouesse JG. Sites of primary malignancies in patients presenting with cerebral metastases. A review of 120 cases. Cancer 1985; 56:880–882.
23. Louis DN, Ramesh V, Gusella JF. Neuropathology and molecular genetics of neurofibromatosis 2 and related tumors. Brain Pathol 1995; 5:163–172.
24. Mirra JM. Bone Tumors. Clinical, Radiologic, and Pathologic Correlations. 1st ed. Philadelphia: Lea & Febiger, 1989.
25. Neumann PHP, Lips CJM, Hsia YE, Zbar B. Von Hippel–Lindau syndrome. Brain Pathol 1995; 5:181–193.
26. O'Neill BP, Illig JJ. Primary central nervous system lymphoma. Mayo Clin Proc 1989; 64:1005–1020.
27. O'Neill BP, Kelly PJ, Earle JD, Scheithauer B, Banks PM. Computer-assisted stereotaxic biopsy for the diagnosis of primary central nervous system lymphoma. Neurology 1987; 37:1160–1164.
28. Petito CK, DeGirolami U, Earle KM. Craniopharyngiomas. A clinical and pathological review. Cancer 1976; 37:1944–1952.
29. Roberts RO, Lynch CF, Jones MP, Hart MN. Medulloblastoma: a population-based study of 532 cases. J Neuropathol Exp Neurol 1991; 50:134–144.
30. Rorke LB. Classification and grading of childhood brain tumors. Cancer 1985; 56:1847–1904.

31. Scheithauer BW. Symptomatic subependymoma. Report of 21 cases with review of the literature. J Neurosurg 1978; 46:689–696.
32. Scheithauer BW, Kovacs KT, Laws ER Jr, Randall RV. Pathology of invasive pituitary tumors with special reference to functional classification. J Neurosurg 1986; 65:733–744.
33. Schneider JH Jr, Raffel C, McComb JG. Benign cerebellar astrocytomas of childhood. Neurosurgery 1992; 30:58–62.
34. Schwechheimer K, Braus DF, Schwarzkopf G, Feller AC, Volk B, Muller-Hermelink HK. Polymorphous high-grade B cell lymphoma is the predominant type of spontaneous primary cerebral malignant lymphomas. Am J Surg Pathol 1994; 18:931–937.
35. Shepherd CW, Scheithauer BW, Gomez MR, Altermatt HJ, Katzmann JA. Subependymal giant cell astrocytoma: a clinical, pathological, and flow cytometric study. Neurosurgery 1991; 28:864–868.
36. Thomas HG, Dolman CL, Berry K. Malignant meningioma: clinical and pathologic features. J Neurosurg 1981; 55:929–934.
37. Wick MR, Swanson PE, Scheithauer BW, Manivel JC. Malignant peripheral nerve sheath tumor. An immunohistochemical study of 62 cases. Am J Clin Pathol 1987; 87:425–433.
38. Winek RR, Scheithauer BW, Wick MR. Meningioma, meningeal hemangiopericytoma (angioblastic meningioma), peripheral hemangiopericytoma, and acoustic schwannoma: a comparative immunohistochemical study. Am J Surg Pathol 1989; 13:251–261.
39. Yasargil MG, von Ammon K, von Deimling A, Valavanis A, Wichmann W, Wiestler OD. Central neurocytoma: histopathological variants and therapeutic approaches. J Neurosurg 1992; 76:32–37.

7

Developmental and Pediatric Neuropathology

I. INTRODUCTION

Developmental/pediatric neuropathology differs from adult neuropathology for three main reasons: the brain and spinal cord are growing, developing and maturing; their responses to injury are usually more limited (and may be different); and the spectrum of "insults" to which the developing nervous system is subject differs from that affecting the mature nervous system. Thus, developmental/pediatric neuropathology constitutes an unusually complex subject.

Historically, malformations of the nervous system have been classified with reference to their morphology. Yet, while certain patterns of malformation are seen reproducibly, many individual malformations show changes that "do not quite fit" into these patterns. Recent advances in molecular biology and developmental neuroscience have elucidated gene defects associated with a few specific malformations (e.g., some forms of lissencephaly), but this analysis has been applicable to only a very small percentage of recognizable malformations; the etiology of most remains obscure. For this reason, most neuropathologists classify developmental lesions with regard to common morphologic patterns while taking into account the presumed disruption of normal processes of central nervous system (CNS) development (i.e., disorders of neuroblast migration, sulcus formation, etc.) that contributed to their pathogenesis.

Understanding developmental/perinatal neuropathology is further complicated by the fact that nervous system malformations can be either primary or secondary (acquired), a distinction that may not always be evident when a specimen is examined. Primary malformations can be either genetically determined or epigenetic (or a combination of the two), while secondary malformations result from destructive processes. However, secondary (acquired) lesions may mimic primary malformations, especially when they are acquired early in intrauterine life.

As the classification of lesions moves from a system that is primarily descriptive to one that incorporates pathophysiologic mechanisms, developmental disorders will be considered in a new light. Advances in the basic science of developmental neurobiology will change the way we evaluate, classify, and consider these complex lesions. A basic understanding of the fundamental processes of development will help the student of neuropathology to understand how these disorders can be meaningfully categorized, and will enable him or her to flexibly integrate advances in developmental neuroscience into a useful system for analyzing nervous system malformations. We will begin this chapter with a brief review of the basic processes involved in brain and spinal cord development.

II. OVERVIEW OF BRAIN AND SPINAL CORD DEVELOPMENT

CNS development requires the complex interplay of a number of coordinated, interdependent processes. First, the neural tube must form and close properly; otherwise neural tube defects will result. The constituent lining cells of the neural tube must proliferate, differentiate, and migrate to their appropriate positions, failing which neuronal migration disorders, disorders of lobar formation and sulcation will result. Neurons must survive in maximally efficient numbers and form (and remodel) appropriate connections. This process of synaptic modeling and remodeling constitutes the essential plasticity of the nervous system, which allows for learning. In addition, the developing nervous tissue must interact in a highly complex mutually inductive fashion with overlying mesenchymal tissues, or else complex malformations (e.g., Arnold-Chiari type II) may occur. Genetic errors, or acquired intrauterine lesions, can affect any or all of these processes, resulting in some of the complex malformative patterns that present to the neuropathologist.

A. Neural Tube Formation

At approximately 4 weeks gestational age, the neural tube forms from the primitive neural streak (Chap. 1). It is covered by simple pseudostratified neuroepithelium, the component cells of which then proliferate around the developing ventricular system. This zone is a mosaic of precursors that will give rise to neurons, astrocytes, oligodendroglia, and ependyma. Neuroblasts and spongioblasts (glial precursors) migrate from the ventricular zone (and subventricular zone) to form the substance of the gray and white matter of the brain and spinal cord. Ependymal cells form from the remaining cells of the ventricular zone.

B. Proliferation and Differentiation

The complex processes of cellular proliferation, determination of cell type, and differentiation are influenced by multiple factors including trophic and growth factors. Growth factors are endogenously synthesized polypeptides which affect fundamental cellular processes by binding to specific receptors on the cell surface. Factors normally present in the developing nervous system include acidic and basic fibroblast growth factor, epidermal growth factor, transforming growth factor beta, platelet-derived growth factor, endothelins, insulinlike growth factor, ciliary neurotrophic factor, and the family of neurotrophic factors which includes nerve growth factor, neurotrophin 3, and brain derived neurotrophic factor. Current molecular neurobiologic research is focused on attempts to elucidate the mechanisms of action of these trophic factors in the developing CNS and to assess their role in plasticity, response to injury, neoplasia, axon guidance, and survival.

Cell surface interactions with other cells and with the extracellular matrix also play a crucial role in these processes. The interactions are guided through cellular adhesion molecules and extracellular matrix receptors. These molecules are transmembrane molecules bearing extracellular domains which bind to molecules on the surface of other cells or in the extracellular matrix. Their intracellular domains, when activated, interact directly with cytoskeletal proteins and trigger the initiation of signal transduction pathways (many of which may act synergistically with the signal transduction pathways initiated by growth factors). The influence of cell surface interactions and trophic factors may be critical in helping precursor cells determine their ultimate cellular fate (e.g., whether to "become" an astrocyte or an oligodendrocyte).

C. Migration

Cells of the developing nervous system must migrate from their original location around the neural tube (ventricular zone region) to assume their appropriate location. A complex combination of migrational patterns allows for the development of a highly organized, three-dimensional nervous system. The primary mode of migration of neuroblasts is along radially oriented glial fibers (radial glia). Radial glia are the first distinct subtype of glial cell to appear during development. They possess cell bodies in the ventricular or subventricular zones and end feet on the pial surface, spanning the entire thickness of the cerebral hemisphere. Radial glia function as a permissive scaffold on which neuroblasts migrate from the ventricular zone to the cortical plate. These radial glia later become astrocytes (and perhaps oligodendrocytes) within the gray and white matter. Neuroblasts can also migrate along axons, essentially using them as guide wires. Finally, some migrating neuroblasts appear not to use either radial glia or axons for guidance. The mechanism(s) guiding this type of migration are still unknown. Recently, several authors have suggested that some neuronal precursors may migrate in closely associated chains.

Glial precursors migrate from the subventricular and ventricular zones to assume their "normal" position within the brain and spinal cord. The mechanisms of their migration are less well understood, but the migration of glial cells occurs over long distances in a highly organized fashion. Migration of neuroblasts to the cerebral cortex occurs in an "inside-out" fashion, as neuroblasts destined for the deepest cortical layers migrate initially, while neuroblasts destined for the more superficial cortical layers migrate past them. The bulk of neuroblast migration occurs between the 7th and 16th weeks of gestation, during which time the cortical plate (future cerebral cortex) is modeled into a six-layered cerebral cortex. Even after this time, however, some neuroblasts continue to migrate through the intermediate zone (future white matter) in a process that can continue up to a few months after birth.

D. Programmed Cell Death, Neuronal Survival, and Making Connections

Programmed cell death (PCD) is an essential mechanism of normal neural development. In normal brain and spinal cord development, there is an overproduction of neuroblasts, many of which will undergo physiological PCD. PCD is an active process involving gene transcription and protein synthesis. It includes, but is not confined to, apoptotic cell death. Glioblasts as well as neuroblasts undergo this process. The initiation of PCD in the absence of trophic factors helps to create a competitive environment for trophic support, ensuring survival of "the best connected neurons."

E. Gyration

As the brain develops, the cerebral cortex changes from a smooth, uniform surface to a highly convoluted, folded structure. This process of gyration dramatically increases the surface area of the cerebral cortex. It is most likely the result of mechanical processes related to differences in size between the cortical plate and the subplate. However, many investigators propose that there is an additional active component to "gyrogenesis." The degree of cortical folding is correlated with the size of the brain.

The first fissures in the brain are seen approx. 16 to 17 weeks in utero. This process of primary gyration continues through 30 weeks. Secondary sulci, which show some characteristic individual variability, begin to appear at approx. 32 weeks, while tertiary sulci, which are the last to appear and show a marked degree of individual variation, are seen at around 36 weeks. Tertiary sulci continue to form postnatally.

F. Myelination and Growth

At birth, the brain weighs approximately 350 g. It increases in mass to approximately 925 g by 1 year, to 1050 g by the age of 2, and to 1240 g by the age of 5. It reaches an adult size of approximately 1350 g by the age of 12. Since the normal complement of neurons is present by the time of birth, what accounts for the increase in brain size and weight? The increase in brain size is due primarily to myelination of the cerebral white matter, which is largely unmyelinated at birth. Myelination begins by approx. 20 weeks in utero and proceeds in a caudal-to-rostral direction. Different tracts within the spinal cord and brain myelinate at different times and rates, which are available in standard tables. As a general rule, the more "fundamental" a tract is for basic function, the earlier it myelinates.

As the brain develops, the most remarkable change is one that is not visible by gross or routine light microscopic examination: the extraordinary synaptic plasticity that allows for learning. Information is encoded and stored, connections are remodeled, and new connections are made as the nervous system develops the remarkable functional diversity which is its *raison d'être*.

III. DEVELOPMENTAL MALFORMATIONS

A. Disorders of Neural Tube Formation and Closure (neural tube defects)

Table 1 summarizes an overview of developmental malformations of the brain and spinal cord.

Neural tube defects are a spectrum of malformations associated with failure of neural tube closure (Fig. 1). Depending on the extent of failure of this process, defects can range from limited asymptomatic forms to clinically devastating conditions.

1. Anencephaly

Anencephaly results from a failure of the anterior end of the neural tube to close. As a consequence, the brain is absent or consists of disorganized islands of neuroglial elements, fibrous tissue, and blood vessels (substantia cerebrovasculosa) (Fig. 2). Frequently there are defects of the overlying cranial vault and scalp (illustrating the complexity of inductive interactions between the neuroectoderm and overlying mesenchymal tissues). Anencephaly may be associated

Table 1 Overview of Developmental Abnormalities of Brain and Spinal Cord

Developmental process		Malformation	
Neural tube formation/closure →	NTD	spina bifida occulta ↕ anencephaly	spectrum
Midline structure formation →	midline defects	arrhinencephaly	
		agenesis of septum pellucidum	
		agenesis of corpus callosum	
Cerebral hemisphere formation →	holoprosencephaly	alobar	
		semilobar	
		lobar	
Organization of cerebral hemispheres			
a) size		micrencephaly	
		megalencephaly	
		hemimegalencephaly	
b) gyral pattern		lissencephaly	
		pachygyria	
		polymicrogyria	
c) gray matter/white matter organization		loss of cortex/white matter demarcation	
		neuronal heterotopia	
d) organization of the cerebral cortex →		cerebral cortical dysplasia	
Formation of posterior fossa →	Arnold-Chiari malformations	type I	
		type II	
Cerebellar formation		Dandy-Walker syndrome	
		cerebellar polymicrogyria	
		cerebellar heterotopia	
		cerebellar aplasia/hypoplasia	
Brainstem formation		aqueduct abnormalities	
		aplasias/heterotopias	
Spinal cord formation (other than NTDs)		syringomyelia	
		diastematomyelia and related lesions	

Abbreviation: NTD = neural tube defect.

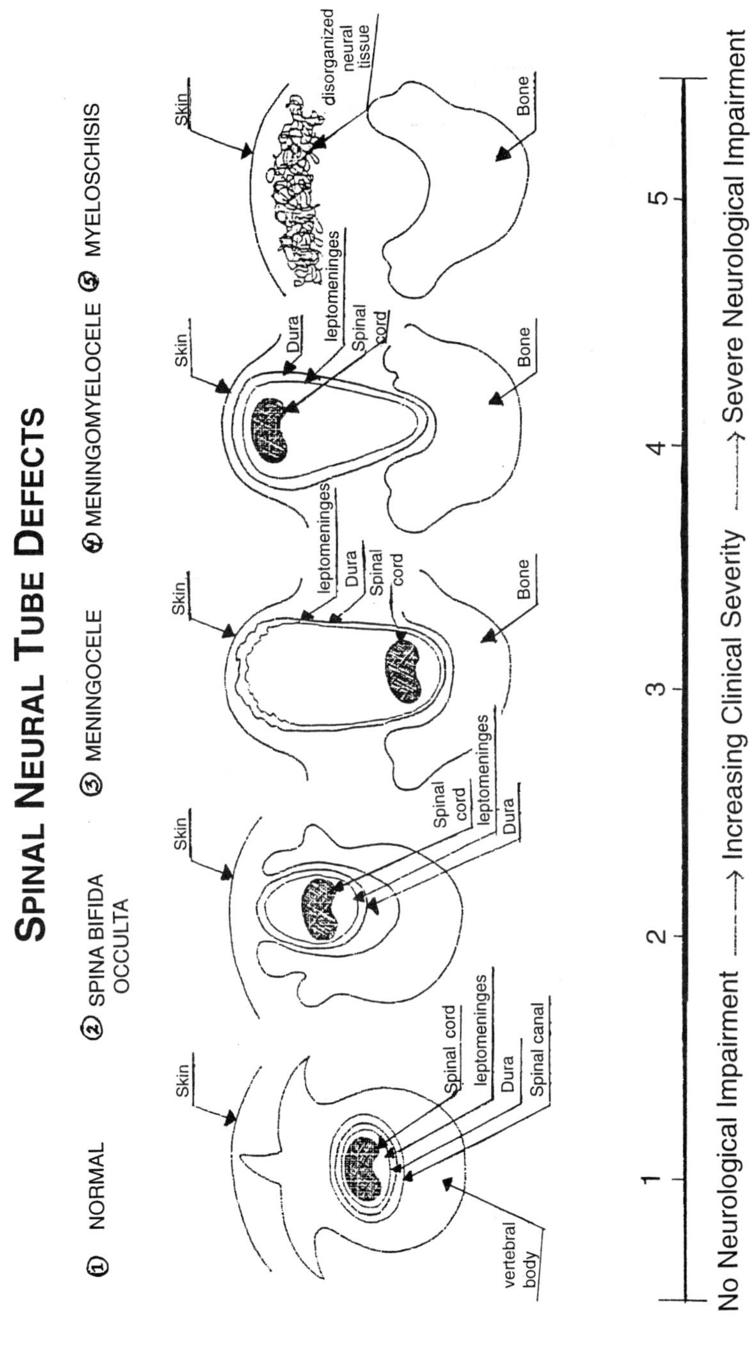

Figure 1 Schematic representation of the spectrum of (spinal) neural tube defects.

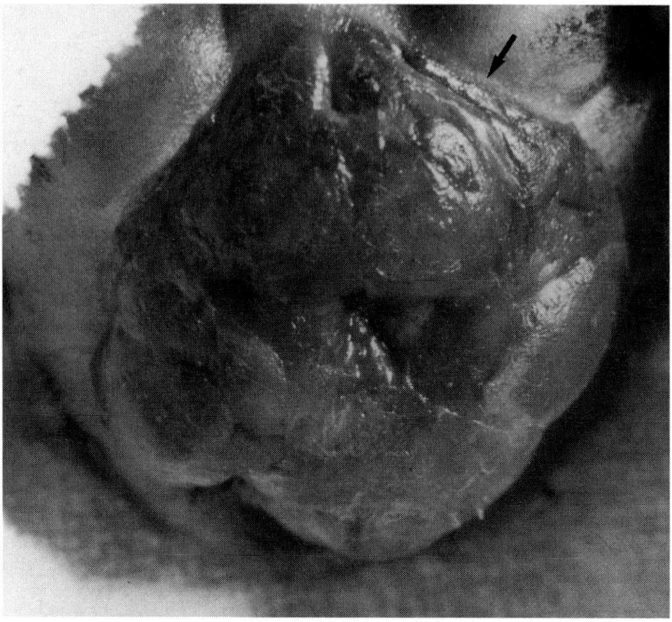

Figure 2 Anencephaly. View from top of the exposed cranial vault (no overlying skull has formed) from an infant with anencephaly. Note the open cranial vault with exposed mass of disorganized neuroglial tissue/substantia cerebrovasculosa (arrow).

with varying degrees of spinal defect, depending on the extent of the failure of neural tube closure, ranging from amyelia (absence of spinal cord) to various forms of spina bifida.

2. *Spina Bifida (cystica)—Including Spinal Meningocele, Menigomyelocele, Myelocystocele, and Myeloschisis*

Spina bifida results from a localized failure of closure of the neural tube, with a resultant failure of normal neuroglial mesenchymal induction. A defect in development of the neuroglial tissue at the site of failure of closure occurs and is frequently accompanied by a defect in the overlying vertebral arch. Spina bifida can take different forms, depending on the extent of the defect.

Spinal meningocele consists of a herniation of the meninges (but not spinal cord) through a defect in the vertebral arch, with protrusion into the skin (Fig. 1). Meningomyelocele refers to a herniation of both spinal cord tissue and overlying meninges through such a defect. Obviously, involvement of the spinal cord itself results in greater neurological disability. Myelocystocele consists of a dilatation of the central canal of the spinal cord and a thinning of the posterior spinal cord. Myeloschisis is a focal loss of the normal spinal cord architecture with replacement by a disc of disorganized neuroglial tissue, fibrotic material, and blood vessels (substantia medullovasculosa). This is the spinal cord equivalent of the substantia cerebrovasculosa seen in anencephaly, and is clinically the most severe form. The characteristic bone changes seen in spina bifida (failure of fusion or absence of vertebral arches) again highlight the complex interdependence of developing neuroglial tissue and mesenchyme.

3. *Spina Bifida Occulta*

Spina bifida occulta occurs when there is a failure of fusion of the overlying vertebral arches, but the spinal cord and meninges remain intact. Usually, there is only a superficial skin defect over the sacral region, with no associated neurologic abnormality. However, occasionally fibrous bands may form between the spinal cord and the bony defect, giving rise to a "tethered" spinal cord, which requires surgical release.

4. *Encephalocele (meningoencephalocele)*

Encephaloceles, or more accurately meningoencephaloceles, are frequently considered part of the spectrum of neural tube defects. However, they are more properly considered as a failure of appropriate mesenchymal formation, since they consist of a herniation of brain tissue and overlying meninges through a defect in the skull, rather than a true neural tube defect. Meningoencephaloceles occur most commonly in the posterior occipital region and may be associated with many dysgenetic syndromes. Pure meningoceles, in which no brain tissue herniates into the sac, may also occur.

Neural tube defects are relatively common, and show extensive variations in prevalence from location to location and within different ethnic groups. They can be routinely screened for in utero by testing the level of maternal (amniotic) alpha fetoprotein, which tends to be elevated in mothers whose fetuses show neural tube defects. This test, while sensitive, is not entirely specific and is used in combination with ultrasound examination as a screening tool for neural tube defects. Their etiology remains unknown, although folate supplementation reduces the risk of neural tube defects. It is unclear whether neural tube defects represent a failure of the neural tube to close, or a reopening of the neural tube due to a focal defect in the neuroepithelium.

B. Disorders of Formation of the Cerebral Hemispheres

1. *Disorders of Formation of Midline Structures*

The anterior aspect of the neural tube (anterior telencephalic wall) is crucial for normal brain development. The anterior *medial* aspect gives rise to the corpus callosum, anterior commissure, hippocampi, fornix, forebrain nuclei, olfactory bulbs and the septum pellucidum, and disturbance of this region early in development leads to a number of midline malformations. Hypoplasia or absence of any of these structures can occur either as an isolated malformation, in a group of midline aplasias, or as part of a more global disturbance of brain development. The clinical severity varies, often depending on the severity of other frequently associated malformations.

a. Arrhinencephaly. This describes congenital absence of the olfactory bulbs. It may be seen as an isolated finding, or in association with other midline abnormalities.

b. Agenesis of the Corpus Callosum. This (Fig. 3) can be complete or partial, depending on the severity of the developmental arrest. Frequently, a bundle of myelinated fibers (bundle of Probst) is present. Usually a large third ventricle fills the space between the cerebral hemispheres, and the cingulate gyrus is absent. Agenesis of the corpus callosum is often found in association with disorders of cerebral hemisphere formation, as well as other malformations including ventricular septal defect, webbed toes, spina bifida, agenesis of the cerebellar vermis, and other somatic abnormalities. It can also be seen in association with mental retardation and seizures. Agenesis of the corpus callosum is also a feature of Aicardi syndrome, an X-linked dominant disease characterized by agenesis of the corpus callosum, chorioretinitis, and infantile spasms. Rarely, agenesis of the corpus callosum is an incidental finding at autopsy.

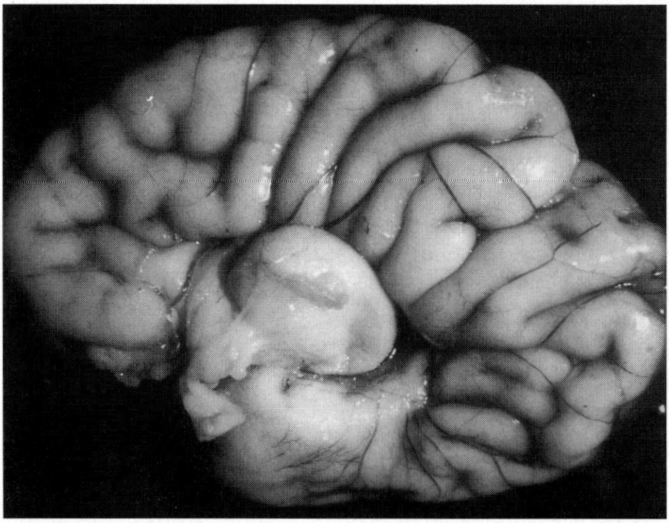

Figure 3 Agenesis of the corpus callosum. Midsagittal section through the brain shows complete absence of the corpus callosum.

c. Agenesis of the Septum Pellucidum. This can occur as an isolated finding or in association with multiple midline abnormalities (Fig. 4). When present with hypoplasia of the optic nerves and disks, it constitutes the syndrome of septo-otic dysplasia, a rare entity associated with endocrine disturbances.

Cavum septum pellucidum (Fig. 5), a pseudomalformation of the septum pellucidum, consists of a cystic cavity between the fornices ("fifth ventricle"). It is more correctly considered a *variant of normal*, since it is normal in the newborn brain and persists relatively frequently in the brains of (neurologically intact) adolescents and adults.

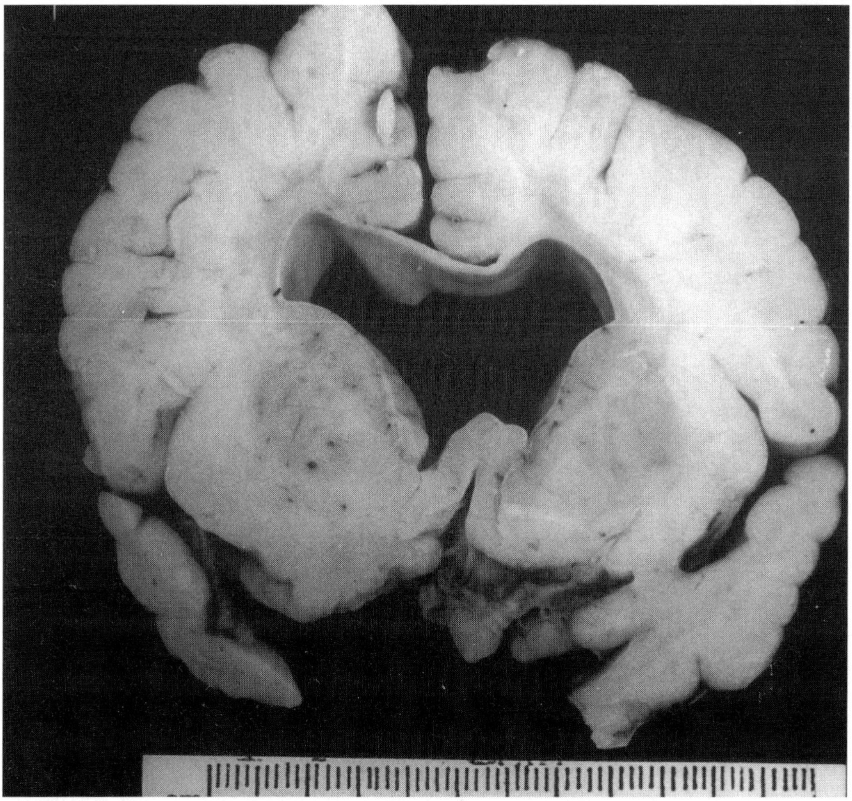

Figure 4 Agenesis of the septum pellucidum in a child with lobar holoprosencephaly. One single, fused ventricle is present. The cerebral hemispheres are separated at this coronal level, but the most anterior portion of the brain had not separated into distinct cerebral hemispheres.

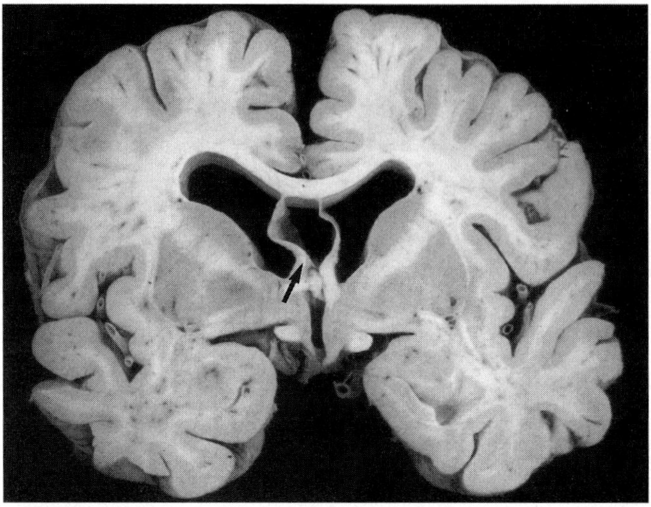

Figure 5 Cavum septum pellucidum. Coronal section through the cerebral hemispheres demonstrates a cystic cavity (cavum septum pellucidum, arrow) above the third ventricle. This pseudomalformation, often present in adult brain, represents a variant of normal.

2. *Disorders of Cerebral Hemisphere Formation* (*lobar formation*): ***Holoprosencephaly***

The anterior telencephalic wall is also critical for the formation of the cerebral hemispheres. During very early embryogenesis, the neural tube provides the structure for the spinal cord and brainstem. However, the paired cerebral hemispheres must develop as outpouchings of the anterior aspect of the neural tube. During the 5th week of embryonic development, paired telencephalic vesicles form as lateral structures from the anterior telencephalic cavity. These vesicles develop into the left and right cerebral hemispheres. Failure of this process results in holoprosencephaly, in which the telencephalon remains as one single bulb, instead of two cerebral hemispheres.

Holoprosencephaly (Fig. 6) is subdivided into three main types, depending on the degree of failure of cleavage.

a. Alobar Holoprosencephaly. In this, the most severe variant, the telencephalon remains as one single mass with a single large ventricle. The ventricle, which may be cystically dilated, is covered by a thin membrane of disorganized neuroglial tissue. The olfactory bulbs are always absent (arrhinencephaly), as are other midline abnormalities (discussed above). Severe craniofacial abnormalities are common, again implying the interdependent role of neuroectoderm

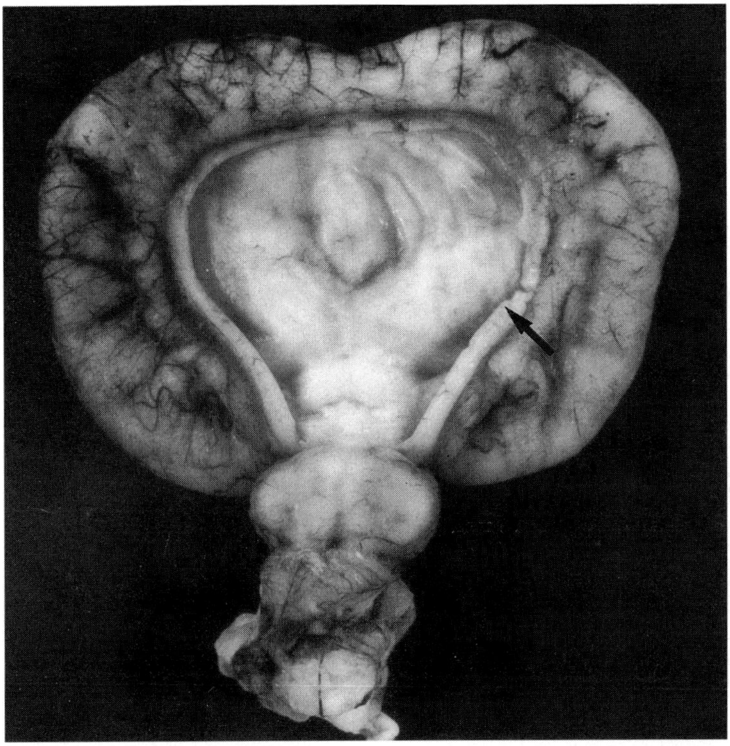

Figure 6 Holoprosencephaly in fetal brain. The telencephalon consists of a single mass with a large single ventricle (arrow) lined by a thin rim of neurological tissue. No interhemispheric fissure is present (alobar holoprosencephaly).

and overlying mesoderm in development. A single or fused double eye ("cyclopia") can sometimes be seen (Fig. 7).

b. Semilobar Holoprosencephaly. In semilobar holoprosencephaly, there is partial lobe formation, which is characterized by an incomplete interhemispheric fissure along the dorsal surface. The frontal aspect of the brain remains one connected bulb, while the posterior/occipital aspect shows cleavage. As expected, craniofacial malformation, absence of the corpus callosum, and arrhinencephaly are also frequently seen. The deep central gray matter structures (basal ganglia and thalami) are frequently fused.

c. Lobar Holoprosencephaly. Lobar holoprosencephaly is characterized by near complete separation of the cerebral hemispheres except for the most anterior aspect. Craniofacial malformations and partial or complete absence of the corpus callosum, and olfactory bulbs are also frequently present (Fig. 4). As a

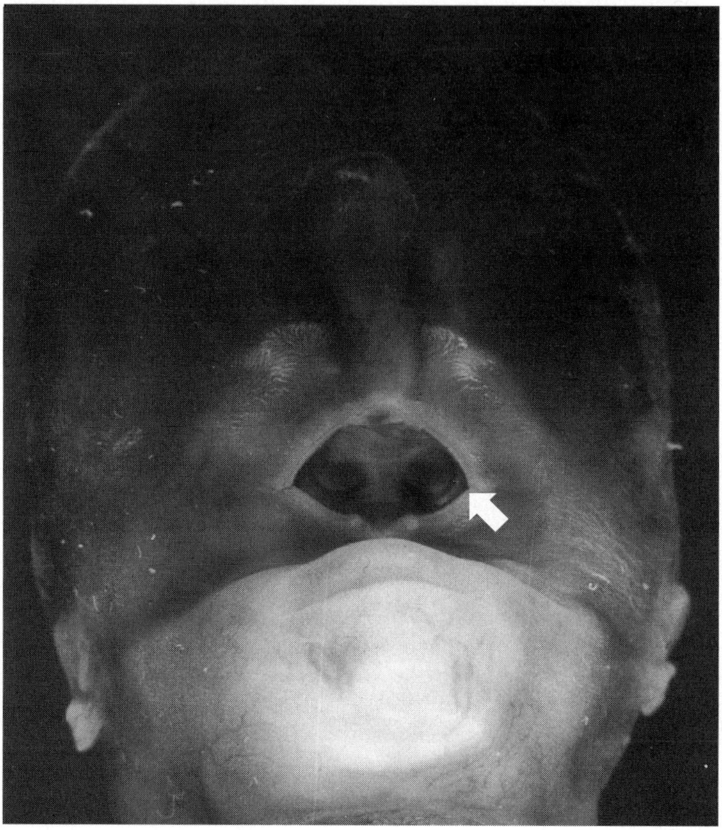

Figure 7 Cyclopia. A single, fused eye (arrow) situated *below* proboscis, as well as severe craniofacial malformation is seen in this photograph of the face of an abortus with holoprosencephaly.

general rule, ocular abnormalities, craniofacial malformations, and even extracranial organ malformations are seen in fetuses with holoprosencephaly.

C. Disorders of Organization of the Cerebral Hemispheres—Neuronal Migration Disorders (cortical dysplasia)

Neuroblasts migrate from their site of origin around the neural tube (ventricular zone) to assume their proper locations within the cerebral hemispheres. They migrate, differentiate, and align themselves appropriately to form the exquisitely organized cerebral cortex. Failure of these processes results in neuronal migration disorders. Initially, abnormalities of organization of the cerebral cortex were referred to largely by their macroscopic characteristics (i.e., lissencephaly, agyria/pachygyria, hemimegalencephaly, microgyria). As neuropathologists discovered the full range of microscopic cortical malformations which produce epilepsy but show no (or relatively mild) gross abnormalities, additional descriptive terms such as "cortical dysplasia" (CD) and "neuronal migration disorder" (NMD) were added to the literature. These disorders of cerebral cortical organization/neuronal migration may encompass disorders of size (i.e., hemimegalencephaly); gyral patterning/sulcation (i.e., lissencephaly, pachygyria, and polymicrogyria [PMG]); gray matter/white matter demarcation (heterotopia); and cerebral cortical organization (CD). These disorders may be grossly discernible, or they may require microscopic evaluation for definitive demonstration. Over 25 different syndromes of abnormal neuronal migration have been described, with various patterns of inheritance, including autosomal-dominant, autosomal-recessive, X-linked, and those with no clear pattern. NMDs have even been noted in association with acquired destructive lesions. Yet these disorders all share basic similarities with regard to process and phenotype. They all reflect abnormalities in the process of neuronal migration and all result in disordered organization and "wiring" of the cerebral cortex. Virtually all produce (often intractable) epilepsy in infants and children.

Some neuropathologists prefer to use a traditional classification of CD/NMDs based largely on gross characteristics of the brain (i.e., lissencephaly, polymicrogyria, neuronal heterotopia), while others, to reflect the conviction that these lesions are related and reflect developmental abnormalities along a continuous spectrum, have chosen to refer to this entire group of lesions as NMDs, CD, or cerebral dysgenesis. The student of neuropathology needs to understand how these classification schemata attempt to use incomplete information to try to meaningfully categorize malformations. The classification and nosology of these complex developmental neocortical malformations will continue to evolve, as understanding of the underlying biology of abnormal brain development at the cellular and molecular levels is acquired.

1. Disorders of Cell Proliferation and Brain Size

a. Micrencephaly. Micrencephaly is a nonspecific descriptive term referring to any brain that is abnormally small (smaller than the mean for age and sex by > 3 SD, or < 900 g in adulthood). In the majority of cases, micrencephaly is secondary to an intrauterine destructive lesion (usually anoxic or infectious), or is seen in association with a more severe cerebral malformation (i.e., holoprosencephaly). True *primary* micrencephaly occurs in families in an autosomal-recessive pattern, and has also been associated with intrauterine irradiation.

b. Megalencephaly. Megalencephaly is a nonspecific term used to describe brains that are large. The term is not strictly defined by size, but usually refers to brains with a weight of > 1600 g. In structurally normal-appearing brains, megalencephaly has been noted in people with both supranormal and subnormal intelligence (in these individuals, the brain is well formed and normally organized). Megalencephaly can also be seen in structurally malformed brains, such as those with features of severe NMD. Other pathologic causes of diffuse enlargement of the brain may occur with cerebral edema, neoplastic proliferations (e.g., gliomatosis cerebri), and degenerative conditions such as Tay-Sachs disease or some leukodystrophies, none of which are true primary pathologic malformations.

c. Hemimegalencephaly. Hemimegalencephaly (HME) (Fig. 8) is a unilateral enlargement of one cerebral hemisphere, with a disorganized malformed cerebral cortex on the affected side. In patients with HME, the gyral pattern is simplified (pachygyria) or shows PMG, or a combination of features. The cerebral cortex is always markedly disorganized on the enlarged side. Affected patients have severe epilepsy, and frequently developmental delays and focal neurologic deficits.

2. *Disorders of Gyral Pattern*

a. Lissencephaly (agyria). As the cerebral cortex develops, it becomes convoluted and folded. This process of gyration and sulcation vastly increases the surface area of the cerebral cortex, and is integral to the formation of a normal brain. Lissencephaly, also called agyria, refers to a brain with a smooth surface, and represents a failure of the normal process of gyration. Rather than the normal cortical convolutions with well-developed secondary and tertiary gyri and sulci, lissencephalic brains are smooth, as seen in brains prior to 16 weeks of gestation, though of larger size. Lissencephaly is often bilateral. Microscopically, the cerebral cortex in these regions is disorganized, and large irregular neurons are frequently present. The term lissencephaly is broadly descriptive, and is associated with a heterogeneous array of microscopic abnormalities. Classic lissencephaly (formerly known as type I) describes a smooth-surfaced brain with no secondary sulci (Fig. 9), which may be characterized by a four-layered neocortex. Classic lissencephaly, when associated with characteristic phenotypic changes including high forehead, hollow temples, and receding chin, is known as Miller-Dieker syndrome. It is transmitted in an autosomal-dominant fashion and is associated with microdeletions in the 17p13.3 region of chromosome 17 in 90% of cases. This region encodes the LIS.1 protein, which is essential for the function of normal axonal growth cones. Other variants of classical lissencephaly show different patterns of inheritance.

Cobblestone (type II) lissencephaly describes a smooth, small brain with an almost total disorder of cortical layer formation. It is often associated with micrencephaly, a small cerebellum, and (frequently) PMG. Cobblestone lis-

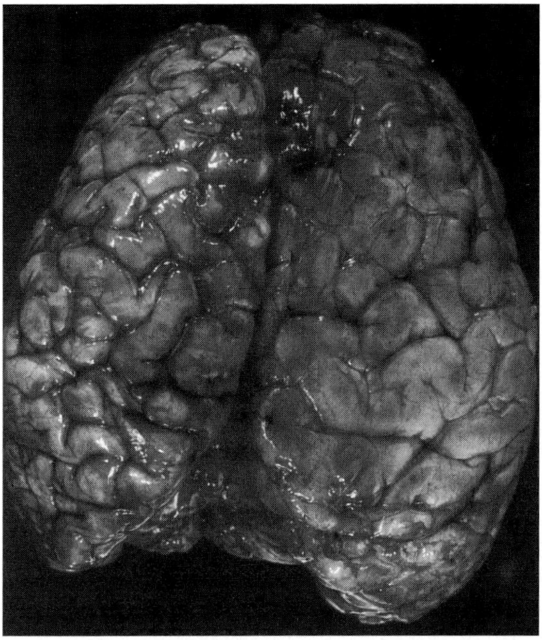

(A)

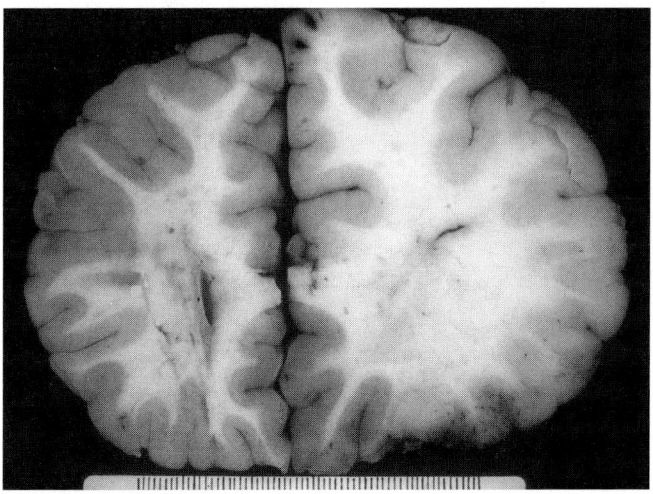

(B)

Figure 8 Hemimegalencephaly. Dorsal view of the brain (A) and coronal section through the cerebral hemispheres (B) from a child with hemimegalencephaly and intractable seizures. Note the markedly enlarged, thickened right cerebral hemisphere.

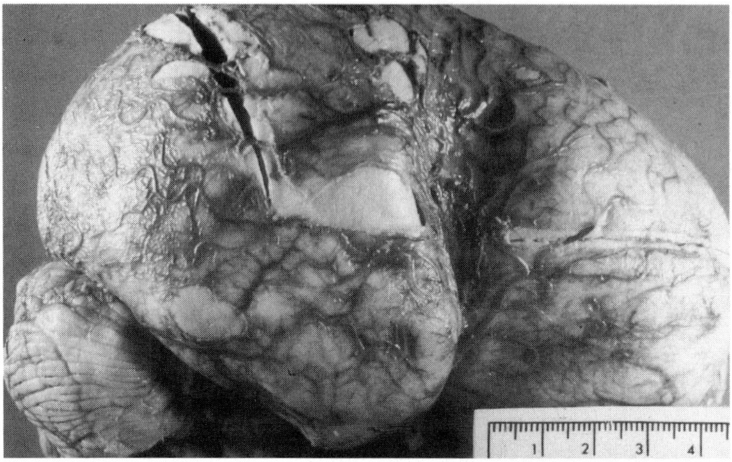

(A)

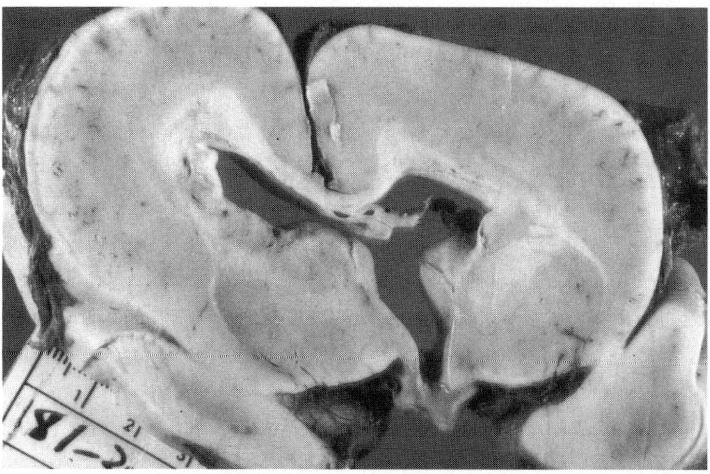

(B)

sencephaly has been associated with a number of autosomal-recessive syndromes, including Walker-Warburg syndrome and Fukuyama-type congenital muscular dystrophy; it has also been seen in association with Zellweger syndrome, which results from a defect in peroxisomal function with an excess of long-chain fatty acids. Some cases of lissencephaly do not seem to fit into any of these well-defined patterns.

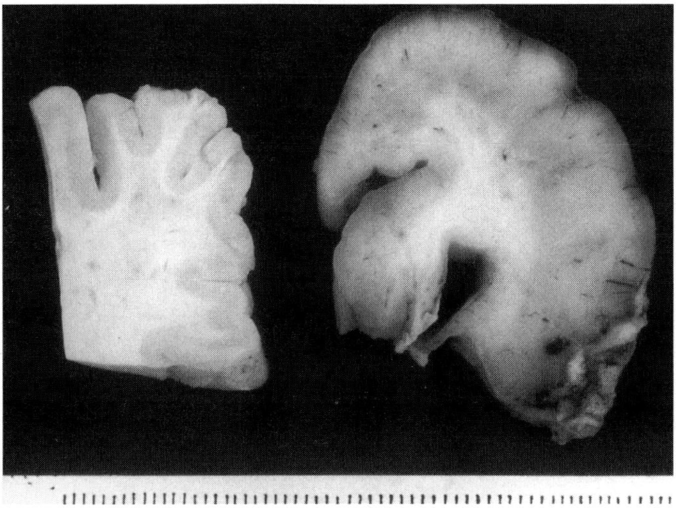

(C)

Figure 9 Lissencephaly. Brain of a child viewed from lateral aspect (A) and in coronal section (B) shows smooth surfaced agyric cortex. On coronal section, note broad cortical band of gray matter and indistinct cortex–white matter junction. (C) Surgical resection specimen from a child with intractable seizures secondary to hemilissencephaly/hemimegalencephaly. Section at right of the panel is from operative specimen, section at left is from (autopsy) control brain. In the resection specimen, note absence of gyri/sulci, markedly widened cortical ribbon, and indistinct cortex–white matter junction. Microscopic features were those of severe cortical dysplasia.

b. Pachygyria. Pachygyria describes a less severe failure of gyration than lissencephaly (agyria). Instead of total absence of gyri, there is a marked decrease in the normal number of convolutions, resulting in broad-based, flattened gyri with greatly reduced numbers of sulci. "Pachygyria" is also a descriptive term rather than a distinct entity. It frequently accompanies other cerebral cortical malformations.

c. Polymicrogyria. Polymicrogyria (Fig. 10) describes small, meandering gyri, often with bridging of the sulci by fusion of the superficial layers. It consists of two histological types. Four-layered PMG is most frequently considered to result from a destructive lesion which occurs at approx. 20 to 24 weeks gestation. An unlayered form is thought to result from an insult earlier in development (approx. 13 to 16 weeks). Whether PMG represents a destructive lesion with secondary malformation, or a primary malformative lesion, continues to be debated, but it is often seen as one feature in a variety of cerebral cortical malformations.

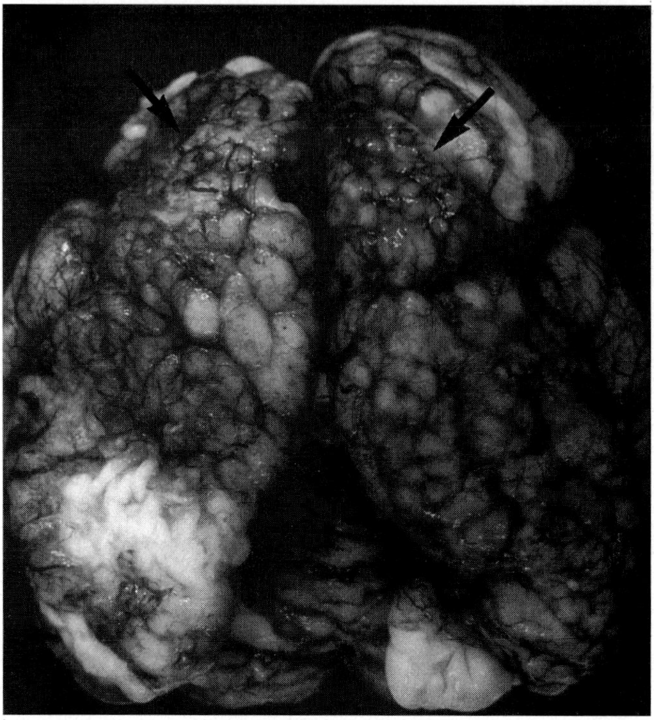

(A)

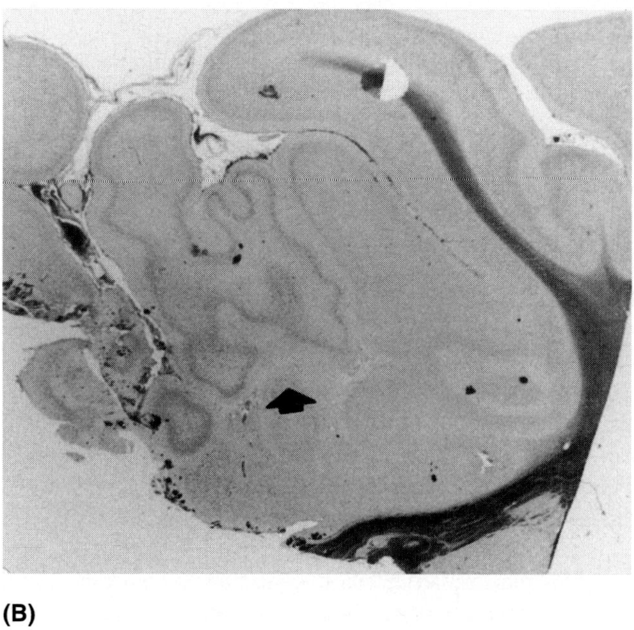

(B)

Figure 10 Polymicrogyria. Dorsal view of the brain from a child with severe bihemispheric polymicrogyria (A). Note the multiple small, irregular, "cobblestone" gyri (arrows). (B) Whole-mount section of a cortical resection specimen from a child with intractable epilepsy. The affected region shows a characteristic pattern of small, fused, meandering gyri (arrow). Kluver-Barrara stain. ([10B] Reproduced, with permission, from reference 25.)

3. *Disorders of Gray Matter/White Matter Demarcation—Loss of Cortex–White Matter Demarcation, Nodular Heterotopia, and Laminar (subcortical band) Heterotopia*

As the brain develops in utero, neurons migrate from the subventricular region to the cortex. Although some neurons are normally present in the subcortical white matter, even in adults, the cerebral cortex and subcortical white matter are usually well demarcated. Loss of the normal cortex–white matter demarcation, with an excess of neurons "entrapped" in the subcortical white matter, is a frequent accompaniment of various developmental malformations of the cortex. Occasionally, large nests or islands of neurons—"neuronal heterotopia"—are present within the subcortical white matter or near the ventricles. Neuronal heterotopia (Fig. 11) may appear as circumscribed nests of gray matter (nodular heterotopia) or may exist in a bandlike pattern in the subcortical white matter (laminar or subcortical band heterotopia). Nodular neuronal heterotopia are frequently seen in malformed brains, suggesting that a whole group of neurons failed to migrate to the surface. Laminar heterotopia (subcortical band heterotopia, SBH) are considerably less common, are usually seen in females, and give the banded appearance known as "double cortex." The gene associated with SBH has been mapped to the chromosome. Mutations in it are associated with laminar heterotopia in females, and lissencephaly in males.

4. *Disorganization of the Cerebral Cortex (cortical dysplasia)*

Microscopically, disorganization of the cerebral cortex (cortical dysplasia; CD) is a feature of almost every neuronal migration disorder. It can take many forms, but usually certain specific microscopic features are present. Neurons of the cerebral cortex appear disoriented or irregularly spaced, and are not organized in the normal six-layered cortical pattern. Neurons of abnormal size and shape may be seen (Fig. 12), some even containing cytoplasmic material which causes them to resemble the neurofibrillary tangles of Alzheimer's disease (see Chap. 8). In very severe cases, large glassy cells which show characteristics intermediate between those of neurons and astrocytes may be seen, suggesting a link between CD and tuberous sclerosis (TSC; see below).

It is important to keep in mind that developmental malformations of the cerebral cortex share basic common features: clinically, they often cause epi-

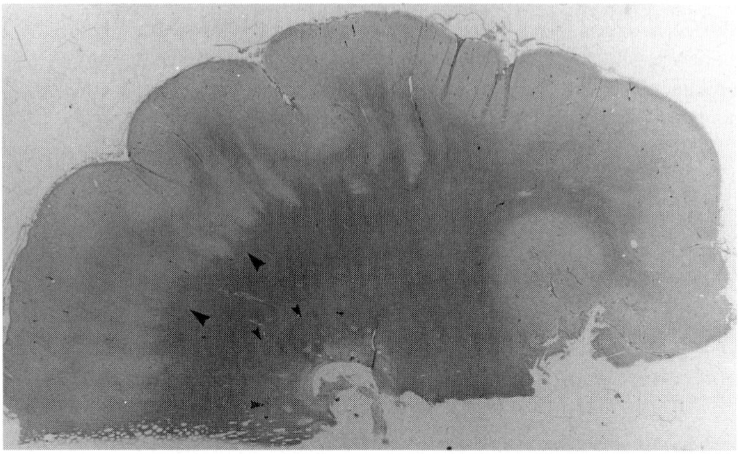

(A)

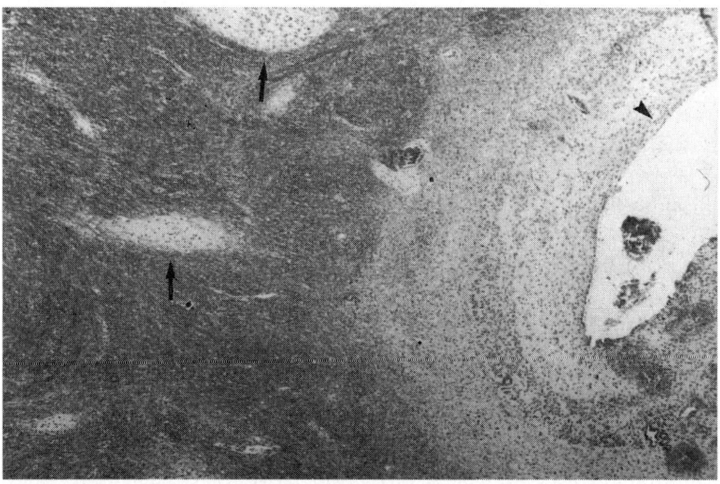

(B)

Figure 11 Neuronal heterotopia. (A) Whole-mount section of a cortical resection specimen from a child with intractable seizures. Pial surface is at top; ventricle is at bottom of the photograph. Note the presence of multiple islands of gray matter (small arrowheads) predominantly around the ventricle (periventricular nodular heterotopia), as well as a band of gray matter (large arrowheads) beneath the cortical surface (laminar heterotopia). (Reproduced, with permission, from reference 25.) (B) Magnified view of the islands of gray matter (arrows) in the white matter surrounding the ventricle (arrowhead) (Kluver-Barrera stain).

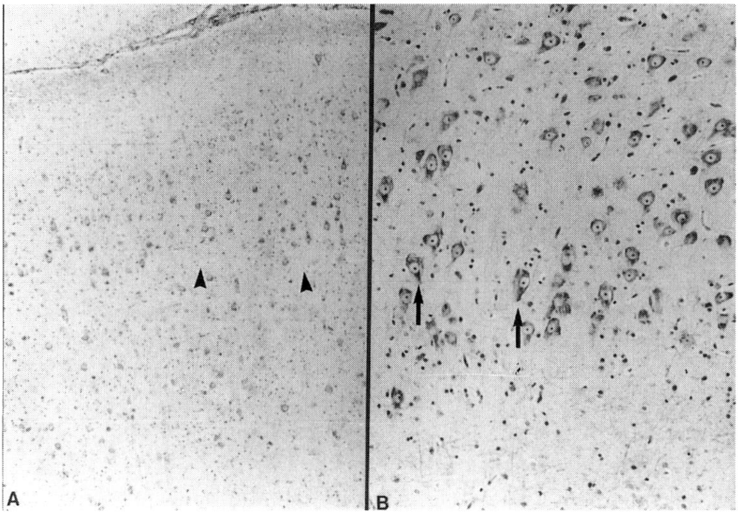

Figure 12 Cerebral cortical dysplasia. Cortical resection specimen from a child with cerebral cortical dysplasia and intractable seizures. (A) Disorganized cortical pattern with irregular clustering of neurons, and prominence of enlarged neurons in the superficial layers (arrowheads). (B) Magnified view shows that many of these abnormally clustered neurons are highly irregular in appearance with dense clumping of the cytoplasm (arrows). H&E stain.

lepsy and mental retardation; they reflect a disturbance in the normal pattern of neuronal migration from germinal matrix to cortex; and they demonstrate a pattern of disorganized cortical architecture. There is often a significant overlap of pathologic features, suggesting the multipotent effects of disruption of the normal processes of brain development.

D. Disorders of Posterior Fossa Formation

1. Arnold-Chiari Malformations

These are complex malformations of the posterior fossa, which underscore the complex interrelationship between the developing neuroectoderm and mesenchyme. There are two clinically important forms:

a. Type I. This consists of a downward herniation of the cerebellar tonsils through the foramen magnum, with minimal distortion of the brainstem. Most of the cases occur in adults and older children and are usually asymptomatic, or incidental findings at autopsy, although syringomyelia (discussed below) may coexist, resulting in significant disability. Also, fibrovascular adhesions may occur around the herniated cerebellar tonsils, resulting in neurologic symptoms. Some neuropathologists do not consider this to be a true malformation, rather a variant of normal, since it may be subclinical.

b. Type II. This is a complex abnormality of the posterior fossa with multiple malformative components and numerous associated features. It results in severe clinical morbidity and mortality. Although its etiology is unknown, evidence points to a failure of interaction between the developing neuroectoderm and mesenchyme. Neuropathologically, Arnold-Chiari type II malformation (Fig. 13) can be divided into four components: cerebellar malformation; brainstem malformation; basocranial bone malformation; and associated features.

The cerebellar component of the Arnold-Chiari type II malformation (Fig. 14) consists of herniated cerebellar tissue arising from the inferior cerebellar vermis. This tissue is distorted and elongated, and no separate cerebellar tonsils or vermis can be clearly identified. This tissue is often attached to the dorsal medulla by fibrovascular adhesions. The cerebellar tissue is gliotic and distorted. The brainstem component consists of elongation and displacement of the medulla, frequently with an S-shaped curve that folds the pons over the inferior olives, and upward displacement of the cervical nerve roots of the spinal cord. The basocranial component of the malformation is highly complex and usually often consists of flattening of the skull base (platybasia), shortening

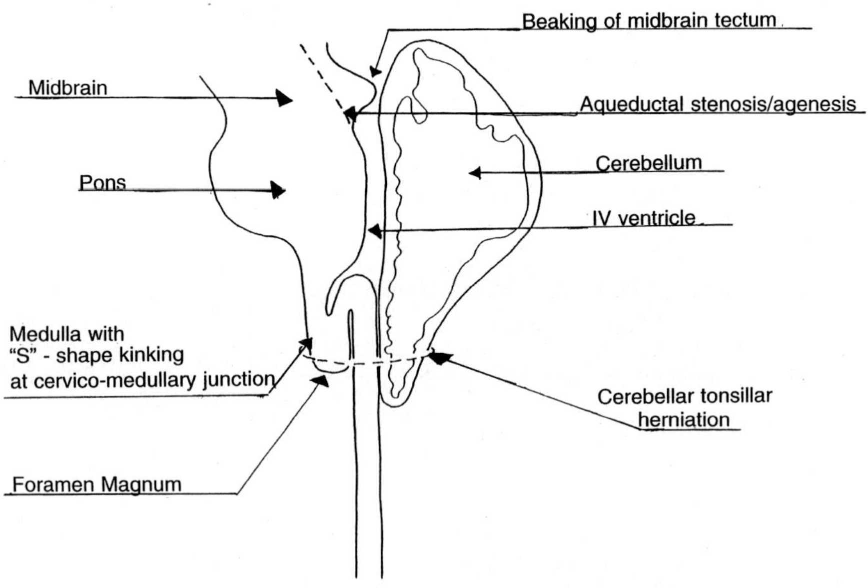

Figure 13 Diagram illustrating the characteristic features of Arnold-Chiari type II malformation.

of the posterior fossa, and occipitoatlantal fusion with or without fusion of several other vertebrae.

The associated abnormalities of Arnold-Chiari type II malformation account for a significant amount of the related morbidity. They include: hydrocephalus; aqueductal stenosis or atresia; meningocele or meningomyelocele (usually lumbar), which is so frequently present that some neuropathologists consider it an essential feature of the malformation; fusion and elongation of the superior and inferior colliculi in the midbrain (tectal beaking); and syringomyelia (discussed below). In addition, neuronal migration disorders of the cerebral hemispheres such as neuronal heterotopia, polymicrogyria, and cortical disorganization are often seen, suggesting a wider disruption of brain development than just that seen within the posterior fossa.

E. Disorders of Cerebellar Development

By the end of the 4th week of intrauterine development, the cerebellum arises from the lateral edges of the alar plates, which become thickened, giving rise to the paired rhombic lips. Proliferating neuroblasts provide precursors for the developing cerebellum and some brainstem nuclei. The rhombic lips fuse by 7.5 weeks of gestation, eventually giving rise to the cerebellar vermis. Neuroblasts migrate along the external surface forming the external granule cell layer. Other neuroblasts from the rhombic lip take a different route, migrating internally, closer to the ventricular surface, to give rise to the Purkinje cells and deep cerebellar nuclei (as well as pontine nuclei and the inferior olivary nuclei). The external granule cell layer is present until 12 to 18 months postnatal; during this time neurons from the external granule cell layer migrate to the internal granule cell layer along radial glial fibers. Disruption of any of these processes results in cerebellar malformations, of which four main types are recognized, as follows.

1. Dandy-Walker Syndrome

Dandy-Walker syndrome (Fig. 15) is a cerebellar malformation of unknown etiology, characterized by three main features: hypoplasia of the cerebellar vermis; cystic dilatation of the fourth ventricle; and enlargement of the posterior fossa. Hydrocephalus is usually seen, and accounts for the most severe morbidity. Other associated abnormalities such as agenesis of the corpus callosum, neuronal heterotopia, and systemic malformations may also be present. The inferior cerebellar vermis is hypoplastic and may be absent. The cyst of the fourth ventricle is lined by a thin layer of disorganized pia-arachnoid and glial tissue. The large cyst sits within an enlarged cranial fossa, and the torcular Herophili (confluence of the sinuses) is displaced upward.

2. Cerebellar Polymicrogyria

Cerebellar polymicrogyria (Fig. 16) describes a pattern of complex small, irregularly fused "ribboning" gyri. These regions are frequently associated with pa-

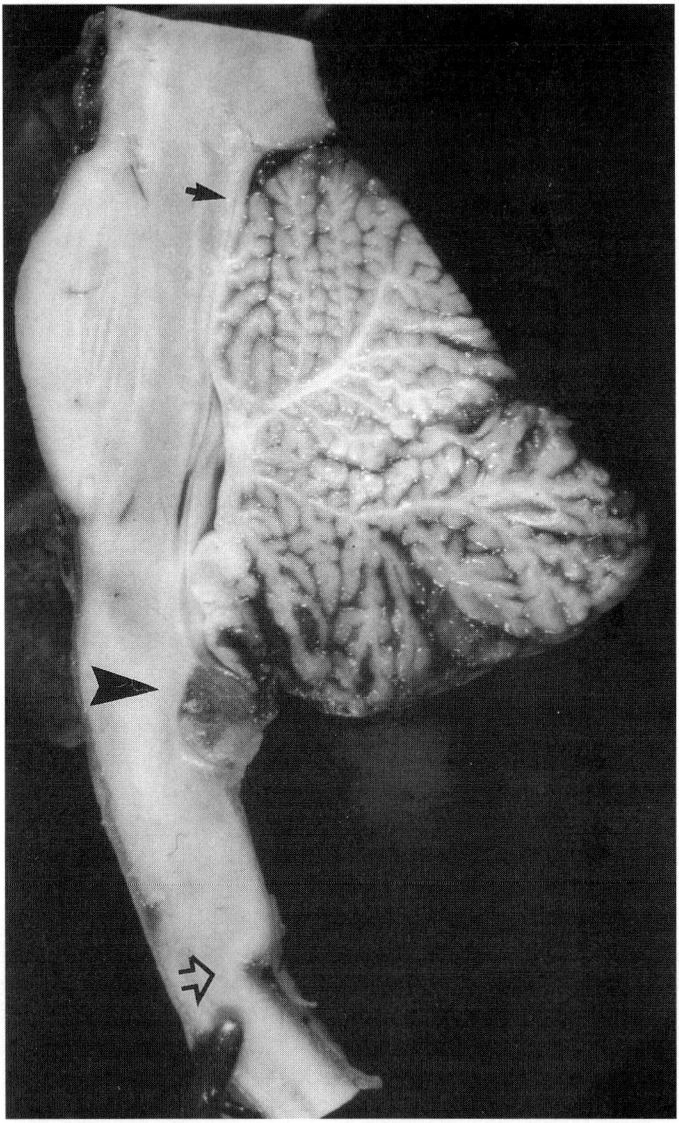

(A)

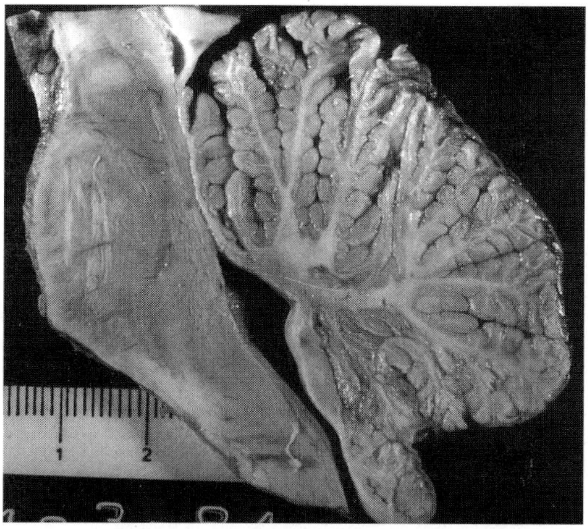

(B)

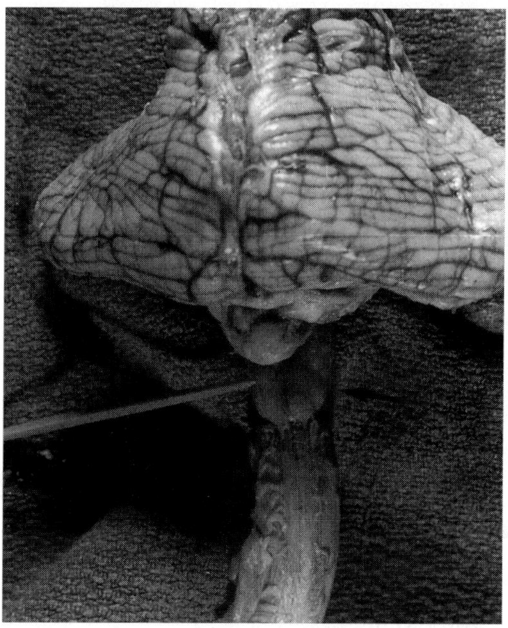

(C)

Figure 14 Arnold-Chiari type II malformation. Sagittal section through the brainstem and cerebellum of a child. (A) Note herniation of the cerebellar tonsils (large arrowhead), S-shape of the cervicomedullary region (open arrow), and apparent stenosis of the cerebral aqueduct (black arrow). (B) Another specimen (sagittal section) shows prominent cerebellar tonsillar herniation and "beaking" of the midbrain tectum. (C) Dorsal view of the cerebellum and spinal cord showing the herniated cerebellar tonsils. A, C reproduced with permission from Vinters HV. In: Batzdorf U, ed. Syringomyelia Current Concepts in Diagnosis and Treatment. Baltimore: Williams & Wilkins, 1991:35–58.

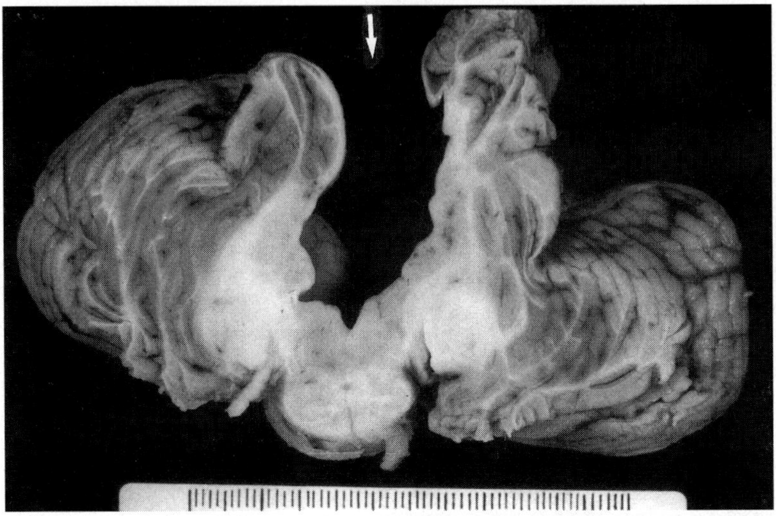

Figure 15 Dandy-Walker malformation. Horizontal section through the brainstem and cerebellum. The cerebellar vermis is absent (white arrow), and the fourth ventricle shows cystic dilatation (the delicate membrane covering the cyst is no longer intact).

chygyric areas of cerebellum. Cerebellar polymicrogyria occurs in association with other cerebellar defects or as an incidental finding, often having produced no symptoms during life. Most cases of cerebellar PMG are associated with destructive lesions, although severe cases may be seen in patients with Walker-Warburg syndrome and Fukuyama-type muscular dystrophy, both of which may be associated with focal cerebral cortical abnormalities such as lissencephaly and polymicrogyria.

3. Cerebellar Heterotopias

Small nests of neurons within the cerebellar white matter or mixed in the Purkinje cell layer or deep cerebellar nuclei (neuronal heterotopia) are often seen in the brains of newborn infants. Most of these disappear with age, and even when persistent appear to be clinically insignificant. Large nodular collections of heterotopic neurons within the cerebellar white matter are rarely seen, but can be present in association with major malformations (i.e., Arnold Chiari type II or Dandy-Walker syndrome), trisomy 13, or, rarely, as an incidental finding.

4. Other Cerebellar Aplasias or Hypoplasias

Hypoplasia or aplasia of the cerebellum may rarely occur, and can involve either the cerebellar vermis or hemispheres. Aplasia of the cerebellar vermis is a rare disorder, differentiated from Dandy-Walker syndrome by the absence of

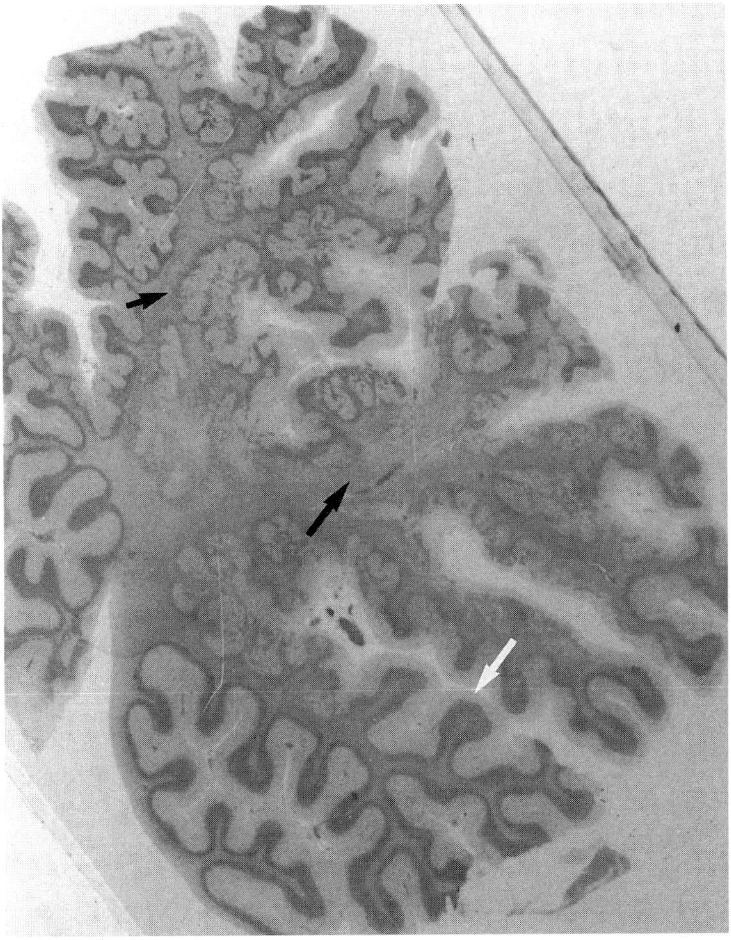

Figure 16 Cerebellar polymicrogyria. Whole-mount midsagittal section. Contrast the small, fused ribboning gyri (black arrows) with the orderly gyral pattern of the normal region of cerebellum (white arrow).

cystic dilatation of the fourth ventricle. Agenesis of the cerebellar vermis, when associated with hyperpnea, abnormal eye movements, ataxia, and mental retardation is known as Joubert syndrome.

Aplasia (or hypoplasia) of one or both of the cerebellar hemispheres may also rarely occur. When associated with abnormalities of the pontine and olivary nuclei, the syndrome is known as neocerebellar (or pontoneocerebellar) aplasia (Fig. 17). Since the cerebellar hemispheres and pontine and olivary nu-

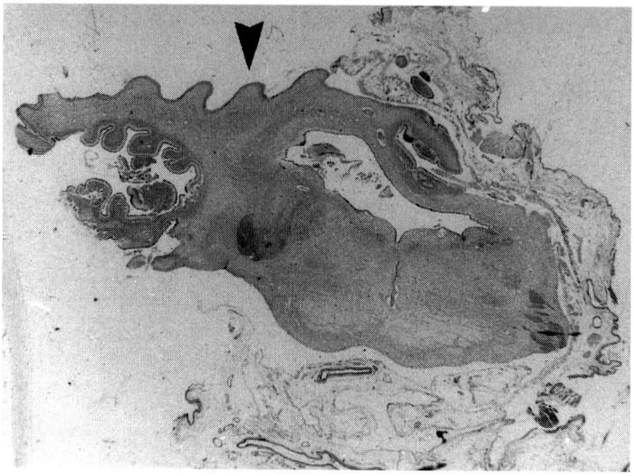

(A)

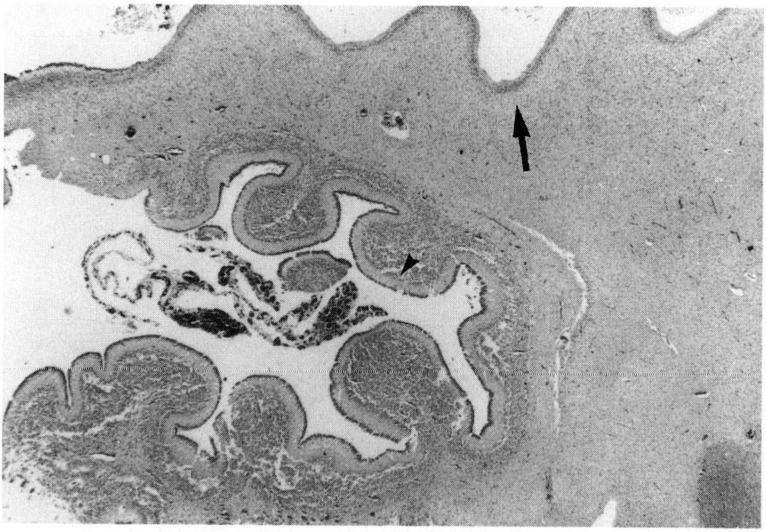

(B)

Figure 17 Pontoneocerebellar hypoplasia in a newborn. (A) Horizontal section through the pons and cerebellum shows a hypoplastic pons (absent pontocerebellar fibers and pontine nuclei) with focal cerebellar hypoplasia. Cerebellum showed absent dentate nuclei, and its dorsomedial portion showed profound Purkinje and granule cell loss (arrowhead) while ventral portions were relatively well preserved. (B) Note contrast between dorsomedial atrophic cerebellum (arrow) and relatively preserved cerebellar cortex (arrowhead). (C) Hypoplastic and (D) intact regions of cerebellum are shown at higher magnification. In (D), note preserved external granule cell layer (arrow) and Purkinje cells (arrowhead).

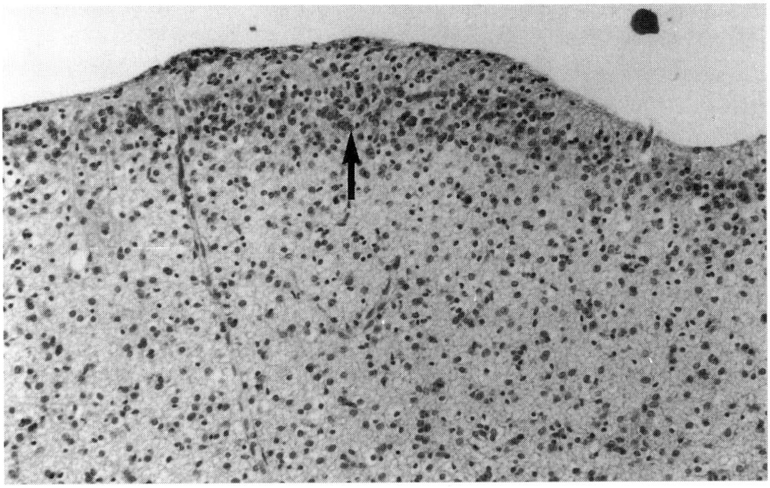

(C)

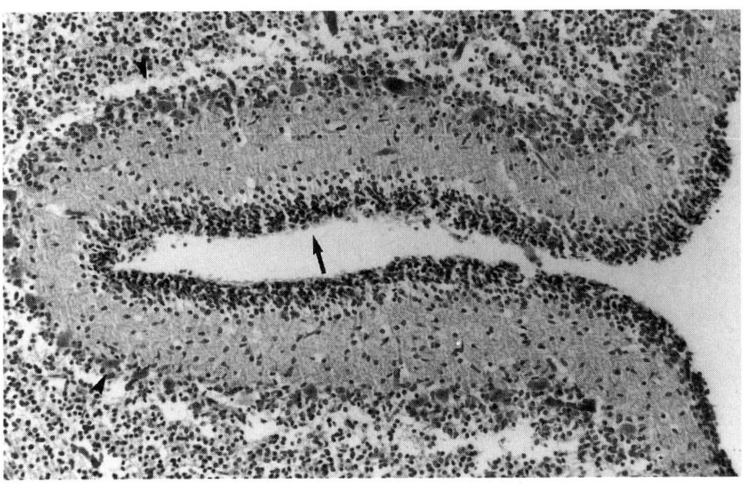

(D)

clei arise from rhombic lip precursors, one can understand how these disruptions are often paired.

F. Disorders of Brainstem Development

1. Developmental Disorders of the Cerebral Aqueduct

The cerebral aqueduct, which serves as a conduit for CSF, allowing it to pass from the third to the fourth ventricles, is a vulnerable site for obstruction. Intrauterine stenosis or obstruction of the aqueduct results in congenital hydrocephalus, with clinically devastating results. True atresia (aplasia or nonformation) of the aqueduct occurs only very rarely. However, four distinct entities associated with narrowing of the cerebral aqueduct have been recognized: aqueductal stenosis, forking of the aqueduct, septum formation, and gliosis of the aqueduct. Aqueductal stenosis (Fig. 18) appears to be a true primary malformation; the other three are secondary disruptions. Isolated aqueductal stenosis is rare, and is characterized by severe narrowing or complete atresia of the aqueduct without gliosis. A hereditary X-linked form has been described, although aqueductal stenosis is more commonly seen in association with other malformations such as Arnold-Chiari type II.

Aqueductal forking results in two smaller channels which may or may not communicate. The whole tectum of the midbrain may be malformed with fusion of the colliculi. Septum formation within the aqueduct rarely occurs, and appears to be a consequence of intrauterine infection rather than a primary malformation. Gliosis of the cerebral aqueduct occurs when the lumen is narrowed by reactive gliosis with disruption of the ependymal layer (granular ependymitis). It appears to occur in response to intrauterine infection, rather than as a primary malformation.

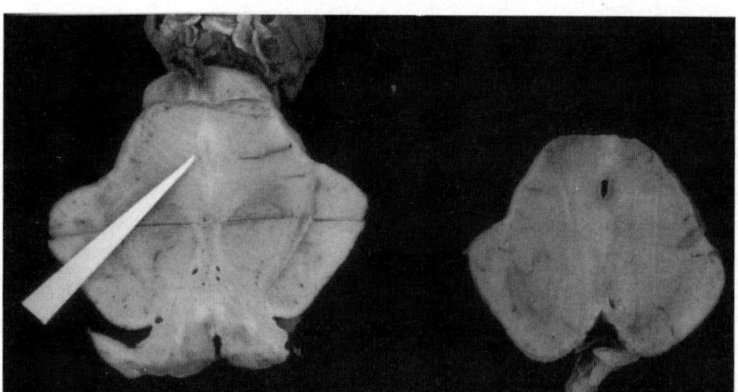

Figure 18 Aqueductal stenosis. Horizontal section through the midbrain of a child with aqueductal stenosis (left side) versus a midbrain section with patent aqueduct.

These lesions of the cerebral aqueduct all lead to hydrocephalus (Fig. 19) presenting at birth or shortly thereafter. In the developing brain, true hydrocephalus must be differentiated from other causes of enlargement of the ventricles, such as a loss of tissue due to destruction (hydrocephalus ex vacuo), or primary failure of growth of the tissue around the ventricles (colpocephaly). True hydrocephalus is an enlargement of the cerebral ventricles due to imbalance between cerebrospinal fluid (CSF) production and absorption. As discussed in Chapter 1, hydrocephalus can result from one of three mechanisms: obstruction to the flow of CSF; increase in the resistance to CSF absorption; or primary overproduction of CSF. In patients with developmental malformations of the brain, hydrocephalus is a common complication, due to direct obstruction to CSF flow. Hydrocephalus is frequently seen in association with midline abnormali-

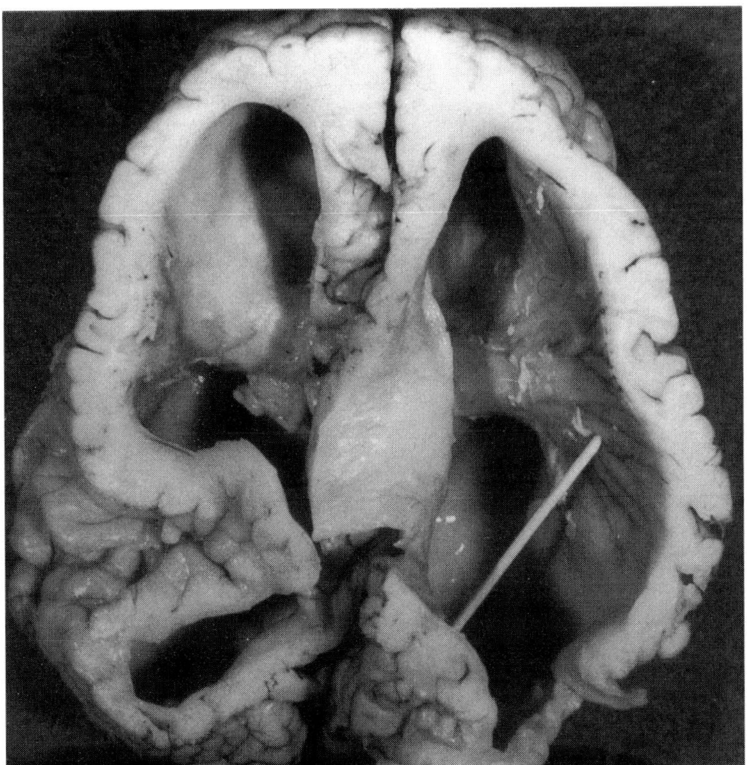

Figure 19 Hydrocephalus. Horizontal section through the cerebral hemispheres showing markedly dilated lateral ventricles.

ties, Arnold-Chiari Type II malformations, and Dandy-Walker malformations, as well as in neonates with malformations of the cerebral aqueduct.

2. *Malformations of Brainstem Nuclei*

Malformations of the brainstem in association with other brain lesions (e.g., Arnold-Chiari type II, pontocerebellar aplasia, etc.) are frequent. Isolated malformations of brainstem nuclei are less common. Heterotopic islands of neurons in and around the inferior olivary nuclei have been noted in association with cerebral cortical malformations such as lissencephaly or pachygyria, and with cerebellar malformations such as Dandy-Walker syndrome. Isolated olivary heterotopias consisting of "stranded" islands of neurons have been noted; these probably represent migrational arrest of neuroblasts originating from the rhombic lip. Abnormalities in the shape of the inferior olivary nucleus may be seen in association with trisomies 13 and 18, holoprosencephaly, and cerebellar aplasias. Much larger-scale derangements of brainstem architecture are seen in the Arnold-Chiari type II malformation (see above).

G. Malformations of the Spinal Cord (other than neural tube defects)

1. *Hydromyelia*

The central canal of the spinal cord becomes obliterated postnatally, leaving behind small nests of ependymal cells. Hydromyelia defines a dilatation of this ependymal lined canal (Fig. 20). It can occur as an incidental finding, or may be associated with other malformations such as Arnold-Chiari type II or neural tube defects.

2. *Syringomyelia*

This term describes a tubular cavitation of spinal cord (Fig. 21), which may extend over multiple levels and into the brainstem (syringobulbia). It is often associated with a specific etiologic condition but may occur de novo or in association with other malformations (e.g., Arnold-Chiari II). Cervical and thoracic segments are most frequently affected. The syrinx (cavity) differs from hydromyelia in that it is not just a dilatation of the central canal, but rather a defect in the substance of the cord with ependymal disruption. The syrinx may be fluid filled and is usually lined by astrocytes (Fig. 22) often with associated Rosenthal fibers. If the central canal becomes incorporated into the cyst cavity or, conversely, the syrinx arises from a hydromyelic cavity (syringohydromyelia), focal areas of ependymal cell lining may be seen. Syringomyelia occurs most commonly in patients who have suffered traumatic spinal cord injury or in patients with tumors, infections (especially arachnoiditis), or ischemia involving the spinal cord. This suggests a pressure-related mechanism in the causation of these defects. Congenital syringomyelia can occur as a primary lesion,

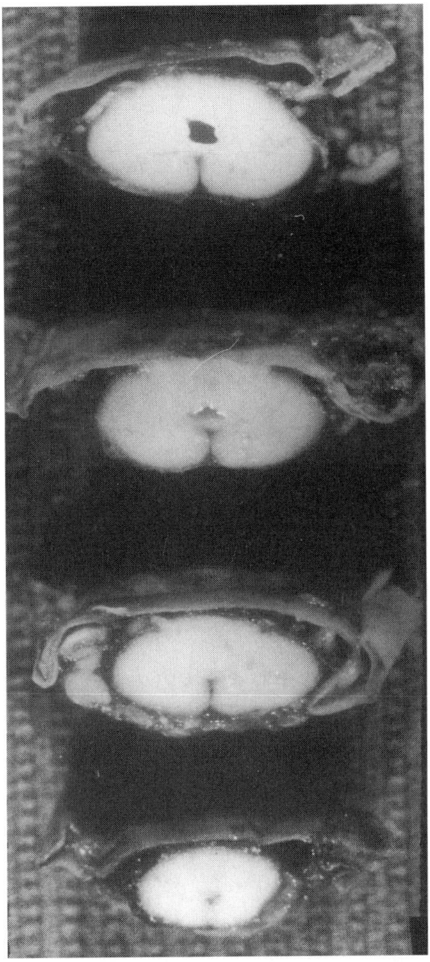

Figure 20 Hydromyelia. Multiple segments of the spinal cord illustrating a fluid-filled enlargement of the central canal.

probably representing a failure of fusion of the alar and basal wings of the developing spinal cord. When a syrinx involves the medulla, it is known as syringobulbia. Syringobulbia usually occurs in association with or as an extension of cervical syringomyelia, but may occur independently.

3. *Diastematomyelia, Diplomyelia, and Dimyelia*

Rarely, the spinal cord may be bifid, or partially bifid. Diastematomyelia occurs when the spinal cord is separated by fibrous tissue or a bony spur, leading to a focally bifid spinal cord. Since it is associated with myelocystocele and mye-

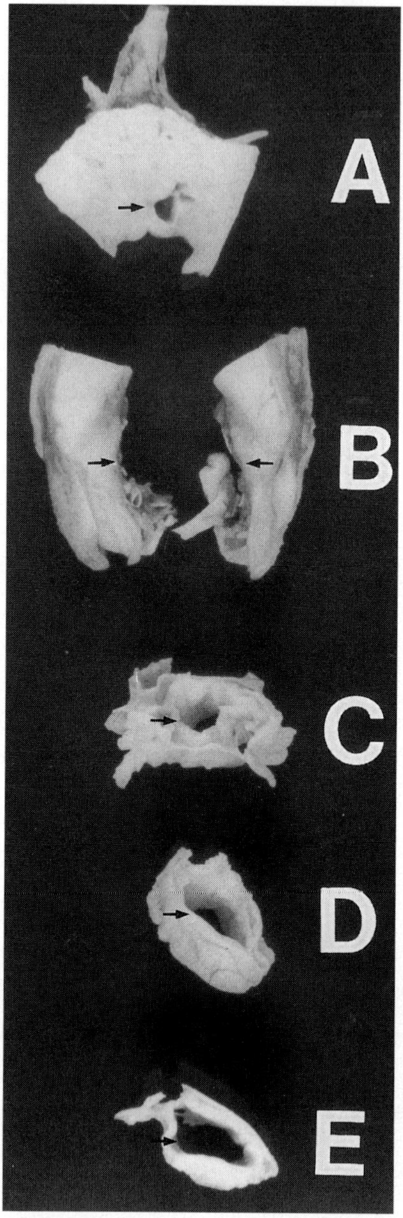

Figure 21 Syringomyelia. Sections through the pons (A), medulla (B), and spinal cord (C, D, and E) in a patient with syringomyelia. A syrinx cavity extends from the spinal cord (syringomyelia), involving the medulla and pons (syringobulbia).

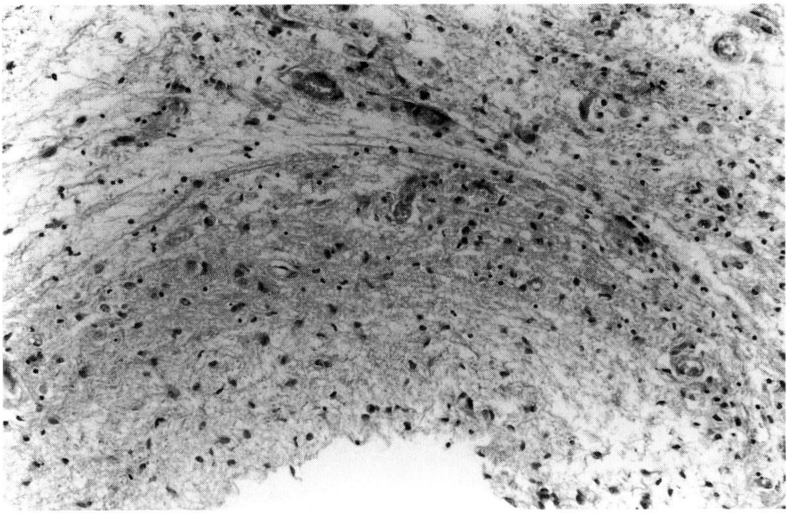

Figure 22 Photomicrograph showing gliotic rim surrounding the syrinx cavity (at bottom).

loschisis in up to 50% of cases, many authors consider it part of the spectrum of neural tube defects. Diplomyelia occurs when there is an isolated accessory spinal cord or partial or complete spinal cord reduplication (Fig. 23), lacking nerve roots, while dimyelia exists when there is a complete duplication of the spinal cord, each one bearing its own set of dorsal and ventral nerve roots.

Table 2 shows incidence figures for selected developmental CNS malformations and chromosomal disorders.

H. Systemic Disorders with Consequences for Brain Development

1. Chromosomal Disorders

a. Down's Syndrome (trisomy 21). This is the most common chromosomal abnormality (approx. 1/800 live births) and represents a common cause of moderate or severe mental retardation. Down's syndrome (DS) is associated with trisomy 21 in 95% of cases, and with a translocation of the long arm of chromome 21 in 4% (the other 1% are mosaic with a mixture of 46 and 47 chromosomes per cell). Clinically, patients with DS have severe mental retardation, bony abnormalities, congenital heart defects, and a characteristic facial appearance. Brains from patients with Down's syndrome show a rounded foreshortened appearance, with a reduction in volume of the frontal lobes and a narrowing of the superior temporal gyrus (Fig. 24). There is an overall reduction

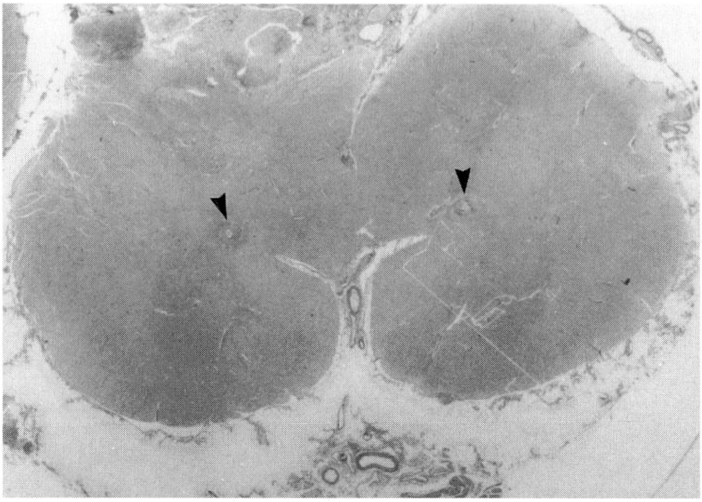

Figure 23. Partial diplomyelia. Horizontal section through the spinal cord showing a focally reduplicated cord. Note two "jerking" ventral median fissures and two central canals (arrows).

of brain size, with the brainstem and cerebellum being relatively smaller in comparison to the cerebral hemispheres. Microscopic changes seen in the brains of young patients with Down's syndrome are subtle and nonspecific.

As patients with Down's syndrome age, their brains accumulate the same neuropathologic abnormalities seen in patients with Alzheimer's disease (senile plaques, neurofibrillary tangles, amyloid angiopathy, neuron and synapse loss).

Table 2 Incidence of Selected Major Congenital CNS Malformations/1000 Live Births[a]

1) *Chromosomal abnormalities*	
a) Down syndrome (trisomy 21)	1.3
b) Edwards syndrome (trisomy 18)	0.125
c) Patau syndrome (trisomy 13)	0.167
2) *Neural tube defects*	0.83–6.63 (vary greatly by region)
3) *Holoprosencephaly*	0.06–0.12
4) *Dandy-Walker malformation*	0.04

[a] Incidence figures vary widely. Most developmental malformations of the brain and spinal cord are so rare that their incidence has not been well characterized. Data for this table adapted from: Buyse ML, ed. Birth Defects Encyclopedia. Cambridge: Blackwell Scientific Publications, 1990; and from: Cotran RS, Kumar V, Robbins SL, eds. Robbins Pathologic Basis of Disease. 5th ed. Philadelphia: W.B. Saunders, 1994.

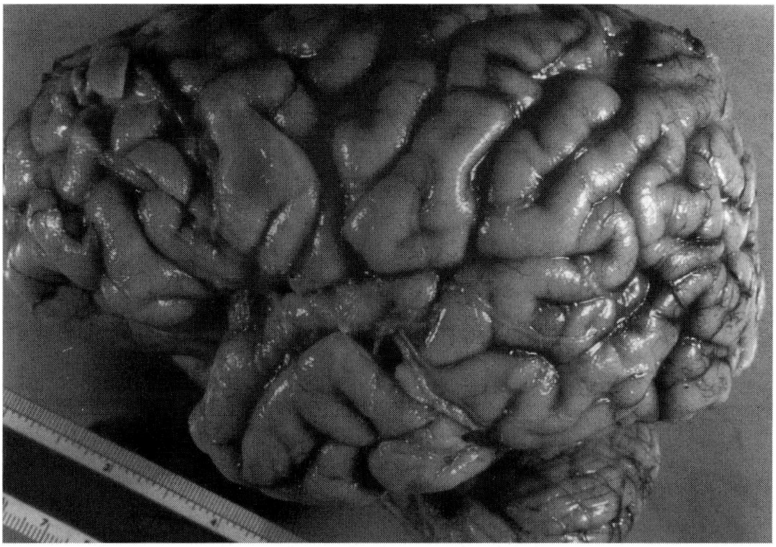

Figure 24 Down's syndrome. Lateral view of the brain illustrates the classic foreshortened appearance.

All DS patients develop Alzheimer changes by the fourth or fifth decade. The amyloid precursor protein which gives rise to soluble beta/A4 protein (implicated in the pathogenesis of Alzheimer's disease) is located on chromosome 21, so that DS patients have an increased copy of this gene.

b. Trisomy 18 (Edwards syndrome). Trisomy 18 (1/8000 births) is characterized clinically by low-birth-weight infants with poor postnatal growth. They have a characteristic appearance with deep-seated ears, micrognathia, and characteristic digit changes. They manifest congenital heart defects and show poor survival. The brains of affected infants exhibit abnormalities in gyration and lobar formation, which can range (in the extreme) to holoprosencephaly. Agenesis of the corpus callosum may be present, and dysplasias of hippocampi, lateral geniculate nuclei, and inferior olivary nuclei are frequent. The cerebellum and gray matter of the pons may also be hypoplastic.

c. Trisomy 13 (Patau syndrome). Trisomy 13 (1/6000 births) is characterized by preterm, small infants with multiple brain and systemic malformations, including microcephaly, microphthalmia, deep-seated ears, cleft palate, polydactyly, rocker bottom feet, cardiac and urogenital defects. Holoprosencephaly and arrhinencephaly are most frequently seen as CNS malformations, in addition to cerebellar heterotopias. Severe craniofacial abnormalities including cyclopia (Fig. 7) may be present.

2. *Gene Defects with Systemic and Developmental Brain Malformations/Hamartomas*

a. Tuberous Sclerosis Complex (TSC). TSC, or Bourneville disease, is an inherited multisystem neurocutaneous disorder characterized clinically by epilepsy and mental retardation (to varying degrees) and associated retinal and skin lesions. Tuberous sclerosis occurs in approximately 1/10,000 individuals and shows a pattern of autosomal dominant inheritance with a high rate of spontaneous mutation. There is a very wide range of disease expression in patients, both clinically and pathologically. Mutations at two gene loci are associated with tuberous sclerosis: one at chromosome 9q34 (TSC1), and the other at 16p13.3 (TSC2).

Pathologically, TSC is characterized by multiple cerebral and systemic malformations and hamartomas (including cardiac rhabdomyomas and renal angiomyolipomas). Although some of the proliferations have the potential to become neoplastic (discussed below), tuberous sclerosis can fundamentally be considered as a developmental brain abnormality, since the characteristic malformations occur during CNS development (Fig. 25). These include cortical tubers (consisting of disorganized cortex with abnormal/"dysplastic" neurons and glia; regions of loss of cortex–white matter demarcation with heterotopic neurons and large "balloon") cells with glassy eosinophilic cytoplasm scattered throughout the subcortical white matter; and subependymal nodules consisting of cells similar to those seen within cortical tubers (these lesions can give rise to subependymal giant cell astrocytomas). The astute reader will notice the similarity of these changes to some of the features described above as NMD/CD, suggesting a potential link between TSC and NMD/CD.

b. Ataxia-Telangiectasia (AT). AT is an autosomal-recessive multisystem disorder characterized by childhood cerebellar degeneration with ataxia, ocular or cutaneous telangiectasias, and a predisposition to cancer (with chromosomal instability and cell cycle abnormalities). The mutated gene is located on chromosome 11q22–23 and encodes a protein similar to phosphatidylinositol-3′ kinase, a crucial factor involved in intracellular signal transduction and cell cycle control. AT is the most common progressive cerebellar ataxia of infants and children, with a prevalence of approximately 1/40,000 children. Pathologically, the cerebellum is atrophic (especially throughout the entire vermis), with a thinning of the molecular layer and a decreased number of Purkinje cells and internal granule cells. Ectopic Purkinje cells within the molecular layer highlight the likelihood of abnormal cerebellar developmental in children with AT.

c. Other "Neurocutaneous Syndromes". A host of other rare conditions characterized by brain and systemic (especially ocular and cutaneous) malformations/hamartomas have been described, highlighting the interrelated development of the nervous system and overlying mesenchyme and ectoderm. Most of

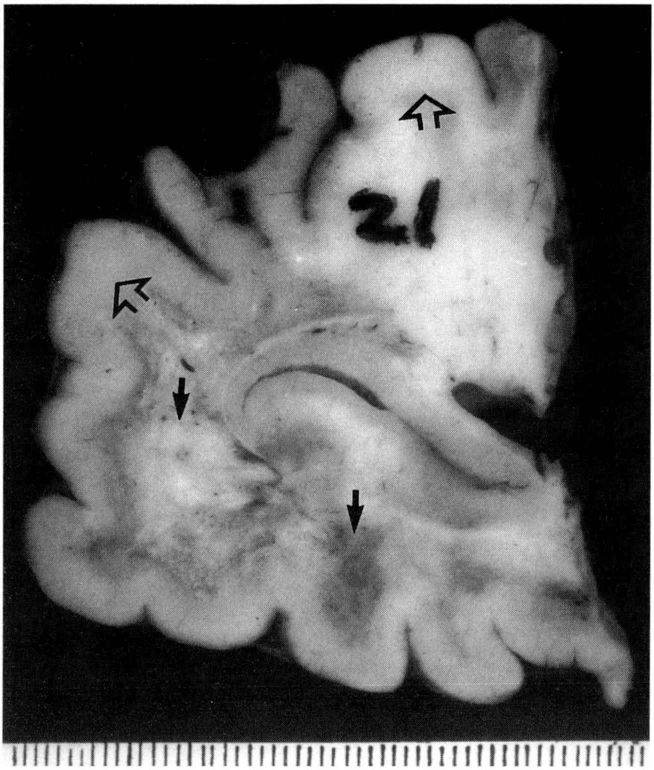

Figure 25 Tuberous sclerosis complex (TSC). Cortical resection specimen. Multiple regions of disorganized appearing white matter (black arrows) which showed, on microscopic sections, disorganized neurons, astrocytes, and balloon cells, with absence of the normal cortex/white matter demarcation (open arrows). Note similarity to the specimen illustrated in Figure 9C.

these syndromes also confer a predisposition for developing tumors. Neurofibromatosis is the most frequent (discussed in Chap. 6). Other, less common syndromes include epidermal nevus syndrome and hypomelanosis of Ito.

3. Sturge-Weber-Dimitri Syndrome

Sturge-Weber-Dimitri syndrome (encephalotrigeminal angiomatosis) is a rare, nonfamilial malformation of unknown etiology characterized by epilepsy, mental retardation, and a facial "port-wine stain" in the distribution of the trigeminal nerve. Intracranial calcification in a "gyriform" pattern on CT or MRI and buphthalmos or glaucoma may also be seen.

CNS changes in this syndrome are characterized by leptomeningeal angiomatosis consisting of dilated and tortuous, thin-walled blood vessels within the subarachnoid space and pia, which may extend into the underlying cerebral cortex and even subcortical white matter. The cerebral cortex and cortical microvessels are heavily calcified (Fig. 26), and cortical atrophy may be extensive. Associated malformations such as PMG, agyria/pachygyria, heterotopias, and cortical disorganization may also be present.

IV. ACQUIRED LESIONS OF THE DEVELOPING BRAIN AND SPINAL CORD—PERINATAL BRAIN INJURY

The perinatal period encompasses the time of intrauterine gestation, birth, and neonatal early-infant life. Since it cannot always be ascertained during which one of these periods an acquired brain lesion occurred, it is useful to group acquired lesions of the CNS into the more inclusive category of perinatal injuries (Table 3).

Perinatal injuries differ significantly from acquired lesions of mature brain in five significant ways:

1. Cells of the developing brain display different patterns of selective vulnerability to insults based on their level of maturation. Mature neurons, as they are "terminally differentiated," are more susceptible to injury than less mature neurons and neuroblasts. Therefore the pattern of neuronal vulnerability tends to correlate with the relative degree of maturation of a particular region. Neurons of the thalamus, basal ganglia, subiculum (transition point between hippocampus and temporal neocortex), cranial nerve nuclei, basis pontis nuclei, and other brainstem nuclei tend to mature earlier than the less mature neurons of the developing cerebral cortex. These earlier-maturing neurons are especially vulnerable to anoxic injury. The morphologic appearance of neurons undergoing anoxic/ischemic change is different in the developing brain than in the brains of older children and adults. Eosinophilic change of neurons, characteristic of severe anoxia in the brains of children and adults, is very uncommon in neonates. Instead, neurons exposed to significant anoxia are characterized microscopically by more subtle findings: cell swelling; central chromatolysis; pyknotic and karyorrhectic changes of the nucleus; and mineralization/ferruginization of dead neurons.

2. Since the vascular supply to the developing brain differs from that seen in the mature brain, the sites subject to lowest oxygen tension in the former are different from those seen in the brains of children and adults. As the brain develops, its blood supply derives from the three major intracranial arteries (anterior, middle, and posterior cerebral), but the anastomotic channels between the cortical penetrating arteries from the cortical surface and deep penetrating arteries from the basal surface are poorly formed. Consequently, a

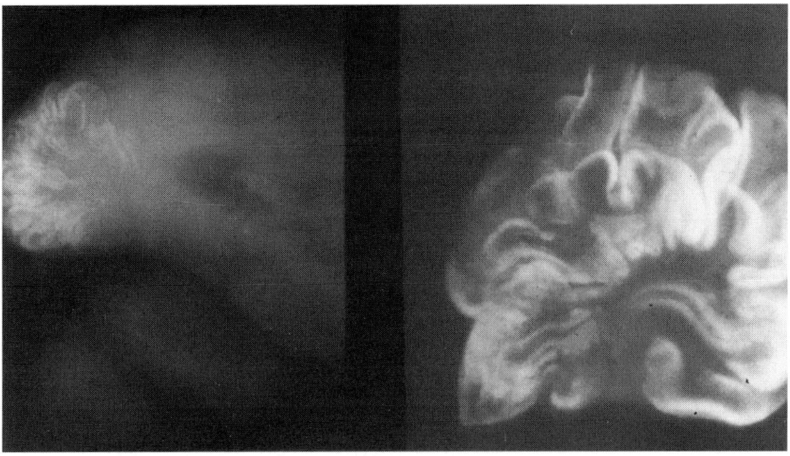

(A)

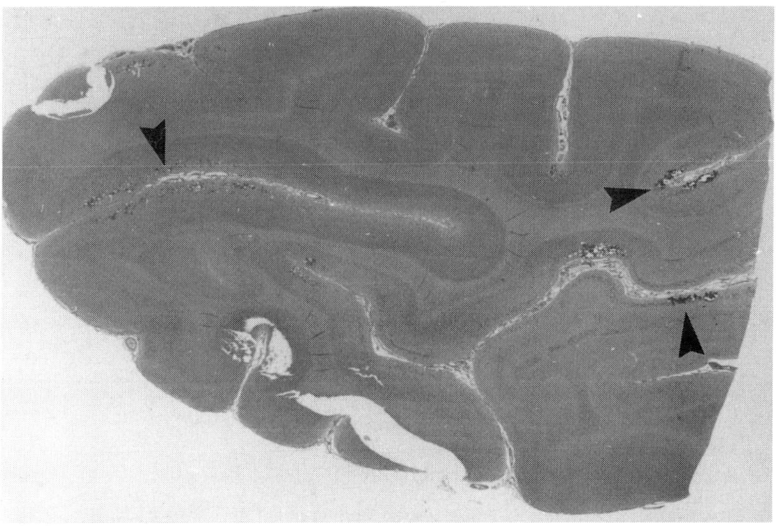

(B)

Figure 26 Sturge-Weber disease (encephalotrigeminal angiomatosis). Neuropathologic features are often best appreciated using soft-tissue radiographs. (A) Lateral view (at left; autopsy specimen, fixed brain) and coronal slice through occipital lobe (at right) both show gyriform "tram track" pattern calcifications in the occipital cortex. (B) Section of brain from another patient shows cortical parenchymal calcifications (arrowheads) in otherwise relatively well formed brain. (Reproduced, with permission, from Vinters HV. In: Duckett S, ed. Pediatric Neuropathology. Baltimore: Williams & Wilkins, 1995:302–333.)

Table 3 Overview of Vascular/Anoxic, Infectious, and Toxic Lesions of Developing Brain and Spinal Cord

Developmental process	Lesion
I. Vascular/anoxic	
Hemorrhages	SEH/GMH
	choroid plexus
	cerebellar
	subarachnoid
	subpial
	intradural
Infarcts	
1) white matter	PVL
2) gray matter	status marmoratus
	pontosubicular necrosis
	ulegyria
	diffuse cortical sclerosis
	hippocampal sclerosis
3) gray and white matter	hydranencephaly
	multicystic encephalopathy
II. Infections	
a) intrauterine	rubella
	CMV
	toxoplasmosis
b) postnatal	bacterial meningitis
	herpes simplex encephalitis
III. Toxic	billirubin encephalopathy
	fetal alcohol syndrome
	other

Abbreviations: SEH = subependymal hemorrhage; GMH = germinal matrix hemorrhage; IVH = intraventricular hemorrhage; PVL = periventricular leukomalacia; CMV = cytomegalovirus.

vulnerable borderzone exists in the periventricular white matter of the developing brain.

3. An intrauterine injury may disrupt fundamental developmental processes, resulting in an appearance that may more clearly resemble a malformation than a destructive lesion. A lesion incurred while cell proliferation, migration, and differentiation are occurring in the developing CNS may have drastic effects on the cerebrum. Therefore, intrauterine "injuries" acquired during the first and second trimesters often tend to appear more like malformations than clearly destructive lesions (i.e., micrencephaly, CMV infection or toxoplasmosis, neuronal heterotopia in response to intrauterine radiation, or polymicrogyria).

4. The glial response to injury changes as the brain develops. GFAP-immunoreactive gliosis, the hallmark of CNS injury in mature brains, is rarely seen before 24 weeks of intrauterine life. Immature astrocytes are not capable of forming the glial scar that is characteristic of injuries in the mature CNS. However, lesions that develop later in intrauterine gestation, during birth, or in the postnatal period will show characteristic patterns of reactive gliosis and more closely resemble destructive lesions. Macrophages are not seen after an injury or necrosis in the early developing brain, although they appear to begin their "scavenging" function in the CNS slightly before astrocytes become capable of reactive change.

5. Since perinatal injuries can result from disturbances within the mother and the placenta, the developing brain is obviously subject to insults not encountered by mature brains.

Perinatal acquired injuries can best be classified into three main categories:

A. Vascular/Anoxic

Perinatal vascular/anoxic lesions can be further subclassified into two broad types: hemorrhages and infarcts (necrotic/cystic lesions).

1. Hemorrhage

Intracranial hemorrhages are the most common lesions in the immature CNS.

a. Subependymal/Germinal Matrix Hemorrhages (SEH/GMH). These are frequent brain lesions (Figs. 27, 28) in low-birth-weight infants (<1500 g). "Germinal matrix" describes the neuroblasts and spongioblasts (glial cell precursors) lining the ventricles (originating from the neuroepithelium of the neural tube), which are destined to migrate to the cerebral cortex (see above). The largest focal mass of germinal tissue overlies the caudate nucleus on each side, rostral to the foramen of Monro, and is referred to as the ganglionic eminence. This zone, which appears during 13 or 14 weeks of intrauterine life, contains

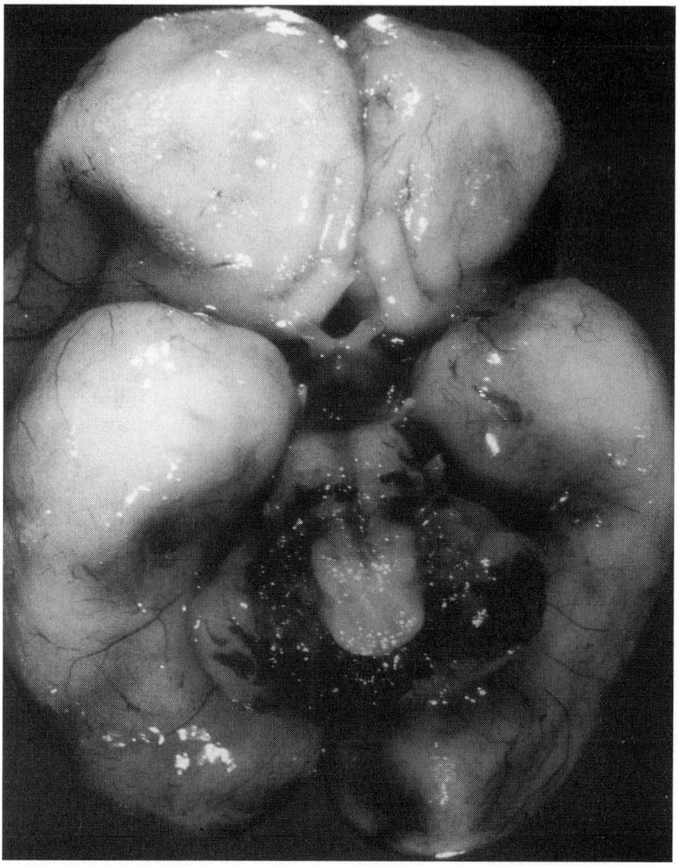

Figure 27 Undersurface of the brain from a premature neonate who developed a large SEH/GMH which ruptured into the lateral ventricles; blood is seen surrounding the cerebellum and brainstem, having extended through the fourth ventricle exit foramina.

neuroblasts destined for the thalamus and basal ganglia, as well as glial cells destined primarily for the subcortical white matter. As the cells migrate to their appropriate locations between weeks 18 and 34 of gestation, the zone diminishes in size, from its maximum size during the second trimester. The germinal matrix contains a rich network of capillaries and large primitive venous channels, which are lined by a single layer of endothelium. These venous channels have poorly and incompletely formed basal lamina and no adventitial connective tissue, so they are highly susceptible to rupture with increased venous pressure. Further, these vessels are frequently congested, and traverse a tortuous

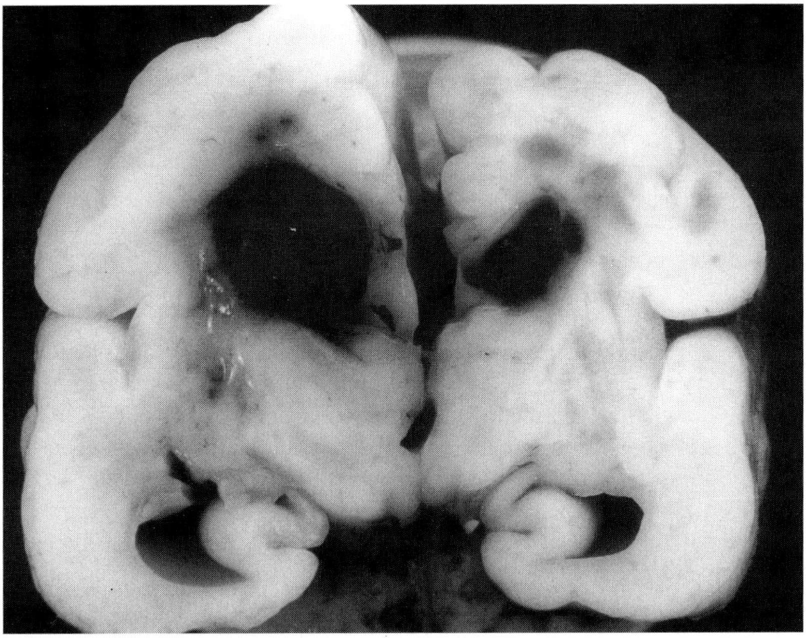

(A)

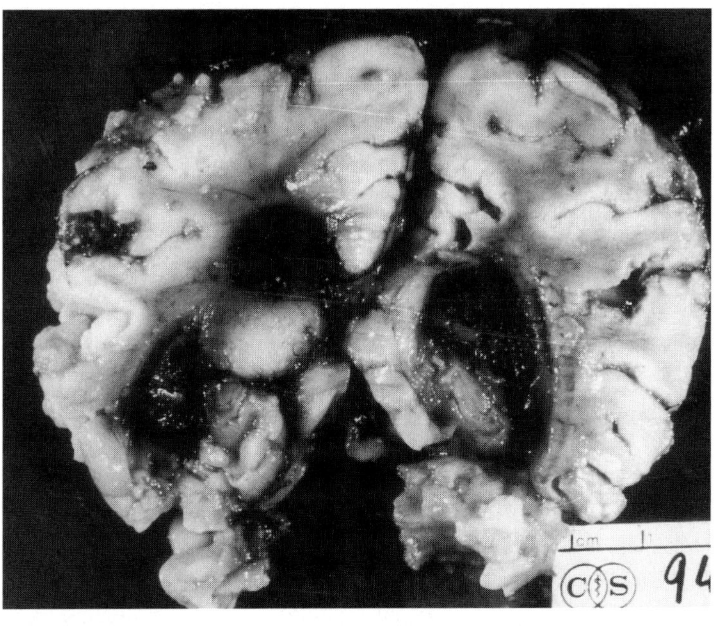

(B)

Figure 28 Large intraventricular hemorrhages (IVH) arising from subependymal/germinal matrix hemorrhages. In both cases, hematomas fill and distend the lateral ventricles, but in (B) there are associated brain parenchymal necrosis and extension of hematoma into the brain substance.

route to their site of drainage. These anatomical factors increase the likelihood of increased venous pressure on the delicate, poorly formed venous channels of the germinal matrix. In addition, since endothelial cells are exquisitely vulnerable to anoxic insults and the basal lamina and connective tissue are poorly formed, endothelial cell necrosis with hemorrhage in the face of anoxia (as is often seen in markedly premature infants) has been suggested as a potential mechanism for these hemorrhages, although the precise pathophysiologic mechanisms of SEH/GMH have not been proven.

The most common site of SEH/GMH is just posterior to the foramen of Monro. The hemorrhages may begin as petechial hemorrhages, but are usually multiple, and frequently confluent, forming a large hematoma (Fig. 28); they are often bilateral. Such hemorrhages may rupture into the adjacent ventricle, especially in infants weighing <1500 g. Intraventicular hemorrhage arising from (GMH) may be sufficiently large to fill the entire ventricular system and extend through the foramina of Magendie and Luschka to give rise to basal subarachnoid hemorrhage (Fig. 27). Clinically, subependymal/germinal matrix hemorrhages are most strongly correlated with prematurity and low birth weight.

Infants who survive the acute hemorrhagic episode may be left with a residual cystic cavity. However, the main complication faced by infants surviving the hemorrhage is posthemorrhagic hydrocephalus. This may occur acutely, as blood fills the basal cisterns obstructing the flow of CSF, or chronically, with organization and fibrosis of the subarachnoid space. Posthemorrhagic hydrocephalus is most frequently associated with early postnatal bleeding and is rarely seen with intrauterine hemorrhages.

b. Intraventricular. Intraventricular hemorrhages (IVHs) usually arise in the context of extension of a SEH/GMH (Fig. 28). IVHs may also arise as an extension of hemorrhage within the choroid plexus and, rarely, from an intraparenchymal hematoma. The risk of intraventricular hemorrhage declines as the age and birth weight of the infant increase. This is due largely to decreased risk of SEH/GMH, but also reflects maturation of the subependymal tissue with formation of the subependymal glial plate.

c. Choroid Plexus Hemorrhage. Choroid plexus hemorrhages are an occasional finding in both premature and term infants. They may coexist with SEH/GMHs or occur independently, often with extension into the ventricles. Choroid plexus hemorrhages are more common in term infants, often in association with congenital heart disease.

d. Subpial Hemorrhage. The subpial regions of the cerebellar and cerebral cortices are vulnerable to small hemorrhages which lift the pia-arachnoid and adherent glial tissue away from the cortical surface. Blood may extend into the subarachnoid space, or remain confined to the subpial region. These small hemorrhages are most often seen over the cerebellar hemispheres and temporal and parietal lobes.

e. Cerebellar Intraparenchymal Hemorrhage. These occur in a significant percentage of premature infants, as many as 20% in one study. They can occur in the cerebellar cortex, white matter, or deep nuclei and are almost always multiple. They may coalesce to form large hematomas, which can be very destructive.

f. Other Intraparenchymal Hemorrhages. Intraparenchymal hemorrhages other than those described are rare in newborns; they usually suggest trauma, bleeding diathesis, or embolic disease.

g. Subarachnoid Hemorrhage. Basal subarachnoid hemorrhages are very common lesions of the perinatal period, usually resulting from extension of an IVH into the basal cisterns and over the convexities of the cerebellum. The most frequent scenario is one in which an SEH/GMH ruptures into the ventricles, and the blood passes through the foramina of Magendie and Luschka to cause the appearance of basal subarachnoid hemorrhage. Subarachnoid hemorrhages may also occur as a consequence of extension of subpial or cerebellar hemorrhage. Subarachnoid hemorrhages can also be seen over the cerebral convexities as an independent finding, or in the setting of trauma or intrapartum hypertension.

h. Intradural Hemorrhages. Intradural hemorrhages into the falx cerebri or the tentorium cerebelli are not infrequent. Small petechial hemorrhages are of no clinical significance and can be seen in premature or mature infants. They may be related to subtle anoxia. Large intradural hemorrhages, on the other hand, strongly suggest antecedent trauma.

2. *Infarcts (necrotic cystic lesions)*

Perinatal nonhemorrhagic vascular/anoxic lesions can be conveniently thought of as lesions involving primarily white matter, lesions involving primarily gray matter, or lesions involving both gray and white matter. They resemble infarcts, but usually show patterns which differ from infarcts in mature brain, although perinatal infarcts resembling those seen in mature brains may also occur.

a. White Matter Lesions. As a consequence of the relatively poorly developed vascular anastomoses between the long penetrating cortical vessels and the deep basal vessels, the deep periventricular white matter is particularly vulnerable to injury, especially in premature infants.

i. Periventricular Leukomalacia (periventricular infarcts). Periventricular leukomalacia (PVL) refers to the presence of regions of necrosis in the periventricular white matter, which usually resolve into cystic cavities (Fig. 29). The lesions are frequently multiple and often bilateral, although not necessarily symmetrical. They may be small or may extend into the centrum semiovale to approach the subcortical white matter. Secondary hemorrhage into a lesion may

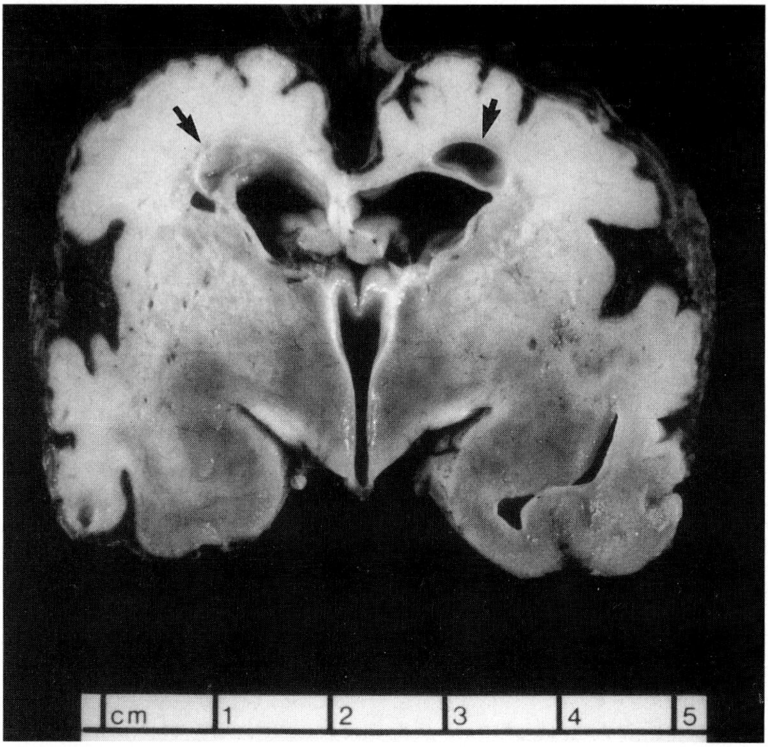

Figure 29 Periventricular leukomalacia. Coronal section through the brain of a child, demonstrating bilateral cystic necrotic lesions (arrows) in the periventricular white matter. Overlying cortex also shows severe atrophy secondary to chronic anoxic/ischemic encephalopathy. (Reproduced, with permission, from HV Vinters, in S Duckett (ed), *Pediatric Neuropathology.* Williams & Wilkins, 1995, pp. 302–333.)

occur. They are most frequently seen anterior to the frontal horns of the lateral ventricles, but also are common at the corners of the lateral ventricles and surrounding their occipital horns.

Although some authors suggest that PVL is clinically seen in association with systemic hypotension (especially in low-birth-weight infants who lack well-developed autoregulation of cerebral blood flow), hyaline membrane disease and cardiac arrest, the most clearly associated pathologic risk factors by rigorous statistical analysis, are endotoxemia (as seen in sepsis), placental abnormalities, and the presence of other associated congenital anomalies.

ii. Periventricular Telencephalic Leukomalacia. This term describes a more subtle and diffuse lesion of the developing white matter of the deep centrum semiovale, in contradistinction to the focal circumscribed lesions of PVL. It is characterized primarily by intense hypertrophic astrocytosis (suggesting it must occur late in intrauterine gestation or intra- or postpartum). Periventricular telencephalic leukomalacia is most strongly associated with endotoxemia. Some authors consider it a subtype of PVL despite the different morphologic substrates of the two types of lesion.

b. Gray Matter Lesions. The selective vulnerability of the gray matter to anoxic/ischemic injury in the developing brain is related to the maturity of its constitutive neurons. Consequently, perinatal gray-matter lesions following anoxic/ischemic insults show a different distribution from that seen in mature brain. The developing neurons of the thalamus, basal ganglia, and brainstem are relatively more mature than the neurons of the cerebral cortex, so they are more vulnerable to selective injury (Fig. 30). However, selective vulnerability is not the only factor that determines injury. Other factors, such as the nature and timing of the insult, the vascular pattern of supply to a given region, and other pathophysiological variables, influence the pattern of injury.

i. Thalamic and Basal Ganglia Lesions (*status marmoratus*). Necrotic lesions within the thalamus and basal ganglia are characterized by neuron loss, astrocyte proliferation, foamy macrophages, and, frequently, mineralization of dead neurons with calcium and iron (ferruginization). Grossly, the thalamus and basal ganglia may show small cysts or, more commonly, a compacted white appearance (due to loss of neurons with reactive gliosis). The term "status

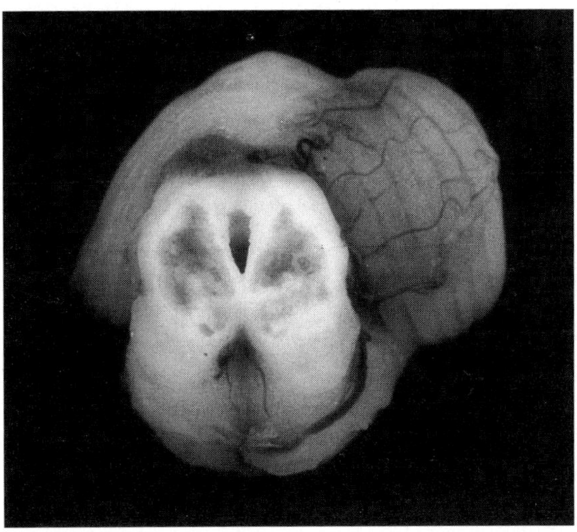

Figure 30 Cystic encephalomalacia in the brainstem of a neonate who had suffered a severe anoxic/ischemic insult.

marmoratus" refers to a marbleized appearance of this region, which is a manifestation of aberrant hypermyelination of disordered axons following injury. This marbled appearance is more commonly described than encountered in practice.

ii. Pontosubicular Necrosis. This describes a loss of the neurons of the basis pontis and the subiculum (the transitional region where the hippocampus merges with temporal neocortex) with associated reactive gliosis. Necrosis of these two separate populations of neurons is often seen together, highlighting their selective vulnerability to anoxic/ischemic injury and their similar vascular supply. Pontosubicular necrosis is usually seen in the clinical setting of infantile respiratory distress, and frequently coexists with other perinatal lesions. The lesions may not be visible grossly. Microscopically, they are characterized by neuron loss with prominent nuclear karyorrhexis (breaking up of the nucleus into clumps) and reactive gliosis.

iii. Necrosis of the Cerebral Cortex: Ulegyria and Diffuse Lobar Sclerosis. Although neurons of the cerebral cortex are relatively less mature than their counterparts in the basal ganglia, thalamus, and brainstem, they are still susceptible to anoxic/ischemic injury. Two main patterns of perinatal injury involving primarily the cerebral cortex are noted: *a*) ulegyria, and *b*) a diffuse pattern of cortical injury (diffuse lobar sclerosis). These patterns can be distinguished on morphologic grounds, although the basic pathophysiology underlying the two cortical lesions is probably similar. For reasons that are not clear, the cerebral cortex appears to be much more vulnerable to anoxic/ischemic injury during the perinatal period than is the cerebellar cortex.

a. Ulegyria. Ulegyria is a localized selective necrosis of neurons of the cerebral cortex; it results in shrunken sclerotic gyri. Involvement is greatest in the depths of gyri with a relative sparing of their crowns, resulting, in its extreme form, in "mushroom gyri" (Fig. 31). Acutely, the lesion may not be grossly apparent. However, it is clearly recognizable in its chronic form. One can postulate that differences in the oxygen tension or neuronal vulnerability between the crown and the depth of the gyrus result in this pattern. The damage is most prominent within cortex, but may extend into the subcortical white matter with attendant reactive gliosis. Microscopically, neuronal necrosis, reactive gliosis, and occasional mineralization of dead neurons are seen. Ulygyria may involve a single gyrus, but it frequently involves a cluster of gyri. It can be unilateral or bilateral, and is most frequently seen in arterial borderzone regions.

b. Diffuse Cortical Injury (diffuse lobar sclerosis). Diffuse injury to the cerebral cortex can occur in neonates in the setting of global anoxia and hypotension (such as occurs with cardiorespiratory arrest). The pathologic changes are similar to those seen in cortical laminar necrosis of mature brains, with the exception that the microscopic alterations reflect the relative immaturity of the developing neocortex. Since the neocortex is not the region of highest selective

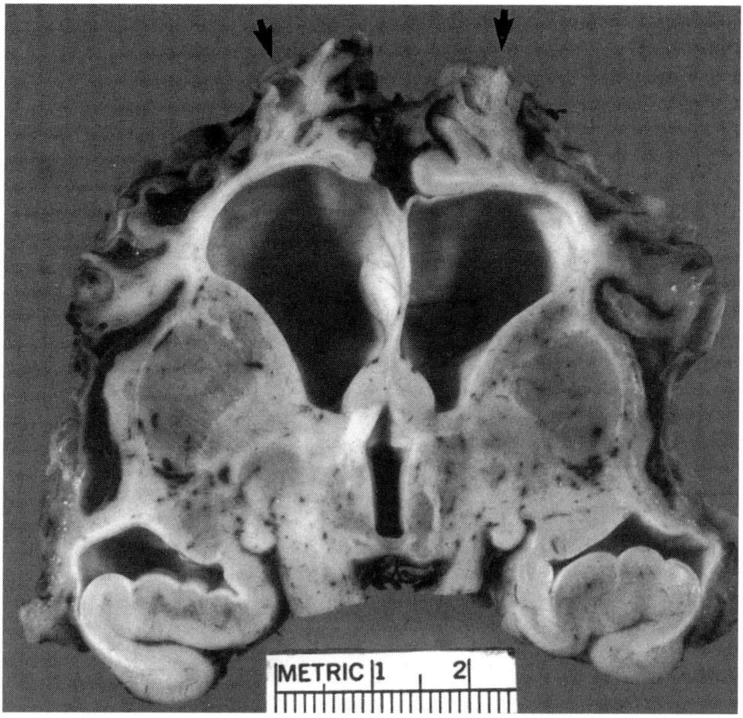

(A)

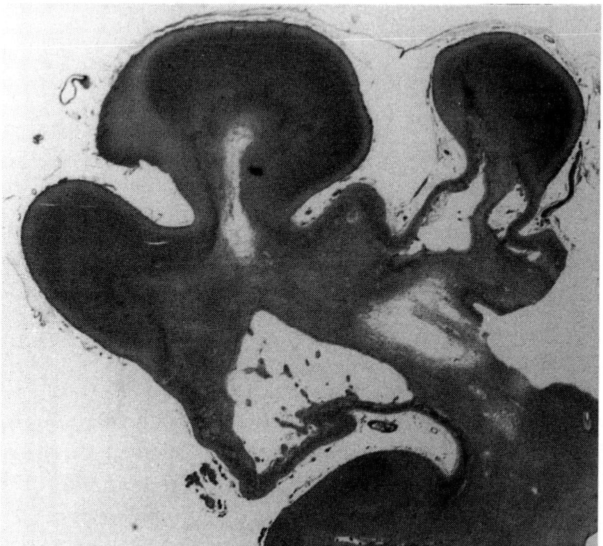

(B)

Figure 31 Ulegyria. After “resolution” of a severe global anoxic/ischemic insult, ulegyria is sometimes seen. Involvement is greatest in the depths of gyri with a relative sparing of their crowns, resulting in “mushroom gyri,” which have the appearance of a mushroom on a stalk. Specimen illustrated grossly in (A) showed severe cortical anoxic injury. (B) Cortical resection specimen from a child with epilepsy.

neuronal vulnerability during the perinatal period, global anoxia usually causes large-scale neuron loss in other neuronal populations as well, such as those within brainstem, thalamus, and basal ganglia. Necrosis of the ventral horns of the spinal cord may also be seen under these circumstances ("hypoxic myelopathy").

iv. Moebius Syndrome. Although neurons of the brainstem are vulnerable to anoxic/ischemic events, the compensatory increased perfusion of the brainstem during global anoxia or hypoperfusion usually protects critical brainstem nuclei such as cranial nerve nuclei. However, neuronal loss within cranial nerve nuclei can develop during the perinatal period, when autoregulation of cerebral blood flow is not fully refined. This level of damage is usually incompatible with survival, but, rarely, patients survive with varying degrees of disability. Moebius syndrome, the best-known clinical example, is a rare syndrome in which patients have facies characterized by drooping corners of the mouth, with some degree of ophthalmoplegia. It results from neuronal necrosis within cranial nerve nuclei VI and VII.

v. Hippocampal Sclerosis. Neurons of the CA1 region of the hippocampus, in addition to those of the subiculum, mature relatively early and are therefore more vulnerable to anoxic/ischemic insults (as well as a variety of other potential insults associated with infantile febrile convulsions). Damage to these neurons can result in hippocampal sclerosis, which is characterized grossly by a shrunken-appearing hippocampus, and microscopically by changes similar to those seen in subicular necrosis (described above). Clinically, hippocampal sclerosis is important as a source of potential seizure activity (causing temporal lobe epilepsy) throughout the patient's life. Although hippocampal sclerosis is by no means unique to the perinatal period, its inclusion in this chapter is warranted by its clinical importance in this age group.

c. Lesions Involving Gray and White Matter. These include a group of cavitary lesions which involve the full thickness of the cerebral hemisphere and arise early in intrauterine development. Vascular territory infarcts involving both gray and white matter in a pattern similar to those seen in mature brains are also included in this category.

i. Cavitary Full-Thickness Lesions Acquired Early in Development

a. Hydranencephaly and Porencephaly. Hydranencephaly (Fig. 32) describes the virtual replacement of the cerebral hemispheres (sparing the basal portions, temporal lobes, and occipital lobes) by a large CSF-containing sac, lined by a smooth, thin arachnoid membrane. Porencephaly is a hydranencephalic cyst in which there is a direct connection between this sac and the ventricular system, with no intervening membrane. Hydranencephaly is an early-acquired destructive intrauterine injury of the cerebral hemispheres in which there is no astrocytic (or other form of reparative) response, and in which development of the adjacent gyri is markedly abnormal. The lesion is frequently bor-

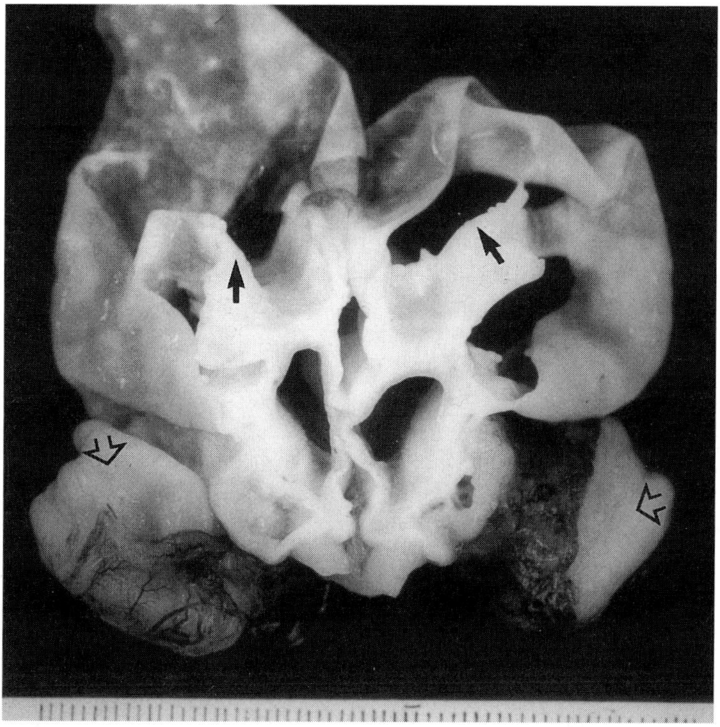

Figure 32 Hydranencephaly. Coronal section through the brain of a premature (31 weeks intrauterine gestation) infant who survived approximately 1 month. The cerebral hemispheres are largely replaced by fluid-filled cystic cavities (black arrows), except for the relatively spared temporal lobes (open arrows).

dered by regions of polymicrogyria and islands of heterotopic neurons, radiating toward the defect. Hydranencephaly is most often seen centered on the middle cerebral artery territory bilaterally, but the zone of destruction frequently extends beyond this. Although the insult inciting hydranencephaly is thought to be anoxic/ischemic, other intrauterine insults, such as viral infections or exposure to toxins, may play a role.

Porencephaly is an older generic term which refers to large, circumscribed, fluid-filled cysts of the cerebral hemisphere resulting from early intrauterine destruction. Porencephalic cysts and hydranencephaly probably represent a spectrum of destruction occurring early in development of the cerebral hemispheres. Similar large cystic lesions of the cerebral hemispheres (as well as micrencephaly) can be seen in fetal-maternal transfusion syndrome, preeclampsia, and twin-twin transfusion syndrome; in the last, one twin does not receive an adequate blood supply from a monochorionic placenta. Schizencephaly is a form of porencephaly in which symmetric clefts exist in place of the primary cerebral fissures. It is also encompassed within the spectrum of intrauterine destructive lesions of the cerebral hemispheres.

b. Multicystic Encephalopathy. This is a destructive process which occurs late in development and therefore is characterized by a glial response. Grossly, the brains of infants with multicystic encephalopathy are small and filled with multiple cystic cavities located primarily in the deep cerebral cortex and subcortical white matter, though the brainstem may be affected (Fig. 30). Lesions are usually in the distribution of the middle and anterior cerebral arteries, with sparing of the middle and inferior temporal gyri. Histologically, the cysts are lined by reactive astrocytes. Residual foamy macrophages can be seen. The cyst cavities are separated by septae of gliotic brain tissue. Multicystic encephalopathy is thought to occur late during intrauterine gestation, during birth or the early postnatal period, and appears to be associated with perinatal anoxia, especially during labor. Multicystic encephalopathy may also be associated with viral infections.

d. Vascular Territory Infarcts. Perinatal infarcts in discrete arterial territories involving the cerebral cortex and subcortical white matter can occasionally occur during the perinatal period. The lesions usually involve the middle cerebral artery territory, and are most frequently secondary to embolic disease. Thrombotic disease in the perinatal period is almost never seen. Rarely, vascular territory infarcts may result from direct trauma to the vessel, or a vascular abnormality such as fibromuscular dysplasia, Moyamoya disease (occlusion of the carotid artery distal to the ophthalmic artery), or a congenital aneurysm. The intracranial venous system in infants is prone to developing venous thrombosis in response to dehydration, sepsis, or congenital heart disease, and hemorrhagic infarcts in the territory of venous drainage may develop as a consequence (see Chap. 2).

B. Infections

Infections of the developing CNS may result in significant lesions of the brain and spinal cord, particularly during the first trimester, since they can cause damage by both direct inflammatory/destructive injury and by disrupting the normal process of development. Fetuses and neonates are at increased risk for infection for three main reasons: they are susceptible to maternal infection (which may be subclinical and undetected); they have an immature immune system; and the birth process itself exposes them to potential infection.

1. Intrauterine Infections

a. Rubella. Rubella is a single-stranded RNA virus which has tropism for vascular endothelial cells in the placenta and developing fetus. A 10% risk of fetal malformations occurs in first-trimester maternal infection. Clinically, it may result in congenital heart anomalies, cataracts, deafness, and mental retardation. Intrauterine infection with rubella is associated with a destructive meningoencephalitis, which results in micrencephaly, polymicrogyria, and frequent degenerative changes of the blood vessels with mineralization.

b. Cytomegalovirus. Cytomegalovirus (CMV) is a double-stranded DNA virus, a member of the family of herpesviruses. Transplacental transmission occurs, resulting in fetal demise, premature birth, or neonatal death. Intrauterine infection during the first trimester results in a number of major acquired malformative lesions. CMV can infect all glial cells and neurons, and it has a predilection for the germinal matrix. Resultant abnormalities include micrencephaly, hydrocephalus, periventricular destruction with mineralization, polymicrogyria, and neuronal heterotopia. Hydranencephaly has also been seen in association with intrauterine CMV infection. Chorioretinitis is a frequent accompaniment. Microscopically, characteristic intranuclear and intracytoplasmic inclusions may be seen (see Chap. 4). CMV infection can also occur late in intrauterine gestation or during the peripartum period, usually with a much better prognosis.

c. Toxoplasmosis. This is a protozoal infection which can result in subclinical maternal infection that may cross the placenta. Intrauterine toxoplasmosis causes a granulomatous meningoencephalitis within the fetus, characterized by multiple foci of necrosis within the cerebral cortex, white matter, basal ganglia, thalamus, brainstem, and spinal cord (the cerebellum is usually spared). Mineralization of the destructive lesions is common, as is associated chorioretinitis. Congenital toxoplasmosis may be associated with some of the same acquired malformations seen with intrauterine CMV infection, including hydrocephalus, polymicrogyria and hydranencephaly. The association of severe acquired malformations with intrauterine toxoplasmosis highlights the role of early intrauterine infection in the disruption of normal developmental processes.

2. *Postnatal Infections*

Newborn infants are susceptible to infections, since their immune systems are immature for the first few weeks of life. Premature infants are at particularly increased risk for all types of infection since they are generally smaller and less mature (with even less well developed immune systems than full-term newborns) and since one of the causes of premature delivery is perinatal infection.

a. Neonatal Bacterial Meningitis. This is most commonly associated with gram-negative bacteria but may also be seen with streptococcal, staphylococcal, and other bacterial infections. Gram-negative infections tend to be most destructive, usually presenting as a purulent meningitis. Necrotizing vasculitis is a frequent accompaniment, resulting in parenchymal infarcts and hemorrhages. Mortality is high (up to 80%), and survivors are usually left with major neurologic consequences, often including hydrocephalus.

b. Neonatal Herpes Simplex Encephalitis. Perinatal infection with herpes simplex virus, which can be acquired during birth from the mother's genital tract, results in a severe necrotizing encephalitis with disseminated visceral herpes infection. Neonatal herpes encephalitis tends to be a diffuse process with gray-matter involvement usually predominating. Vascular congestion is a prominent feature, as are multiple petechial hemorrhages scattered throughout the cerebral cortex. Characteristic intranuclear inclusions can usually be identified in neurons and glia. Neonatal herpes encephalitis is a devastating but preventable cause of severe perinatal injury.

3. Toxic

Maternal exposure to many different compounds may be associated with abnormalities of fetal development; the field of teratology is devoted to this topic. Although the list of substances that may have potential adverse effects on neural development is long, we will focus on two well-defined entities.

a. Bilirubin Encephalopathy (kernicterus). Bilirubin is formed from the breakdown of blood and is normally taken up by the liver and conjugated with glucuronic acid so that it may be excreted by the kidneys. Abnormal accumulation of bilirubin in the neonatal setting occurs under two main circumstances:

1. Hemolytic anemia or erythroblastosis fetalis in the setting of Rh antigen or blood group incompatibility
2. Disorders of hepatic conjugation of bilirubin (i.e., Crigler-Najjar and Gilbert's syndrome)

Mild hyperbilirubinemia associated with breast feeding does not pose a significant risk of bilirubin encephalopathy. The incidence of bilirubin encephalopathy has markedly decreased since the 1950s, with the advent of exchange transfusion and with the continued development of modern approaches to the treatment of Rh incompatibility and neonatal jaundice. There is a distinct pattern of neuronal vulnerability to bilirubin. Involved regions include the neurons of subthalamic nuclei, pyramidal cell layer of the hippocampus, globus pallidus, and cranial nerve nuclei of the brainstem. Occasional involvement of the thalamus, caudate, and putamen occur. Grossly, these regions tend to appear slightly yellowish in the fresh state; formalin-fixed brains lose this discoloration. Microscopically, there are neuronal necrosis, pyknosis (shrinkage and hyperchromasia of the nucleus), chromatolysis, and even eosinophilic degeneration; however, the bilirubin pigment itself is lost in formalin-fixed, paraffin-embedded sections.

b. Fetal Alcohol Exposure. Knowledge of the potentially harmful effects of fetal alcohol exposure has triggered a behavioral change in many expectant mothers. Despite this, the specific effects of alcohol on the developing brain and the amount of exposure required to cause damage remain somewhat obscure. Laboratory data suggest that alcohol may affect basic brain developmental processes such as neuronal migration. A wide spectrum of abnormalities has been associated with maternal consumption of alcohol, including a higher rate of fetal demise, premature birth, low birth weight, postnatal growth retardation, and malformations (comprising the "fetal alcohol syndrome"). Clinically, fetal alcohol syndrome is associated with characteristic facial anomalies, mental retardation, seizures, and cerebellar dysfunction. A range of neuropathologic abnormalities have been associated with fetal alcohol syndrome, including holoprosencephaly, spina bifida, agenesis of the corpus callosum, neuronal heterotopias, and hydranencephaly. More subtle and indefinite changes have also been described. The precise role and mechanism of alcohol in the development of fetal malformations remains to be fully clarified.

Table 3 presents an overview of acquired perinatal lesions of the brain and spinal cord.

V. COMMON SYNDROMES WITH VARIABLE STRUCTURAL CNS COMPONENTS

A. Mental Retardation

This is arbitrarily defined as an IQ of <70. It is not a specific entity, but rather an "end point" that can occur in association with 1. chromosomal disorders; 2. systemic disorders with single or polygenic inheritance with *associated* mental retardation (e.g., TSC or inborn errors of metabolism such as Tay-Sachs disease); 3. primary malformations; and 4. perinatal destructive lesions arising from vascular/anoxic, infectious, or toxic injuries. Very rarely, severe maternal iodine deficiency may result in mental retardation (cretinism). Chromosomal disorders associated with mental retardation include Down's syndrome, trisomy 13, trisomy 18 and the fragile X syndrome. Unfortunately, the specific cause of mental retardation may not be clearly ascertainable in nearly 50% of cases. Improved ultrasound diagnosis, amniocentesis, and chorionic villus sampling have helped identify some cases of mental retardation prenatally, by identifying chromosomal or genetic defects, or structural lesions.

B. Cerebral Palsy

This is a clinical term which defines a constellation of symptoms that may arise from a number of different etiologies. Cerebral palsy is characterized as a generally nonprogressive motor disorder of infancy or early childhood which arises in the prenatal, peripartum, or (occasionally) postnatal state. It is characterized by spastic paraparesis and dyskinesia. Depending on the location and extent of the destructive injury, mental retardation and seizures may also occur. Cerebral palsy results from perinatal injury to the pyramidal system, the extrapyramidal system, and even the cerebellum. Pathologically, it is associated primarily with destructive lesions of the vascular/anoxic (i.e., any of the hemorrhagic or necrotic cystic lesions), infectious, or toxic type, as described above. Cerebral palsy was initially attributed to "birth injury," although it appears that most cases occur during the prenatal period.

C. Sudden Infant Death Syndrome (SIDS)

This is defined as the unexplained sudden death of an infant less than 1 year old, in whom no other cause of death can be found, even after complete autopsy examination and assessment of the scene of death. A number of brain abnormalities have been found in infants dying of SIDS, including enlarged hypoglossal nuclei, increased brain weight, small pineal gland, and abnormal concentrations of catecholamines and neuropeptides. The most significant associated finding to date has been that of selective hypoplasia of the arcuate nuclei (paired structures in the ventral medulla which facilitate chemosensitivity to carbon dioxide and hydrogen ion) in a number of cases. This discovery suggests a possible mechanism for the failure of normal response to cardiopulmonary stimuli in infants dying of SIDS.

VI. CONCLUSION

By keeping in mind the normal pattern of brain and spinal cord development, disruptions of this process can be more meaningfully understood and classified. By thinking of these diverse disorders of brain development in terms of simple pathophysiologic processes and their effects on normal development, the student of neuropathology can develop a "conceptual scaffold" on which to evaluate CNS lesions in infants and children. Further, by flexibly integrating the rapidly progressive discoveries arising in basic developmental neuroscience, the student will be in a position to assess novel data on CNS development into a "global" view, including cellular/molecular aspects of normal/abnormal brain development.

REFERENCES

1. Allen WC, Volpe JJ. Periventricular-intraventricular hemorrhage. Pediatr Clin North Am 1986; 36:47–63.
2. Barth PG. Prenatal clastic encephalopathies. Clin Neurol Neurosurg 1984; 86:65–75.
3. Barth PG. Disorders of neuronal migration. Can J Neurol Sci 1987; 14:1–16.
4. Cameron RS, Rakic P. Glial cell lineage in the cerebral cortex: a review and synthesis. Glia 1991; 4:124–137.
5. des Portes V, Pinard JM, Smadha D, Motte J, Boespflug-Tanguy O, Moutard ML, Desguerre I, Billuart P, Carrie A, Bienvenu T, Vinet MC, Bachner L, Beldjord C, Dulac O, Kahn A, Ponsot G, Chelly J, Dominant X linked subcortial laminar heterotopia and lissencephaly syndrome (XSCLH/LIS): evidence for the occurrence of mutation in males and mapping of a potential locus in Xq22. J Med Genet 1997; 34:177–83.

6. Dobyns WB, Truwit CL. Lissencephaly and other malformations of cortical development: 1995 update. Neuropediatrics 1995; 26:132–147.
7. Ellis RE, Yuan JY, Horvitz HR. Mechanisms and functions of cell death. Annu Rev Cell Biol 1991; 7:663–698.
8. European Chromosome 16 Tuberous Sclerosis Consortium. Identification and characterization of the tuberous sclerosis gene on chromosome 16. Cell 1993; 75:1305–1315.
9. Filiano JJ, Kinney JC. Sudden infant death syndrome and brainstem research. Pediatr Ann 1995; 24:379–383.
10. Friede RL. Ponto-subicular lesions in perinatal anoxia. Arch Pathol 1972; 94:343–354.
11. Friede RL. Developmental Neuropathology. 2nd ed. Berlin: Springer-Verlag, 1989.
12. Gilles FH. Perinatal neuropathology. In: Davis RL, Robertson DM, eds. Textbook of Neuropathology. 2nd ed. Baltimore: Williams and Wilkins, 1991:281–330.
13. Gomez MR. Tuberous Sclerosis. 2nd ed. New York: Raven Press, 1988.
14. Grafe MR. The correlation of prenatal brain damage with placental pathology. J Neuropathol Exp Neurol 1994; 53:407–415.
15. Hori A. A review of the morphology of spinal cord malformations and their relation to neuroembryology. Neurosurg Rev 1993; 16:259–266.
16. Johnson EM Jr, Deckwerth TL. Molecular mechanisms of developmental neuronal death. Annu Rev Neurosci 1993; 16:31–46.
17. Kinney HC, Filiano JJ, Sleeper LA, Mandell F, Valdes-Dapena M, White WF. Decreased muscarinic receptor binding in the arcuate nucleus in sudden infant death syndrome. Science 1995; 269:1446–50.
18. Kwiatkowski DJ, Short MP. Tuberous sclerosis. Arch Dermatol 1994; 130:348–354.
19. Larroche JC. Fetal encephalopathies of circulatory origin. Biol Neonate 1986; 50:61–74.
20. Leviton A, Gilles FH. An epidemiological study of perinatal telencephalic leukoencephalopathy in an autopsy population. J Neurol Sci 1973; 18:53–66.
21. Leviton A, Gilles FH. Acquired perinatal leukoencephalopathy. Ann Neurol 1984; 16:1–8.
22. Lois C, Garcia-Verdugo JM, Alvarez-Buylla A. Chain migration of neuronal precursors. Science 1996; 271:978–981.
23. Martin R, Roessmann U, Fanaroff A. Massive intracerebellar hemorrhage in low-birth-weight infants. J Pediatr 1976; 89:290–292.
24. McLone DG, Knepper PA. The cause of Chiari II malformation: a unified theory. Pediatr Neurosci 1989; 15:1–12.
25. Mischel PS, Nguyen LP, Vinters HV. Cerebral cortical dysplasia associated with pediatric epilepsy. Review of neuropathologic features and proposal for a grading system. J Neuropathol Exp Neurol 1995; 54:137–153.
26. MRC Vitamin Study Research Group. Prevention of neural tube defects: results of medical research council vitamin study. Lancet 1991; 338:131–137.
27. Nakamura Y, Okudera T, Hashimoto T. Vascular architecture in the white matter of neonates: its relationship to perventricular leukomalacia. J Neuropathol Exp Neurol 1994; 53:582–589.

28. Nelson KB, Ellenberg JH. Antecedents of cerebral palsy. N Engl J Med 1986; 315:81–86.
29. Norman MG, Ludwig SK. Congenital malformations of the nervous system. In: Davis RL, Richardson DM, eds. Textbook of Neuropathology. 2nd ed. Baltimore: Williams and Wilkins, 1991:207–280.
30. Norman MG, McGillivray BC, Kalousek DK, et al. Congenital Malformations of the Brain. Pathologic, Embryologic, Clinical, Radiologic and Genetic Aspects. New York: Oxford University Press, 1995.
31. Okazaki H. Fundamentals of Neuropathology. 2nd ed. New York: Igaku-Shoin, 1989.
32. Rakic P. Principles of neural cell migration. Experientia 1990; 46:882–891.
33. Richardson EP Jr. Pathology of tuberous sclerosis. Neuropathologic aspects. Ann NY Acad Sci 1991; 615:128–139.
34. Roessmann U, Gambetti P. Pathological reaction of astrocytes in perinatal brain injury. Acta Neuropathol 1986; 70:302–307.
35. Rorke LB. Anatomical features of the developing brain implicated in pathogenesis of hypoxic-ischemic injury. Brain Pathol 1992; 2:211–221.
36. Ross ME, Allen KM, Srivastava AK, Featherstone T, Gleeson JF, Hirsch B, Harding BN, Andermann E, Abdullah R, Berg M, Czapansky-Bielman D, Flanders DJ, Buerrini R, Motte Mira AP, Scheffer I, Berkovic S, Scaravilli F, King RA, Ledbetter DH, Schlessinger D, Dobyns WB, Walsh CA. Linkage and physical mapping of X-linked lissencephaly/SBH (XLIS): a gene causing neuronal migration defects in human brain. Hum Mol Genet 1997; 6: 555–62.
37. Sarnat HB, Cerebral Dysgenesis: Embryology and Clinical Expression. New York: Oxford University Press, 1992.
38. Sherwood AJ, Smith JF. Bilirubin encephalopathy. Neuropathol Appl Neurobiol 1983; 9:171–285.
39. Skoff RP, Knapp PE. The origins and lineages of macroglial cells. In: Kettennmann H, Ransom BR, eds. Neuroglia. New York: Oxford University Press, 1995:135–148.
40. Takashima S, Tanaka K. Development of cerebrovascular architecture and its relationship to periventricular leukomalacia. Arch Neurol 1978; 35:11–16.
41. Tarby TJ, Volpe JJ. Intraventricular hemorrhage in the premature infant. Pediatr Clin North Am 1982; 29:1077–1104.
42. Walsh C, Cepko CL. Cell lineage and cell migration in the developing cerebral cortex. Experientia 1990; 46:940–947.
43. Weidenheim KM, Bodhireddy SR, Nuovo GJ, Nelson SJ, Dickson DW. Multicystic encephalopathy: review of eight cases and etiologic considerations. J Neuropathol Exp Neurol 1995; 54:268–275.
44. Willinger M, James LS, Catz C. Defining the sudden infant death syndrome (SIDS): deliberations of an expert panel convened by the National Institute of Child Health and Human Development. Pediatr Pathol 1991; 11:677–684.
45. Venes JL, Linder S. Sturge-Weber-Dimitri Syndrome. Encephalotrigeminal Angiomatosis. In: Edwards MSB, Hoffman HJ, eds. Cerebral Vascular Disease in Children and Adolescents. Baltimore: Williams and Wilkins, 1989:337–341.

8

Neurodegenerative Diseases

I. INTRODUCTION

Degenerative diseases of the nervous system are among the most biologically baffling and clinically challenging. Given that many of them (for example, Alzheimer's disease) increase in incidence with advancing age and that the population as a whole is "aging," in the coming decades many neurodegenerative conditions will become an even greater public health problem than they are at present. Apart from their impact on public health, these diseases bring tragic consequences to the persons they afflict and their families: individuals previously capable of robust independent living slowly become incapable—either physically or mentally, or both—of caring for themselves, much less those around them. The frustration of dealing with these conditions has, however, led to unique neurobiological approaches aimed at understanding their pathogenesis and suggesting clues to their prevention and eventual treatment.

Neurodegenerative diseases constitute an extremely heterogeneous group of disorders that share certain unifying features:

1. In most cases, their etiology is unknown, though this is rapidly changing as many are proven to have a specific genetic and/or metabolic basis.

2. They all show selective involvement of specific groups of neurons and/or fiber tracts; affected neurons and tracts may be widely distributed in the CNS (as in the case of Alzheimer's disease) or fairly well localized (Parkin-

son's disease). The seminal pathologic event in their onset/progression is usually *loss* of such neurons and/or fiber tracts, with resultant development of scarring or astrocytic gliosis (see Chap. 1). With progression of the disease over time, this relatively selective loss of neurons/fibers may have downstream (anterograde) or retrograde effects on other tracts, tract systems, or groups of neurons—the mechanisms of Wallerian, retrograde and transsynaptic degeneration discussed in Chapter 1 thus come to take on a practical importance for understanding disease pathogenesis and progression. In some neurodegenerative diseases, characteristic nuclear or cytoplasmic inclusions and abnormalities of the cytoskeleton or neuropil may develop. These often serve as diagnostic structural "markers" for the specific disease (and are usually demonstrable using special stains and/or immunocytochemistry), though they may not always be informative about its etiology or pathogenesis.

3. Though they may develop at any age, most are relentlessly (though often slowly) progressive over months or years. Death from a neurodegenerative illness may result not from the neurologic disorder itself, but be secondary to intercurrent problems, especially infections, to which a bedridden and incapacitated individual is especially prone.

4. Clinically, neurodegenerative diseases present with dementia (here defined as a global decline in higher intellectual functions including abnormalities of memory storage and retrieval, and personality changes), or abnormalities of the motor and sensory systems (with extremely variable manifestations) or both. The presentation of a given disorder, together with the tempo of disease progression, usually leads the neurologist to a specific diagnosis, one usually supported by characteristic neuroimaging and electrodiagnostic studies. Rarely, a brain biopsy is performed to confirm a specific diagnosis (e.g., that of Alzheimer's disease), especially in a patient with a puzzling dementia; however, since the neuropathologic features of many conditions in this broad category are relatively banal (consisting of slowly evolving neuron loss and proliferation of reactive astrocytes) and sometimes found in neuroanatomic areas not easily accessible to a biopsy needle, the reader can surmise that the results of such an invasive procedure may often not be helpful and may in fact, on occasion, be somewhat misleading.

Table 1 summarizes the prevalence and genetic features of some of the most common forms of neurodegenerative disease.

II. APPROACHES TO RESEARCH ON CNS AGING AND DEGENERATION

Few biologic phenomena have intrigued biomedical scientists so profoundly as those associated with cell aging or senescence, and (eventually) cell death. In the nervous system, these phenomena are especially poignant and of great con-

Table 1 Incidence and Genetics of Selected Neurodegenerative Conditions

Disease	Prevalence	Genetics
AD/SDAT	5–10% 65 yr + 20–40% 80 yr + 10% familial, usually autosomal-dominant	Approx. 10% familial Various mutations: APP (chrom 21) . . . 670/671 692 693 (HCHWA-D) 717 PS-1 (chrom 14) Various PS-2 (chrom 1) Various ApoE 4 is a "risk factor" gene
PD	30–90/100,000 Rarely familial	Pending
MND/ALS	5/100,000 10% familial, usually autosomal-dominant	10–20% of familial cases show SOD1 mutations Other mutations rare
HD (chorea)	4–7/100,000	Autosomal-dominant, 4p (CAG)n trinucleotide repeat encoding huntingtin
OPCA/MSA	2/100,000	Various genes . . . most trinucleotide (CAG)n repeats SCA1 (chrom 6p22–23) SCA2 (chrom 12q23–24) SCA3 (chrom 14q32) SCA4 (16q24) SCA6 (19p)
FA	Rare	Autosomal-recessive chrom 9 (frataxin/GAA trinucleotide repeat)
DRPLA	Rare	Trinucleotide repeat (CAG)n chrom 12p

AD/SDAT = Alzheimer's disease/senile dementia of Alzheimer type; PD = Parkinson's disease; MND/ALS = motor neuron disease/amyotrophic lateral sclerosis; HD = Huntington disease/chorea; OPCA/MSA = olivopontocerebellar atrophy/multisystem atrophy; FA = Friedreich ataxia; DRPLA = dentatorubropallidoluysian atrophy; APP = amyloid (A4) precursor protein; HCHWA-D = Dutch form of familial cerebral amyloid angiopathy, thought to be an autosomal-dominant variant of AD with predominantly CAA (rather than senile plaques or neurofibrillary tangles) as the primary microscopic abnormality; PS = presenilin; ApoE = apolipoprotein E; SOD1 = superoxide dismutase 1.

sequence because the major pool of cells associated with "higher" cortical and sensorimotor functions (i.e., neurons) constitute a terminally differentiated and largely nonrenewable resource within the CNS. General theories concerning cellular mechanisms of aging have focused on two major approaches:

1. Cell senescence as a "wear and tear" phenomenon, whereby cytoplasmic or nuclear accumulation of waste products, increasing posttranslational modifications of proteins, or damage caused by free radicals gradually leads to irreversible degeneration of the cell.

2. "Genome-based" theories, which explain cell and tissue aging and death on the basis of occurrences such as a finite doubling time of normal diploid cells (likely to be of minimal relevance for the CNS, since most neurons or neuronal precurors have stopped dividing years or decades prior to their death), somatic (nongermline) mutations, and programmed cell death.

The explosion of research on neurodegenerative diseases has been predicated on several key developments in the understanding of their biological basis. It is worth remembering and emphasizing that detailed descriptions of their associated neuropathologic changes formed the basis for mechanistic research aimed at deciphering molecular and genetic events significant in their etiology and progression. Key developments in this area have been the following:

1. The recognition that many neurodegenerative conditions that occur (for the most part) sporadically also often have a genetic/familial form or variant which is frequently inherited in an autosomal-dominant fashion. This has allowed for identification of disease-associated genes using classic linkage analysis and testing of candidate genes as well as positional cloning. Understanding the biology of how these genes work and the proteins they encode then provides important clues to sporadic forms of an illness. Inserting disease-associated genes into transgenic mice has been especially valuable in (potentially) understanding the basis of motor neuron disease (amyotrophic lateral sclerosis) and Alzheimer's disease. Cell biologic approaches to deciphering the molecular basis for expression or OVERexpression (within CNS) of unique or characteristic disease-associated proteins (e.g., Alzheimer's beta/A4 amyloid) represent a further vital contribution of basic research to solving the riddle of these mysterious illnesses.

2. The discovery in the early 1990s that some degenerative conditions affecting the peripheral and central nervous system develop from mutations resulting from unstable expansion of triplets of nucleotides within portions of the genome has led to reclassification of several genetically determined conditions as "trinucleotide/triplet repeat" diseases; this phenomenon will be considered more fully in a discussion of Huntington's disease/chorea and spinocerebellar degenerations.

3. Biochemical processes fundamental to the function of all cells (e.g., the posttranslational modification that occurs with protein phosphorylation) may

be deranged in a variety of conditions that result in the death of neurons. Unraveling the unique metablic functions and needs of the CNS is an integral part of this process. Mutations in the mitochondrial genome (mtDNA), for example, may cause defects in oxidative phosphorylation that could result in Parkinson's disease. Defective mitochondrial energy production may also increase levels of free radicals, which have been implicated in the causation or progression of several conditions under review in this chapter. Lipid peroxidation may generate reactive oxygen species that can indirectly impair membrane transport proteins crucial for neuronal function, including sodium/potassium-ATPase and glucose transporter. Many neurodegenerative conditions manifest neuronal cytoplasmic "inclusions" that reflect profound abnormalities of normal neuronal cytoskeletal components.

4. The discovery over the past 10 to 20 years of novel "infectious" agents that can produce progressive neurodegenerative diseases without causing classic neuropathologic stigmata of infection (i.e., "slow virus" or, more recently, "prion" diseases) has led to a redefinition of both groups of disorders and an evolving interface of research between them (see also Chap. 4).

5. The concept of excitotoxicity that has evolved with the recognition that glutamate, an excitatory neurotransmitter, has the potential to destroy neurons via activation of ionotropic receptors, has led to the recognition that neurons may literally be "stimulated to death" in the course of acute or subacute hypoxic/ischemic, hypoglycemic, or traumatic CNS injury. Neurons may also be more vulnerable to glutamate-induced damage when their energy metabolism becomes impaired, suggesting that excitotoxic injury may (indirectly) lead to worsening/progression of diseases characterized by chronic, rather than only acute/subacute, neuronal injury. Excitotoxic injury results from overstimulation of the N-methyl-D-aspartate (NMDA) receptor and is probably mediated by excessive calcium influx into the cell, which in turn mediates activation of nitric oxide synthase (NOS), leading to production of nitric oxide, and stimulates phospholipases or calcium ion overload of mitochondria, an event that generates potentially toxic superoxide anion.

6. Rediscovery of the occurrence of programmed cell death (PCD; apoptosis) in both normal development of, and disease affecting, the brain has led to a search for excessive apoptosis as one mechanism that might represent a "final common pathway" for various neurodegenerative conditions. Recent experiments utilizing cortical neurons, for example, suggest that their exposure to short durations or low concentrations of NMDA in the presence of the free-radical peroxynitrite leads to neurotoxicity resulting in apoptosis, whereas intense exposure to high concentrations of NMDA (or peroxynitrite) triggers necrotic neuronal death. Various genes (p53, bax, bcl-2, and bcl-X) and their respective proteins mediate PCD—e.g., bax as a cell death-*promoting* protein and bcl-2 as an apoptosis-*blocking* molecule.

On this background we will consider several neurodegenerative diseases from the perspective of their clinicopathologic features and how these might fit into an etiologic/pathogenetic neurobiological framework.

III. ALZHEIMER'S DISEASE/SENILE DEMENTIA OF ALZHEIMER TYPE

First described in 1907 by Alois Alzheimer and believed, until the 1960s, to be a rare cause of (usually) presenile dementia, Alzheimer's disease (AD) is now recognized as the single most common cause of both presenile and senile dementia (presenile dementia is defined here as occurring in patients under the age of 65 years; senile dementia as occurring in patients 65 years or older). AD occurring at 65 years or older is usually described as senile dementia of Alzheimer type (SDAT) but from a neuropathologic viewpoint, they probably represent the same entity—accepting the fact that patients with the established *clinical* diagnosis of AD/SDAT show significant histopathologic heterogeneity at autopsy and yet may still fall within the neuropathologic "definition" of AD/SDAT.

Recognition that AD/SDAT was the commonest neuropathologic substrate of dementia followed upon simple, yet fundamentally important, observations by Blessed, Tomlinson, and Roth in the late 1960s. These investigators examined, at autopsy, a large number of brains from patients who had been either demented or not demented during life, and found that the majority of those with dementia had "excessive" numbers of senile plaques and neurofibrillary tangles (to be discussed below) in comparison to age-matched controls. Almost immediately "senility," which had previously been vaguely attributed to small "strokes" or decreased cerebral blood flow in the elderly, was reconfigured as Alzheimer's disease.

A. Clinicopathologic Features

AD/SDAT probably occurs in all races, though it has been most thoroughly studied in Caucasians. In this population, severe dementia is present in as many as 5% to 10% of patients over the age of 65 years, and *some* degree of dementia may be present in twice this number. Among persons over the age of 80, at least 20% are estimated to have severe dementia. Of those who are demented, over 50% have AD/SDAT. AD/SDAT usually presents with insidious onset of memory disturbance (especially short-term memory), personality change, and speech abnormalilties, with (in the early stages of disease) sparing of the motor, sensory, and visual systems. Psychiatric symptoms (e.g., paranoia) may also be an early manifestation of AD. Speech initially sounds "empty" or devoid of meaningful contact, and eventually difficulties in comprehension develop though fluency is relatively preserved until late stages of the disease. Problems with visuospatial skills may develop. The disease generally progresses for 8 to 10 years or even longer, at the end of which affected patients are usually bedridden, mute, and unable to recognize even close family members.

Patients who present clinically with a dementing illness are commonly worked up with a view to excluding "treatable" conditions that may mimic dementia (e.g., hypothyroidism, drug-induced encephalopathy, respiratory insufficiency, brain tumor [especially a frontal lobe glioma or meningioma], chronic subdural hematoma). This having been done, the clinical diagnosis of AD/SDAT is supported by evidence of cortical atrophy on CT or MRI scans, and parietotemporal hypoperfusion on positron emission (PET) or single-photon emission computed tomographic (SPECT) scanning, as well as detailed neuropsychologic testing. It has recently been suggested that further evidence *favoring* the diagnosis of AD/SDAT is to be found by assaying CSF levels of various AD-associated proteins (e.g., beta/A4, tau) and defining a given patient's ApoE genotype [see below], though the "predictive value" of these techniques has yet to be standardized against autopsy results. Nevertheless, the clinical diagnosis of AD/SDAT is approximately 85% to 95% accurate. The only way to make the *definitive* diagnosis, however, is by brain biopsy or autopsy.

The brain of a patient with AD/SDAT may appear grossly normal or it may show diffuse atrophy, with significant widening of the sulci and shrinkage/atrophy of gyri (Fig. 1). Sections of fixed brain usually confirm the presence of atrophy and may show enlargement of the lateral ventricles secondary to brain shrinkage, i.e., hydrocephalus ex vacuo (Figs. 1, 2), to be distinguished from hydrocephalus resulting from obstruction of CSF flow or failure of its normal resorption in the arachnoid granulations.

How best to confirm the diagnosis of AD/SDAT using microscopic sections of brain has generated significant debate among Neuropathologists for several years. One problem arises because all of the microscopic lesions of AD/SDAT *may* occur, to a modest degree and extent, in the brains of mentally normal and neurologically intact elderly people. In one way, therefore, the diagnosis of AD/SDAT is a quantitative or semiquantitative one—though in practical terms not all laboratories have either the time or manpower to "quantify" AD brain microscopic lesions. The microscopic lesions that are overrepresented in the brain of a patient with AD/SDAT are illustrated schematically in Figure 3. As indicated, one of the lesions, granulovacuolar degeneration (of Simchowicz), occurs primarily and most often exclusively in the pyramidal cell layer of the hippocampus, whereas the other three—senile "neuritic" plaques (SPs), neurofibrillary tangles (NFTs), and cerebral amyloid angiopathy (CAA)—are widely distributed throughout the cortex. SPs and NFTs may occur within deep central gray-matter structures (hypothalamus and basal ganglia) and (especially NFTs) within the brainstem. Two of the lesions, SPs and NFTs, are best appreciated on silver stains (e.g., Bodian,

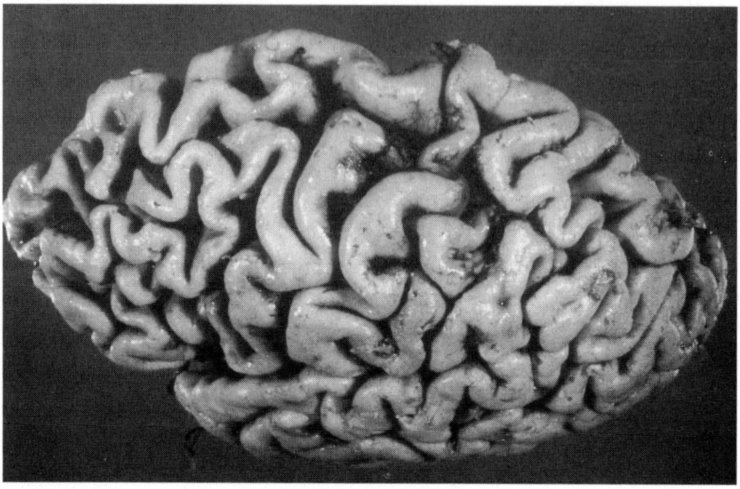

(A)

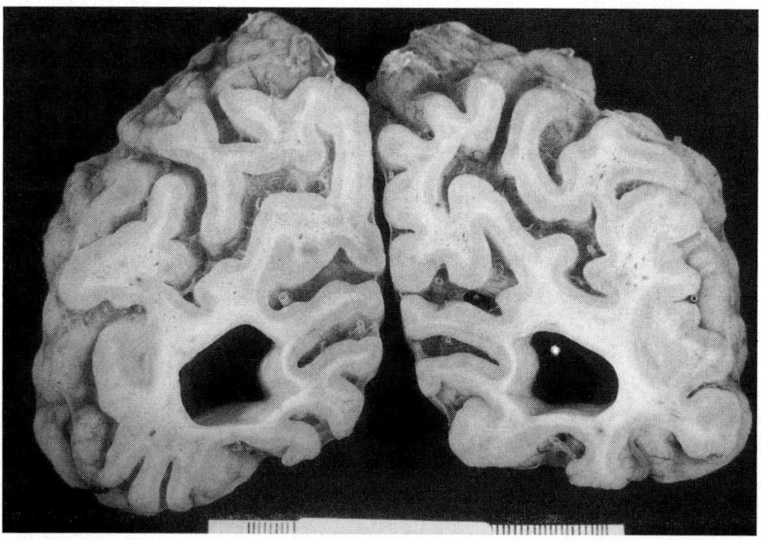

(B)

Figure 1 Alzheimer's disease. (A) External view of one cerebral hemisphere from fixed brain, showing striking diffuse atrophy of cerebral cortex, with widening of the sulci. (B) Coronal section, posterior parietal. Note pronounced widening of sulcal spaces between gyri, which (in a normal individual) would be hardly visible.

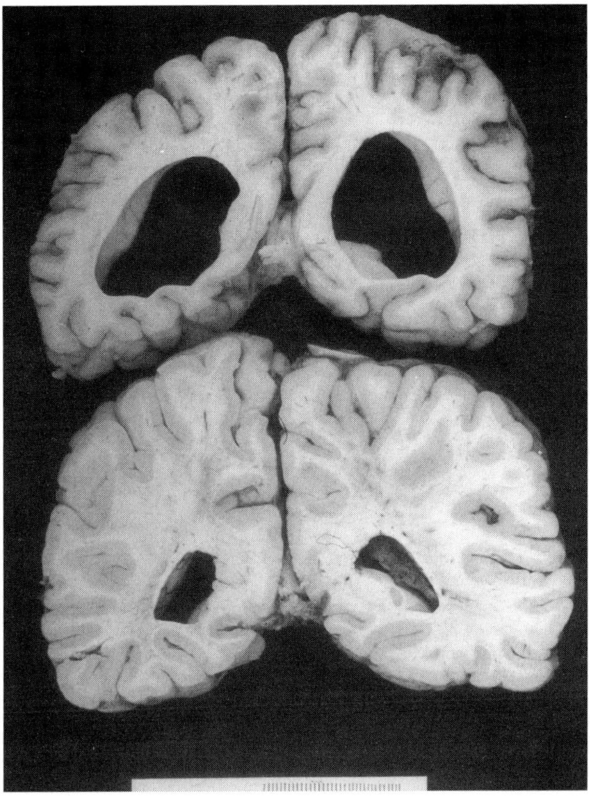

Figure 2 Alzheimer's disease. Coronal sections through comparable planes of a control (normal) brain (bottom) and brain from an AD patient (top) show cortical atrophy in the AD specimen, with pronounced enlargement of the lateral ventricles, a phenomenon described as hydrocephalus ex vacuo.

Bielschowsky), whereas CAA is most easily recognized on Congo red-stained sections viewed under polarized light, or using an immunohistochemical technique (see below). SPs and CAA may be dramatically highlighted in thick sections of brain stained with the Campbell-Switzer technique (Fig. 4). A few words about each lesion before we consider how they should be assessed to arrive at a neuropathologic diagnosis of AD/SDAT, and what they tell us about the neurobiology of age-related CNS degeneration:

1. Granulovacuolar Degeneration (GVD)

GVD is a good descriptor for this neuronal lesion, found predominantly in the pyramidal cell layer of the hippocampal formation. The neuronal cytoplasmic

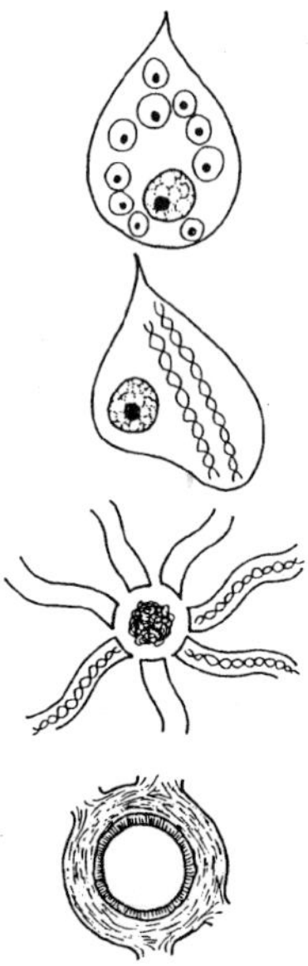

LESION	AMYLOID	NEOCORTEX	HIPPOCAMPUS
Granulovacuolar degeneration (intraneuronal)	NO	NO	+++
Neurofibrillary tangle (intraneuronal)	YES	++	+++
Senile "neuritic" plague (extraneuronal)	YES & NO	+++	+++
Amyloid angiopathy (extraneuronal)	YES	+++	+

Figure 3 Schematic diagram showing microscopic lesions (and their distribution within brain) which, when present in excessive numbers, correlate with the clinical diagnosis of AD/SDAT. All of these microscopic abnormalities are frequently observed, though to a lesser extent, in the brains of mentally normal, elderly patients.

Nissl substance becomes displaced by clear vacuoles of variable size, each containing a basophilic granule. GVD is quite easily recognized on H&E-stained sections. Granulovacuolar change may represent proliferation within neuronal cell cytoplasm of complex lysosomes. Though GVD is almost a "forgotten lesion" in AD research, it is worth remembering that some studies have shown that the numbers of neurons affected by GVD in the brains of some demented AD patients correlate with the *duration* of dementia.

2. *Neurofibrillary Tangles (NFTs)*

NFTs are, like GVD, intraneuronal lesions but with a markedly different light microscopic, ultrastructural, immunohistochemical, and molecular profile, and are (usually) more widespread within the neocortex. Though visible with routine stains, they are highlighted using silver stains (such as the modified Bielschowsky or Gallyas techniques) (Fig. 5) or immunocytochemical stains utilizing primary antibodies to the microtubule-associated protein (MAP) tau, a protein of MW 50,000 to 64,000 Daltons which has several isoforms that arise

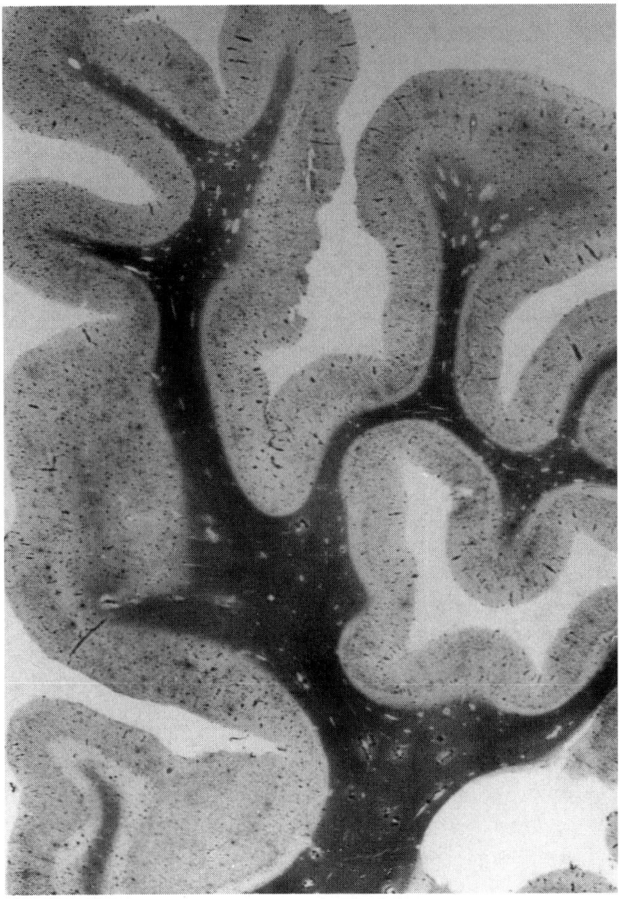

Figure 4 Cortical lesions of AD/SDAT seen in a 100-μm-thick section of brain stained by the Campbell-Switzer technique. The "speckled" appearance in the cortex results from the presence of abundant (amyloid-rich) SPs and severe CAA; normal cortex would appear uniformly pale. (Preparation courtesy of Professor Heiko Braak, Frankfurt, Germany.)

from a single gene by alternative mRNA splicing. In AD/SDAT, there is evidence for abnormal phosphorylation of tau with its conversion into the subunits of AD paired helical filaments (PHFs), a characteristic ultrastructural feature of NFT (Fig. 6). PHFs (earlier described as bifilar helices) consist of tightly adherent pairs of helical 10-nm-wide protofilaments wound about each other such that the maximum width of a PHF is 20 to 24 nm and its half-periodicity is approx. 80 nm. NFTs also often contain straight filaments that vary in diameter from 10 to 20 nm.

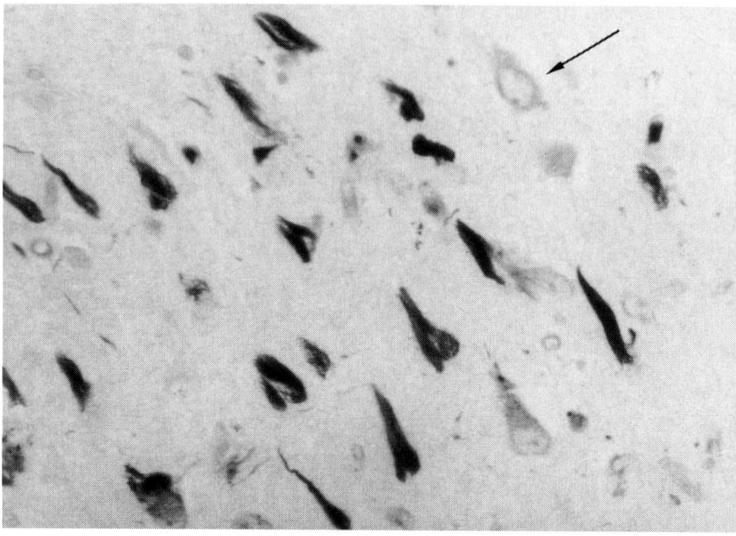

Figure 5 Gallyas-stained section of AD brain showing numerous flame-shaped neurofibrillary tangles within cortical pyramidal neurons. By contrast, rare pale neurons (arrow) represent uninvolved cells.

Though NFTs may be seen in viable neurons with "healthy"-appearing nuclei, they may persist in the neuropil after the NFT-containing neuronal cell body dies; these are described as "ghost tangles." In particularly severe AD/SDAT, NFT may (rarely) be identified in neurons of the granule cell layer of the hippocampus. Some investigators (e.g., see Braak et al., 1996, Ref. 3), have stated that a progression of NFT change can be used to establish a neuropathologic "staging" for AD/SDAT—the earliest NFT neuronal alterations being in the transentorhinal region, subsequent changes affecting the adjoining cortical and subcortical components of the limbic system, and finally (in advanced disease) NFT neuronal change extending into the cerebral neocortex. As a practical guide, a neocortical brain biopsy for dementia which shows the presence of *any* NFTs allows for the relatively certain diagnosis of AD.

3. *Senile "Neuritic" Plaques (SPs)*

SPs are perplexing microscopic lesions that, when "fully mature," have both a neuronal (neuritic) and an extraneuronal component. Key events in their evolution are the subject of much debate. "Diffuse" plaques, thought to represent the earliest stage in their development, are essentially invisible on routine stains and represent ill-defined areas of wispy immunoreactivity with antibodies to Alzheimer beta/A4 (Aβ) protein (see below) in the neocortex; such beta/A4

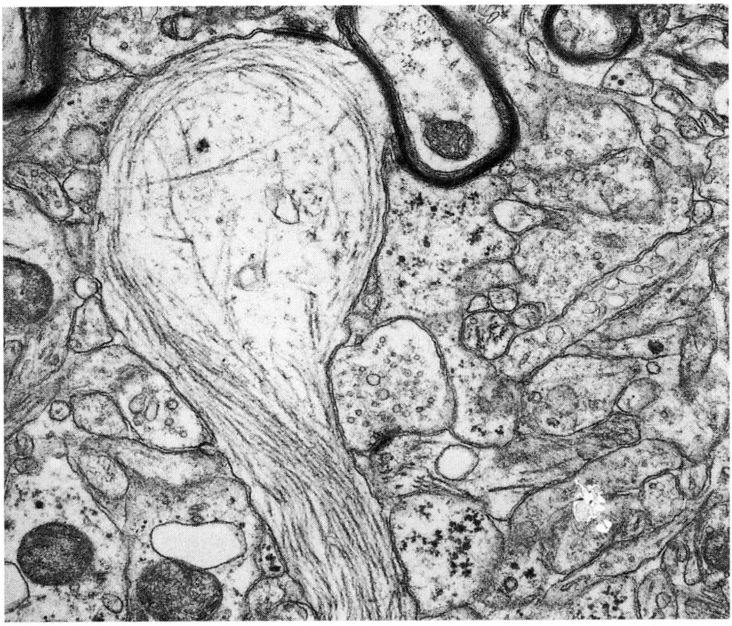

Figure 6 PHF, characteristic of NFTs and neurites of SPs, are present in abundance in a neuronal process (at left) seen on electron microscopic examination of a brain biopsy from an AD patient. Elsewhere, synapses and unmyelinated and myelinated neuronal processes are identified.

immunoreactivity does NOT imply the presence within cortical neuropil of fibrillar amyloid. More "advanced" SPs have a neuritic component, which includes injured, dying, or dead neuronal processes usually showing PHFs within them. In "mature" SPs, a large hyaline eosinophilic core is present at the center of a neuritic "corona" (Fig. 7). This "core" has staining properties of beta/A4 amyloid, and beta/A4 immunoreactivity also often extends into the region around the amyloid core. SPs with a significant neuritic and amyloid component are visible on routine histologic stains but are particularly easy to visualize with various silver stains (Fig. 7).

Obviously the SP is a complex structure with various components; it may also be associated with significant microglial and astrocytic proliferation in the surrounding neuropil, though whether these cellular events contribute to *formation* of the SP or represent a cellular *reaction to it* is at present unresolved. The presence of inflammatory cells (i.e., microglia) within, or in close proximity to, one of the key microscopic brain lesions associated with AD has suggested anti-inflammatory medications as one possible treatment for, or prophylaxis against, AD/SDAT. Since debates about plaque evolution and maturation at

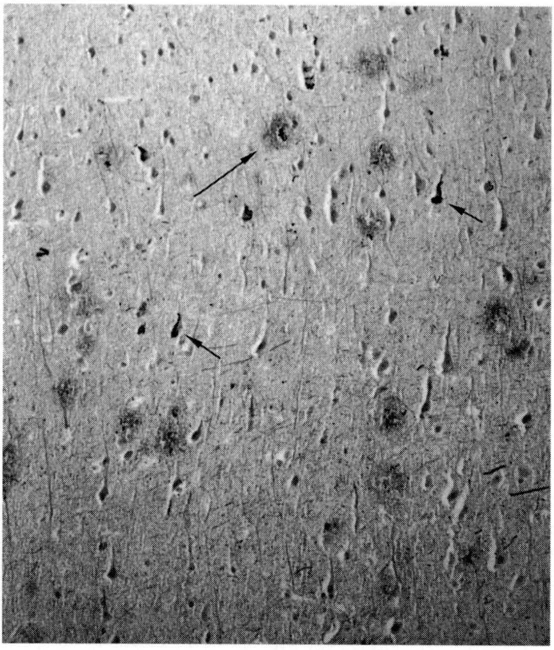

(A)

Figure 7 Brain biopsy from an AD patient (A,B). (A) Section stained by a silver (Bielschowsky) technique shows abundant SPs with both a neuritic and amyloid core component (long arrow). Short arrows indicate NFTs. (B) Parallel section stained with an anti-beta/A4 antibody shows many SPs to have beta/A4 immunoreactivity. (C) Magnified view of an SP (AD brain, autopsy specimen) stained with the Campbell-Switzer technique, showing both the neuritic "corona" and amyloid core of the plaque.

present must be based on inferential arguments based on human biopsy and autopsy material, the recent development of transgenic mouse models of AD in whose brains plaquelike amyloid deposits are found *predictably* is likely to help resolve issues about the primacy (or lack thereof) of beta/A4 amyloid or neuritic change in the pathogenesis and neurobiologic significance of the SP.

4. Cerebral Amyloid Angiopathy (CAA)

Also known as congophilic angiopathy or cerebrovascular amyloidosis, CAA represents a cerebral microvascular amyloidosis that (like other AD-associated lesions) occurs in the absence of AD/SDAT, but is often especially severe in AD patients. There is debate as to whether a sporadic age-related form of CAA may produce cerebral hemorrhage in the *absence* of clinical dementia. Micro-

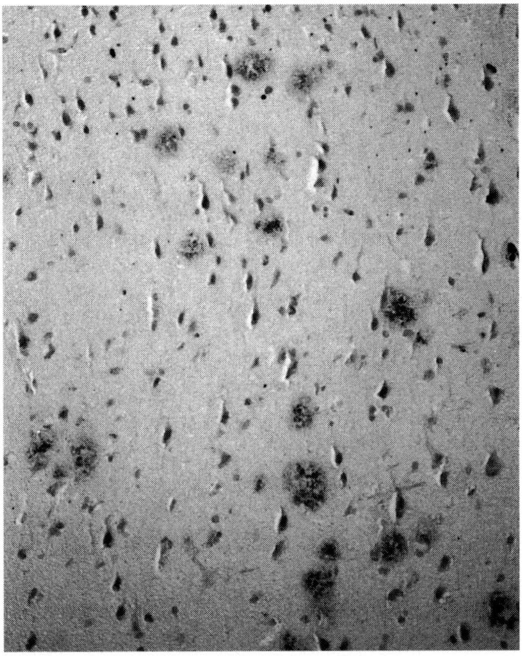

(B)

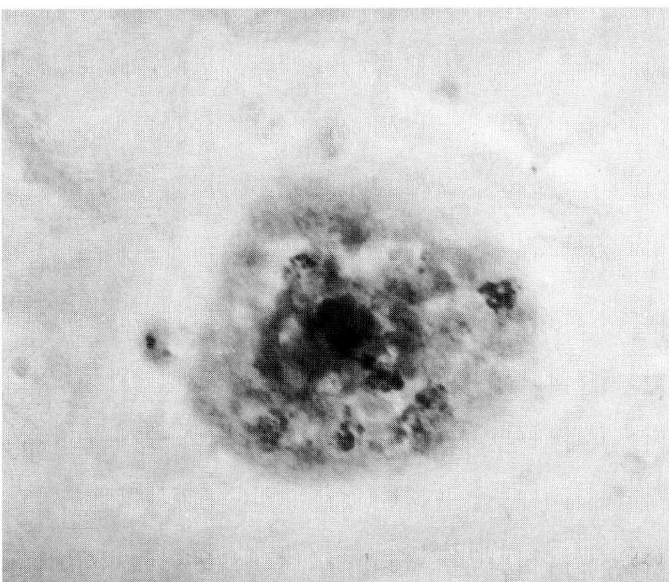

(C)

scopically, CAA is identified as an effacement of normal arteriolar (smooth muscle cell rich) media (Fig. 8) with its replacement by a hyaline/glassy eosinophilic material that has typical staining properties and immunohistochemical features of beta/A4 amyloid (Fig. 9; see also Chap. 2).

Amyloid may also be seen in the walls of capillaries and venules. Larger meningeal arteries may have amyloid deposits localized more prominently on their adventitial surfaces. Just as SP amyloid can be demonstrated immunohistochemically using primary antibodies to the beta/A4 protein, so CAA associated with aging/AD is "decorated" using this antibody (Fig. 9), though biochemical studies suggest that SP and CAA beta/A4 amyloid may not always be identical in length. The role of CAA and associated microangiopathies in the pathogenesis of stroke (especially cerebral hemorrhage) is discussed in Chapter 2, as are hereditary forms of CAA found in Icelandic and Dutch patients which produce *primarily* stroke and are less consistently associated with dementia (Fig. 10).

5. *Other Lesions*

Other lesions have been implicated in the pathogenesis of AD/SDAT. Rodlike bodies of Hirano are bullet- or rod-shaped, brightly eosinophilic structures iden-

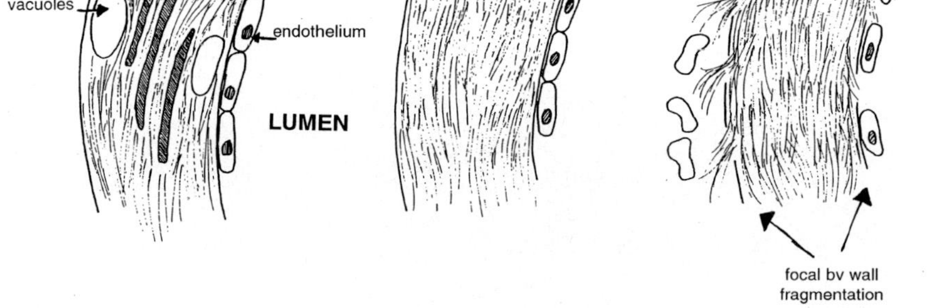

Figure 8 CAA, schematic diagram. This lesion affects cerebral arterioles and capillaries. Diagram illustrates mild, moderate, and severe degrees of CAA, which are thought to result (in arterioles) from progressive degeneration of the media as fibrillar 7- to 10-nm diameter amyloid accumulates in the vessel wall. Eventually, amyloid fibrils may extend into the surrounding brain parenchyma (panel at right). See Chapter 2 for a discussion of stroke-related complications of CAA.

tified in the neuropil, usually of the hippocampus. Though they are associated with changes of brain aging and AD/SDAT, they have no convincing role in disease causation. Neuropil threads (NTs), found in abundance in the neocortex of AD patients, represent cell processes of NFT-bearing neurons that contain PHF and are immunolabeled with antibodies to phosphorylated tau, just as NFTs are. Some investigators maintain that *all* of the above microscopic lesions associated with AD represent biologically intriguing epiphenomena that have little to do with onset or progression of the dementing illness. Rather, these workers believe that gradual but progressive loss of neocortical synapses (secondary to as yet incompletely defined deficiencies of neurotrophic "maintenance" factors) correlates best with the neuropsychologic abnormalities of AD/SDAT. As well, loss of neurons from basal forebrain (cholinergic) nuclei—e.g., the nucleus basalis of Meynert—is a prominent feature of the neuropathology of AD/SDAT.

B. Making/Confirming the Clinical Diagnosis of AD/SDAT

Though an abundance of the previously described microscopic lesions (Fig. 3) throughout the neocortex and hippocampus would seem to render the neuropathologic diagnosis of AD/SDAT relatively straightforward, nagging issues about its nosology remain. Is the *clinical* diagnosis of dementia necessary in a patient for the *neuropathologic* diagnosis to be made? Put differently, do the neuropathologic findings only serve to support the clinical diagnosis, or are the neuropathologic features sufficiently characteristic that they allow for a definitive diagnosis regardless of the presence/absence of well-documented dementia?

Considering only neuropathologic criteria, what numbers of microscopic lesions are sufficient for the diagnosis of AD/SDAT and how many may be present as a function of "normal" aging? Can one type of microscopic lesion predominate (at the expense of others) and still produce the clinical syndrome of AD/SDAT? For example, can a patient have predominantly SPs OR NFTs OR CAA and still develop clinically typical AD? The heterogeneity of AD-related lesions is striking when large numbers of brains from demented individuals with this disorder are examined. Essentially all patients with Down's syndrome who survive into middle age (the fourth or fifth decade) show AD microscopic alterations within their brains.

To resolve such troublesome issues, various sets of consensus criteria have been developed to guide the pathologist in arriving at a reasonable certainty as to the diagnosis of AD/SDAT based on a thorough brain examination. The most widely used of these are currently the CERAD criteria, developed by the Consortium to Establish a Registry for Alzheimer's Disease (see Mirra SS et al., 1991, Ref. 30). This group recommends that a minimum of seven tissue

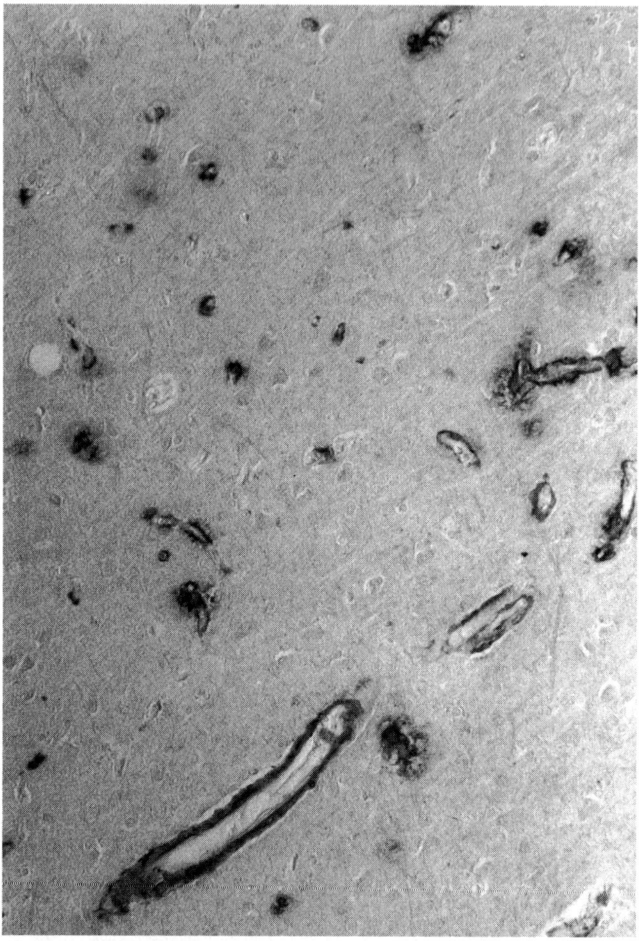

(A)

Figure 9 CAA and SP amyloid immunolabeled using immunohistochemical technique incorporating anti-beta/A4 antibody. (A) Low-magnification view with arteriolar and capillary beta/A4 amyloid. (B) Magnified view showing CAA-affected arterioles cut in cross section and a large SP (arrow), possibly centered on a capillary.

sections be taken from the brain to include middle frontal, superior and middle temporal, inferior parietal and anterior cingulate cortex, hippocampus (at the coronal level of the lateral geniculate nucleus), entorhinal cortex with amygdala, and midbrain to include the substantia nigra. The cortical sections should be stained with a silver technique (e.g., modified Bielschowsky) and a method to demonstrate amyloid (e.g., Congo red). Immunohistochemistry of sections

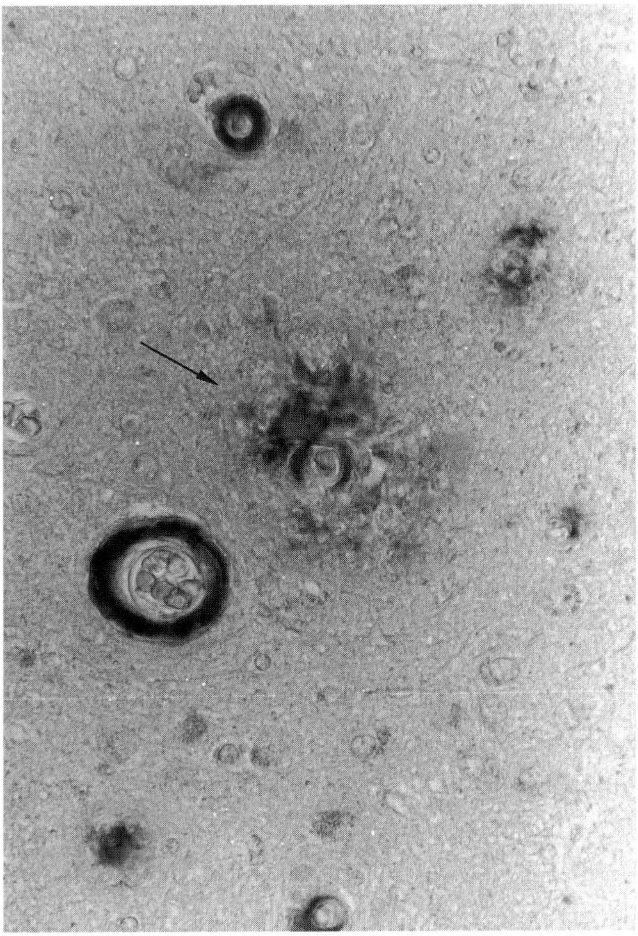

(B)

using antiubiquitin antibodies (to optimally demonstrate Lewy bodies; see below) should be carried out when available. Using a template available from CERAD, the various lesions are graded as being absent, mild/sparse, moderate, or severe/frequent. Based on the score obtained following this semiquantitative assessment, a final diagnosis of "normal brain," possible, probable, or definite AD is made.

C. Molecular Pathogenesis and Genetics

The modern era of AD research began with Glenner and Wong's isolation and preliminary characterization (in 1984) of the amyloid protein that is (see above)

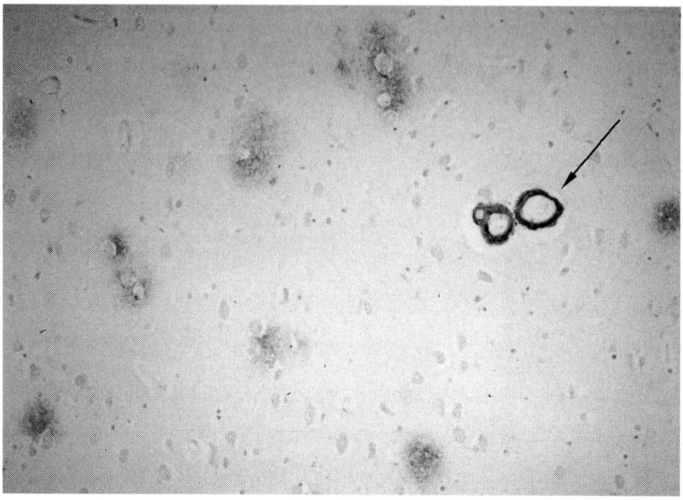

Figure 10 Dutch form of CAA resulting from a codon 693 mutation of the APP gene. Section has been immunostained with an anti-beta/A4 1-42 antibody. Note especially prominent labeling of arteriolar walls (arrow), and patchy diffuse beta/A4 immunoreactivity in the adjacent parenchyma. (Preparation courtesy of Drs. Marion Maat-Schieman and Raymund A. C. Roos, Leiden, The Netherlands.)

an integral component of both SPs and CAA. Eventually named the Alzheimer beta/A4 protein, this is a small, 39 to 43 amino acid peptide with a unique sequence. It is cleaved from a larger protein, the A4, or amyloid precursor protein (APP), a membrane-spanning protein encoded by a gene on chromosome 21 with a large N-terminal extracellular component and a small intracellular C-terminal segment. Beta/A4 is constituted by a 28 amino acid extracellular segment and an 11 to 15 amino acid intramembrane component. APP itself has several isoforms (of 695, 751, and 770 amino acid residue length) that result from alternately spliced APP transcripts, the two longest isoforms including a 56 amino acid domain that shows homology with Kunitz type protease inhibitors. APP can probably be synthesized by a variety of cell types, including neurons and microvascular smooth muscle cells.

Abundant beta/A4 can be demonstrated immunohistochemically in brain tissue sections from AD/SDAT patients (Figs. 7, 9), and, as expected, smaller numbers of immunoreactive lesions may be present in the CNS of mentally normal elderly individuals. Beta/A4 deposits are found in SPs and CAA but usually not in the cytoplasm of NFT-bearing neurons or neurons showing GVD. What (if anything) does brain parenchymal or microvascular beta/A4 deposition have to do with the onset or progression of AD/SDAT?

Families with inherited AD (usually of early, i.e., presenile, onset and inherited as an autosomal-dominant trait) sometimes show mutations in the gene encoding APP, often within the beta/A4 coding domain or very close to it. The best-characterized of these are (using the APP770 numbering system) a familial AD (FAD) "double" mutation involving amino acids 670 and 671 (just N-terminal to the start of beta/A4), a FAD mutation at amino acid 717 (just C-terminal to the end of beta/A4), and two mutations (Dutch and Flemish) within the beta/A4 coding region at, respectively, amino acids 693 and 692. The APP693 mutation determines a phenotype which is dominated by CAA (see also Chap. 2), with relatively little in the way of parenchymal beta/A4 deposition and rare NFTs. Neuropathologic features of the APP692 mutation are as yet not fully known, there having been few brain biopsies or autopsies of affected patients, though they have (as in HCHWA-D) both dementia and cerebral hemorrhages secondary to severe CAA and prominent parenchymal and microvascular beta/A4 deposits within the cortex. Cultured cells derived from some patients with FAD mutations show abnormalities of APP processing in vitro that may explain some patterns of beta/A4 deposition in the brain.

Beta/A4 appears to be a soluble product of cellular processing of APP which is detectable, using sensitive methods, within the CSF. An alpha-secretase (as yet unidentified) cleaves APP between amino acids 16 and 17 of the beta/A4 sequence, yielding a NON-beta/A4 containing fragment of APP that, presumably, is incapable of forming insoluble beta/A4. An alternate route by which APP can be processed results from action of a beta-secretase, which "cuts" APP at the N-terminal end of beta/A4, and subsequent action of a gamma-secretase at the C-terminus of beta/A4. The latter, beta/A4-generating process, may also occur within the cell's endosomal-lysosomal compartment. How (or even whether) the generation of beta/A4 causes the neuronal cytoskeletal abnormalities that result in formation of NFTs is not known.

And the genetics of AD/SDAT become yet even more complex! Within the past 5 years, other FAD mutations have been discovered on chromosomes 14 and 1. The chromosome 14 mutations occur in a gene that encodes presenilin-1 (PS-1), an integral membrane protein, while the chromosome 1 mutations are in a gene that encodes presenilin-2 (PS-2). PS-1 appears to be the major gene for familial presenile dementia. The presenilins share a similar size (approx. 450 amino acids) and have >65% amino acid sequence homology. At the time of this writing, there is feverish research activity aimed at understanding where the presenilins are found in normal and AD brain, what their cellular function is, and how mutations in genes encoding them might produce disease—especially, do they interact with APP or beta/A4? Preliminary evidence suggests that PS mutations are associated with beta/A4 overproduction.

To complete the extraordinarily complex portrait of the genetic influences on AD/SDAT, it needs to be mentioned that an important "susceptibility gene" for AD is that which encodes the $\epsilon4$ isoform (as opposed to $\epsilon2$ or 3) of apolipoprotein E (ApoE). The ApoE4 genotype is hugely overrepresented among AD/SDAT patients in comparison to the general population, and the ApoE locus may account for as much as 50% of susceptibility to AD/SDAT.

How all of these molecular, genetic, and biochemical factors come together to "cause" AD/SDAT is still . . . a mystery, though the basic data that have been generated are of immense importance in allowing one to conceptualize this tragic and very common condition. Yet the role of the pathologist in piecing together bits of the puzzle should not be underestimated. The phenotype determined by a given mutation is in most instances more interesting than the mutation itself—how the latter leads to the former can only be meaningfully sorted out by an investigator who understands or can interpret what is occurring in the tissue itself! The value of careful genetic/pathologic correlative studies cannot be overstated.

IV. NON-ALZHEIMER DEMENTIAS

By comparison with AD/SDAT, other forms of dementing illness are comparatively rare, though the relative frequency of some may have been underestimated in the past. Estimates of their relative frequency tend to be variable and frequently change because the various clinicopathologic syndromes that may cause dementia are periodically redefined, and different centers with an academic interest in specific types of dementia tend to study disproportionately large numbers of patients with those disorders. Patients who are thought on clinical grounds to have AD/SDAT during life are often found at autopsy to have another disorder, or another disease *superimposed on* AD (e.g., "stroke" related to cerebrovascular disease). One large autopsy study published in 1992 (see Mendez et al., 1992, Ref. 29) found that of 650 patients diagnosed during life as having AD/SDAT, at autopsy approx. 80% had AD with or without other neuropathologic abnormalities. For the remainder, the most common neuropathologic diagnoses (in roughly decreasing order of frequency) were Parkinson's disease, "nonspecific degenerations," Pick disease, and multiple cerebral infarcts. Of interest, 11 of 650 patients had no significant neuropathologic abnormality. We shall now consider the pathologic conditions most likely to mimic the clinical picture of AD/SDAT—indeed, some of them may be related to AD.

A. Multi-Infarct Dementia

Multiple infarcts (and microhemorrhages) are frequently found in the brains of patients with otherwise typical changes of AD/SDAT. Dementia then presumably results from mixed parenchymal/ischemic brain alterations. The infarcts/hemorrhages may result from longstanding (hypertensive) cerebral microvascular disease, (large-vessel) atherosclerosis, or cardiogenic or other emboli (see

Chap. 2). The clinical implication of this is that multi-infarct/ischemic vascular dementia is to some extent treatable or preventable. Patients will often have experienced "stroke" symptoms during life, unless the ischemic/hemorrhagic lesions are very small—for example, the size of lacunes or even smaller scars within the neocortex. The relationship between multiple small ischemic lesions in the CNS and Binswanger's subcortical leukoencephalopathy is also discussed in Chapter 2, as is the more recently described symdrome of CADASIL.

Relatively "pure" multi-infarct or ischemic-vascular dementia (MID/IVD) is probably quite rare, though in the absence of rigorous prospective clinicopathologic studies using (for example) modern neuroimaging techniques, its true incidence is unknown. A pathologist faced with the autopsy brain of a patient in whom this is the suspected diagnosis must rigorously rule out parenchymal disease as a contributing factor to the dementia, and needs to document the anatomic loci in which ischemic lesions are found, as well as their size and causal vascular disease. Recently, elderly patients with dementia have been found frequently to show evidence of hippocampal pyramidal cell layer neuron cell loss in a pattern not unlike that seen with hippocampal sclerosis found in patients with temporal lobe epilepsy. Cell loss and gliosis in this anatomical structure, which has important functions in memory storage and retrieval, could certainly further worsen a dementing illness caused by either cerebral infarcts or AD/SDAT.

B. Frontotemporal Dementia(s)

This represents a rather heterogeneous group of dementing illnesses, not a single entity. Some investigators suggest that, as a group, these disorders constitute (after AD/SDAT) the second largest category of parenchymal dementias, though this will need to be confirmed in prospective studies of this recently defined (or redefined) constellation of diseases.

1. Clinicopathologic Features

Subserved by the term frontotemporal dementia (FTD) are the following disorders: Pick disease, primary progressive aphasia, frontal lobe or frontotemporal degeneration, dementia associated with motor neuron disease (MND), and, possibly, corticobasal degeneration; the last will briefly be discussed in this section. Primary progressive aphasia is a clinically defined rather than neuropathologic entity—neuropathologic studies of affected individuals indicate structural abnormalities that fall into one of the FTD categories to be described. It is vital for clinicians to recall that non-FTD conditions may present with primarily frontal lobe signs/symptoms; this is well documented in patients with AD/SDAT, in those with spongiform encephalopathy, in rare stroke patients with thalamic infarcts, and in those harboring frontal lobe (intra-axial or extra-axial) neoplasms.

FTDs often present clinically in a pattern that differs substantially, however, from that encountered with AD/SDAT patients. Deterioration of personality and social skills and graces is a dominant feature of these dementias, as are lack of insight, neglect of personal hygiene, inflexible thinking, and impaired judgment. A decline in speech is characteristic and aphasia may be the main feature. Lack of social tact with the commission of antisocial acts and misdemeanors (such as careless driving) are noted, but memory functions may remain relatively intact. Physical examination reveals various speech disturbances, and "release" signs characteristic of frontal lobe lesions. Patients who have MND-associated dementia also obviously show signs of MND (amyotrophic lateral sclerosis; discussed below). Disease onset is usually in the early- to mid-50s, and duration to death ranges from 8 to 11 years. Some (though not all) series report a female predominance of FTDs, and 30% to 50% have a strong hereditary component.

Neuropathologic features that characterize FTD in general and allow categorization into various subtypes are fairly subtle and largely dependent on immunohistochemical staining of brain sections with a variety of commercially available antibodies (see Table 2). The unifying feature of these entities is the existence of selective (sometimes regional) atrophy of the frontal and temporal lobes, visible on high-resolution neuroimaging studies and readily apparent at the time a fixed brain is examined and cut. Neuropathologic features of the specific disease patterns are as follows:

a. Pick Disease. Atrophy in this relatively rare form of FTD—also described as "circumscribed lobar sclerosis"—can be very severe, and asymmetrical between the right and left cerebral hemispheres. In the most pronounced cases, atrophy can result in an affected gyrus taking on a knife-edge appear-

Table 2 Neuronal Inclusions Associated with Neurodegenerative Disorders

Disease	Inclusion	Tau	Ubiq	Cryst	NF (p)
AD/SDAT	NFT	+++	++	−−−	+
Pick dis	Pick body	+++	++	++	−−−
LB dis	LB	+(a)	+++	+	+
MND (D)	"Inclusion"	−−−	+++	−−−	−−−
(SpCd)	"Inclusion"	−−−	+++	−−−	−−−
CBD	Balloon cell	++	+/−	+++	+++

See also notes for Table 1 (disease abbreviations).
Ubiq = ubiquitin; Cryst = alpha beta-crystallin; NF(p) = phosphorylated neurofilament; LB dis = Lewy body disease, including DLBD, Parkinson's disease; MND (D) = motor neuron disease/ALS with dementia (cortex); MND (SpCd) = motor neuron disease primarily affecting spinal cord anterior horn cells; CBD = corticobasal degeneration; (a) tau immunoreactivity observed in cortical LB only.

ance. Though frontal and temporal lobes (including hippocampi) are affected, the temporal lobe usually shows a characteristic pattern of involvement of the middle and inferior temporal gyri (Fig. 11), while the superior temporal gyrus shows involvement (atrophy) of its anterior one-third but relative sparing of its posterior two-thirds. On microscopic examination of affected gyri, there is usually neuron loss with astroctyic gliosis, sometimes of a profound degree; gliosis may extend into the subcortical white matter, which may also show (secondary) demyelination. Striatal atrophy may be present.

The most typical microscopic feature of Pick disease is the existence of "Pick bodies" (Fig. 12), large argentophilic neuronal cytoplasmic inclusions that are also immunoreactive with antibodies to tau, ubiquitin, and alpha beta-crystallin. Ultrastructurally, Pick bodies are composed of non-membrane-bound disorganized collections of filamentous material. On H&E stains, Pick bodies may be difficult to detect—they have the appearance of swollen neurons, though the "filamentous skein" substructure of a Pick body may be detectable. Swollen (chromatolytic-appearing) neuronal cell bodies lacking argentophilic inclusions are, as it happens, also a histologic feature of Pick disease. Pick bodies most commonly occur in neurons of the hippocampus (both granule and pyramidal cell layers), but are also detectable in the neocortex and even within deep central grey matter structures—e.g., the hypothalamus and striatum. Perhaps in deference to the recognition that Pick disease was the "original" FTD to be well characterized as a distinct clinicopathologic entity, some have suggested that the FTD group of disorders be renamed the "Pick complex."

b. Dementia Associated with MND. A relatively small subset of patients with MND/ALS, in addition to having classic neuromuscular features of the disorder (see below), show dementia of the frontal lobe type. Gross and microscopic features are as for that disorder (see below). An additional feature in MND-associated dementia is the presence throughout atrophic neocortex (especially lamina II) and hippocampal dentate granule cells of scattered swollen or "ballooned" (nonargentophilic) neurons, which are immunoreactive for ubiquitin, but not tau and only rarely for alpha beta-crystallin (Table 2).

c. Frontotemporal Dementia/Frontal Lobe Degeneration. Affected brains show, on gross inspection, symmetrical convolutional atrophy in the anterior temporal and frontal lobes, though (unlike with Pick disease) this is neither knife-edge in severity nor circumscribed. Enlargement of frontal portions of the lateral ventricles is noted. The striatum, amygdala, and hippocampal formations are usually spared the "destructive" or atrophic process. Microscopic changes are best seen in regions of grossly visible atrophy as well as the anterior cingulate gyrus, with conspicuous sparing of the superior temporal gyrus. The changes include spongy change or microvacuolization, with astrocytic gliosis, affecting the superficial cortical layers (I to III) (Fig. 13). The gliosis can be

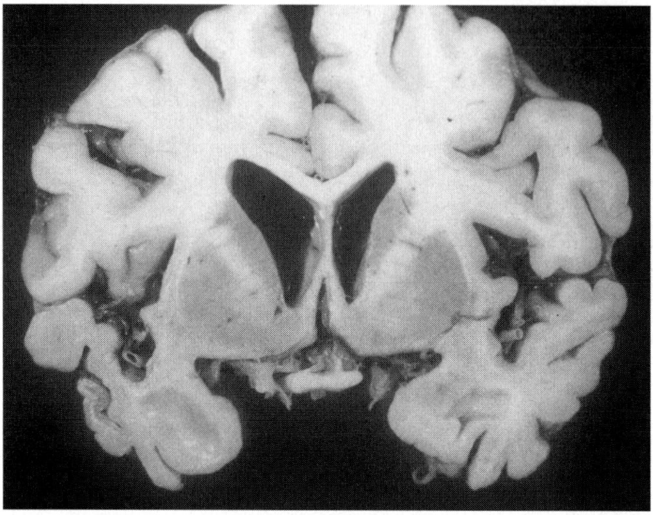

(A)

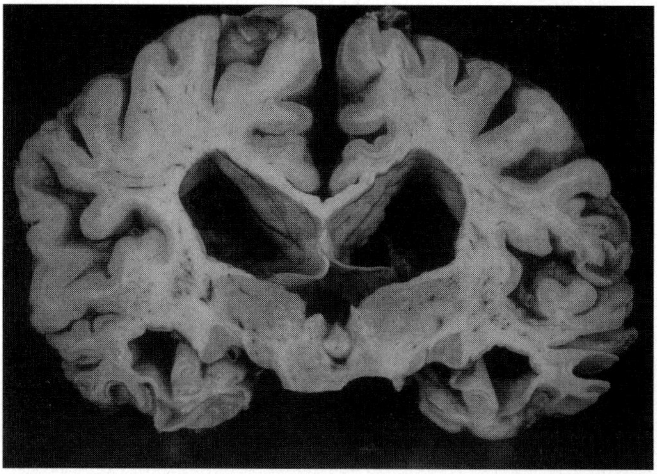

(B)

Figure 11 Pick disease; coronal sections of brain from two patients. Panel B shows more severe degree of atrophy (with hydrocephalus ex vacuo) than panel A. However, both cases illustrate preferential atrophy (amounting to knife-edge atrophy in panel B) of the middle and inferior temporal gyri, with relative sparing of the superior temporal gyrus. In panel A, the middle and inferior temporal atrophy is more severe on the left than the right.

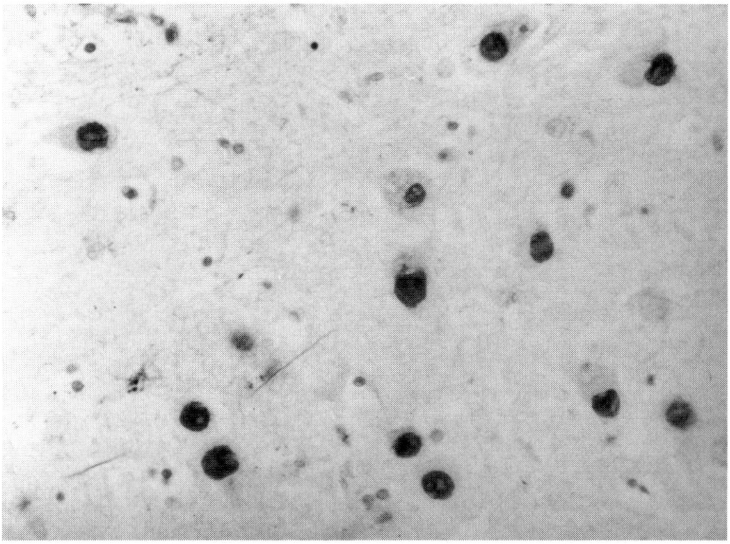

(A)

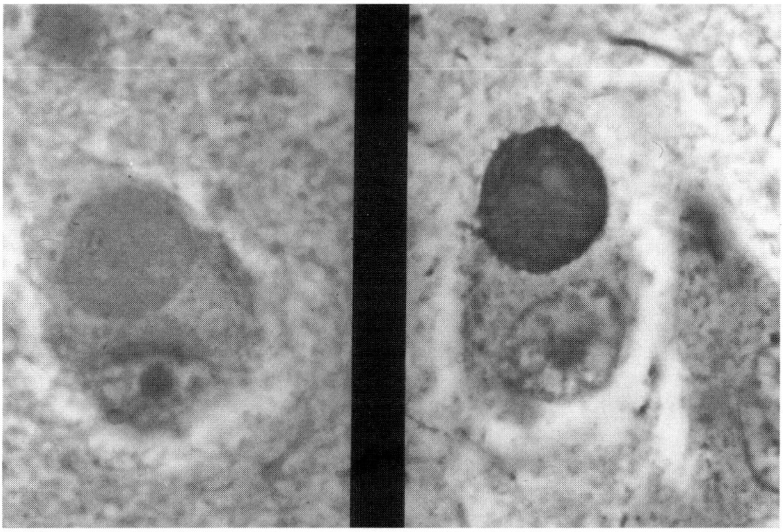

(B)

Figure 12 Pick bodies. (A) Silver-stained section shows numerous argyrophilic neuronal cytoplasmic inclusions; neuronal nuclei are barely visible. (B) Magnified views of Pick body-bearing neurons stained with H&E (left panel) and a silver technique (right panel). Though Pick body is visible even on H&E staining as a cytoplasmic skein of fibrillar material, appearance is dramatically highlighted with the silver stain.

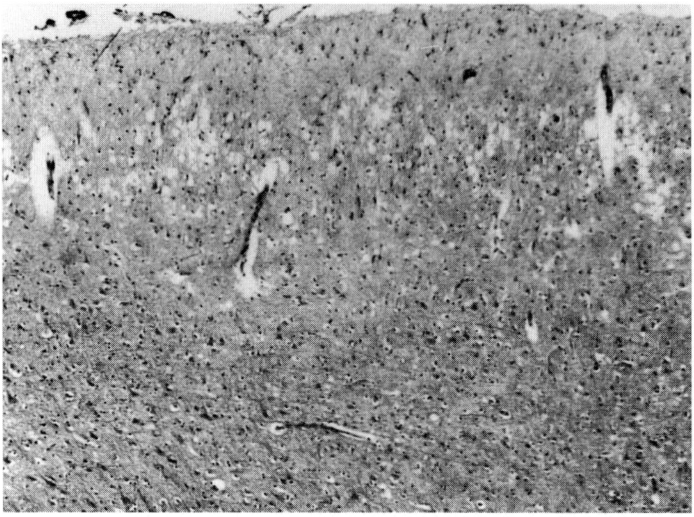

(A)

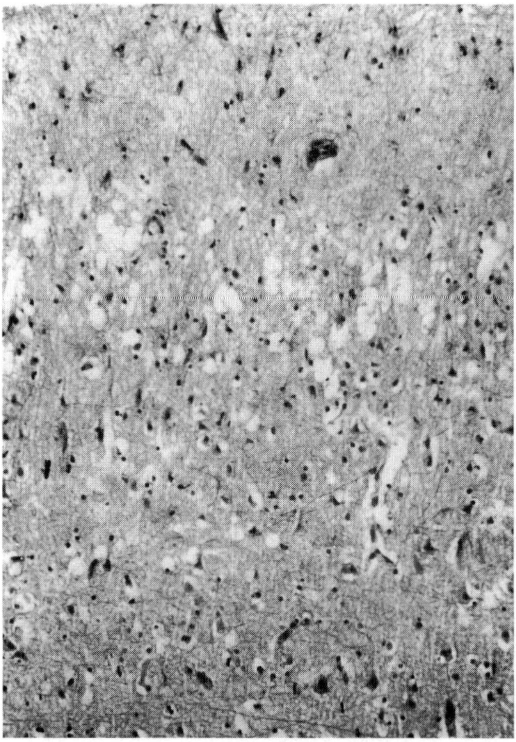

(B)

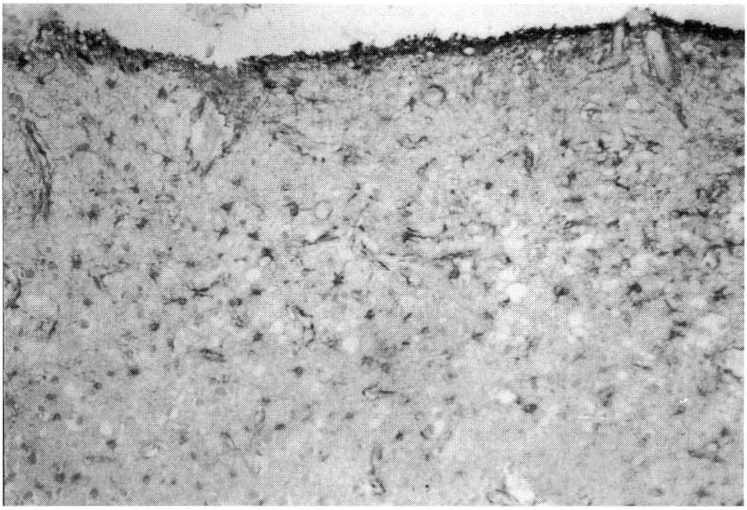

(C)

Figure 13 FTD, microscopic appearance of cortex. Note the diffuse spongy appearance of the superficial cortex. (A,B), with associated pronounced astrocytic gliosis, highlighted with the use of anti-GFAP immunohistochemistry (C). Unfortunately, this appearance, while characteristic of FTD brain, is also sometimes seen in AD/SDAT.

effectively demonstrated using anti-GFAP immunohistochemistry (Fig. 13). Neuron loss is noted in cortical layers II and III, and neurons of layer V are noted to be atrophic though present. (NB: It should be noted that this superficial cortical spongy change is also sometimes seen in the neocortex of patients with otherwise typical AD/SDAT.) Typified by their absence in this "purest" form of FTD are Pick bodies, swollen neurons, and Lewy bodies; immunohistochemistry using primary antibodies to tau, ubiquitin, and alpha beta-crystallin is unrevealing.

d. Corticobasal Degeneration (CBD). Synonyms for this disease include corticodentatonigral degeneration with neuronal achromasia and corticobasal ganglionic degeneration. Affected patients present in the sixth or seventh decade with extremely complex symptomatology that includes a slowly progressive condition characterized by a unilateral tremulous, akinetic, rigid, and apraxic limb held in a fixed dystonic posture. The linkage of CBD to FTDs has been suggested because of neurobehavioral similarities; i.e., CBD patients may show aphasia and behavior characteristic of a frontal lobe disturbance. Kinship between this condition and other predominantly extrapyramidal disorders has also been suggested.

CBD may be a difficult diagnosis neuropathologically as well as clinically. Sections of affected brain show basophilic neuronal cytoplasmic inclusions (not unlike NFTs of AD), multifocal neuron loss, and astrocytic gliosis. Ballooned/swollen neurons showing tau, alpha beta-crystallin, and phosphorylated neurofilament (but minimal ubiquitin) immunoreactivity are characteristically present, especially in neocortical layer II. The substantia nigra shows variable neuron loss.

2. *Molecular Pathogenesis and Genetics*

As mentioned, FTDs have a strong hereditary component. Hence there has been feverish activity aimed at discovering a responsible gene or group of genes. Though there is no universal agreement on a unique locus that is associated with FTD, linkage to chromosome 17 has been suggested (see also the discussion of DDPA below).

C. Diffuse Lewy Body Disease (DLBD)

This entity is in competition with the "FTD family" and multi-infarct or ischemic vascular dementia as the second most common form of dementing illness. Its biology and neuropathologic features are inextricably linked with those of idiopathic Parkinson's disease. There is also still considerable debate as to whether this constitutes a distinctive nosologic entity or represents a variant of AD/SDAT or of Parkinson's disease see discussion below. One result has been the evolution of competing nomenclatures for this group of conditions; the following are among the descriptive terms (in addition to DLBD) that have been applied to slightly different or even identical forms of the same disease: Lewy body variant of AD, senile dementia of Lewy body type, and diffuse cortical Lewy body disease (Lewy body dementia). The all-encompassing term Lewy body disease may be used to describe conditions associated with the presence of these structures in the cortex, brainstem, or both. For a lucid discussion of the controversy surrounding issues of nomenclature and terminology with this group of conditions, see Hansen and Galasko (1992), Ref. 13.

1. *Clinicopathologic Features*

Variable numbers of Lewy bodies (LBs) occur in the neocortex of the vast majority of patients who meet neuropathologic criteria for the diagnosis of idiopathic Parkinson's disease (PD) (for discussion of this entity and a description of Lewy body structure, see below). Recognition of this fact resulted from the widespread use of modern immunohistochemical techniques that optimize the pathologist's ability to detect LBs in the neocortex, where they can otherwise be difficult to visualize (Fig. 14). However, some patients may have abundant and widely distributed cortical LBs (temporal lobe, insular cortex, and cingulate gyrus seem to be sites of predilection) whereas others have only relatively few.

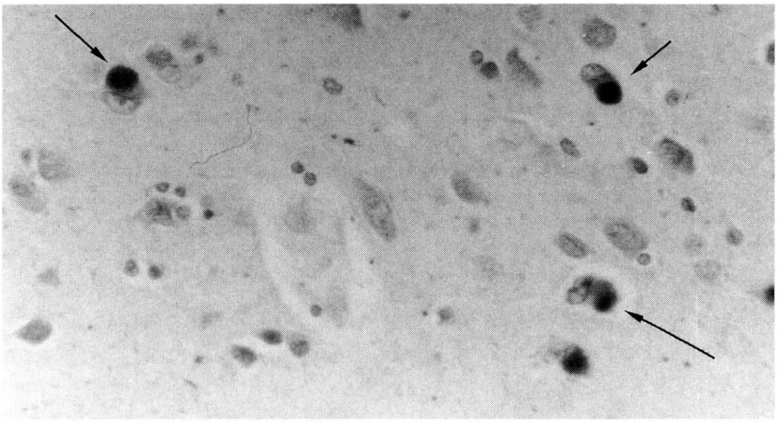

Figure 14 Neocortical LBs (arrows), highlighted using antiubiquitin immunohistochemistry. See also Figure 16.

A small minority of patients have what might be considered "pure" DLBD, with widely distributed cortical LBs and an absence of AD neuropathologic change. As well, such patients' symptoms are usually those of an extrapyramidal disorder rather than dementia.

Among Lewy body disease patients who present with dementia, however, only a minority have, as their neuropathologic substrate, LBs restricted to the brainstem with only scattered LBs in the cortex—i.e., neuropathologic features of idiopathic PD. As many as 60% of PD patients also have pathologic features of AD/SDAT. AD-related neuropathologic change is less pronounced in DLBD patients than in those with the pure form of AD/SDAT (if such exists!). Specifically, relatively fewer NFTs are present in DLBD patients than in those with AD/SDAT and while SP densities may be comparable between AD/SDAT and DLBD, a larger proportion of SPs in DLBD are of the diffuse type; i.e., they lack neuritic change. This suggests that such DLBD patients may have a relatively earlier stage of concomitant AD/SDAT. As Hansen and Galasko (1992) (Ref. 13) have stated, "AD pathology in Lewy body disease cannot . . . be the result of coincidental 'normal aging' superimposed upon a neurodegenerative process driven exclusively by . . . Lewy bodies."

It appears that the spectrum of "Lewy body disease" has both a clinical and a neuropathologic aspect: clinically, disease in affected patients ranges from an extrapyramidal disorder in which bradykinesia and rigidity are prominent, to one characterized more by dementia than extrapyramidal features; pathologically, the continuum encompasses (at one end) classic features of idiopathic PD with pigmented neuron loss, gliosis, and LBs in the brainstem (pigmented nuclei) and at the other widespread neocortical LBs, *usually* with an admixture of AD changes with especially prominent SPs. DLBD patients have a dementia that in many respects is similar to that which characterizes AD/SDAT. However, fluctuations in cognitive ability may cause diagnostic confusion with ischemic-vascular dementia. Psychiatric features (delusions, hallucinations, depression) tend to be more common than in AD, and extrapyramidal manifestations are less pronounced than in PD, usually with an absence of the typical resting ("pill-rolling") tremor.

D. Other Causes of Dementia

The disorders described above account for the vast majority of patients with dementia. Rare conditions include progressive subcortical gliosis (of Neumann), a dementing illness characterized by widespread astrocytic gliosis involving (as the name implies) subcortical and deep white matter, as well as various "deep gray matter" structures including thalamus and the inferior olivary nuclei. Of biologic interest is the recent finding, within a familial form of the disease, of prion protein (see Chap. 4) in affected brain and linkage of the disorder to chromosome 17 (see also the possible role of chromosome 17 in FTDs, discussed above). It has been suggested that chromosome 17-linked dementia may constitute a distinct disease. Its clinical characteristics include disinhibition, dementia, parkinsonism, and amyotrophy (hence the abbreviation DDPA), while the associated neuropathologic features include neuron loss, gliosis, and spongiform change in limbic neocortex as as well as neocortical association areas and subcortical nuclei (including the substantia nigra) and argyrophilic neuronal inclusions with distinct histochemical and ultrastructural features. Even rarer causes of dementia include a condition described as "intranuclear inclusion body disease."

Other neuropathologic conditions that may have dementia as a major or presenting symptom are discussed elsewhere in this book. Multiple sclerosis patients may, for example, develop dementia though clinical presentation in this way is extraordinarily rare. Patients may become demented after experiencing an episode or repeated episodes of anoxic/ischemic encephalopathy—e.g., in the course of cardiopulmonary arrest with resuscitation. In one such patient we have studied, bilateral hippocampal pyramidal cell neuron loss with gliosis was the only significant neuropathologic finding, though the patient had experienced a "dementing" illness after several intraoperative episodes of severe hypotension preceding the onset of his neurologic difficulties. Various diffusely infiltrating neoplasms can present as a dementing illness and, in the absence of a well-defined tumor mass, may be misdiagnosed as a "parenchymal" dementia until the time of brain biopsy or autopsy; three rare ones are gliomatosis cerebri, widely infiltrating primary CNS lymphoma, and disseminated intravascular lymphomatosis (previously referred to as intravascular angioendotheliosis). Infectious disorders that can present with dementia, including CNS infections with agents having unusual biological properties (spongiform encephalopathies) are discussed in Chapter 4. Though rare as a disease entity, this must always be relatively prominent in the differential diagnosis of any patient who undergoes brain biopsy for a rapidly progressive dementia; the likelihood of this diagnosis becomes greater when the patient has experienced myoclonic jerks and is known to have characteristic EEG abnormalities. Metabolic disorders (e.g., ceroid lipofuscinosis) may not manifest until relatively late in life, at which time they present as dementia.

V. PARKINSON'S DISEASE

We take leave now of diseases that present primarily/exclusively with dementia, to consider several entities that have major motor/sensorimotor components.

Idiopathic Parkinson's disease (PD), the commonest form, is inextricably linked with the biology of the Lewy body (LB) (first described in the early 1900s) and hence DLBD, which is discussed extensively above. A much less common form of PD, the postencephalitic variant, will be reviewed briefly. Described in the early 1800s by Parkinson as "the shaking palsy" and amplified later in the century by Charcot, PD came to be recognized as a disorder affecting the substantia nigra and striatonigral pathways in the early decades of this century.

A. Clinicopathologic Features

PD presents as a slowly progressive neurologic disorder characterized by tremor, rigidity, and bradykinesia. Masklike (expressionless) facies, postural instability, and a festinating gait are often seen. Clinically, the differential diagnosis includes rare conditions such as striatonigral degeneration (SND), progressive supranuclear palsy (PSP), and multiple system atrophy (MSA; see below). Disease onset is generally in the early seventh decade of life, and patients survive, according to one large recent study, for a mean of 13 years; i.e., death usually occurs in the mid-eighth decade, with a very broad range for all of these figures, e.g., the diagnosis of idiopathic PD has been made in individuals as young as 30 years. Effective treatment of the illness with levodopa and DOPA decarboxylase inhibitors has increased survival among PD patients by as much as 3 to 6 years. PD patients most commonly present with asymmetric tremor, though up to one-fifth of affected patients may have absence of a resting tremor. Dementia occurs in over 40% of patients; the controversy over whether this is due to concomitant AD/SDAT, the presence of neocortical LBs, or both, is discussed above. Of interest, in some large necropsy series, as many as one-third of PD patients have concomitant striatal pathologic changes, including, most commonly, lacunar infarcts or SPs that may contribute to the symptoms.

Postencephalitic parkinsonism, seen rarely now, was thought to be a consequence of the pandemic of encephalitis lethargica that occurred predominantly in 1917 to 1925. Neuropathologic features of affected patients included severe pigmented neuron loss in the substantia nigra (SN) with the presence of neurofibrillary tangles in remaining neurons and elsewhere throughout the brain. This rare condition is of historical interest in that examination of the brains of affected individuals clearly implicated the SN as a major site of neuropathologic change in patients with a classic parkinsonian syndrome.

Neuropathologic features of PD include characteristic gross, microscopic, and immunohistochemical components. At brain cutting, the SN and locus ceruleus (LC), the most prominently pigmented nuclei of the brainstem, show loss of their normal dark appearance (Fig. 15). Microscopic diagnosis is based on the finding of depletion of pigmented neurons in the SN and LC with LBs in at least some of the remaining neurons (Fig. 16). LBs, quite readily identified on routine H&E-stained sections, may also be seen in nonpigmented neurons throughout the brainstem and basal forebrain nuclei and within neocortex,

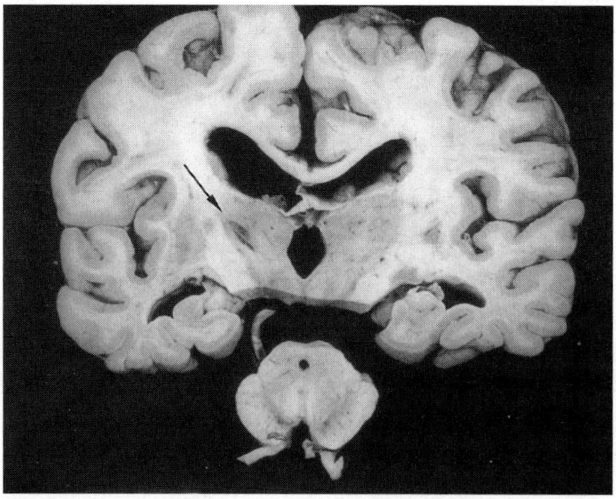

Figure 15 Parkinson's disease. Midbrain (bottom of figure) shows marked pallor of substantia nigra, especially its lateral portions. Coronal section of cerebral hemispheres shows a linear scar in the thalamus (arrow), representing a stereotactic thalamotomy carried out years prior to the patient's death. This was one treatment for severe tremor in PD patients. A more recent form of surgical intervention, effective in some PD patients, is stereotactic pallidotomy.

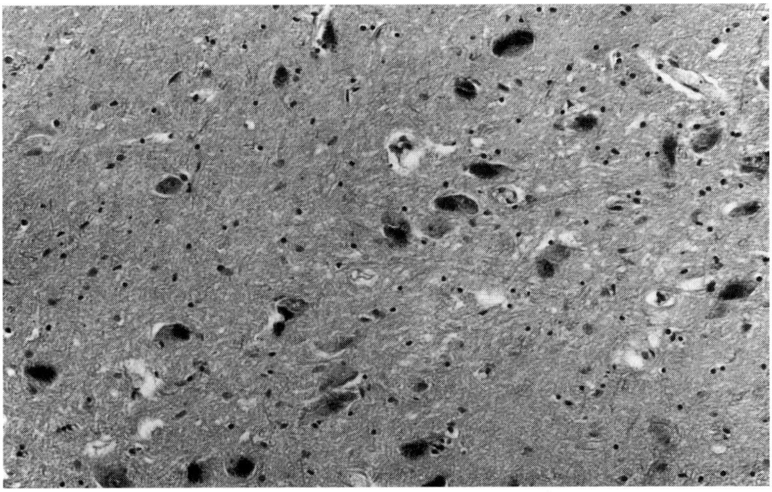

(A)

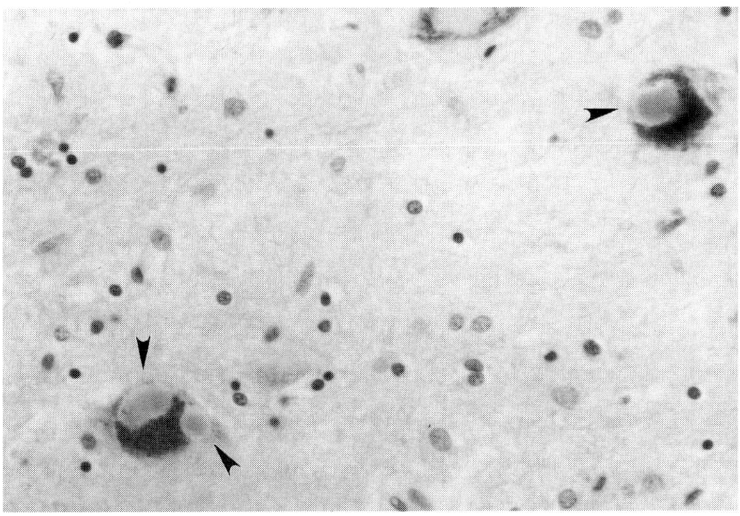

(B)

Figure 16 (A) Microscopic appearance of normal substantia nigra, showing neurons containing abundant cytoplasmic neuromelanin. In PD (idiopathic or postencephalitic), there is severe loss of such pigmented neurons; in idiopathic PD, many residual neurons contain cytoplasmic Lewy bodies (arrows, panel B). These are (on H&E stain) eosinophilic or magenta-colored cytoplasmic inclusions with a surrounding halo. Multiple LBs of varying size may be present in an affected neuron, as in the cell at lower left (double arrowhead).

where they are dramatically highlighted using ubiquitin immunohistochemistry (see Fig. 14). Though anti-ubiquitin antibodies label LBs, they also stain NFTs and SP neurites; i.e., ubiquitin immunostains must be evaluated in the anatomical context of the lesion(s) under evaluation. Multiple LBs may be seen in an affected neuron. Variable astrocytic gliosis may be present within (especially) the SN, and neuromelanin may be seen in an extracellular location in the neuropil ("pigment incontinence") or having been ingested by macrophages.

Shy-Drager Syndrome describes a rare condition defined by parkinsonian features and profound autonomic instability (e.g., severe orthostatic hypotension). Neuropathologic findings in affected patients include degeneration of pigmented nuclei (but LBs are found only rarely) and degeneration of CNS neurons that are components of the autonomic nerous system—e.g., dorsal motor nucleus of the vagus n., intermediolateral cell columns of the thoracic spinal cord.

B. Molecular Pathogenesis and Genetics

The diagnosis of PD depends on the finding of LBs in (especially) the SN and locus ceruleus. Although—as in the case of other intraneuronal cytoplasmic "inclusions"—they may represent a marker for the disease rather than a specific clue to its pathogenesis, and rare LBs are sometimes found in asymptomatic elderly patients—they have been the subject of intense investigation. Biochemical, ultrastructural, and immunohistochemical studies indicate that they are composed of a central (electron-dense by electron microscopy) core surrounded by radiating thick and thin filaments, which include various cytoskeletal components, including neurofilaments that have undergone changes such as phosphorylation, ubiquitination, crosslinking, and proteolysis. Tau is *not* present. LBs are also immunoreactive for a form of amyloid found in a Finnish variant of familial amyloidosis, which results from mutation of a gene encoding gelsolin, an actin-modulating protein. Thus, mechanistic hypotheses as to the mode of LB formation have included (cytoskeletal) protein aggregation followed by subsequent biochemical modifications (see review by Pollanen et al., 1993; Ref. 34). Ubiquitin itself is a polypeptide involved in nonlysosomal, ATP-dependent degradation of abnormal cellular proteins (hence its prevalence in AD as well as the Lewy body diseases).

One of the more recent insights into possible pathogenetic mechanisms important in PD—especially as regards the apparent "selective vulnerability" of the SN—occurred by means of an unfortunate "misadventure of nature." Recreational intravenous drug users in the San Francisco Bay area were found to develop a parkinsonian syndrome that apparently results from contamination of "home-made" batches of drugs with the powerful neurotoxin MPTP. This has led to development of a primate animal model of PD, which develops SN neuropathologic changes that are similar to, but not identical with, alterations that occur in the human disease. Toxic/environmental theories of PD pathogenesis currently dominate the literature, as do ideas about the possible importance of free radicals and oxidative stress. Rare families with PD are under intense scrutiny with the hope that, analogous to work in AD/SDAT, a responsible gene might be isolated in some patients, which would then provide neurobiologic insights to the disorder in ALL patients.

VI. HUNTINGTON'S DISEASE

Unraveling the molecular genetics of this autosomal-dominant disorder (HD; also described as Huntington's chorea, HC) within the past 15 years has represented a triumph of interdisciplinary—not to mention multinational and intercontinental—collaborative research involving dozens of clinicians and basic neuroscientists and geneticists. The apparent disease-producing mechanism—that of a trinucleotide or triplet repeat expansion within the genome—serves as the paradigm by which numerous other neurodegenerative conditions are coming to be understood.

A. Clinicopathologic Features

HD has a prevalence of 4 to 7/100,000, while the heterozygote frequency is approx. 1/5000. Though sporadic cases are described, inheritance is usually as an autosomal-dominant trait. Age of onset is variable; patients may present with late onset (over 50 years of age, representing one-fourth of cases and associated with maternal transmission), in the range of 20 to 49 years (referred to as early or midlife, respectively), or as juvenile disease (10% of cases, especially linked to paternal transmission, associated with a more fulminant course, and most likely to present with rigidity or akinesia). Defining signs and symptoms of the disease include chorea, rigidity, and neuobehavioral abnormalities that eventually lead to dementia.

Overall, the hyperkinetic form—presenting with chorea—is the most prevalent. Cognitive decline may, however, precede and overshadow the movement abnormalities. Survival after diagnosis can be for as long as 15 to 20 years. The differential diagnosis is most difficult in patients who present with dementia (in whom the differential includes any of the presenile dementias; see above) or the rigid/akinetic form (in whom other considerations are juvenile PD, Wilson's disease, or other metabolic abnormalities that involve the brain). There is no effective treatment for HD.

Neuropathologic features include, grossly, cerebral atrophy, especially involving cortex but also subcortical white matter, and, usually, more profound atrophy of the caudate nucleus (Fig. 17), putamen, and globus pallidus. The micro-

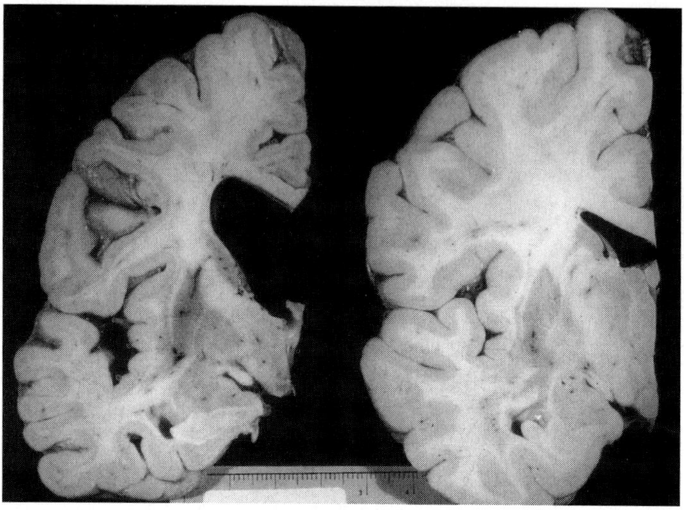

Figure 17 Huntington's disease. Coronal hemisection of brain from an affected patient (left side of figure), in contrast with a control/normal hemisection from the same plane (right). Note diffuse cortical atrophy, with especially prominent shrinkage of the caudate and lentiform nucleus, both of which showed neuron loss and astrocytic gliosis. There is resultant enlargement of the left lateral ventricle.

scopic correlate of ganglionic atrophy is neuron loss and astrocytic proliferation (gliosis). Neurons involved earliest in the disease include GABA-ergic cells and those producing several other peptide neurotransmitters (e.g., substance P, enkephalin), while late in the disease neurons containing somatostatin, neuropeptide Y, and nitric oxide (NO) synthase are affected. The neocortical changes may be difficult to appreciate in the absence of immunohistochemical study; large pyramidal neurons are lost, but the degree of gliosis can be surprisingly minimal. Juvenile-onset patients may show cerebellar atrophy with loss of Purkinje cells.

B. Molecular Pathogenesis and Genetics

Early in the 1980s, based on study of a large South American kindred of affected patients, the HD gene was localized to chromosome 4p. The gene has been found to contain a long repeat of the trinucleotide/triplet sequence CAG. In normals, CAG repeats range from 9 to 35 (mean 19), whereas in HD-affected patients the comparable figures are 37 to 120+ (mean around 45 to 50). This has led to a highly sensitive and specific molecular diagnostic test for HD, though there is slight overlap in the number of CAG repeats between affected and unaffected individuals. The gene encodes a protein, *huntingtin*, with as yet unknown function or pathophysiologic significance despite the finding that the gene and its protein are widely expressed in both the CNS and viscera. Thus, a leading set of hypotheses predicts that HD may result from interaction of huntingtin with a protein or group of proteins which shows a more circumscribed expression pattern, explaining the "selective vulnerability" of certain neuronal groups within the brains of affected patients.

Neuronal cell death in HD appears to involve inappropriate apoptosis. CAG triplet repeat expansion encodes a protein with polyglutamine stretches of varying lengths, which in turn influence proteolytic cleavage of the huntingtin molecule—although huntingtin cleavage occurs to some extent with CAG repeats of "wild-type" size in the course of apoptosis. Put differently, the CAG repeat expansion may enhance a normal cellular function. Other proteins (e.g., glyceraldehyde-3-phosphate dehydrogenase [GAPDH], ubiquitin-conjugating enzyme) may interact with huntingtin to produce neuronal injury/death. These novel observations pertinent to the mechanism of action of huntingtin have been made largely in tissue culture experiments. The challenge to clinical and experimental neuropathologists will be to test their relevance in human tissues, and to assist with development and validation of an appropriate animal model for HD, which has not yet been achieved.

HD also shows "anticipation" within families; i.e., successive generations tend to have an increasingly early age of disease onset. This may be explained by the finding that later generations with the disease tend to have increasing lengths of CAG repeats, since the greater the number of such triplet repeats, the younger is the age of disease onset and the more rapid its rate of progression.

VII. PROGRESSIVE SUPRANUCLEAR PALSY (PSP)

Also known as Steele-Richardson-Olszewski syndrome in honor of the physicians who first described and defined this disorder in Toronto during the early 1960s, this rare condition—which has extrapyramidal, brainstem, and neurocognitive components—must be in the differential diagnosis for any patient with these major groups of clinical signs and symptoms.

A. Clinicopathologic Features

PSP is a relatively rare, nonfamilial condition, occurring with roughly equal frequency in men and women, showing clinical onset at age 55 years and beyond, usually in the mid- to late 60s or 70s. Disease duration to death is usually from 3 to 10 years. Patients may present with one or more features from a constellation of clinical abnormalities, the most commonly observed of which are bradykinesia, rigidity, gait difficulties, and postural tremor—a picture quite similar to that seen in PD. A distinguishing finding in PSP patients is the presence of supranuclear gaze palsy or ophthalmoplegia. Patients with ophthalmoplegia are much more likely than those without to develop dementia.

Neuropathologic features observed grossly may be relatively nonspecific. Atrophy may be (but often is not!) visualized in the basal ganglia, subthalamus, and brainstem (especially midbrain) (Fig. 18), with associated dilatation of the third ventricle and cerebral aqueduct. Pigmented brainstem nuclei (i.e., SN and LC) may appear pale. Microscopic sections of brain show neuron loss and gliosis, together with abundant intraneuronal neurofibrillary tangles and neuropil threads, throughout multiple sites of the deep central gray matter, brainstem, and cerebellar nuclei. Structures especially likely to show changes include globus pallidus, subthalamic nucleus, and nucleus basalis of Meynert and

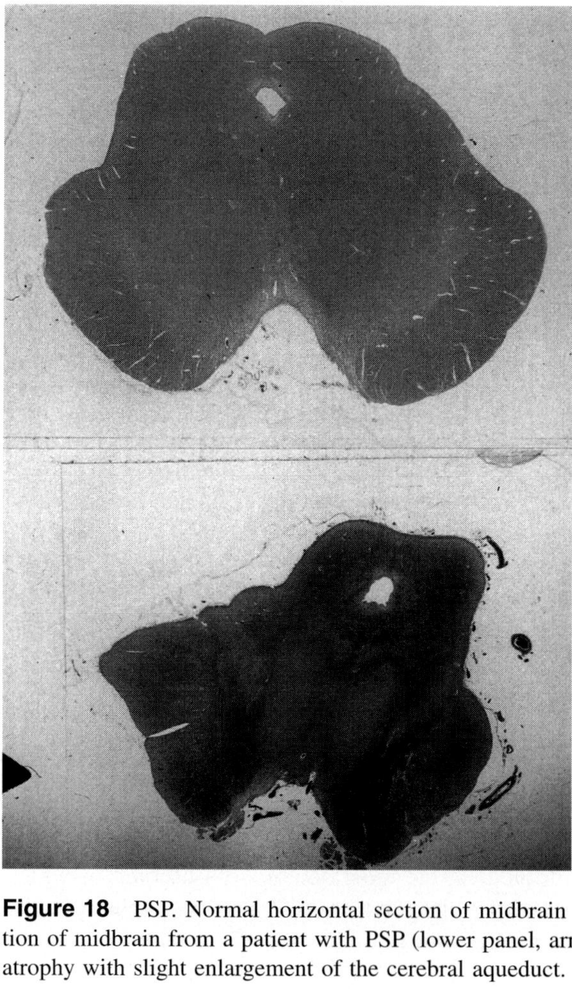

Figure 18 PSP. Normal horizontal section of midbrain (top panel) in contrast to section of midbrain from a patient with PSP (lower panel, arrowhead). Note mesencephalic atrophy with slight enlargement of the cerebral aqueduct.

(within brainstem and cerebellum) the colliculi, SN, red nucleus, nuclei of cranial nerves III and IV, dentate nucleus of the cerebellum, pontine, and inferior olivary nuclei. NFT (but relatively scarce SP) are seen in the neocortex (which may also show neuron loss, gliosis, and atrophy), especially laminae III to VI, hippocampus, and parahippocampal region. Tau immunohistochemistry effectively demonstrates the NFT change and neuropil threads and immunostains some neurons that do not show obvious NFT cytoskeletal alterations.

NFT of PSP differ from AD-associated NFT (see above) by:

1. A more "globose/globular" intracytoplasmic configuration, possibly imposed on them by the distinctive shapes of neurons in which they occur (Fig. 19)
2. Relative absence of PHF but presence of 12- to 15-nm-diameter straight filaments on ultrastructural examination
3. Different tau isoforms

It may be safe to conjecture that the cellular pathogenesis of PSP hinges on derangements of the normal neuronal cytoskeleton, its assembly, transport, or breakdown.

Clinical considerations aside, the *neuropathologic* differential diagnosis includes (previously described) postencephalitic PD, which PSP closely mimics morphologically, and an entity described among patients in Guam by the term parkinsonian-dementia complex. As the name of the latter implies, affected patients consistently show dementia and manifest widespread neurofibrillary pathology in basal and brainstem structures as well as the neocortex—a picture almost identical to that of PSP and postencephalitic PD.

VIII. MOTOR NEURON DISEASE (MND)/AMYOTROPHIC LATERAL SCLEROSIS (ALS)

The names MND and ALS are used, respectively, in the United Kingdom and the U.S., to describe a constellation of degenerative diseases characterized by progressive loss of motor neurons (in the brainstem and spinal cord) and degeneration of the corticospinal tracts (CSTs). Though the terms are used somewhat interchangeably, the authors prefer the designation of MND.

A. Clinicopathologic Features

Included in this group of diseases are patients who present primarily with bulbar palsy (e.g., manifest as dysphagia), motor weakness ("spinal muscular atrophy") including muscle wasting and fasciculations, and spastic paraparesis ("primary lateral sclerosis"). Onset is extremely variable, though usually in the fifth or sixth decade of life. Most series report an approximately twofold male predominance, and survival beyond 5 years after diagnosis is rare. Dementia, when it occurs, is of the FTD type (see above). Findings at the time of presenta-

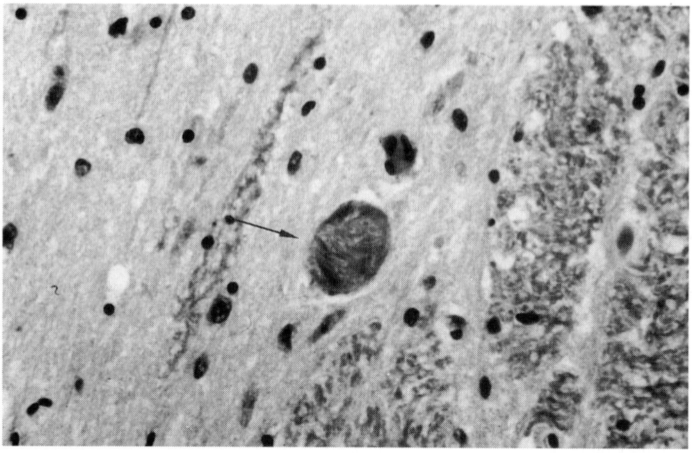

(A)

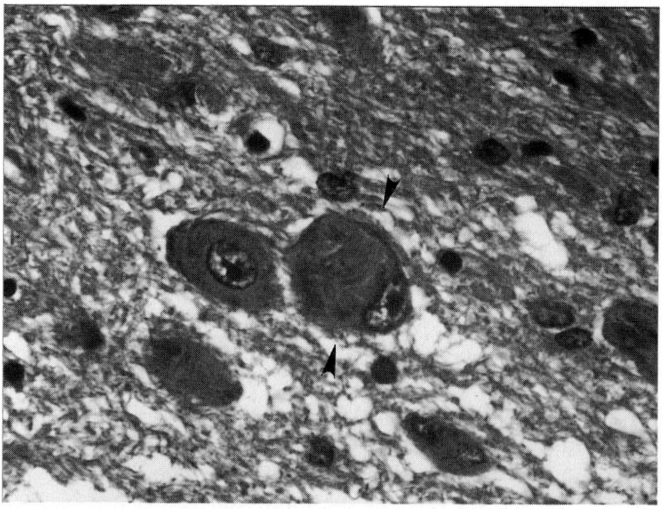

(B)

Figure 19 "Globose" NFTs in brainstem neurons, of the type seen in PSP. Note fibrillar material filling the cytoplasm (arrows). These structures can often be visualized on H&E stains, but are highlighted using silver stains and tau antibodies. Contrast appearance with that of cortical NFT seen in AD/SDAT (Fig. 5) and Pick bodies (Fig. 12).

tion usually include a combination of abnormalities pointing to both upper and lower motor neuron disease. No effective treatment is currently available, though in view of pathogenetic theories (see below), candidate drugs include antioxidants, glutamate receptor antagonists, and various neurotrophic factors.

Neuropathologic features, as expected, involve both the neuromuscular system and the CNS. Skeletal muscle shows changes of severe denervation atrophy. CNS alterations have been described in several elegant papers, but probably never more thoroughly than in the study of Brownell et al. (1970), Ref. 4. Grossly visible abnormalities may be minimal, consisting of varying degrees of cortical atrophy (see discussion of MND-FTD) and shrinkage of ventral roots of the spinal cord. Variable neuron loss (with associated astrogliosis) is noted in several motor nuclei of the lower brainstem (especially the hypoglossal) and throughout the anterior horn cell population of the spinal cord, with relative sparing of autonomic nuclei (Fig. 20). Pyramidal tract degeneration is often most prominent in the spinal cord, but may be seen at any level, including the internal capsule and within brainstem (Fig. 21).

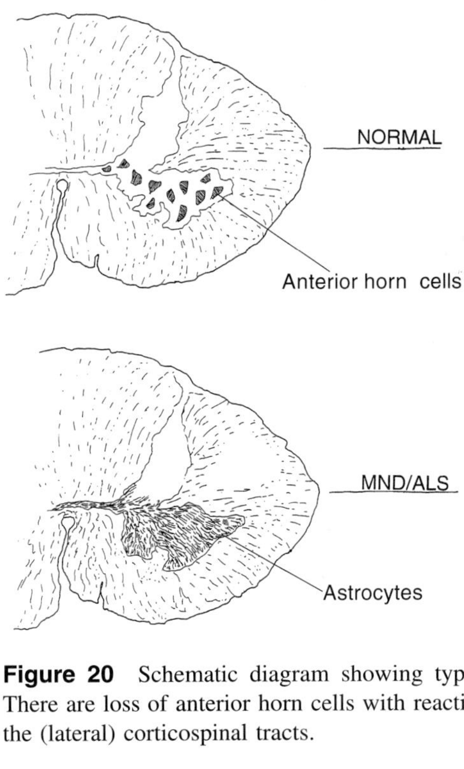

Figure 20 Schematic diagram showing typical spinal cord features of MND/ALS. There are loss of anterior horn cells with reactive astrocytic gliosis, and degeneration of the (lateral) corticospinal tracts.

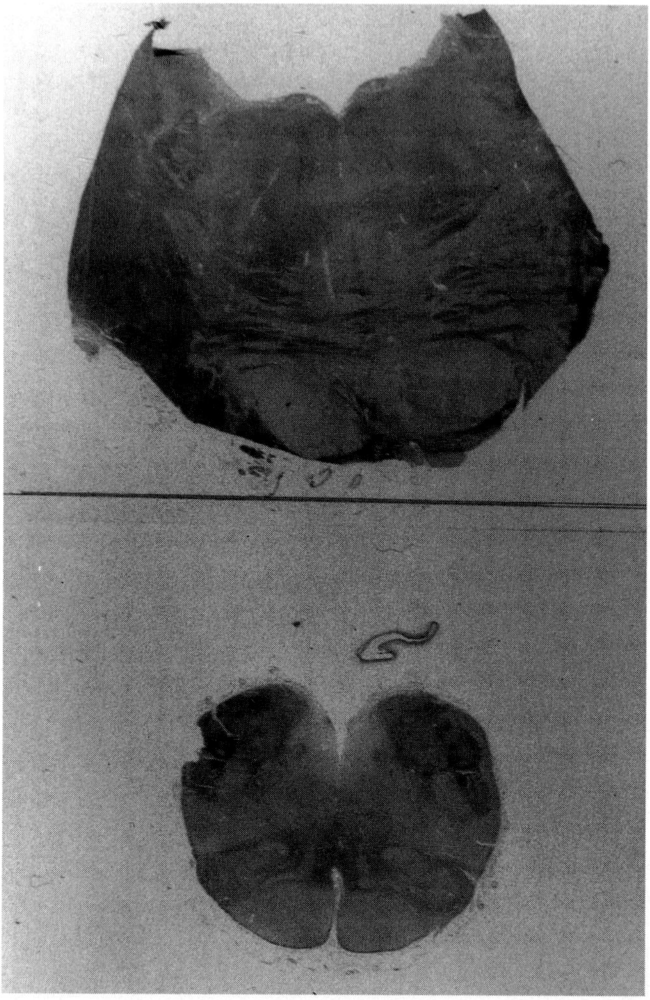

(A)

Figure 21 Myelin-stained sections of pons and medulla (upper and lower segments, panel A) and spinal cord (panel B) removed at autopsy from a patient with MND/ALS. Note severe pallor of corticospinal tracts at all levels. In the spinal cord, both ventral and lateral corticospinal tracts are affected; dorsal columns stand out by their relatively robust normal pattern of staining.

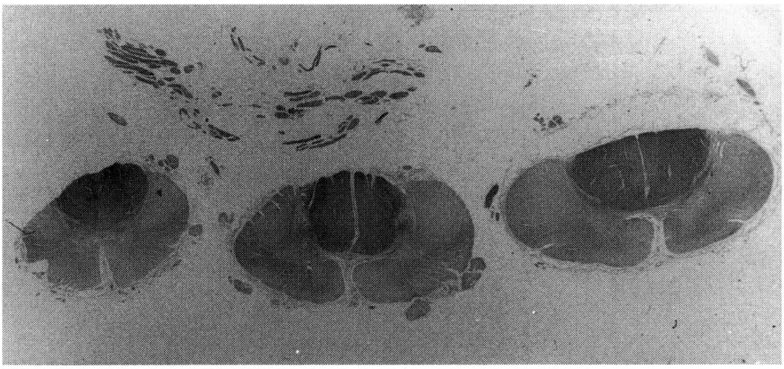

(B)

Neuropathologic examination of the CNS from a patient with end-stage MND/ALS provides few clues to how and why motor neurons die/disappear. Neuronophagia is encountered among a few neurons, the rarity of this phenomenon hardly surprising in a condition that extends over many years. Chromatolysis of residual motor neurons is infrequently observed, though slight microvacuolization of the neuronal cytoplasm may be present. Inflammatory changes seen in exceptional cases suggest (in these few patients) an autoimmune or "infectious" etiology. A variety of neuronal cytoskeletal abnormalities and inclusions have been described in MND/ALS, usually within the cytoplasm of anterior horn cells, including Bunina bodies (round or elongated eosinophilic structures 1 to 10 μm in diameter), various spheroidal or hyaline inclusions, and even Lewy- and Hirano-like bodies. In a Guamanian variant of ALS, granulovacuolar degeneration has been noted within spinal cord anterior horn cells. By immunohistochemistry, neurofilament and ubiquitin epitopes may be localized to these inclusions, and their filamentous ultrastructure is confirmed by electron microscopy. Neurofilament accumulations may extend into the somewhat swollen proximal axons of residual anterior horn cells.

B. Molecular Pathogenesis and Genetics

Etiologic theories of this disorder have centered on atypical infectious (especially viral) agents, environmental toxins, heavy metals, and autoimmune and genetically determined mechanisms. Approximately 5% to 10% of cases of MND/ALS are familial (usually inherited as an autosomal-dominant trait), with an earlier age of onset than for sporadic patients and neuropathologic change that may involve more extensive degeneration of long tracts other than the CSTs (e.g., spinocerebellar tracts). Recently, approx. one in five cases of familial MND/ALS (FALS) have been associated with a mutation in the gene encoding Cu,Zn superoxide dismutase (SOD-1), an enzyme that normally converts the superoxide free radical anion into hydrogen peroxide. At least 40 different missense mutations in SOD-1 have been found in early-onset FALS families. Autosomal-recessive forms of MND/ALS (RFALS) have been identified in Tunisia and Pakistan; some of these variants manifest disease onset in childhood or adolescence. Recessive variants may show predominantly lower motor neuron involvement, while others show primarily upper motor neuron signs and symptoms; by the time of endstage disease, most forms "converge" to the point of showing both upper and lower motor neuron abnormalities clinically and manifestations thereof at autopsy. One form of X-linked bulbar and spinal muscular atrophy (Kennedy's disease) is localized to chromosome Xq21.3-q22 and appears to result from trinucleotide repeats in the gene that encodes the androgen receptor.

Transgenic mice carrying some of the SOD-1 mutations develop features akin to those observed in human MND/ALS and show anterior horn cell loss in the spinal cord at sacrifice. As well, structural abnormalities within affected anterior horn cells are such as to suggest glutamate-induced neurotoxic effects. At this time, however, precise cellular pathogenetic mechanisms operant in patients with SOD-1 mutations are unknown. Likely "final common pathways" by which these mutations cause disease will involve either a loss of normal enzyme function or gain of an adverse function. Though there is no evidence for linkage of human MND/ALS to mutations in genes encoding neurofilament proteins, transgenic mice overexpressing some neurofilament subunits or mutant forms of neurofilament develop weakness and neurogenic muscular atrophy, as in the human disease.

IX. MULTIPLE SYSTEM ATROPHY (MSA)/ SPINOCEREBELLAR DEGENERATIONS

A historical perspective on this heterogeneous, comparatively rare group of disorders is instructive. While most of them have long been recognized as having a familial/genetic component, prior to the era of molecular genetics they were subclassified based on subtle variations of clinical symptomatology and/or neuropathologic findings. Frequently, clinical and neuropathologic overlap of syndromes was observed. Syndromes were frequently named after the individuals who first described them—leading to eponymous descriptions that twisted the tongues of medical students and trainees in clinical neuroscience more often than they illuminated pathogenetic mechanisms.

Within the past 5 to 10 years, there has been a "landslide" of molecular and neurogenetic information pertinent to many of these entities. It is a testimonial to the speed with which the molecular basis for these disorders is emerging that this section of the chapter is likely to be out of date before the manuscript goes to press, much less appears in print! We will therefore provide a cursory description of the relevant clinical and morphoanatomic characteristics that tend to "unify" these diseases and comment briefly on genetic abnormalities as they are currently understood—with strong advice to the reader that this is intended *only* to provide a framework for understanding them. Well-defined entities within this group will be described briefly in greater detail.

A. Clinicopathologic Features

Characteristic of essentially all of the MSAs is presentation at varying ages with some combination of ataxia, motor and extrapyramidal abnormalities, and dementia, with variably rapid progression of signs and symptoms over many months, years, or even decades; i.e., they share some similarities with (previously described) conditions such as PSP, PD, and Lewy body disease, though ataxia is a more prominent feature of MSAs, especially the olivopontocerebellar atrophies.

1. Olivopontocerebellar Atrophy/Degeneration (OPCA)

These disorders can be thought of as being of autosomal-dominant inheritance, of autosomal-recessive inheritance, or sporadic. Their prevalence is around 2/100,000. In familial OPCA there is a male predominance, whereas in sporadic OPCA males and females tend to be affected in equal numbers. Age of onset is extremely variable, ranging from infancy to advanced age, though familial cases are more likely to begin in the third decade, while sporadic examples more commonly present in the sixth decade and beyond. Disease duration ranges from a few months to decades. Defining clinical features include cerebellar dysfunction often with gait ataxia (frequently with identifiable cerebellar atrophy on appropriate imaging studies), usually pyramidal tract symptoms and ocular movement abnormalities, and one or more of a variety of other neurologic findings including (but not restricted to) dementia, abnormalities of sphincter function, dementia and dysphagia. Epileptic seizures and resting tremor are generally not part of the clinical constellation, though myoclonus may occur in late stages.

Examination of the brain (grossly) reveals marked atrophy of the cerebellum and brainstem (especially pons and inferior olivary nuclei of the medulla) (Fig. 22), with relative preservation of supratentorial structures, though in the spectrum of MSA shrinkage of the basal ganglia may be noted. Microscopic examination shows loss of cerebellar Purkinje cells and often granule cells, but relative preservation of the dentate nucleus. Pontine nuclei of the basis pontis show neuron loss with astrocytic proliferation (gliosis), which may be noted as well in the inferior olivary nuclei. Loss of some neurons may represent a "transsynaptic degenerative" phenomenon in consequence of "primary" loss of

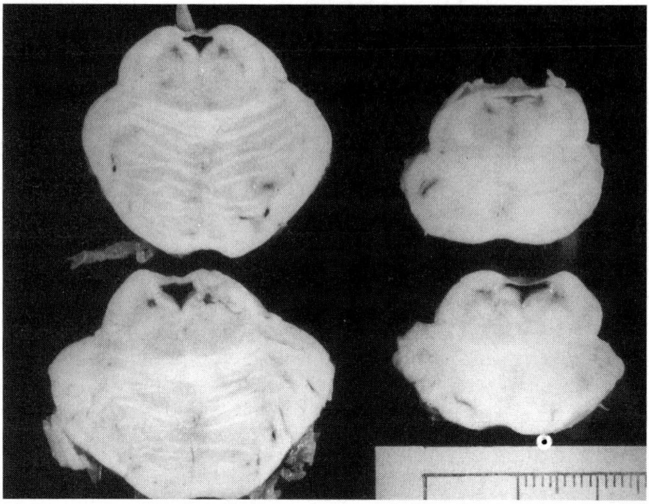

Figure 22 OPCA/MSA. Normal sections of pons (left side of figure) in contrast to comparable sections from a patient with severe OPCA (right side). In section from the affected individual, there is profound atrophy with especially prominent shrinkage of the basis pontis. Slight depigmentation of the locus ceruleus is also noted.

a well-defined group of cells. However, defining the neuron population initially affected can be a daunting, sometimes impossible task. Neuron loss within basal ganglia is variable from case to case. Argyrophilic inclusions may be seen within the cytoplasm of neurons and oligodendrocytes, especially in sporadic OPCA.

2. *Molecular Pathogenesis and Genetics*

Studies in the 1970s and 1980s documented enzyme and neurotransmitter abnormalities in some of these disorders, many of which were subsequently found to be nonspecific. More recently, genetic "lesions" have been discovered as the basis for several MSA/OPCAs. An important caveat to this information: Defining a genetic mutation underlying a disease does not always explain cellular pathogenesis, though it has major implications for molecular diagnostics relevant to previously mysterious illnesses. Clinical and experimental neuropathologists are likely to be key players in deciphering specific information as to how the genes actually cause lesions within the CNS.

Recent classification of the MSA/OPCAs based on identified mutations has revealed the following genetic loci to be of importance:

OPCA type I (gene SCA1) maps to chromosome 6p22-23; the mutation appears to determine an unstable trinucleotide/triplet repeat, CAG, similar to that observed in HD. The encoded protein is ataxin-1.

Gene SCA2 is localized on chromosome 12q23-24.1. Again, a CAG repeat has been observed, and the encoded protein is ataxin-2.

Gene SCA3, associated with Machado-Joseph disease, maps to chromosome 14q32.1. A CAG repeat is associated with the protein ataxin-3.

Two other genes, SCA4 (on chromosome 16q) and SCA6, on 19p are associated with phenotypes that include ataxia and sensory neuropathy.

The triplet/trinucleotide repeat disorders share pathogenetic features with HD (e.g., anticipation, worse prognosis as a function of larger number of repeats).

3. Friedreich Ataxia (*FA*)

This autosomal-recessive degeneration should more properly be considered a systemic disease than one that involves only the nervous system. Affected patients often have cardiomyopathy, pes cavus, skeletal abnormalities, hypertrophic cardiomyopathy, and endocrine abnormalities. Presentation is generally before puberty, usually with ataxia in the lower limbs. Neuropathologic features include degeneration of the dorsal columns and corticospinal and spinocerebellar tracts. Patients also often show degeneration of dorsal root ganglia with a resultant axonal neuropathy.

FA is also a triplet repeat disorder, but the trinucleotide expansion is of GAA rather than CAG. The abnormal gene maps to chromosome 9 and encodes the protein frataxin. The exact molecular pathogenesis of this trinucleotide repeat disorder appears to differ from that of the previously described entities, in which CAG repeats predominate.

4. Dentatorubropallidoluysian Atrophy (*DRPLA*)

This is an extraordinarily rare neurodegenerative disorder characterized by pathologic abnormalities in (as the name suggests) pallidofugal and dentatorubral pathways and the subthalamic nucleus, though other neuronal populations may be affected. It is of neurogenetic interest insofar as it represents yet another example of disease determined by CAG (trinucleotide) repeats in a gene on chromosome 12.

5. Striatonigral Degeneration

There is debate as to whether this represents a distinct disease. Patients present, usually in the fifth or sixth decade, with extrapyramidal features (sometimes including orthostatic hypotension); i.e., clinical features mimic PD or Shy-Drager syndrome. At autopsy, neuron loss and gliosis are widespread within the basal ganglia, substantia nigra, pons, and cerebellum (Fig. 23).

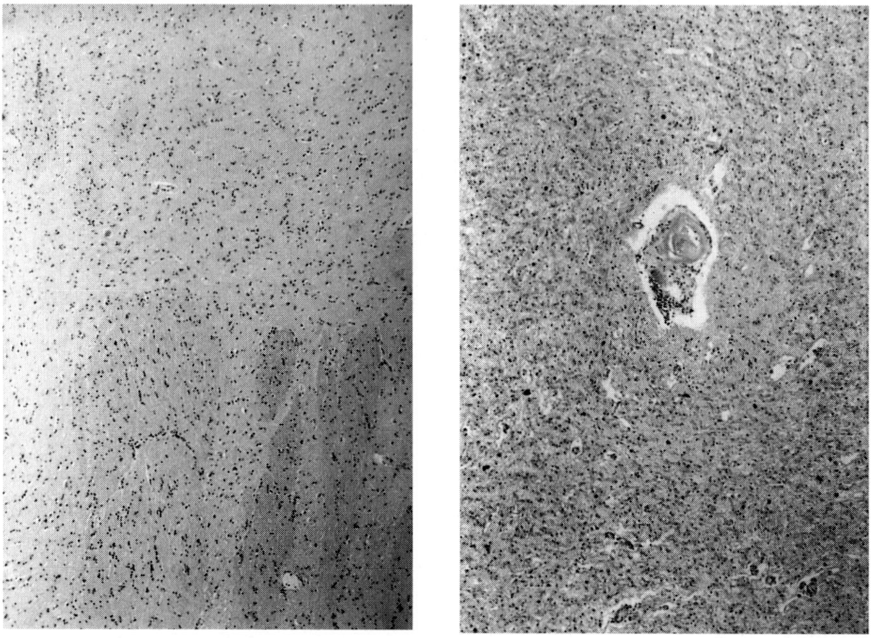

(A) (B)

Figure 23 Striatonigral degeneration. Autopsy specimen shows control/normal striatum (A) contrasted with severely gliotic striatum from comparable region in an affected patient. (B) Increase in cell density is the result of astrocyte proliferation. (C) Section (at slightly higher magnification) of affected striatum immunostained with anti-GFAP highlights the prominence of reactive astrocytes. (D) Substantia nigra contains residual intact neuromelanin-containing neurons and areas with pigment incontinence (arrows)—i.e., fragmented melanin that is extracellular or within macrophages.

6. Neuroaxonal Dystrophy (NAD) Hallervorden-Spatz Disease (HSpD)

This group of disorders, usually of autosomal-recessive inheritance, is typified by the presence, widely distributed throughout the CNS, of neuroaxonal spheroids in addition to neuron loss and astrocytic proliferation. Some regard the spectrum of NAD as including HSpD, infantile and juvenile NAD, and neuroaxonal leukodystrophy. Clinically HSpD patients present with a motor/extrapyramidal disorder that usually includes choreoathetotic or tremulous movements and dementia. Disease duration from onset to death is in the range of 10 to 15 years. Microscopic lesions (neuron loss, gliosis, axonal swellings, and neuroaxonal spheroids) are most abundant (in the case of HSpD) within globus

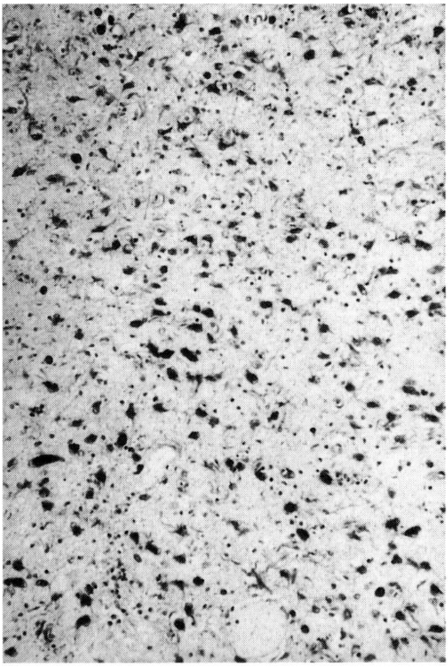

(C)

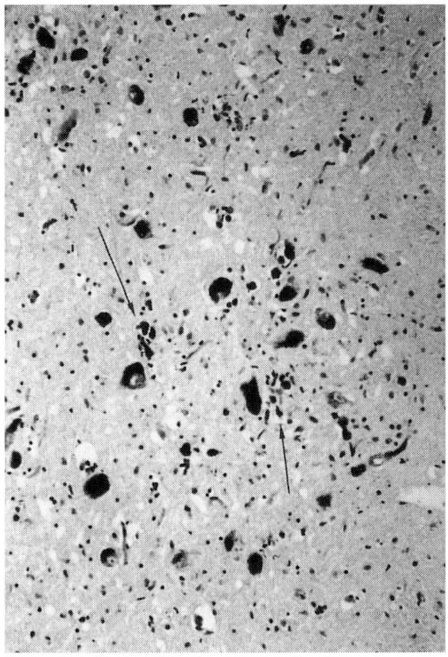

(D)

pallidus, SN (especially its pars reticulata component), nuclei of the posterior columns, and (less commonly) other regions of the CNS. Iron pigment may accumulate locally at sites of neuropathologic abnormality, leading to their taking on a rusty brown appearance at the time of brain cutting. In the case of juvenile and infantile NAD, the neuroaxonal changes are more widely distributed throughout the brain.

X. ACQUIRED (PARANEOPLASTIC) DEGENERATIONS OF THE NERVOUS SYSTEM

Though research on degenerative diseases of the CNS has a predominantly molecular genetic flavor, a group of rare disorders that arise as complications of systemic cancer may mimic familial neurodegenerative diseases: they present with progressive neurologic dysfunction, and a frequently observed neuropathologic correlate is the loss of selected neuronal populations in the CNS or PNS. Paraneoplastic syndromes may involve the brain, spinal cord, nerve, neuromuscular junction, or skeletal muscle. One intriguing feature of these conditions is that neurologic deterioration may set in and significantly progress before the primary malignancy has declared itself or metastasized, though the onset of new neurologic symptoms in a patient with a known primary cancer usually heralds metastasis of the neoplasm to brain parenchyma and/or the subarachnoid space. If a patient comes to autopsy with a rapidly progressive neurodegenerative condition occurring in the absence of a family history, toxin exposure, or other apparent etiology, the pathologist must undertake a thorough search for an occult malignancy. Some common paraneoplastic syndromes are described below.

A. Paraneoplastic Cerebellar Degeneration

Affected patients develop rapidly progressive symptoms of pancerebellar dysfunction over weeks or months, and at autopsy show severe loss of Purkinje (and sometimes granule) cell neurons with associated Bergmann astrogliosis. Implicated primary malignancies most commonly encountered are gynecologic tumors, breast or lung cancer, and lymphoma. Paraneoplastic cerebellar degeneration is further substratified, using serologic criteria, into:

1. That found in patients who produce an anti-Yo antibody which reacts with 34- and 62-kD proteins expressed within the cytoplasm of both Purkinje cells and the tumor (most often breast or gynecologic, though variants associated with Hodgkin's disease and squamous cell lung carcinoma are described).
2. A type in those who have anti-Ri antibody and (in addition to cerebellar degeneration) opsoclonus, dementia, and myoclonus.
3. A variant in patients with anti-Hu antibodies who have an associated paraneoplastic encephalomyelitis—again, with many neurologic signs other than those of "pure" cerebellar degeneration.

B. Paraneoplastic Encephalomyelitis

Patients develop dysfunction involving multiple loci within the CNS and at autopsy have variably extensive microglial nodules, neuronophagia, and perivascular lymphocyte cuffing—features that mimic viral encephalomyelitis (see Chap. 4), though no responsible virus has been consistently isolated from the nervous system. Many affected individuals also have sensory neuropathy. In the large majority of affected patients, bronchial (squamous cell) carcinoma is the cause. Variants of this rare syndrome occur in patients who manifest predominantly limbic changes, motor neuron dysfunction, and/or cerebellar or brainstem degeneration.

C. Paraneoplastic Opsoclonus-Myoclonus

This is most commonly associated with neuroblastoma (in children) or breast and lung cancer (especially of squamous cell type).

D. Paraneoplastic Necrotizing Myelopathy

This is seen in the presence of various carcinomas and lymphoma. The disorder begins clinically in the thoracic region, whence it descends and/or ascends. (Paraneoplastic conditions that affect peripheral nerve and skeletal muscle will be considered more fully in Chapter 10.)

Because of the strong (though not exclusive) association of many of these rare conditions with circulating antibodies to neuronal components, they may provide a neuroimmunologic "window" on focal CNS degeneration and constitute an interesting research interface among fields concerned with autoimmunity, neoplasia, and neuronal degeneration.

REFERENCES

1. Beal MF. Mitochondria, free radicals, and neurodegeneration. Curr Opin Neurobiol 1996; 6:661–666.
2. de Belleroche J, Orrell RW, Virgo L. Amyotrophic lateral sclerosis: recent advances in understanding disease mechanisms. J Neuropathol Exp Neurol 1996; 55:747–757.
3. Braak H, Braak E, Yilmazer D, de Vos RAI, Jansen ENH, Bohl J. Pattern of brain destruction in Parkinson's and Alzheimer's diseases. J Neural Transm 1996; 103:455–490.
4. Brownell B, Oppenheimer DR, Hughes JT. The central nervous system in motor neurone disease. J Neurol Neurosurg Psychiatry 1970; 33:338–357.
5. Brun A. Frontal lobe degeneration of non-Alzheimer type. I. Neuropathology. Arch Gerontol Geriatr 1987; 6:193–208.
6. Constantinidis J, Richard J, Tissot R. Pick's disease. Histological and clinical correlation. Eur Neurol 1974; 11:208–217.
7. Cooper PN, Jackson M, Lennox G, Lowe J, Mann DMA. Tau, ubiquitin, and alpha beta-crystallin immunohistochemistry define the principal causes of degenerative frontotemporal dementia. Arch Neurol 1995; 52:1011–1015.
8. Cruts M, Hendriks L, Van Broeckhoven C. The presenilin genes: a new gene family involved in Alzheimer disease pathology. Human Molec Genet 1996; 5:1449–1455.
9. Dalmau J, Graus F. Paraneoplastic syndromes. In: Samuels MA, Feske S, eds. Office Practice of Neurology. New York: Churchill Livingstone, 1995.
10. Daniel SE, de Bruin VMS, Lees AJ. The clinical and pathological spectrum of Steele-Richardson-Olszewski syndrome (progressive supranuclear palsy): a reappraisal. Brain 1995; 118:759–770.
11. Forno LS. Neuropathology of Parkinson's disease. J Neuropathol Exp Neurol 1996; 55:259–272.
12. Gearing M, Mirra SS, Hedreen JC, Sumi SM, Hansen LA, Heyman A. The Consortium to Establish a Registry for Alzheimer's Disease (CERAD). Part X. Neuropathology confirmation of the clinical diagnosis of Alzheimer's disease. Neurology 1995; 45:461–466.

13. Hansen LA, Galasko D. Lewy body disease. Curr Opin Neurol Neurosurg 1992; 5:889–894.
14. Hardy JA, Higgins GA. Alzheimer's disease: the amyloid cascade hypothesis. Science 1992; 256:184–185.
15. Hauw J-J, Daniel SE, Dickson D, et al. Preliminary NINDS neuropathologic criteria for Steele-Richarson-Olszewski syndrome (progressive supranuclear palsy). Neurology 1994; 44:2015–2019.
16. Hendriks L, van Broeckhoven C. The betaA4 amyloid precursor protein gene and Alzheimer's disease. Eur J Biochem 1996; 237:6–15.
17. Hsiao K, Chapman P, Nilsen S, et al. Correlative memory deficits, Abeta elevation, and amyloid plaques in transgenic mice. Science 1996; 274:99–102.
18. Hughes AJ, Daniel SE, Blankson S, Lees AJ. A clinicopathologic study of 100 cases of Parkinson's disease. Arch Neurol 1993; 50:140–148.
19. Ikonomidou C, Turski L. Excitotoxicity and neurodegenerative diseases. Curr Opin Neurol 1995; 8:487–497.
20. Jackson M, Lowe J. The new neuropathology of degenerative frontotemporal dementias. Acta Neuropathol 1996; 91:127–134.
21. Joachim CL, Selkoe DJ. The seminal role of beta-amyloid in the pathogenesis of Alzheimer disease. Alzheimer Dis Assoc Disorders 1992; 6:7–34.
22. Kosik KS. Alzheimer's disease: a cell biological perspective. Science 1992; 256:780–783.
23. Kosik KS. The molecular and cellular biology of tau. Brain Pathol 1993; 3:39–43.
24. La Spada AR, Paulson HL, Fischbeck KH. Trinucleotide repeat expansion in neurological disease. Ann Neurol 1994; 36:814–822.
25. Lee MK, Borchelt DR, Wong PC, Sisodia SS, Price DL. Transgenic models of neurodegenerative diseases. Curr Opin Neurobiol 1996; 6:651–660.
26. Lund and Manchester Groups. Clinical and neuropathological criteria for frontotemporal dementia. J Neurol Neurosurg Psychiatry 1994; 57:416–418.
27. Martin JB. Molecular genetics in neurology. Ann Neurol 1993; 34:757–773.
28. McKeith IG, Galasko D, Kosaka K, et al. Consensus guidelines for the clinical and pathologic diagnosis of dementia with Lewy bodies (DLB): report of the consortium on DLB international workshop. Neurology 1996; 47:1113–1124.
29. Mendez MF, Mastri AR, Sung JH, Frey WH II. Clinically diagnosed Alzheimer disease: neuropathologic findings in 650 cases. Alzheimer Dis Assoc Disorders 1992; 6:35–43.
30. Mirra SS, Heyman A, McKeel D, et al. The Consortium to Establish a Registry for Alzheimer's Disease (CERAD). Part II. Standardization of the neuropathologic assessment of Alzheimer's disease. Neurology 1991; 41:479–486.
31. Nasir J, Goldberg PJ, Hayden MR. Huntington disease: new insights into the relationship between CAG expansion and disease. Human Molec Genet 1996; 5:1431–1435.
32. Orr HT. Unstable trinucleotide repeats and the diagnosis of neurodegenerative disease. Hum Pathol 1994; 25:598–601.
33. Petersen RB, Tabaton M, Chen SG, et al. Familial progressive subcortical gliosis: presence of prions and linkage to chromosome 17. Neurology 1995; 45:1062–1067.

34. Pollanen MS, Dickson DW, Bergeron C. Pathology and biology of the Lewy body. J Neuropathol Exp Neurol 1993; 52:183–191.
35. Roses AD. The Alzheimer diseases. Curr Opin Neurobiol 1996; 6:644–650.
36. Siddique T, Deng H-X. Genetics of amyotrophic lateral sclerosis. Human Molec Genet 1996; 5:1465–1470.
37. Sima AAF, Defendini R, Keohane C, et al. The neuropathology of chromosome 17-linked dementia. Ann Neurol 1996; 39:734–743.
38. Tomlinson BE, Blessed G, Roth M. Observations on the brains of demented old people. J Neurol Sci 1970; 11:205–242.
39. Trojanowski JG, Schmidt ML, Shin R-W, Bramblett GT, Rao D, Lee VM-Y. Altered tau and neurofilament proteins in neurodegenerative diseases: diagnostic implications for Alzheimer's disease and Lewy body dementias. Brain Pathol 1993; 3:45–54.
40. Van Broeckhoven C. Presenilins and Alzheimer disease. Nature Genet 1995; 11:230–232.
41. Verbeek MM, Eikelenboom P, de Waal RMW. Differences between the pathogenesis of senile plaques and congophilic angiopathy in Alzheimer disease. J. Neuropathol Exp Neurol 1997; 56:751–761.
42. Verity MA, Wechsler AF. Progressive subcortical gliosis of Neumann: a clinicopathologic study of two cases with review. Arch Gerontol Geriatr 1987; 6:245–261.
43. Vinters HV, Miller BL, Pardridge WM. Brain amyloid and Alzheimer disease. Ann Intern Med 1988; 109:41–54.
44. Vinters HV, Wang ZZ, Secor DL. Brain parenchymal and microvascular amyloid in Alzheimer's disease. Brain Pathol 1996; 6:179–195.
45. Warren ST. The expanding world of trinucleotide repeats. Science 1996; 271:1374–1375.

9

Metabolic Abnormalities

I. INTRODUCTION

An enormous number of metabolic disorders affect the nervous system, and a basic knowledge of biochemistry and more recently of genetics is required to more fully appreciate the complexities of these conditions. Therefore, this chapter takes a somewhat less conventional approach to metabolic disease in that the basic function each of the cytoplasmic organelles is discussed as a prelude to a basic discussion of the diseases that arise as a result of genetic and biochemical perturbations in the particular organelle.

II. PEROXISOMAL DISEASE

Peroxisomes are membrane-bound cytoplasmic organelles present in virtually all cells and which through a variety of anabolic and catabolic pathways play a key role in intermediary metabolism in man. Peroxisomes have an average diameter of 0.2 to 1.0 μm, but the number and size of individual peroxisomes vary according to cell type. Key catabolic reactions include degradation of very long-chain fatty acids, catabolism of L-pipecolic acid, substrate oxidation with resultant formation of H_2O_2 which is converted to H_2O by peroxisomal-based catalase, and possibly also a role in degradation of phytanic acid. Key anabolic reactions that occur within the peroxisome include the preparation of ether lipids involved in the synthesis of plasmalogen, which is a component of cell membranes including myelin; partial involvement in bile acid synthesis; and possibly also involvement in cholesterol synthesis.

Peroxisomal disorders may be attributed to either a failure of peroxisome biogenesis or to deficiency of single enzymes involved in peroxisomal function. Unlike mitochondria, peroxisomes do not have their own DNA and are dependent on the importation of nuclear-encoded proteins for their synthesis. Thus, a defect in the importation of peroxisomal matrix proteins will give rise to incompletely formed or defective peroxisomes. Such defective peroxisomes may be difficult to visualise in involved cells. In the absence of peroxisomes there is a deficiency of multiple peroxisomal-based enzymes. Not all of the genes involved in peroxisome biogenesis have been identified. Failure to assemble normal peroxisomes is characteristic of Zellweger syndrome (ZS).

The second large group of peroxisomal disorders consists of those in which peroxisomes are structurally normal but are deficient in a single enzyme. Typical of this group of peroxisomal disorders is adrenoleukodystrophy (ALD).

Adrenoleukodystrophy (ALD) (80%), Zellweger syndrome (7.8%), and neonatal adrenoleukodystrophy (NALD) (4.0%) comprise over 90% of all known peroxisomal disorders. Neurologic involvement is present in virtually all peroxisomal disorders. Neurologic features are age-dependent, and in the neonatal period hypotonia and craniofacial dysmorphism are typical. Later (6 months plus) there is developmental delay with seizures, sensory neural deafness, and more obvious dysmorphic features. Behavioral change with intellectual deterioration is another important clinical feature and in the presence of a peripheral neuropathy or myelinopathy is suggestive of an underlying peroxisomal disorder. Nonneurologic clinical clues include hepatomegaly, features of malabsorption, and retinopathy.

The considerable variation in phenotypic expression of peroxisomal disorders has led to the development of genetic techniques such as complementation analysis in order to determine distinct subgroups which might have a common genetic basis. The technique is based on the principle that fibroblasts from two patients, deficient in differing peroxisomal enzymes, will, when fused with each other, have the deficiency corrected by the other patient's normal enzyme. Thus cells that complement each other in this way represent distinct genotypes. Some 16 complementation groups and by inference genotypes have been shown to be associated with clinical manifestations of peroxisomal assembly disorders.

Systemic pathologic features of generalised peroxisomal disorders (ZS, infantile Refsum's disease, NALD) include micronodular cirrhosis, renal cyst formation, and ophthalmic involvement including cataract formation, pigmentary retinopathy, and optic atrophy. Adrenal atrophy is a typical feature of ALD and adrenomyeloneuropathy (AMN), the latter also having testicular atrophy.

Ultrastructurally, the generalized peroxisomal disorders are characterized by the presence of lysosomes containing trilaminar spicules which are thought to represent altered lamellar lipid. The single enzyme peroxisomal disorders are characterised by either single or fused cytosolic lamellae.

A. Neuropathology of Specific Peroxisomal Disorders

Zellweger's syndrome is characterized by disorders of neuronal migration which include heterotopic nodules in the cerebral white matter, pachygyria-polymicrogyria in the Sylvian region, and dysplasia of the inferior olives. Developmentally abnormal neurones may contain membranous cytoplasmic bodies as may astrocytes. Golgi studies have demonstrated abnormal dendritic branching and poor spine development. The cerebral white matter may show varying degrees of loss, which is particularly well seen on MRI. Periventricular cysts may be seen in newborn infants. The neuropathology of other generalized peroxisomal disorders such as rhizomelic chondrodysplasia punctata and NALD is limited to isolated case reports, some of which include descriptions of abnormal neuronal migration. Presumably very long chain fatty acids (VLCFA) interfere in the normal interactions between migrating neurons and radial glia (see also Chap. 7).

ALD is characterized neuropathologically by widespread confluent inflammatory demyelination which begins in the occipital region and spreads anteriorly to eventually involve all of the subcortical white matter (Figs. 1, 2). In

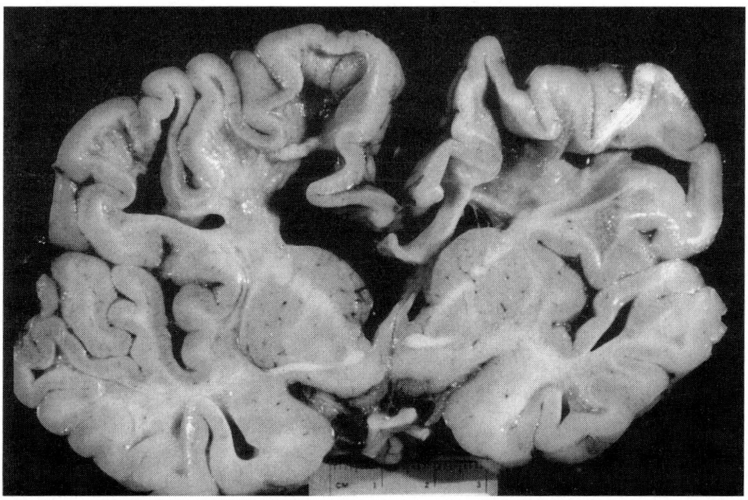

Figure 1 Coronal section of brain from a 5-year-old boy with fatal adrenoleukodystrophy, showing widespread cavitary change within centrum semiovale, with relative preservation of both deep central and cortical gray matter.

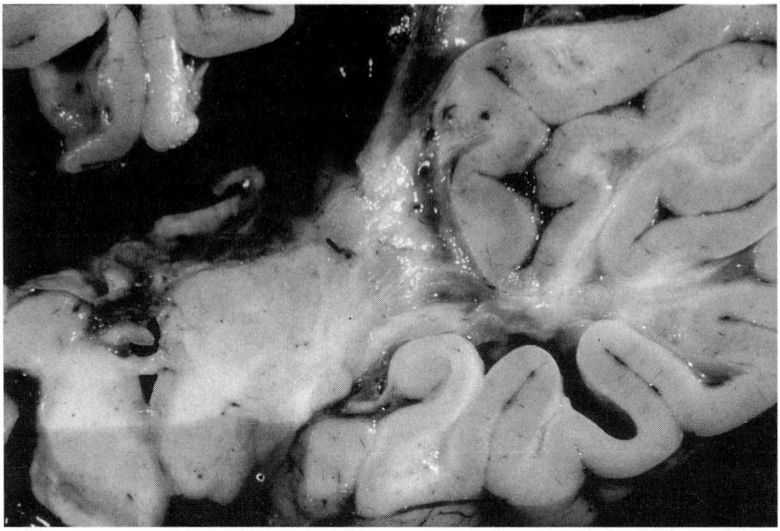

Figure 2 Magnified view of brain shown in Figure 1 (at a different coronal level) to demonstrate almost total loss of subcortical white matter.

the terminal stages of the illness, there may be extensive axonal loss with cystic cavitary change. The cerebellar white matter may also be involved as may the brainstem, but the spinal cord is rarely if ever involved. Microscopically there is an accumulation of macrophages containing laminar-lipid profiles. An intense lymphocytic and plasma cell infiltrate may also be present. Typically the lymphocytes and plasma cells are found behind the advancing edge of the demyelinated area, in contrast to MS, where the lymphocytic infiltrate is present in relatively normal white matter ahead of the area of demyelination. It has been proposed that the myelin is inherently unstable because of the accumulation of VLCFA. The unstable myelin undergoes degradation and the breakdown products stimulate astrocytes, microglia, and lymphocytes to proliferate. Cytokine release contributes further to myelin destruction.

Adrenomyeloneuropathy (AMN) is characterized by spinal tract degeneration with secondary myelin loss. Lymphocytes and plasma cells are sparse. Axonal spheroids and axonal atrophy, features of an axonal degenerative process, may be present. Involvement of hemispheric white matter is minimal when compared with ALD. The mechanisms whereby VLCFA result in extensive confluent myelin loss in ALD and a relatively pure axonal degenerative process in AMN are unclear.

ALD is characterized by an impaired ability to metabolise VLCFA which results in their accumulation. Lignoceroyl coenzyme A, a peroxisomal based coenzyme involved in VLCFA metabolism, is impaired. The ALD gene is mapped to Xq28 and it encodes a 745 amino acid protein which belongs to a family of ATP-binding transporter proteins, which are used to provide energy for substrate transport across membranes. Analysis of the ALD protein (ALDP) gene has demonstrated that the majority of families have mutations occurring at a mutational hotspot or elsewhere in the gene. The mechanism whereby a mutation in the ALDP results in impaired VLCFA CoA ligase activity in peroxisomes remains to be determined.

III. LYSOSOMAL DISEASE

The history of lysosomal storage disorders (LSDs) has evolved from initial clinicopathological descriptions through chemical identification of the abnormal storage products followed by identification of the related metabolic defects and finally culminating in identification of the underlying gene defect(s). Lysosomes are membrane-limited cytoplasmic organelles whose function is to degrade complex lipids, carbohydrates, proteins, phosphates, complex glycoproteins, and glycolipids. Lysosomal dysfunction may result from deficiency of a lysosomal enzyme or its subunit or because there is a deficiency of an activator protein. Less commonly, lysosomal dysfunction may develop because there is deficiency of a lysosomal carrier protein required to participate in the export of degraded material or because of a failure to target and transfer nuclear encoded lysosomal protein into lysosomes.

All lysosomal storage disorders have in common the presence of an enzyme deficiency or inactivation coupled with the accumulation of metabolites within a variety of cell types, but particularly within the nervous system. Virtually all of the genes coding for lysosomal enzymes, activator proteins, and other transport proteins have been cloned. Identification of specific mutations associated with each disease type has facilitated diagnosis of these conditions. The days of attempting to establish a tissue diagnosis of a particular storage disorder based on the ultrastructural characteristics of the accumulated metabolite are past. Listed in Table 1 are the more frequently encountered lysosomal storage diseases. The conditions are listed by name together with the abnormal storage metabolite, the metabolic defect, and its genetic basis.

IV. SPHINGOLIPIDOSES

Sphingolipids have a backbone of ceramide or N-acylsphingosine to which are attached phosphocholine and galactose or glucose molecules. A cerebroside consists of a molecule of glucose or galactose linked to the sphingosine moiety of ceramide. The gangliosides have several glucose or galactose molecules

Table 1 Lysosomal Storage Disorders

Disease	Accumulated metabolite & relevant enzyme	Neuropathology	Metabolic defect (enzyme deficiency)	Gene and locus	Gene defect
Gaucher Types 1, 2, 3 Only types 2 and 3 involve nervous system	Glucocerebroside (cerumide + glucose) gluocerebrosidase catalyzes hydrolytic cleavage of glucocerebroside to ceramide and glucose	Perivascular lipid-filled cells and neuronophagia, mechanism of neuronal injury not fully determined	Glucocerebrosidase deficiency	7604-bp gene at 1q21 encoding 497 amino acid protein	36 mutations described to date
			Lack of saposin activator	Chromosome 10	
Niemann-Pick A and B; brain not involved in type B	Sphingomyelin accumulates because deficiency of sphingomyelinase results in failure to catalyze the hydrolytic cleavage of sphingomyelin to ceramide and phosphocholine	Neuronal cytomegaly with pallor and vacuolotion, lamellated membrane bound inclusions.	Sphingomyelin-phosphodiesterase 1 deficiency	11p15.1-p15.3 Gene cloned	12 mutations and 2 deletions
		Progressive atrophy	Absence of saposin D activator protein		
Niemann-Pick C and D	Excessive intracellular unesterified cholesterol	Neuronal cytomegaly due to pleomorphic loose lipid lamellae	Impaired esterification of exogenous lipoprotein-derived cholesterol	18q11-q12 though probably polygenic	Not determined

Krabbe	Galactocerebroside (ceramide/galactose)	Myelin loss from subcortical white matter with perivascular mononuclear globoid cells, later becoming mulinucleate. Curved or straight tubular profiles. Peripheral nerve demyelination but no globoid cells	Galactosylceramidase (GALC) 669 amino acid residues	GALC located 14q21-q31; contains 17 exons spanning about 60 kb of genomic DNA	5 missense mutations described, 1 deletion, and 1 patient with multiple mutations
Metachromatic leukodystrophy	Sulfatide (ceramide + galactose + sulfate) Arylsulfatase A saposin B (SAP-1)	Myelin loss with PAS macrophages which show brown metachromasia with toluidine blue or acidified eresyl violet. Also present in Schwann cells	Arylsulfatase A deficiency (ARSA) deficiency saposin B (SAP-1) required as heat-stable activator	ARSA 22q13.31 SAP-1 10q22.1	31 amino acid substitutions, 1 nonsense mutation, 3 deletions identified
Fabry	Ceramide trihexoside (ceramide + glucose + galactose + galactose)	Vascular accumulation of PAS + /Sudan black + binefringent material which leads to luminal occlusion and ischemia in brain or nerve. Concentric or parallel lipid lamellae	α-Galactosidase A	Xq21.33-q22	15 GLA gene rearrangements, 3 mRNA processing defects, and 31 GLA point mutations described

Table 1 Continued

Disease	Accumulated metabolite & relevant enzyme	Neuropathology	Metabolic defect (enzyme deficiency)	Gene and locus	Gene defect
Tay-Sachs	GM2 ganglioside (ceramide + glucose + galadose + n-acetyl galactosamine actosamine + n-acetyl neuraminic acid)	Megalencephaly (depending on disease stage), ballooned neurones containing Luxol fast blue-positive material which is PAS-positive on frozen section. Membranous cytoplasmic bodies with parallel or concentric lamellae	Hexosaminidase A (one α and one β subunit)	α-subunit located 15q23-24 and β-subunit located 5q11.2-13.3	Multiple mutations described in α-subunit gene
AB variant of Tay-Sachs	As above	As above	GM2 activator required for hexosaminidase A function	5q32-q33	3 mutations described
Sandhoff	GM2 ganglioside asialo GM2	As above	Hexosaminidase A and B both deficient (Hex B contains two β-subunits)	5q13	10 mutations described in Hex B gene on 5q13
GM1-gangliosidosis	GM1 ganglioside (ceramide + glucose + galactose + n-aceyl galactosamine + n-acetyl neuraminic acid + galactose)	Neuromal cytomegaly with slightly granular cytoplasm and membranous bodies similar to Tay-Sachs. Striatum shows preferential involvement	β-Galactosidase Lysosomal Protective Protein	3p21.33 Chromosome 20	17 mutations described

attached. Sphingolipids are important components of cell membranes, particularly in neurones. Failure to degrade sphingolipids results in accumulation of ceramide in affected cells.

This section will only focus on the neurologic manifestations of the LSDs. The sphingolipidoses may involve gray matter, white matter, or peripheral nerve. Typically, gray matter neurones show enlarged cell bodies with swollen axons and dendrites. Seizures, visual impairment, and regression with loss of acquired skills is typical. Leukodystrophies are characterized by loss of myelin and may be accompanied by accumulation of the abnormal metabolite in macrophages located within the area of demyelination. In the PNS, Schwann cell dysfunction arising from accumulation of lysosomal storage products may result in peripheral neuropathy.

A. Gaucher Disease

There are three types of Gaucher disease, two of which involve the central nervous system and are characterized by brainstem involvement with supranuclear gaze palsies, difficulty with respiration and swallowing, and progressive motor system dysfunction and cognitive impairment. The brain shows perivascular accumulation of lipid-filled cells. Surprisingly, microglial nodules with neuronophagia are a striking feature.

B. Niemann-Pick Diseases

The Niemann-Pick group of diseases includes four categories. Types A and B are associated with marked deficiency of sphingomyelinase and accumulation of sphingomyelin in multiple organs. The brain is not involved in type B. Patients with type A Niemann-Pick disease typically show delayed motor milestones with progressive intellectual deterioration. There is usually marked hypotonia. Hepatosplenomegaly provides a major clinical clue as does the presence of cherry-red spots in the macula. The brain shows large, distended pale neurones filled with lamelated cytoplasmic inclusions.

Types C and D show dramatic differences both in clinical presentation and in the underlying biochemical defect. Patients with type C Niemann-Pick typically show supranuclear gaze palsies with ataxia and movement disorders. Epilepsy is common. Brainstem involvement may lead to aspiration. Neuropathologic descriptions are infrequent, but typically there is neuronal distension and axonal swelling due to accumulation of granular material which by electron microscopy consists of pleomorphic loose lipid lamellae (Fig. 3). The molecular defect underlying Niemann-Pick type C is unknown. However, given the number of steps involved in the endocytosis and processing of low-density lipoprotein cholesterol-ester, it is likely that the disease will demonstrate genotypic heterogeneity.

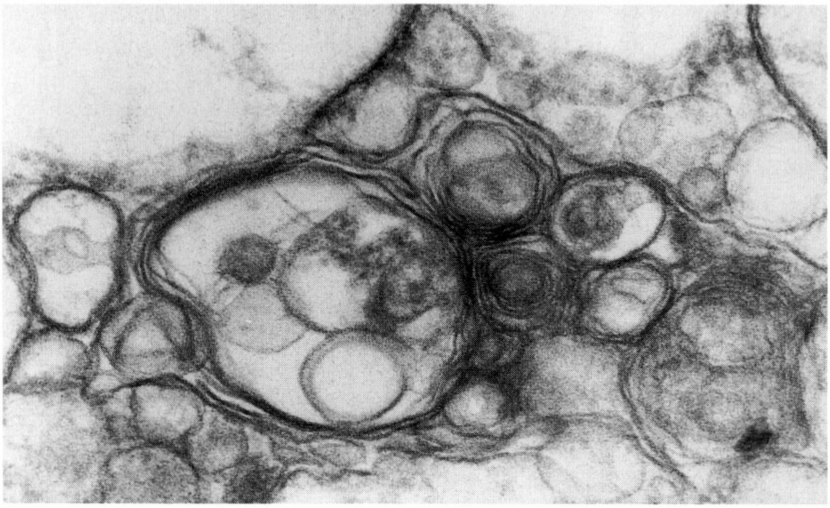

Figure 3 Brain biopsy obtained from a 9-year-old girl with dementia, seizures, and ataxia, showing intraneuronal pleomorphic loose lipid lamellae typical of Niemann-Pick disease type C. (Mag ×50,000.) Skin fibroblasts showed prominent accumulation of unesterified cholesterol in perinuclear vesicles, together with markedly impaired intracellular esterification of exogenous lipoprotein-derived cholesterol. (Micrograph courtesy of Dr. Marie T. Vanier.)

C. Krabbe Disease (globoid cell leukodystrophy)

Krabbe disease is due to a deficiency of galactocerebrosidase, which is required for the hydrolysis of the galactosyl molecule from ceramide. Typically Krabbe disease begins in infancy and manifests as a leukodystrophy with progressive degeneration of white matter, which shows extensive replacement by large perivascular distended globular multinucleated cells (Fig. 4).

D. Metachromatic Leukodystrophy

In the sulfatide lipidoses there is an accumulation of cerebroside sulfate because of deficiency of sulfatidase or on occasion because of a reduction in the levels of SAP-1, an activator protein required as a cofactor by sulfatidase. At least seven sulfatidase enzymes have been identified, the majority of which are involved in mucopolysaccharide degradation. Arylsulfatase, which is deficient in MLD, has five natural substrates. MLD may set in in childhood or adulthood. Clinically, the infantile form is characterized by mental deterioration, progressive motor system degeneration with a gait disturbance together with dystonia, and occasionally choreoathetosis. Peripheral neuropathy may also be present.

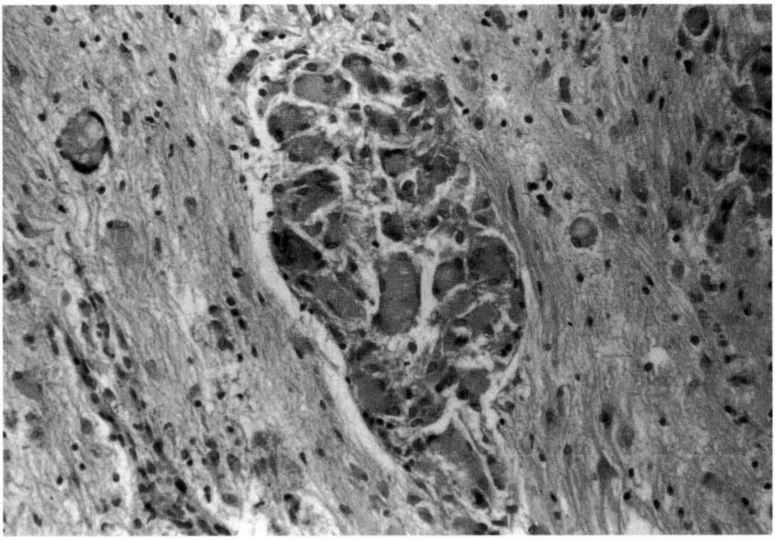

Figure 4 Autopsy brain from a patient with Gaucher's disease showing large globular perivascular and occasionally multinucleated cells.

Pathologically there is marked loss of cerebral and cerebellar myelin which is associated with axonal injury and loss as the disease progresses. Intrafascicular oligodendroglia are reduced and gliosis may be severe. Globular granular deposits lying free in the white matter and located within macrophages are typical. These bodies stain positively with PAS and are brown when stained with 1% amplified cresyl violet. Under polarized light the granules exhibit green-yellow birefringence. Ultrastructurally the granules contain stacks of irregular lamellar profiles. Peripheral nerve may show segmental demyelination and the granules may be present in Schwann cells. In addition to accumulation of cerebroside sulfate, other sulphate containing compounds such as cholesterol sulfate, heparan sulfate, and dermatan sulfate may accumulate. Psychiatric symptoms are common in the adult form of MLD, which is characterized by less widespread metachromatic material. Arylsulfatase A in the presence of an activator protein (SAP-1) catalyzes the degradation of sulfatides to cerebroside and sulfate. SAP-1 deficiency may also result in typical MLD. Reduction in arylsulfatase activity without accompanying sulfatide accumulation is typical of pseudodeficiency of ARSA and is a common polymorphism in which certain mutations cause low levels of enzyme activity without obvious clinical dysfunction. The arylsulfatase A gene is located on chromosome 22q13.31 region, and is 3.2 kb in length. Multiple mutations and occasional deletions have been described in association with differing residual levels of ARSA activity. Additionally deficiencies of SAP-1, an activator protein required by arylsulfatase A, may give rise to MLD. SAP-1 is derived from prosaposin, the gene for which is encoded on chromosome 10. At least four mutations associated with MLD have been described in the SAP-1 domain of the prosaposin gene.

E. Fabry Disease

Alpha-galactosidase A deficiency is an X-linked recessive disorder in which there is an accumulation of glycosphingolipids with terminal galactose molecules. Neurologic involvement results from vascular deposition of the undigested substrate together with accumulation in neurones, especially of the autonomic neurones in the gut. Microvascular involvement leads to occlusion and resultant focal cortical ischemia. Deposition in brainstem nuclear groups may also occur as may accumulation in peripheral sensory neurones and Schwann cells. The accumulated substrate may be seen as PAS and Sudan black-positive birefringent material in endothelial cells. Concentric or parallel stacked lamellae may be seen ultrastructurally (Fig. 5). Alpha-galactosidase A is encoded on the X chromosome at q21.33-q22. The gene has been completely sequenced. The GLA gene has a high level of polymorphism. Multiple gene rearrangements together with a large number of point mutations have been described in association with Fabry's disease.

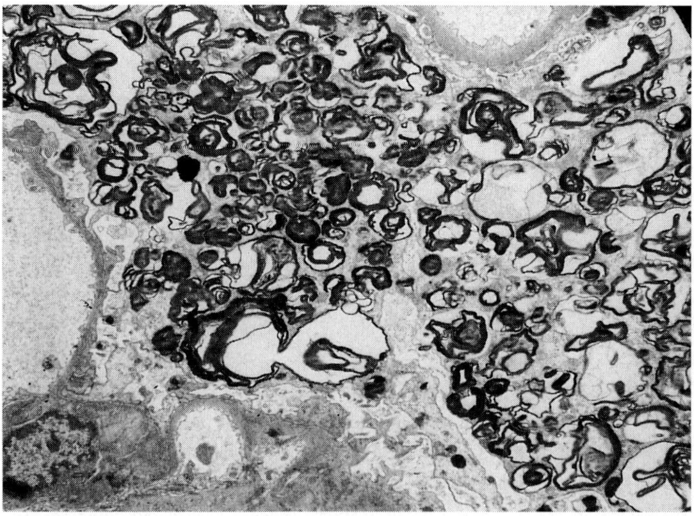

Figure 5 Renal biopsy from a patient with Fabry disease, which demonstrates numerous electron-dense concentric lipid lamellae. (Mag ×3,500.)

V. GANGLIOSIDOSES (See table 1)

A. Tay-Sachs Disease

Tay-Sachs is the most important of the gangliosidoses, and in this condition defective or deficient hexosaminidase-A results in a failure to cleave N- acetyl-galactosamine residue from the GM2 ganglioside. A GM2 activator protein is required for this reaction. Ballooned neurones containing PAS and Luxol fast blue-positive fine cytoplasmic material are characteristic of Tay-Sachs (Fig. 6). Autonomic neurones show similar change. White matter shows myelin loss and reactive gliosis. Membranous cytoplasmic bodies having a lamellar configuration are present on ultrastructural examination. They may also be present in peripheral nerve and skin. GM2 ganglioside is the major storage material.

Typically infants show progressive intellectual decline with seizures and blindness while later-onset cases tend to show a more prolonged course. The presence of a cherry-red retinal spot is virtually diagnostic. Presentation with isolated anterior horn cell involvement may result in a motor neurone diseaselike condition in adults. There are two forms of lysosomal hexosaminidase. Hexosaminidase A is composed of one α-subunit and one β-subunit, while hexosaminidase B contains 2 β-subunits. The α-subunit gene is present at 15q23-24 and the β-subunit gene is present at 5q11.2-13.3. They are structurally similar. A small transport protein binds to the GM2 ganglioside and promotes access of hexosaminidase A to this substrate complex. Deficiency of both hexosaminidase A and B results in Sandhoff disease (Fig. 7), while the AB variant refers

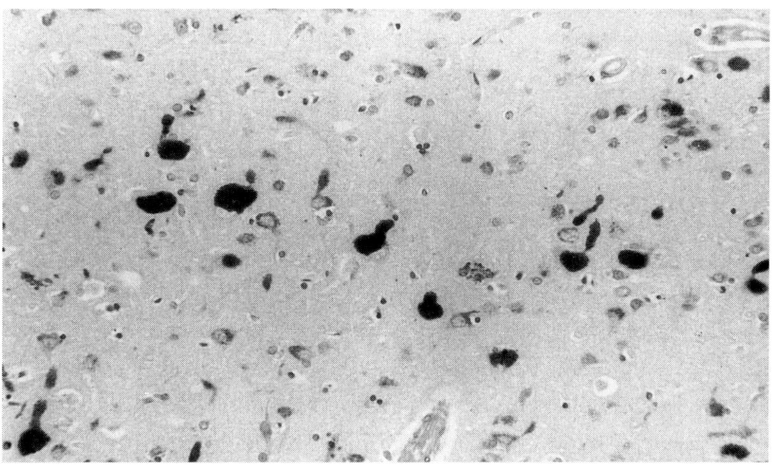

Figure 6 Section of autopsy-derived cerebral cortex from a patient with Tay-Sachs disease showing ballooned neurons stained positively with Luxol fast blue.

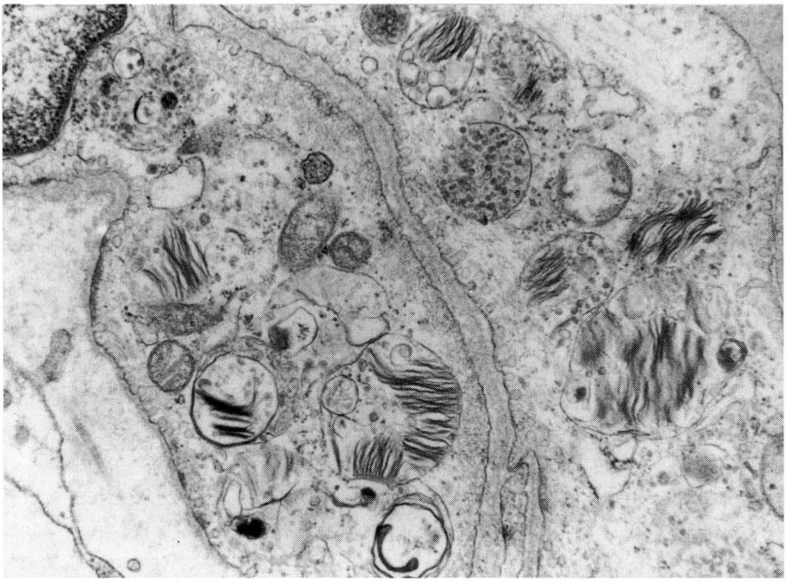

Figure 7 Conjunctival biopsy showing membranous cytoplasmic bodies typical of the type seen in Sandhoff disease and other gangliosidoses. (Mag $\times$10,000.)

to patients with normal activity of hexosaminidase A and B but who lack the activator protein necessary for degradation of the GM2 ganglioside by hexosaminidase A. Multiple mutations have been described involving the α-subunit, some of which are particularly common among Ashkenazim. Mutations affecting the β-subunit are much less common. Improved carrier screening and prenatal diagnosis has resulted in a dramatic decrease in the prevalence of Tay-Sachs disease. Testing is based on gene product screening (enzyme testing) together with DNA based mutation analysis.

B. GMI Gangliosidosis

Beta galactosidase deficiency causes GMI gangliosidosis and also Morquio B disease. GM1 ganglioside accumulates in neurones, particularly those in the striatum. Involved neurones are large and pale and have lightly granular cytoplasm with membranous bodies visible on ultrastructural examination. The β-galactosidase gene is located at 3p21.33, and multiple mutations have been reported to cause GM1 gangliosidosis of differing phenotype. The particular phenotypic expression of the disease, as in all lysosomal disorders, depends on the level of residual activity and on whether one or both alleles are mutated.

VI. MUCOPOLYSACCHARIDOSES

In the mucopolysaccharidoses (MPS) there is an inherited deficiency of one or more enzymes involved in the catabolism of glycosaminoglycans (GAGs), as a result of which there is widespread visceral accumulation of GAGs. GAGs, which are linked to a protein core, are polymers that contain amino sugars linked to uronic acid. The amino sugar is either n-acetyl-glucosamine or n-acetyl-galactosamine attached to either glucuronic or iduronic acid. The GAGs are also sulfated. Thus the GAGs may be classified on the basis of the differing sugars attached and on the degree of sulfation (Table 2).

Several lysosomal enzymes may be required to completely degrade an individual GAG. The GAGs are widely distributed in all tissues, particularly in connective tissues. The MPS disorders are characterized by failure of enzymatic cleavage of either a sugar or a sulfate molecule during normal GAG degradation. The presence of similar sulfate linkages and similar uronic acids in different GAGs frequently leads to the accumulation of more than one GAG when a particular sulfatase or uronidase is deficient. Conversely, as more than one enzyme is required for degradation of certain GAGs, a particular MPS phenotype may result from more than one enzyme deficiency. At least four variants of Sanfilippo are described in which four distinct enzymes are deficient. The MPS disorders are characterized by massive excretion of GAGs in the urine, and, while identification of the particular GAG will contribute to establishing a specific diagnosis, measurement of individual enzymes is required to establish a definitive diagnosis. The majority of genes that code for individual enzymes involved in GAG degradation have been cloned. Multiple mutations involving the genes coding for these enzymes have been and are being described with increasing frequency. Increased availability of mutation analysis will lead to improved carrier detection and identification of at-risk individuals who might benefit from treatments such as bone marrow transplantation. Improved genotype-phenotype correlation should lead to a better understanding of the MPS group of conditions.

Neurologic involvement is present in all of the MPS disorders with the possible exception of MPSI-S and MPSVI (Table 3). The severity of neuropathologic involvement varies within and between particular subtypes. MPSI-H or Hurler shows the most severe change. The skull is large, hyperostotic, and deformed; the spine may show a kyphosis which progresses to gibbus formation. The meninges are thickened and opaque due to increased numbers of macrophages and collagen. The brain may show hydrocephalus. Widened perivascular spaces due to accumulation of distended macrophages may be visible to the naked eye and are recognizable on MRI. Neurons are distended, and pale and frozen sections stain positively for PAS, Luxol fast blue, and oil red O, reflecting the secondary accumulation of lipid. Demonstration of GAGs within

Table 2 Glycosaminoglycans

Glycosaminoglycan	Amino sugar	Hexuronic acid	Sulfate
Chondroitin-4-sulfate	N-acetylgalactosamine	Glucuronic acid	4-OSO_3
Chondroitin-6-sulfate	N-acetylgalactosamine	Glucuronic acid	6-OSO_3
Dermatan sulfate	N-acetylgalactosamine	Glucuronic acid and iduronic acid	4-OSO_3 2-OSO_3
Heparan sulfate	N-acetylglucosamine	Glucuronic acid and iduronic acid	2-OSO_3 6-OSO_3
Keratan sulfate	N-acetylglucosamine	Galactose	6-OSO_3

neurons in formalin-fixed sections is extremely difficult, but some metachromasia may be observed in toluidine blue-stained frozen sections. Biochemical analysis, however, demonstrates large amounts of the relevant GAG within brain. EM studies reveal large membrane-bound vacuoles. Membranous cytoplasmic bodies similar to those seen in the gangliosidoses may be present. Lamellae may be arranged in parallel, giving rise to the term zebra body. The EM appearances are not diagnostic of a particular MPS subtype. The remaining MPS subtypes show less severe but essentially similar changes, none of which are diagnostic for a particular subtype.

Table 3 Mucopolysaccharidoses

Disease	Accumulated glycosaminoglycan	Enzyme deficient	Gene locus
MPS I	Dermatan sulfate and Heparan sulfate	α-L-iduronidase	4p16.3
Hurler IH			
Scheie IS	Dermatan sulfate		
Hurler/Schie IH/IS	Dermatan sulfate		
MPS II Hunter	Dermatan sulfate and Heparan sulfate	Iduronate sulfalase	Xq28
MPS III Sanfilippo	Heparan sulfate		
A		Sulfamidase	17q25.3
B		α-N-acetylglucosaminidase	17q21
C		Acetyl CoA: α-glucosaminide: N-acetyl transferase	14
D		N-acetylglucosamine-6-sulfate sulafatase	12q14
MPS IV Morquio's	Keratan sulfate	N-acetylgalactosamine-6-sulfate sulafatase	16q24.3
MPS VI Maroteaux-Lamy	Dermatan sulfate	N-acetylgalactosamine-4-sulfatase	5q11-q13

VII. GLYCOGEN STORAGE DISEASES (GSDs)

This section will deal only with the disorders of glycogen metabolism that present clinically with major neurological findings. Glycogen is most abundant in liver and muscle. Anaerobic glycolysis accounts for very little of the energy requirements of muscle but is an important energy source during isometric muscular contraction and other high-intensity muscular efforts, when it is mobilized into the aerobic pathways. Brain glycogen levels are much lower than those in muscle. There are 11 steps involved in glycogen synthesis and breakdown, with a close symbiotic relationship between the enzymes involved in glycogen synthesis and those involved in glycogen degradation. GSDs may affect muscle alone or in combination with brain or liver or other organs. The pattern of involvement is determined by the presence of distinct tissue specific isoenzymes. Different proteins/enzymes having the same substrate are encoded at different loci. Conversely, other involved enzymes may be composed of multiple subunits; the relative proportions of these subunits in different organs will determine the severity of that particular organ involvement. The GSDs involving muscle are characterized by exercise intolerance and muscle cramps. A properly executed forearm ischemia test is an essential part of the investigation but requires good patient cooperation, which may be difficult to achieve in childhood. Muscle necrosis may result in myoglobinuria. Progressive muscle weakness may occur in the absence of obvious exercise intolerance. The presence of excess glycogen in the muscle biopsy provides a clue to the presence of a GSD, but there are many examples where the amount of glycogen as assessed by the PAS stain is not excessive. It is not possible to distinguish the different GSDs on muscle histology alone. Muscle histochemistry is essential but is inadequate in isolation for accurate diagnosis. It is advisable to obtain biochemical confirmation when a GSD is suspected, and this can be carried out on frozen muscle. The genetic basis of many of the GSDs has been established, and it is clear that there is a very high level of genetic heterogeneity even in conditions such as McArdle disease, which has a relatively stereotyped clinical picture. Nevertheless, it can be anticipated that genetic diagnosis will become more readily available in the near future. The GSDs with major neurologic involvement are summarized in Table 4. Some of the other disorders, particularly those caused by defects in terminal glycolysis, may involve muscle. However, these conditions are exceptionally rare.

A. Acid Maltase Deficiency (GSD-II)

The infantile form is characterized by deposition of glycogen in liver, heart, and skeletal muscle, resulting in organomegaly and profound muscle weakness. Involvement of respiratory muscle and cardiac failure may be fatal. The child-

Table 4 Glycogen Storage Diseases (GSDs) with Major Neurologic Involvement

Disorder	Enzyme deficiency; gene and defects	Organ involvement	Major clinical presentation	Neuropathology
GSD-II Acid maltase or Pompe disease	Lysosomal α-glucosidase Gene sequenced and assigned to 17q21-23 10 + missense mutations and deletions	Muscle $\pm$ liver and heart	Infantile—Hypotonia and organomegaly Childhood—Muscle weakness and calf hypertrophy Adult—Myopathy and respiratory muscle weakness	Vacuolar myopathy. Glycogen in lysosomes and free in cytoplasm. Anterior horn cell involvment in infantile form
GSD-III Cori-Forbes	Debrancher 1p21 Gene defects not yet well characterized but 124bp deletion in one family	Liver and muscle	Hepatomegaly with dysfunction and late-onset myopathy (variable severity)	Vacuolar myopathy. Glycogen in sarcoplasm.
GSD-V McArdle	Myophosphorylase (MPH) Gene sequenced and assigned to 11q13 10+ mutations and rare deletions	Muscle	Exercise intolerance with muscle pain and cramps	Variable glycogen accumulation and absence of MPH staining
GSD-VII Tarui	Phosphofructokinase Muscle isoenzyme (PFK-M) 7 + missense mutations and a few frameshift and splicing error mutations	Muscle	As in GSD-V: exercise intolerance with muscle pain and cramps	Variable glycogen accumulation with absence of PFK staining by histochemistry

hood form sets in later and has a more protracted but fatal course. The adult form is restricted to skeletal muscle and, unusually for a myopathy, may present with respiratory failure secondary to intercostal and diaphragmatic involvement. Muscle biopsy in each type demonstrates a vacuolar myopathy with PAS-positive glycogen, best demonstrated in sections that have not been processed to paraffin or through water-based solutions. Ultrastructurally, the glycogen is present within lysosomes and lying free between myofibrils. An unusual vascular pathology consisting of vacuolar degeneration of small and large arterial blood vessels may be seen in the brain in the adult form. Using cell lines from the three phenotypes it has been demonstrated that there is a good correlation between the level of residual α-glucosidase activity and disease type. Patients with the severest infantile form have hardly any residual enzyme activity. Multiple mutations and a few deletions involving the α-glucosidase gene at 17q21-23 have been reported in GSD-II, but correlation between the phenotype and genotype remains to be defined. Although a probable diagnosis may be obtained with muscle biopsy, confirmation must be obtained by direct measurement of α-glucosidase levels in lymphocytes or fibroblasts. Prenatal diagnosis can be obtained by measuring levels of α-glucosidase in chorionic villi.

B. Debrancher Enzyme Deficiency (Cori-Forbes disease; GSD-III)

Although debrancher enzyme deficiency primarily involves liver in childhood, muscle weakness with wasting may occur in some patients. This may be associated with cardiac involvement. The muscle biopsy appearances are not different from those in McArdle disease.

C. Myophosphorylase Deficiency (McArdle disease; GSD-V)

Although McArdle disease is the prototype GSD, it is in fact extremely rare. Typically the disease sets in in adulthood and is suggested by a history of exercise-induced cramps, particularly following episodes of isometric muscular contraction or more commonly following sustained exercise such as vigorous walking. Should the patient persist in exercising through the cramps, muscle necrosis may develop and result in myoglobinuria. Some patients do not give a history of cramps and instead present with progressive weakness indistinguishable from other causes of muscle weakness. A rare fatal form which presents with neonatal weakness has been described. Muscle biopsy may demonstrate increased glycogen deposition, but this is variable and in some instances the PAS reaction may be normal. However, histochemical demonstration of absent myophosphorylase activity in muscle fibers and not in endomysial or perimysial blood vessels, which serve as internal controls, is the most important finding.

Western blot demonstrates absence or a marked reduction of myophosphorylase levels in the majority of patients. Mutations of several different types have been reported in the myophosphorylase gene at 11q13, with a nonsense mutation at codon 49 being the most frequent. This nonsense mutation impairs protein synthesis, while some of the other missense mutations give rise to functionally inactive myophosphorylase. Genetic investigations should always be initiated in this unusual myopathy as there is still much to be learned about genotype-phenotype correlations.

D. Phosphofructokinase Deficiency (Tarui disease; GSD-VII)

Phosphofructokinase (PFK) deficiency has a similar clinical presentation to GSD-V and is particularly common in Ashkenazi Jewish patients. A hemolytic anemia may be present. The muscle biopsy shows similar changes to McArdle's, though glycogen is less likely to be found in lysosomes. PFK deficiency is demonstrated histochemically. PFK is a tetrameric enzyme of which the muscle (M) component is encoded by a gene on chromosome 1. A variety of mutations have been described in the PFK-M gene, but genotype-phenotype correlations are in the process of being established.

VIII. MITOCHONDRIAL DISEASES

The spectrum of mitochondrial disease has broadened enormously in the past 5 years. While brain and muscle are the organs most frequently affected by mitochondrial dysfunction, there is increasing awareness that other diverse diseases, such as cardiomyopathy, diabetes mellitus, aplastic anemia, and renal tubular acidosis, may have a mitochondrial basis. Though controversial, there is some evidence that mitochondrial dysfunction may play a role in aging (see Chap. 8) and in certain neurodegenerative diseases. Mitochondria are unique in that they possess their own DNA, a situation which developed as mitochondria were endosymbiotically incorporated into cells in the early stages of plant evolution. Mitochondria have the ability to replicate and to transcribe and translate their own DNA. Mitochondrial DNA (mtDNA) is a circular, closed, double-stranded molecule which consists of 16,569 nucleotides encoding protein subunits as well as the structural RNA required to translate these subunits. There are a number of features by which mtDNA and nuclear DNA differ. MtDNA is maternally inherited through the oocyte cytoplasm; thus, maternal inheritance is a feature of many mitochondrial diseases.

MtDNA is inherently unstable because repair mechanisms are poor and because there are few introns present. Mutations are frequent and are particularly likely to be induced by oxygen free radicals generated during the key mitochondrial process of oxidative phosphorylation (OXPHOS). Development of a new mutation results in a mixture of mutant and normal (wild-type) mtDNA within a cell, a process known as heteroplasmy. During successive cell divisions there is a gradual drift toward a situation where some cells possess entirely normal or entirely abnormal mtDNA (a process known as homoplasmy), and some cells retain a mixture of normal and abnormal mtDNA (heteroplasmy). The consequences for a cell or organ in terms of reduced energy output will depend on the proportions of wild-type to mutant mtDNA present. Organs vary in their bioenergetic requirements, with brain, retina, and muscle (both cardiac and skeletal) being most dependent on mitochondrial-derived ATP; it is these organs/tissues that are most often involved in mitochondrial disease. As a consequence of heteroplasmy, phenotype variability is a characteristic feature of mitochondrial disease. A bioenergetic deficit, if severe enough, will lead to cell death, and if nonreplicating cells, such as neurones or retinal ganglion cells are involved, there will be devastating neurological consequences.

Mitochondria do not function independently of nuclear control. MtDNA codes for only 13 of the more than 80 polypeptides distributed among the five multiple enzyme complexes (I–V) involved in the OXPHOS pathway. It is therefore apparent that the nucleus has by far the dominant role in OXPHOS. Nuclear-encoded polypeptides must be assembled in the cell cytoplasm and imported into the mitochondrion prior to final assembly into a functional unit. Very little is known of diseases due to defects in the importation of nuclear-encoded polypeptides into the mitochondrion.

To generate energy, mitochondria utilize the metabolic products of glycolysis (pyruvate) and fatty-acid metabolism which are transported into the mitochondrial matrix. Here they are oxidized to acetyl CoA, which in turn is oxidized in the Krebs cycle. The reducing equivalents (NADH and $FADH_2$) thus generated are subsequently oxidized by complex I and complex II, respectively. Electrons are carried along this chain of proteins to ubiquinone and via a common pathway comprising complex III, cytochrome C, and complex IV to the final hydrogen acceptor, which is molecular oxygen. In this process a proton-motive force is generated that is used by complex V to synthesize ATP. Uncoupling of oxidation and phosphorylation is an extremely rare clinical event, but, interestingly, it provided the basis for one of the first clinical descriptions of mitochondrial disease by Luft in 1962.

Classification of mitochondrial diseases is clinically difficult because of phenotype variability and because the presence of age-related, nonpathogenic somatic mutations in mtDNA can hamper precise genotyping. Current laboratory screening of patients suspected of having a mitochondrial disease is based on demonstration of altered lactate:pyruvate ratios in blood or CSF and on the demonstration of morphologic and functional alterations in mitochondria in accessible tissue such as muscle. Where diseased tissue is not available, it is possible, in certain well-characterized mitochondrial disease syndromes, to demonstrate a specific mutation or rearrangement in mtDNA obtained from peripheral blood. The limitations of this approach in a patient not conforming to the classical disease descriptions are obvious.

The cardinal histologic feature of mitochondrial disease is the ragged-red fiber (RRF), recognized in muscle cells by subsarcolemmal granular red-brown staining using the modified Gomori trichrome stain (Fig. 8). Electron microscopic examination of this area reveals an increased number of mitochondria with bizarre paracrystalline mitochondrial forms sometimes present. The histochemical demonstration of diminished or absent cytochrome oxidase (COX) activity complemented by enhanced succinic dehydrogenase (SDH) activity in sections of fresh frozen muscle is also a very useful screening test for mitochondrial dysfunction. COX is encoded by mtDNA, and as a consequence of a mutation in mtDNA its expression may be downregulated. SDH is encoded by nuclear DNA and undergoes compensatory upregulation in the presence of diminished COX activity. It is not possible to devise an all-inclusive classification system for mitochondrial disease which readily encompasses their genetic, biochemical, pathological, and clinical features. Attempts to classify mitochondrial disease on a biochemical basis, while conceptually useful and therapeutically important, are not applicable to clinical practice. The biochemical expression of an underlying mtDNA mutation may be impossible to determine if the

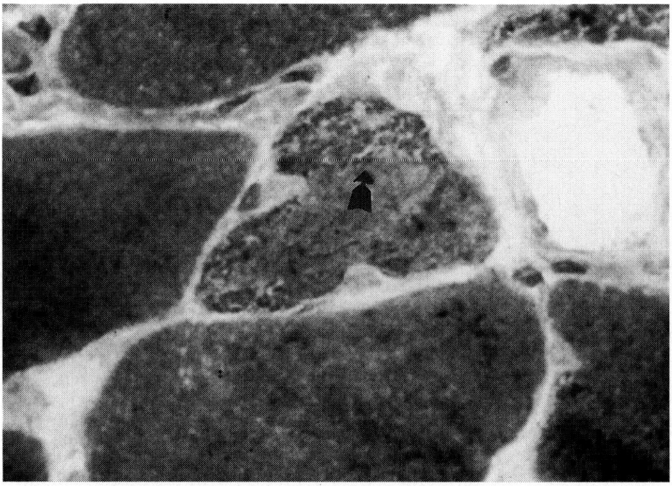

Figure 8 Transverse section of skeletal muscle stained with modified Gomori trichrome technique to show subsarcolemmal accumulation of granular dark material (arrow) indicative of ragged-red fiber formation. (See also Chap. 10.)

condition is selectively expressed in inaccessible tissue such as heart, brain, or retina. Similarly, the demonstration of a particular mutation in mtDNA need not necessarily be associated with disease expression if the ratio of mutant to wild-type mtDNA lies below a critical threshold for disease expression.

Neuropathologic features include the presence of ragged-red fibers and areas of cerebral cortical necrosis accompanied by capillary proliferation. While these features are relatively stereotyped, they are not specific for particular mitochondrial disorders. Currently, the best operational classification of mitochondrial disease is one based on the recognition of particular phenotypes associated with specific mitochondrial point mutations or deletions, or with presumptive mutations in nuclear DNA, which may or may not induce secondary effects in mitochondrial DNA. It is vital to remember that the syndromes listed below show considerable variability of clinical expression both within and between individual families. It is easy to overlook the possibility of a mitochondrial cause when a patient presents with only one of these features—e.g., epilepsy, myopathy, neuropathy, deafness, or visual impairment (Table 5).

A. Point Mutations

1. MELAS (mitochondrial myopathy, encephalopathy, lactic acidosis, and strokelike episodes)

Typically MELAS presents in young adults as stroke, migraine, or epilepsy. Deafness and diabetes mellitus may be present. An important clue is the observation that areas of cerebral cortical infarction lie outside a major vascular territory (Fig. 9). Some families may show overlap with other mitochondrial syndromes including chronic progressive external ophthalmoplegia (CPEO) and myoclonic epilepsy with ragged-red fibers (MERRF). Skeletal muscle involvement is reflected in the presence of ragged-red fibers (RRFs), though the number of RRFs may vary enormously with some patients having none. The clinical course is variable but areas of cerebral infarction may be so extensive as to result in death. Over 80% of MELAS cases are associated with $A \rightarrow G$ transition at position 3243 in the mitochondrial $tRNA^{Leu(UUR)}$ gene. A number of other point mutations involving $tRNA^{Leu(UUR)}$ genes at positions 11084, 3252, 3256, 3271, and 3291 have been reported. Deficiencies of complexes I, III, and IV have been described in MELAS patients. The mechanism whereby the point mutation results in reduced activity of the respiratory chain enzymes is uncertain, but interference with transcription termination is a possibility. There is poor correlation between the levels of mutant mtDNA and the presence or absence of disease in particular families. The presence of disease-modifying mutations in other areas of mtDNA may explain this variability in disease expression.

Neuropathologic studies of MELAS are sparse. The brain typically shows areas of necrosis which, depending on their duration, may demonstrate cavita-

Table 5 Classification of Mitochondrial Disorders with Major Involvement of the CNS/PNS

Mutations in mtDNA	Disease group	Gene mutated	Major biochemical defect	Common abnormality in mtDNA
A. Point mutations	MELAS	$tRNA^{LeuUUR}$	Complex I reduced	A-G 3243
	MERRF	$tRNA^{lyx}$	Complexes I and IV	A-G 8344
	LHON	ND1; ND2; ND4; ND5; ND6; COl	Complex I, III, or IV	G-A 11778; 3460 or 14484
	NARP	ATPase 6	Not characterized	T-G 8993
	Leigh disease (some cases)	ATPase 6 and El alpha subunit of PDHC and possibly nuclear genes	Complex I or IV or PDHC	A-G 8344; T-C/G 8993
B. Deletions	KSS and CPEO	All deletions involve loss of multiple genes encoding respiratory chain subunits		4977bp Δ + multiple Δ's ranging 2.0–7.0 kb
	Myopathy (sec Chap. 10)			
	Pearson syndrome			4.9 kb Δ + other Δ's ranging 9–14 kb in length
	Wolfram syndrome	Partial cytochrome oxidase deficiency		8.5kb Δ + 4p16
	MNGIE			Multiple deletions
	Neuropathy			Two populations deleted mtDNA-not characterized

C. Postulated nuclear DNA mutations	Leigh disease (some cases) Myopathy (some cases)		
D. Depletion of mtDNA	mtDNA depletion syndromes		Cytochrome oxidase deficiency
E. Acquired mitochondrial dysfunction	Aging Drug induced (antiviral nucleoside analogues) Oxidative stress Neurodegenerative disorders		

Note: For abbreviations, see text.

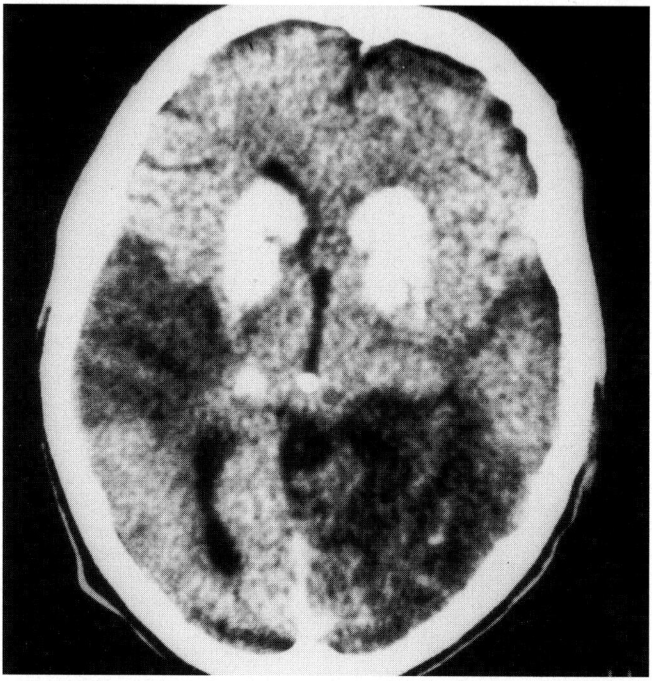

Figure 9 Axial non-contrast-enhanced CT brain scan which demonstrates a large region of low-density change in right occipital region and a similar area in left parietal region, originally attributed to "simple" ischemic infarcts. Patients also had short stature, deafness, and an A→G mutation at position 3243 in mtDNA, typical of MELAS syndrome. Note bilateral basal ganglionic calcification, which may also be present in this disorder.

tion (Fig. 10). There is intense proliferation of capillaries but in reality it is not possible to make a microscopic distinction between infarction due to vascular causes and necrosis due to an energy deprivation state. The occipital cortex is the most frequently involved area, but all areas may ultimately be affected. Skeletal muscle shows variable numbers of RRFs and interfiber mosaicism for COX/SDH.

2. *MERRF* (*myoclonic epilepsy with ragged-red fibers*)

The complete clinical expression of MERRF includes myoclonus, epilepsy, myopathy, and ataxia. Additionally, dementia, optic atrophy, and spasticity may be present. Some families demonstrate overlap with MELAS. Onset may be in childhood or adulthood. Neuropathologic descriptions are limited to a few case

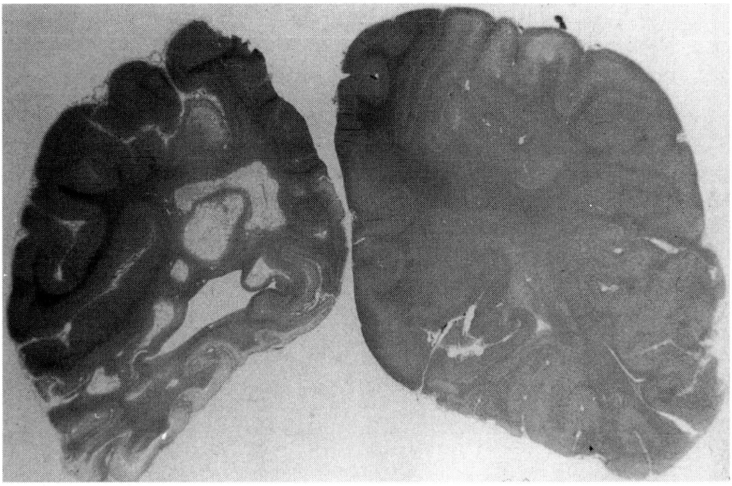

Figure 10 Whole-mount (coronal plane) section of cerebral hemispheres from a patient with MELAS showing large area of cavitary change in left occipital region. Microscopic examination showed capillary proliferation, astrocytic gliosis, and occasional surviving neurons in regions of gliosis.

reports. Microscopic examination shows loss of neurons and gliosis affecting the globus pallidus, substantia nigra, red nucleus, dentate nucleus, inferior olivary nucleus, cerebellar cortex, and the spinocerebellar tracts of the spinal cord. Some patients have demonstrated bilateral symmetrical involvement of the thalami, the colliculi, and the pontine and medullary tegmentum, a distribution of changes similar to that observed in Leigh disease. Abnormal mitochondria may be observed in brain if tissue preservation is adequate. MERRF and the Ramsay-Hunt syndrome (cerebellar dyssynergia) share certain clinical features. Over 90% of MERRF cases are associated with an A-G transition in the $tRNA^{lys}$ gene at position 8344 in mtDNA which gives rise to deficiencies in enzyme complexes I and IV of the respiratory chain. Transfer of mtDNAs carrying the 8344 mutation to human cell lines devoid of mitochondrial DNA causes a severe defect in mitochondrial translation in the recipient cells, which is independent of nuclear background. This implies that the tRNA mutation is sufficient to cause the disease. A T$\rightarrow$C transition in the $tRNA^{Lys}$ gene at position 8356 has also been described in MERRF.

3. Leber's Hereditary Optic Neuropathy (LHON)

LHON is the most common cause of midlife visual loss (Fig. 11). Although more than 15 different mtDNA mutations have been reported in LHON, over

90% of patients have one or another of three G→A point mutations at position 11778, 3460, or 14484. LHON mutations involve polypeptides in complex I, III, or IV. Visual loss may occur simultaneously in both eyes or sequentially. Progression of visual loss may be rapid or slow. Unusually for mitochondrial disease, some patients may show recovery of vision. The severity, rate of disease progression, and likelihood of recovery are linked to particular mutations with 11778 patients having the worst and those with the 14484 mutation having the best prognosis. Disease associations include cardiac conduction defects, sensory peripheral neuropathy, and a multiple-sclerosis-like syndrome in females with the 11778 mutation. A severe progressive striatal disorder has been described in a Swedish 11778 family. While alcohol- and tobacco-induced optic injury may cause diagnostic confusion with LHON, the issue is resolved by detection of an LHON-associated mtDNA mutation. There is no good evidence that either excess alcohol or tobacco alters the expression of a LHON-associated mutation.

Not all patients with LHON have a family history, and not all relatives of an affected patient having a mutation will express the disease. Other, missense or secondary mtDNA mutations at positions 3394, 4216, 4917, 7444, 13708, and 15812 may be present and influence the disease expression in an

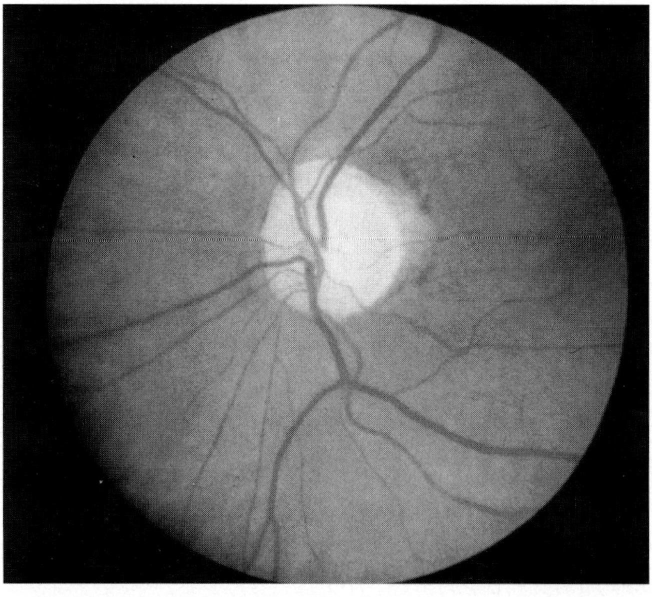

Figure 11 Funduscopic examination showing severe optic atrophy in a patient with Leber hereditary optic atrophy.

at-risk family member. The bias toward male patients has led to a suggestion that an X-linked gene may exert an influence but no such X-linked gene has been reported. There are no effective treatments to alter disease outcome. Ophthalmologic examination reveals peripapillary telangiectasia, microangiopathy without fluorescein leakage, vascular tortuosity, and, ultimately, optic atrophy. Detailed pathologic descriptions of the disease in the early stages are not available.

4. Neuropathy, Ataxia, and Retinitis Pigmentosa (NARP)

NARP is an extremely rare condition in which a sensorimotor neuropathy is accompanied by developmental delay, dementia, ataxia, and retinitis pigmentosa. A T→G point mutation at position 8993 in subunit 6 of mitochondrial ATPase is present. There are no detailed pathologic descriptions of NARP.

5. Leigh Disease (LD)—Subacute Necrotizing Leukoencephalopathy

LD is the prototype childhood mitochondrial disorder. Clinical presentation and course vary considerably, and several adult-onset cases have been reported. Similarities between the pathology of LD and Wernicke's encephalopathy prompted a search for evidence of involvement of the pyruvate dehydrogenase complex (PDHC). Defects in PDHC, cytochrome C oxidase, complex I, and complex IV activity have all been described in LD patients. Depending on the series reported, either complex IV or complex I deficiency is the most common biochemical defect. Point mutations involving T→G and T→C transitions at position 8993, or A→G transition at position 8344 have been reported in LD. There is no correlation between the phenotype and either the mutation or biochemical defect. Defects in nuclear DNA have been reported in isolated patients. Clinical presentation in childhood is usually at around 1 year and includes developmental delay or regression with failure to thrive. Eye movement disorders, optic atrophy, dystonia, pyramidal or extrapyramidal signs, or respiratory insufficiency are frequently present. Brainstem swelling and cranial nerve involvement may lead to an erroneous diagnosis of brainstem glioma. The clinical course is one of fairly rapid progression leading to death. Pathologically the lesions are characterized by a relatively stereotyped pattern of distribution and by striking vacuolation, macrophage infiltration, gliosis, intense capillary proliferation, and some neuronal loss. The presence of surviving neurons in the center of an area of intense capillary proliferation and gliosis eliminates vascular-based ischemia as a diagnostic possibility. Gray and white matter are involved, and myelin loss may be severe in the centrum semiovale.

Typically, the brainstem shows symmetrical lesions involving the periaqueductal gray matter and substantia nigra, the pontine and medullary tegmentum, and several cranial nerve nuclei (Fig. 12). The cerebellar dentate nucleus,

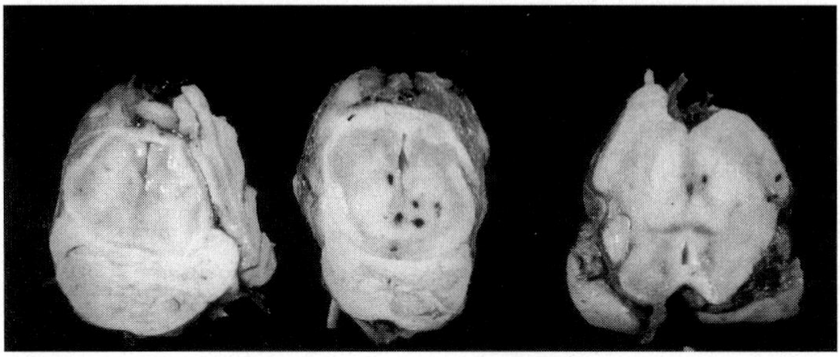

Figure 12 Transverse sections of brainstem from a patient with Leigh disease. At autopsy the brainstem appeared swollen and on sectioning (after fixation) revealed tegmental petechial hemorrhages and periaqueductal softening with pallor.

thalamus, and striatum (Fig. 13) [but not the mamillary bodies] are usually involved. Involvement of the inferior olives is correlated with the loss of Purkinje cells in the cerebellar cortex and may be due to selective loss of climbing fibers causing increased firing activity of Purkinje cells leading to excessive calcium ion entry. Myelin involvement may be characterized by cavitation or at least by microscopic spongy change. Topographical variations in disease severity are frequent. In spite of the capillary proliferation, hemorrhage is not present—another feature which distinguishes LD from Wernicke's. Biotinidase deficiency may result in a LD like pathology.

Much work remains to be done on the correlation of the genotype and phenotype. In autopsy cases, it is crucial to harvest fresh brain tissue with minimal or no delay from all areas of brain, brainstem, cerebellum, and spinal cord so that respiratory chain enzymes and mitochondrial DNA can be analyzed and the results correlated. Germ-line DNA should also be obtained.

B. Deletions Involving mtDNA

1. Kearns Sayre Syndrome (KSS)—Chronic Progressive External Ophthalmoplegia (CPEO)

CPEO and KSS are considered together as disorders in which there is progressive impairment of extraocular eye movements. KSS, which is distinguished from CPEO by the presence of systemic involvement, usually sets in before 20 years of age and is characterized by external ophthalmoplegia, pigmentary retinopathy, and at least one of ataxia, cardiac conduction defect, and raised CSF protein. Patients with KSS may go on to develop diabetes mellitus, deafness, or Pearson's syndrome. The phenotypes of KSS and CPEO are typically associated with deletions of mtDNA. All large deletions remove tRNA and protein-coding areas with the result that mitochondrial protein translation is im-

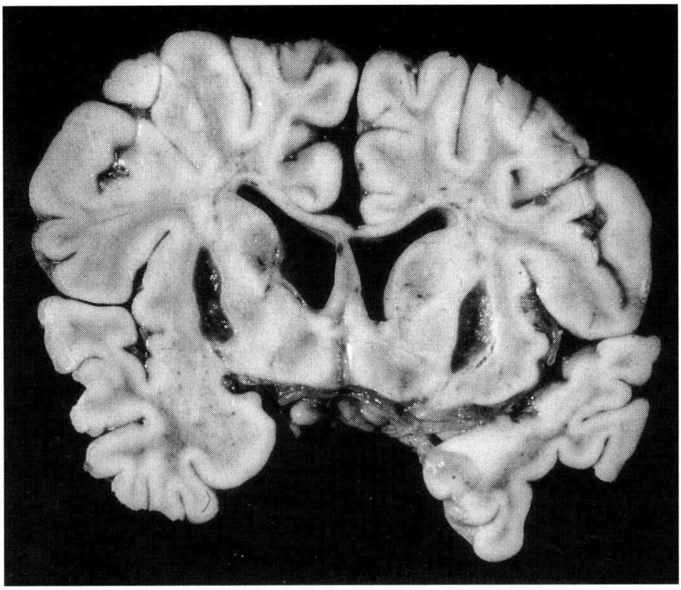

Figure 13 Coronal section of brain from same patient as shown in Figure 12, demonstrating bilateral symmetrical areas of tissue loss in region of the putamen. The brainstem and striatal appearances are typical of Leigh disease.

paired. Several deletions have been characterized, with loss of a 4977bp sequence the most common. The 4997bp deletion is also found in Pearson's syndrome where high levels of the mutant mtDNA are found in all tissues, while in KSS high levels of mutant mtDNA are confined to brain and muscle (skeletal, cardiac, and eye) and in CPEO, high levels are probably confined to eye muscle only. Some patients with KSS may have multiple mtDNA deletions. There is increasing evidence of genetic heterogeneity in CPEO and KSS. In addition to deletions, mtDNA duplications have been reported in KSS but not in CPEO. Autosomal-dominant CPEO has been linked to chromosome 10q in a Finnish family and to 3p in Italian kindreds, while a recessive form of CPEO has been characterized in related Arab families, factors which indicate a significant role for nuclear DNA. The size and site of the deletion do not correlate with the severity of the disease.

Deletions involving mtDNA are probably generated as a result of replication errors. Replication of the two strands of mtDNA commences from two widely separated origins and progresses asymmetrically. Thus during replication, single strands of mtDNA may be briefly exposed, allowing time for short repeated and complementary sequences, normally present on both strands at different loci, to inappropriately fuse with resultant exclusion of any intervening DNA between the repeated segments.

Skeletal muscle shows ragged-red fibers together with depletion of cytochrome oxidase and the accumulation of structurally abnormal mitochondria. There may be extreme variability of cytochrome oxidase staining. In patients with pure CPEO, biopsy of skeletal muscle is unlikely to be rewarding, but the orbicularis oculi muscle or other extraocular muscle will show identical features; however, these muscles are unlikely to be available for diagnostic purposes. Detailed neuropathologic descriptions of KSS are rare but, white matter vacuolation has been reported as to have spinal cord changes similar to those seen in Leigh disease.

2. *Pearson Marrow-Pancreas Syndrome* (*PMPS*)

PMPS is a rare fatal disorder of infancy in which pancytopenia is accompanied by pancreatic exocrine insufficiency. Some patients go on to develop KSS. Most patients have a 4.9-kb mtDNA deletion, but deletions may range in size from 9 to 14 kb and are located between tRNACyst and the D-loop. Duplications may also be present; 3-methylglutaconic aciduria was detected in a few patients with PMPS.

3. *Wolfram Syndrome* (*WS*)

WS is a rare progressive neurodegenerative disorder transmitted in an autosomal-recessive manner and characterized by optic atrophy, diabetes mellitus, diabetes insipidus, neurosensory hearing loss, urinary tract abnormalities, and neurological dysfunction. Evidence that this multisystem disorder is linked to mitochondrial dysfunction is increasing. A heteroplasmic 8.5-kb deletion in mtDNA has been reported in a family with WS. Recently, Wolfram syndrome has been linked to markers on chromosome 4p16, a finding that suggests a role for nuclear-encoded genes whose products might interact with mtDNA.

4. *Mitochondrial Neurogastrointestinal Encephalomyopathy* (*MNGIE*)

MNGIE is another rare syndrome of probable mitochondrial origin which is clinically characterized by gastrointestinal symptoms including recurrent nausea, vomiting, and intestinal dysmotility with diarrhea. Eye movement abnormalities and peripheral neuropathy may be present. Neuroimaging reveals widespread white matter changes. Ragged-red fibers may be present, and a partial defect of cytochrome c oxidase activity has been demonstrated in several patients. Multiple deletions in mtDNA have been described in affected patients.

5. *Neuropathy*

A mixed-demyelinating peripheral neuropathy without central nervous system involvement but with a major deletion in mtDNA has been described in an Irish family, but such cases of pure neuropathy of mitochondrial origin are exceptionally rare.

C. Defects in Nuclear DNA Resulting in Mitochondrial Disease

It is easy to forget that over 90% of mitochondrial proteins are encoded by nuclear DNA, synthesized on cytoplasmic ribosomes, and imported into the mitochondrion via a complex series of steps which involve recognition of addresses on the outer aspect of the mitochondrion by leader proteins. Within the mitochondrion, nuclear and mitochondrial-encoded proteins are assembled into a functional complex. Very little is known about defects in the nuclear control of mitochondrial function. However, it can be anticipated that there will be increased recognition of mitochondrial diseases which demonstrate Mendelian rather than maternal inheritance. Such diseases will likely fall into one of four categories as a result of defects in nuclear genes which code for tissue or non-tissue-specific proteins or which code for proteins involved in transmitochondrial membrane transport or for proteins which are involved in establishing communications between nuclear DNA and mtDNA.

D. Depletion of mtDNA

Some young patients with COX deficiency have been shown to have ratios of mitochondrial to nuclear DNA in skeletal muscle which are below the norm for age matched controls. This decline in mtDNA levels is paralleled by a decline in human mitochondrial transcription factor, which is an important regulator of mtDNA transcription and replication; whether this is a primary or secondary event is as yet unclear.

E. Acquired Mitochondrial Dysfunction

In the absence of good repair mechanisms, mtDNA is vulnerable to the development of acquired mutations. The tendency for such mutations to increase with aging has important implications, particularly for age-related neurodegenerative disorders such as Parkinson's disease (PD) (see Chap. 8). Aging is associated with a decline in respiratory chain capacity in a wide variety of tissues, and this is reflected in the increased number of COX-depleted muscle fibres as well as an increased number of ragged-red fibers in muscle from aged patients. These alterations in skeletal muscle are associated with an increased number of mtDNA deletions. Thus, in the presence of these naturally occurring changes, it is extremely difficult to establish a diagnosis of mitochondrial myopathy in the elderly.

The accumulation of acquired somatic mtDNA mutations in different parts of the brain, when combined with inherited germ-line mutations, may be sufficient to impair mitochondrial transcription and translation. If the ratio of mutant to wild-type mtDNA exceeds a critical threshold, oxidative phosphorylation (OXPHOS) may be compromised to such an extent that a bioenergetic crisis develops. In a nonreplicating cell such as a nigral neurone, this may be sufficient to cause cell death. Additionally, impairment of OXPHOS is itself likely to lead to further mtDNA injury through the generation of free radicals. It is attractive to try to explain selective neuronal vulnerability, a key feature of neurodegenerative disorders, on the basis of differential ratios of mutant to wild-type mtDNA in certain neuronal subgroups. Unravelling the interplay among defects in energy metabolism, oxidative damage, and possibly excitotoxic injury is beyond the scope of this section, but the evidence that these factors have a major role to play in the neurodegenerative disorders is increasing.

There has been considerable interest in the mechanism whereby the antiviral nucleoside analogs (ANAs) such as zidovudine (AZT) induce mitochondrial injury. In addition to hematologic, cardiac, and hepatic toxicity, AZT induces a severe myopathy characterized by ragged-red fibers and a partial deficiency of cytochrome c oxidase activity. These changes regress on discontinuance of the AZT. The mechanism of mitochondrial toxicity probably involves inhibition of DNA-polymerase-γ. The ANAs are being increasingly used to establish animal models of mitochondrial disease which will help to clarify mechanisms of mtDNA replication.

IX. LIPID DISORDERS OF MUSCLE AND BRAIN

These disorders, though infrequent, are included here for the purposes of continuity. Reference will be made to this section from the section on muscle disease. Fatty acids play a crucial role in energy production. Before fatty acids can be oxidized in mitochondria to yield acetyl-CoA, they must first be freed by hydrolysis from triacylglycerols in tissues, transported attached to albumin in the plasma, and freed for transport across cell membranes to the mitochondria. Fatty acids are converted to CoA thioesters through the actions of short-, medium-, and long-chain acyl-CoA synthetases. The transport of esterified free fatty acids or fatty-acyl-CoA across the mitochondrial membrane is dependent on the presence of carnitine, which acts as a carrier molecule or shuttle by accepting the fatty-acyl group, a reaction catalyzed by carnitine palmitoyltransferase I (CPT I), located on the outer mitochondrial membrane. Fatty-acylcarnitine is transported across the inner mitochondrial membrane where the fatty-acyl group is donated to intramitochondrial CoA under the influence of carnitine palmitoyltransferase II (CPT II). Thus, intramitochondrial fatty-acyl-

CoA becomes the substrate for beta-oxidation. Fatty-acid oxidation involves a series of dehydrogenation steps which are catalyzed by acyl-CoA dehydrogenases (ACADs), each specific for a given length of fatty acid. The ACADs contain nicotinamide and flavine adenine dinucleotide molecules which act as electron acceptors. The ultimate goal is the production of acetyl-CoA (which enters the Krebs cycle) and the reduced forms of nicotinamide and flavine adenine dinucleotide (NADH and $FADH_2$), the oxidation of which yields electrons which in turn are transported along the respiratory chain to produce ATP.

Disorders of fatty-acid metabolism may involve muscle in isolation or in conjunction with other systemic organs with, in certain cases, secondary involvement of brain through associated metabolic defects. Fatty acids may accumulate in liver or heart. Undegraded acyl-CoA esters are toxic and may in turn inhibit other mitochondrial enzymes. Investigation of patients with fatty-acid oxidation defects is complex, but, at the very least, patients suspected of having disease in this pathway should undergo measurements of plasma fatty acids, urinary organic acids, and acylglycines, which are formed through combination of acyl-CoA esters and glycine. Individual enzymes including the various acyl-CoA dehydrogenases, CPT I, CPT II, and carnitine itself may be measured but require a tissue source such as muscle or cultured fibroblasts.

A. Short-Chain Acyl-CoA Dehydrogenase Deficiency (SCAD)

This extremely rare condition may present with infantile or adult muscle weakness. A metabolic acidosis may be present. While a number of animal models of SCAD deficiency exist, there are few additional clinical or pathological data available.

B. Medium-Chain Acyl-CoA Dehydrogenase Deficiency (MCAD)

By contrast, MCAD is a relatively common condition which presents as an intermittent illness characterized by episodes of coma or even a Reye-like syndrome, with sudden death in some cases. Even if the diagnosis is established, some survivors may show mental retardation. Pathologic examination in fatal cases may demonstrate cerebral edema with accumulation of fat in liver and muscle. The MCAD gene is located on chromosome 1. The majority of cases are due to an A985G mutation in exon 11. The heterozygote carrier state is as high as 1/52 in some countries, but the disease has an estimated prevalence of 1/10,000, indicating a high number of asymptomatic homozygotes. However, because of the importance of MCAD deficiency as a cause of sudden death, neonatal screening is now offered in many countries.

C. Long-Chain Acyl-CoA Dehydrogenase (LCAD)

LCAD deficiency is very rare and is characterized by similar intermittent episodes of coma precipitated by fasting-induced hypoglycemia or by hepatomegaly and cardiomegaly with failure, especially in the first months of life. A very long chain acyl-CoA dehydrogenase (VLCAD) deficiency has also been reported and may present with hypoketotic hypoglycaemia or cardiac disease. Each of the above disorders should also be considered as a potential cause in cases of sudden adult death.

D. Carnitine Deficiency

Deficiency of carnitine may be systemic or restricted to skeletal muscle and may arise as a result of dietary deficiency or an inherited metabolic defect. Carnitine may be lost due to failure of renal tubular reabsorbtion. Deficiency of other enzymes involved in the transport of fatty acids across the mitochondrial membrane may lead to secondary carnitine deficiency. Deficiency leads to reduced transport of long-chain fatty acids into mitochondria with their secondary accumulation in liver, muscle, and other organs. Blockade of fatty-acid oxidation leads to dependence on glucose metabolism for energy production. A diet low in carbohydrate and rich in lipid may precipitate an acute crisis with hypoglycemia. This episode may simulate Reye's syndrome. The pathology of carnitine deficiency is characterized by lipid droplets in affected organs. Death during an acute crisis may be associated with cerebral edema.

E. Carnitine Palmitoyltransferase (CPT)

Deficiency of CPT I and II, located respectively on the outer and inner mitochondrial membranes, may lead to episodes of coma, hypoglycemia, and hepatomegaly with increased liver fat. An alternative presentation with muscle cramps, weakness, and even myoglobinuria is described. The CPT I and CPT II genes are located on chromosomes 11q and 1p32, respectively.

F. Reye's Syndrome (RS)

RS is included in this section as many of the features associated with RS may be present in patients with disorders of fatty-acid and organic-acid metabolism. Typically, there is a prodromal period in which a severe upper respiratory tract infectionlike picture is followed by onset of a deteriorating level of consciousness, vomiting, and coma. Abnormal liver function tests, particularly ammonia, are typical. The mortality is high if treatment is delayed, and even with early treatment mortality may reach 80%. In fatal cases the liver shows microvesicular fatty change while the brain shows severe edema. Ischemic changes which have a laminar distribution may also be present. Enlarged mitochondria may be seen in the brain and liver and have led to suggestions of a defect in mitochondrial metabolism.

Aspirin and valproic, isovaleric, and other organic acids have been implicated in the pathogenesis of RS. There is experimental evidence that these substances may interfere with mitochondrial permeability translation (MPT). The incidence of RS has fallen slightly, but whether this is due to a decline in aspirin consumption in children is undetermined.

X. INBORN ERRORS OF METABOLISM (IEM)

An in-depth review of the inborn errors of metabolism is beyond the scope of this chapter. While neurologic involvement is a frequent finding in the majority of these conditions, the neuropathologic features are relatively nonspecific. Introduction of mass neonatal screening for the most common disorders has resulted in a dramatic decline in the number of cases with profound mental handicap and major neuropathologic change. It is not possible to devise a classification that encompasses the diverse clinical, biochemical, and genetic features of these conditions. There is no place for a morphologic approach to classification. Diagnosis is based on a combination of clinical and biochemical findings with genetic investigation of increasing importance and of increasing usage. Broadly, the IEM can be grouped into organic acidemia, urea cycle disorder, defects of branched-chain amino acid metabolism, and single amino acid disorders such as phenylketonuria (PKU).

Shared characteristics of these diseases include the inheritance of an enzyme deficiency, accumulation of potentially toxic compounds proximal to the enzyme defect, failure to synthesize essential metabolites, and development of secondary metabolic derangements such as hypo- and hyperglycemia, hyperammonemia, and ketonuria. Essential investigations include measurement of urinary amino and organic acids, serum ammonia, and glucose, lactate, and pyruvate levels.

A. Organic Acidemia (OA)

Important OAs include propionic acidemia, methylmalonic acidemia, and glutaric acidemia.

1. Propionic Acidemia (PA)

PA is caused by deficiency of propionyl-CoA carboxylase which is a biotin-dependent mitochondrial enzyme required for the conversion of propionyl-CoA to D-methylmalonyl-CoA. Important precursors of propionyl-CoA include threonine, methionine, valine, and isoleucine. As a result of the enzyme defect, there is excretion of propionyl-CoA in the urine and decreased levels of D-methylmalonyl-CoA. The enzyme consists of six α and six β subunits, the α gene being located on chromosome 13 and the β gene on chromosome 3. Multiple defects on both genes have been described. The disease is invariably fatal. Neuropathologic descriptions are rare but include white matter vacuolation, especially in the white matter tracts of the striatum together with vascular and parenchymal mineralization. One patient with PA has been shown to have had acute hemorrhagic lesions in the basal ganglia with foci of neuronal loss. Vascular proliferation and swollen endothelial cells were also seen in the basal ganglia and were interpreted as evidence of possible blood-brain barrier breakdown.

2. *Methylmalonic Acidemia* (*MMA*)

MMA is caused by deficiency of methyl-malonyl-CoA mutase which is a B_{12}-dependent enzyme that catalyzes the conversion of methyl-malonyl-CoA to succinyl-CoA. The gene is on chromosome 6. Methylmalonate is excreted in the urine. Deficiency of the active B_{12} derivative results in the impaired enzyme activity. Some patients are B_{12}-responsive. The neuropathology includes bilateral symmetrical areas of neuronal loss in the globus pallidus and mild to moderate delay in myelination.

3. *Glutaric Aciduria Type I* (*GA I*)

GA I is an organic acidemia in which there are striking neuropathologic abnormalities. Glutaric acid is formed as a result of lysine, hydroxylysine, and tryptophan metabolism. Glutaryl-CoA dehydrogenase (GCDH), a mitochondrial matrix enzyme, is involved in their metabolism. The GCDH gene is mapped to 19p13.2. Mutation analysis is at an early stage, but multiple mutations have been reported in Amish families. Deficiency of GCDH results in large amounts of glutaric acid appearing in the urine, and causes a neurologic disorder with wide clinical variation ranging from an acute infantile encephalopathy to dystonia and spastic paraparesis. In fatal cases the brain may demonstrate frontotemporal atrophy with widening of the Sylvian fissures, which appear as opened opercula on MR scanning. Striatal necrosis or striatal neuronal loss and gliosis may be present and appear on MR as hypodense areas (Fig. 14). Bilateral arachnoid cysts have also been described. Glutaric aciduria type II is included in the disorders of branched-chain amino acids.

B. Urea Cycle Defects (UCDs)

Urea formation from ammonia, bicarbonate, ornithine, citrulline, and arginine requires completion of six enzymatic reactions in the liver (Fig. 15). Three

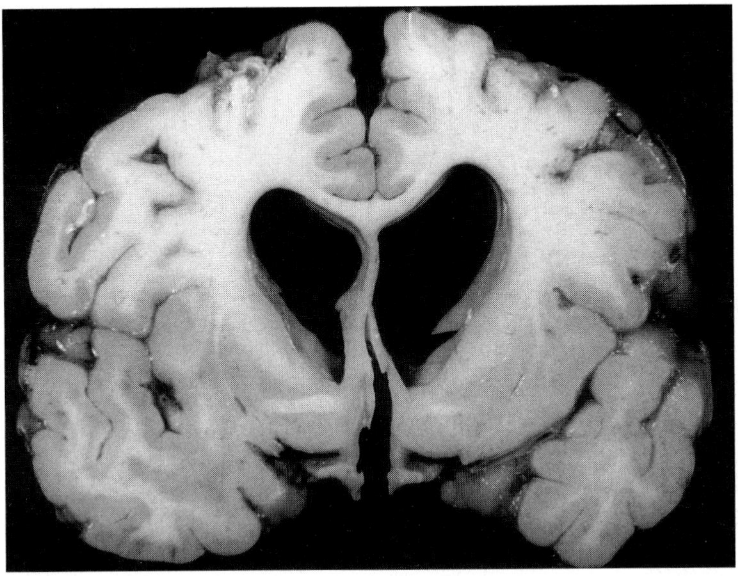

Figure 14 Bilateral symmetrical atrophy in caudate nuclei (and possibly also putamens) in a patient with glutaric aciduria type 1. Opercular widening (also typical of this disorder) is not present.

of the enzymes involved—argininosuccinate synthase (ASS), argininosuccinate lysate (ASL), and arginase—are located within the mitochondrial matrix; the remaining three, ornithine transcarbamylase (OTC), carbamylphosphate synthase (CPS), and N-acetylglutamate synthase (NAGS), are located in the cytosol.

Hyperammonemia is the cardinal biochemical manifestation of UCDs and is one of the mechanisms whereby these disorders cause neurologic injury. The nonionized form of ammonia crosses the blood-brain barrier. Different areas of brain respond with varying degrees of sensitivity to ammonia. Brain utilizes α-ketoglutarate and ATP to remove ammonia. Reduction in either could impair energy metabolism. Ammonium ions inhibit glutaminase and may alter levels of glutamate and other neurotransmitters. Proliferation of Alzheimer type II astrocytes is reflective of the elevated ammonia brain levels and is present in all UCDs. Additional neuropathologic changes may also be present in each of the six defects. The earlier recognition of UCDs followed by treatment, which may include protein restriction, replacement of deficient urea cycle components, and enhancement of alternative pathways to dispose of toxic metabolites, has reduced the prevalence of severe end-stage cases with gross neuropathologic

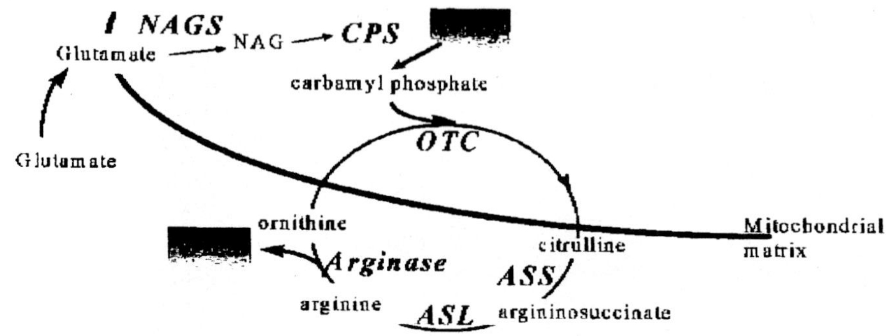

Figure 15 Diagram showing the "urea cycle."

abnormalities. Clinical presentation varies but is characterized in the neonatal period by vomiting, seizures, and hyperammonemic coma. Later, the presentation may be episodic and be precipitated by infection or diets rich in protein. The three cytosolic enzymes are CPS, OTC, and NAGS.

CPS catalyzes the synthesis of CP from ammonia and bicarbonate. CPS deficiency may be lethal in infancy or cause seizures in later years. The effects of hyperammonemia are as in the other UCDs. In fatal longstanding cases the brain may show diffuse atrophy with spongy degeneration. The gene for CPS has been assigned to 2q34-q35.

OTC deficiency, the only X-linked disorder of the six, may be associated with large destructive areas of brain necrosis which are often diagnosed as stroke or infarcts clinically and pathologically (Fig. 16). The OTC gene is mapped to Xp21.1 and is about 73 kb long. Numerous mutations and deletions have been reported; some of these involve the leader peptide, which is responsible for incorporation of the protein into the mitochondrial matrix.

NAGS catalyzes the formation of n-acetyl glutamate (NAG) from glutamate and acetyl-CoA. NAG is an important activator of CPS. NAGS deficiency is rare but in the neonatal period may cause uncontrollable movements, visual impairment, and hyperammonemic coma. There are no detailed descriptions of the neuropathology.

The three mitochondrial matrix enzymes are ASS, ASL and arginase.

ASS deficiency (citrullinemia) may cause neonatal irritability, seizures, and coma or present later with mental retardation in childhood or even in adulthood with episodic behavioral or psychiatric symptoms. The neuropathologic findings are clearly different at each stage. Cerebral edema may be dominant in the neonatal period with diffuse cerebral atrophy and spongy degeneration present in older fatal cases. The ASS gene is mapped to chromosome 9q34, but

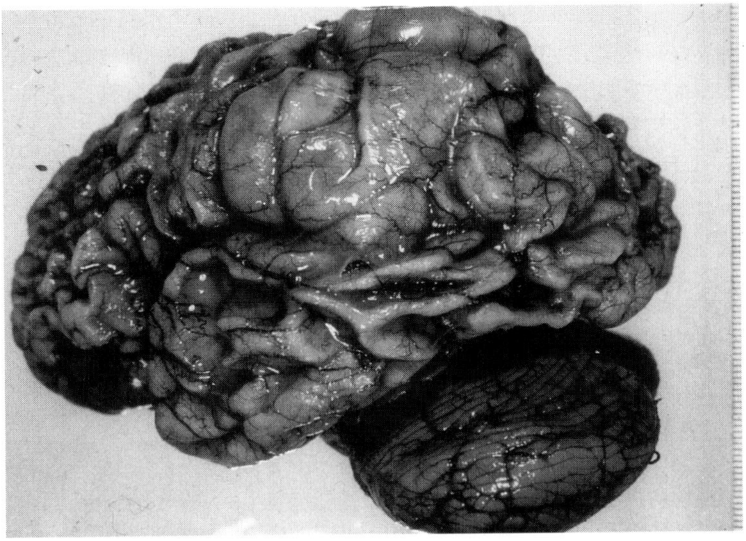

Figure 16 Large areas of focal cortical atrophy involving the frontotemporal regions of cerebral hemispheres in a patient with ornithine transcarbamylase deficiency.

several pseudogenes are located on other chromosomes. As in many of the other UCDs, multiple mutations have been described in the ASS gene.

ASL deficiency also results in neonatal and later-onset disease. The presence of trichorrhexis nodosa or dry brittle hair with nodules helps to distinguish this UCD from the others. The neuropathology in the neonatal period or later is not different from that in ASS deficiency. The ASL gene is approximately 35 kb long and is mapped to 7q11.2, and again a number of different mutations have been reported.

Arginase deficiency is extremely rare and results from mutations in one or the other of two arginase genes (ARG I and ARG II). The neurologic disease includes coma, spastic paraparesis, and seizures. Postmortem descriptions are limited and do not show any specific pathology.

C. Disorders of Branched-Chain Amino Acid (BCAA) Metabolism

The branched-chain amino acids (leucine, isoleucine, and valine) have a branched methyl group at the 3 or 4 position and undergo degradation in a series of three steps—reversible transamination, oxidative decarboxylation, and dehydrogenation. In the cytosolic transamination step, there is coupling of the relevant branched amino acid to α-ketoglutarate to form a branched-chain ketoacid (BCKA). The BCKA is transported across the mitochondrial membrane, where it undergoes decarboxylation by a large enzyme complex (BCKAD complex). Dehydrogenation of the branched acyl-CoA derivatives is carried out by one of two acyl-CoA dehydrogenases. The oxidation products derived from this series of reactions are utilized as energy sources or in fatty-acid and cholesterol synthesis. Given the complex nature of the enzymatic steps involved, it is not surprising that there are multiple clinical deficiency states, the most notable from a neurologic point of view being maple syrup urine disease (MSUD), its variants, and glutaric aciduria type II (GA II). Prominent clinical features include mental retardation coupled with metabolic disturbances such as hypoglycemia and acidosis.

1. Maple Syrup Urine Disease (MSUD)

MSUD is due to failure of the second, or decarboxylation, step in degradation of BCAAs which is dependent on the functional integrity of the BCKAD enzyme complex. This complex is composed of three subunits—a branched-chain α-ketoacid decarboxylase (E1), a dihydrolipoyl transacyclase (E2), and a dihydrolipoyl dehydrogenase (E3)—together with various subunits and additional regulatory enzymes. The genes for each of the enzymes have been mapped and cloned. The functioning of this enzyme complex is analogous to the pyruvate dehydrogenase complex. The molecular genetics of MSUD indicates considerable variability, which is reflected in the differing subtypes. Classically there is onset of seizures, spasticity and altered respiration in the neonatal period. The tell-tale odor is best detected in the urine. Without treatment, there is progression to death or survival with severe mental retardation, dystonia, and eye movement disorders. Intermittent and thiamine-dependent forms may also occur. Examination of the brain in the acute phase may reveal edema. The brain may show diminished myelination, though MR has failed to show any significant abnormalities of the white matter in treated cases. Spongy change and the presence of crystalline deposits in unfixed sections have been reported in the older literature. There are no detailed recent neuropathology descriptions of MSUD.

2. Glutaric Aciduria Type II (GA II)

GA II is typical of a defect in the third stage in BCAA degradation in which deficiency of differing mitochondrial electron-transferring flavoproteins leads to defective dehydrogenation with consequent failure to transfer electrons from acyl-CoA dehydrogenases down the mitochondrial electron transport chain. The gene for the α-subunit of flavoprotein is located on 15q23-q25. A number of GA II-associated point mutations have been described in this gene. There is increased urinary excretion of isobutyric, isovaleric, acid and 2-methylbutyric acids; the metabolites of valine, leucine, and isoleucine as well as excretion of glutaric acid. Examination of the brain in fatal cases demonstrates cortical dysplasia with pachygyria. Other organs may demonstrate fatty change.

D. Single Amino Acid Disorders

Widespread neonatal screening for the more common amino acid disorders when combined with dietary and other treatments has virtually eliminated these disorders as causes of mental handicap. Most neonatal screening includes tests for phenylketonuria, galactosaemia, hypothyroidism, and maple syrup urine disease. Three of the more common single amino acid disorders associated with neurologic disease are discussed below.

1. Phenylketonuria (PKU)

Classic PKU, the most common metabolic cause of mental retardation, results from a deficiency of phenylalanine hydroxylase (PAH), which is required for the conversion of phenylalanine to tyrosine. In its absence there is accumulation of phenylalanine, which is converted to phenyl pyruvate and phenylacetate. Other hyperphenylalaninemic syndromes are described in which PAH activity is reduced but not completely absent. Tetrahydrobiopterin is an important cofactor for PAH activity and is in turn dependent on a number of critical steps for its synthesis. PKU patients have severe mental handicap often with microcephaly, spastic paraparesis, and extrapyramidal signs. Seizures are common. Neuropathologic descriptions are based on old case studies but include spongy degeneration of white matter with varying degrees of cortical neuronal loss. Gliosis and neuronal loss may be present in the thalamus and globus pallidus and in the lateral geniculate body. The mechanism of gray and white matter injury is not a simple toxic effect of excess phenylalanine, but rather the result of competition between phenylalanine and other amino acids for entry into brain across the blood-brain barrier. The PAH gene is located on chromosome 12q. Multiple mutations have been reported. There are considerable differences in the frequency of different mutations in differing populations. Defects in biopterin metabolism may lead to partial PAH deficiency with resultant hyperphenylalaninemia and also to impairment of tryptophan metabolism, for which it is also an important cofactor.

2. Galactosemia

Galactose is an important source of energy for newborn infants but must first undergo conversion to glucose through the actions of galactokinase (GALK), galactose-I-phosphate-uridyltransferase (GALT), and UDP-galactose-4-epimerase. Classic galactosemia is characterized by a deficiency of GALT, the gene for which is located on 9p13. Untreated classic galactosemia is fatal; when treatment is delayed, irreversible neurologic injury may occur and manifest as early onset of cataract formation, mental handicap, and delayed brain growth. Long-term survivors may show a spastic gait with ataxia and postural tremor. MR images of brain demonstrate increased signal in the periventricular white matter. Neuropathologic findings in longstanding cases include cerebral atrophy, myelin loss, Purkinje cell loss, excessive neuronal lipofuscin, and neuroaxonal-spheroid-like structures in the thalamus. GALK and epimerase deficiency are extremely rare, less severe, and less likely to have neurologic symptoms.

3. *Homocystinuria*

The majority of patients with homocystinuria are deficient in cystathionine β-synthase (CBS), a pyridoxal 5′-phosphate (PLP) enzyme involved in the conversion of methionine to cysteine through the transsulfuration pathway. Methionine is an important precursor of homocystine, and defects in B_{12} and folate metabolism may also lead to homocystinuria. The human CBS gene maps to chromosome 21q22.3 and encodes the CBS subunit of 551 amino acid residues. CBS deficiency is inherited as an autosomal-recessive trait, the prevalence of which varies in different areas of the world. Typical clinical features of homocystinuria include ectopia lentis, osteoporosis, mental handicap, and an increased risk for development of atherosclerosis and thromboembolic disease. Not all patients have mental handicap. Some patients deficient in CBS may respond to pyridoxal. Neuropathologic findings in homocystinuria include sagittal sinus thrombosis and multiple cerebral infarcts of varying sizes and ages. Patients with severe mental handicap may show cerebral atrophy and diffuse myelin loss.

XI. CEROID LIPOFUSCINOSES (CLNs)

The CLNs are among the most common inherited and fatal neurodegenerative disorders and are characterized by the progressive intraneuronal accumulation of autofluorescent lipofuscin pigment. They are broadly characterized by progressive intellectual decline, retinal degeneration, and seizures. Classification is based on age at onset and is further defined by reference to clinical, neurophysiological, and pathological findings (Table 6). The various subtypes are referred to by a plethora of eponyms. The validity of these phenotypes is under active reassessment, as the genetic basis for the majority of subtypes has been ascertained. However, as yet, there is no test which replaces light microscopic and ultrastructural examination of skin, rectal mucosa (Fig. 17), conjunctiva, or brain in order to demonstrate lipofuscin pigment. The CLN lipopigment must be distinguished from conventional lipofuscin by the presence of curvilinear profiles (Fig. 18) or granular osmiophilic deposits (GRODs), and, in some cases, by the presence of yellow autofluorescence (Fig. 19).

Table 6 Summary of Main Clinical, Pathological, and Genetic Features of the Ceroid Lipofuscinoses

Designation	CLN1	CLN2	CLN3	CLN4	CLN5
Eponym	Infantile Santavuori disease, Finnish variant	Late infantile type Jansky-Bielschowsky disease	Juvenile-type Batten disease; Vogt-Spielmeyer disease	Adult-type Kufs disease	Variant late infantile type
Gene locus	1p32 gene encoding palmitoyl protein thioesterase (PPT)	Not determined	16p12.1 1.02 kb deletion present in majority	Not determined	13q21.1-q32
Age of onset	8–20 months	2–4 yr	4–9 yr	30 yr +	4–5 yr
Main clinical features	Dementia, seizures, visual failure	Epilepsy, dementia, myoclonus	Visual impairment, rigidity	Dementia, ataxia	Mental retardation, ataxia, and myoclonic epilepsy
Vacuolated lymphocytes	No	No	Yes	No	No
Storage products	Granular osmiophilic deposits	Curvilinear or fingerprint profiles	Curvilinear or fingerprint profiles	Fingerprint and granular profiles	Curvilinear bodies and fingerprint profiles
Subunit c Mitochondrial ATP synthase	Not increased	Not increased	Increased	Increased	Not determined

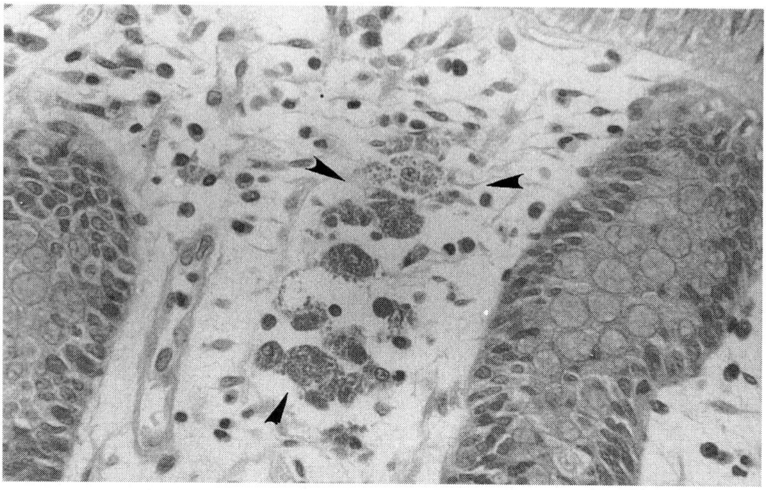

Figure 17 Rectal mucosal biopsy in which there are numerous PAS-positive macrophages (arrows) distended with granular material typical of the ceroid lipofuscinoses.

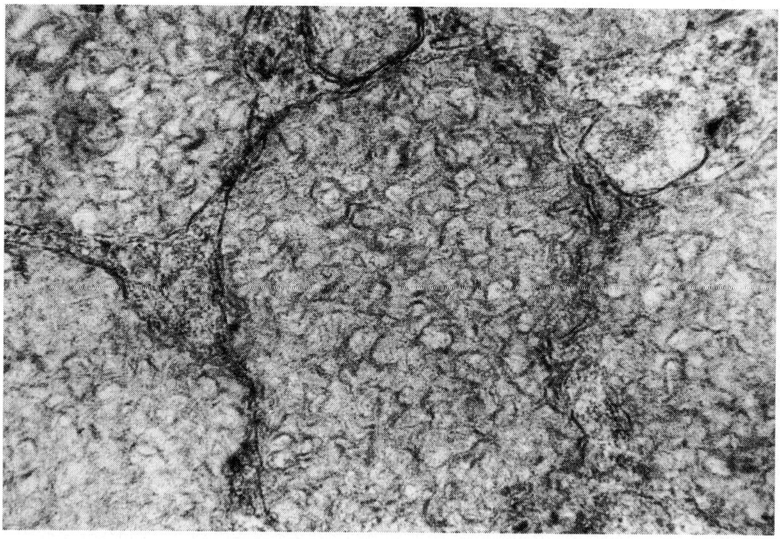

Figure 18 Brain biopsy showing distension of neuronal cytoplasm by typical curvilinear profiles, from a patient with CLN 3. (Mag $\times 10{,}000$.)

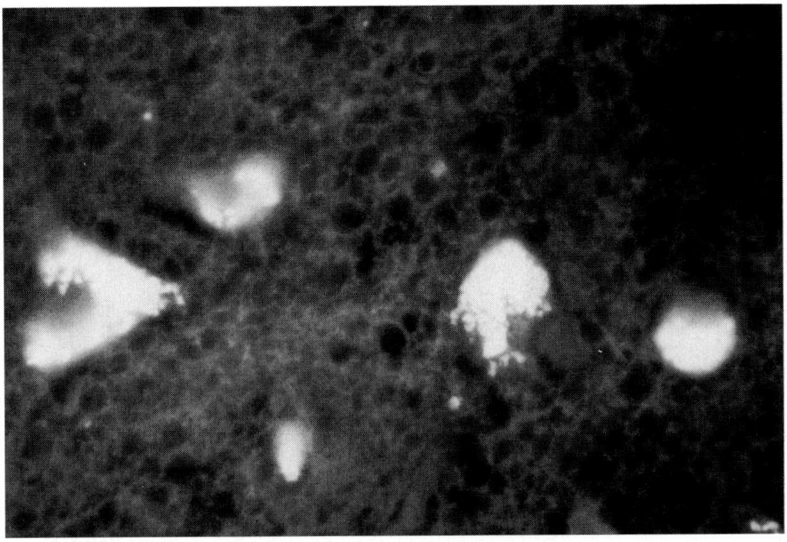

Figure 19 Unstained section of brain viewed under ultraviolet light to demonstrate autofluorescence (which was yellow) in a patient with Kufs disease (CLN 4).

As well as the classic forms outlined above, there is increasing recognition of variant forms that do not conform to these phenotypes. The CLNs vary in the degree of systemic involvement, but in general all, with the possible exception of CLN4, involve the rectal mucosal ganglion cells. Skin, muscle, and conjunctivae may be used for diagnosis but in less experienced hands are difficult to interpret. A brain biopsy may be required if CLN4 is suspected, as there is variability in the degree to which systemic organs are involved in this form. Chorionic villi may be used for prenatal diagnosis. The lipopigment causes minimal neuronal distension and exhibits bright yellow autofluorescence which contrasts with the brown autofluorescence of normal lipofuscin. There is strong PAS positivity and, with the exception of the infantile form, there is bright blue cytoplasmic staining with Luxol fast blue. These staining reactions are unaffected by formalin fixation or by processing to paraffin. Ultrastructurally the stored material consists of GRODs in the infantile form and in the late-infantile variant consists of curvilinear bodies. In the juvenile form there may be fingerprint inclusions as well as curvilinear profiles. All three types of inclusion have been described in the adult form (Figs. 20, 21). In general a rectal biopsy that includes ganglion cells should be the first and, in the majority of cases, the definitive diagnostic test. The gross appearance of the brain will be determined by the stage of the disease at which death occurs. In the late stages the brain is atrophic and there is variable neuronal loss which may be paralleled

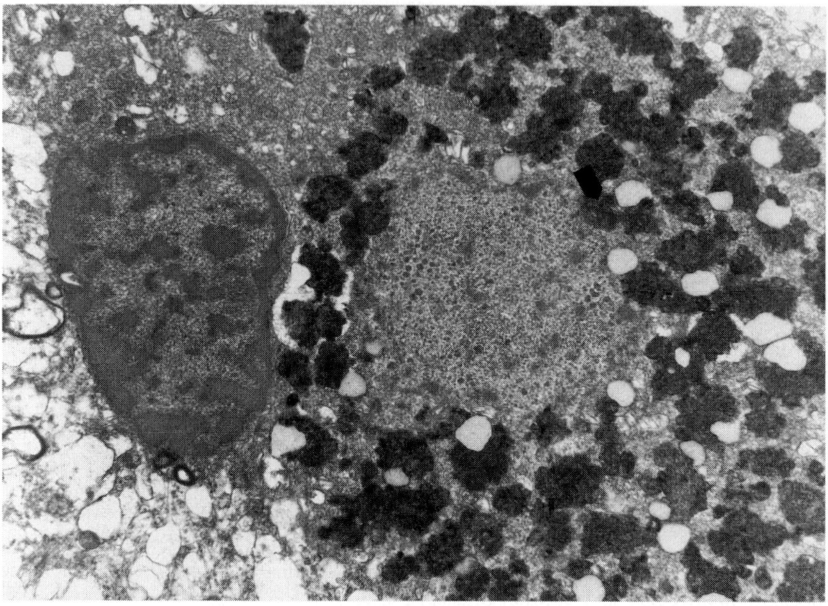

Figure 20 Brain biopsy from patient with Kufs disease, in which cytoplasmic granular osmiophilic deposits are present (arrow). (Mag ×40,000.)

by myelin loss. All areas of brain are involved. The degree of cortical atrophy may be minimal in the adult form.

XII. MISCELLANEOUS METABOLIC DISORDERS

A. Canavan Disease (CD)

Alternatively known as spongy degeneration of the nervous system, CD is a progressive degenerative disorder characterized by onset within the first 6 months of life, developmental regression, hypotonia, visual loss, and characteristic megalencephaly. Congenital, infantile, and juvenile forms have been described, though whether they all share identical biochemical abnormalities is unknown. Until recently, diagnosis was made on the basis of megalencephaly and MR evidence of a diffuse white matter disorder coupled with biopsy or autopsy evidence of spongy degeneration of white matter. Typically the brain demonstrates widespread spongy degeneration of white matter with variable myelin loss and proliferation of astrocytes. In long-term survivors the degree of white matter vacuolation tends to diminish. Recently patients with CD have been shown to have elevated urinary N-acetylaspartic (NAA) acid levels due to

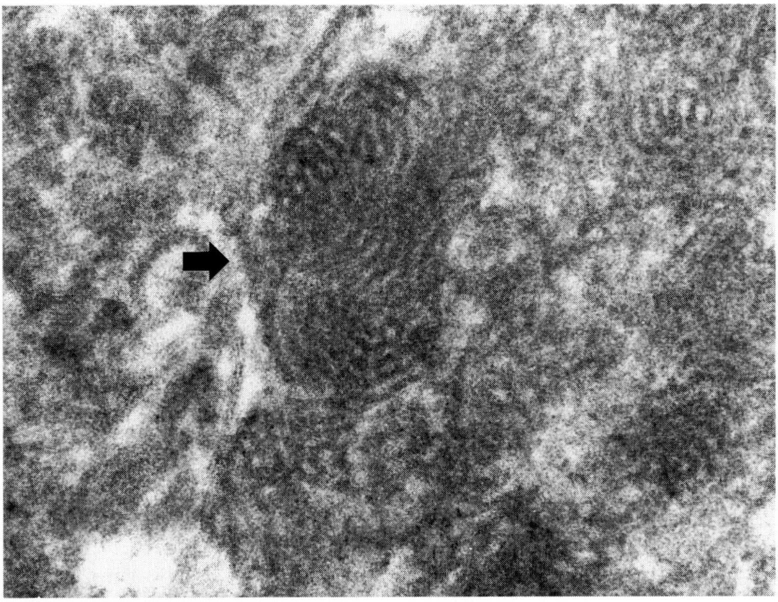

Figure 21 Brain biopsy from sister of the patient whose brain tissue is illustrated in Figure 19. Note fingerprint inclusions (arrow) present within neuronal cytoplasm. (Mag $\times$100,000.)

a deficiency of aspartoacyclase (ASPA), the enzyme responsible for the hydrolysis of N-acetylaspartic acid to L-aspartic acid and acetate. The mechanism whereby the elevated NAA results in white matter degeneration is undetermined. The human ASPA gene has been localized to human chromosome 17p13. Three mutations in this gene have been found to account for virtually all of the CD patients of Ashkenazi-Jewish origin. The genotype of non-Jewish European patients is more diverse, with as many as nine mutations described—all occurring in a hot spot located in exons 4–6 of the ASPA gene. Measurement of NAA levels is unreliable for identification of carriers.

B. Alexander Disease (AD)

AD is a poorly understood condition which shares the clinical feature of megalencephaly with CD. Onset may be at anytime from birth to early childhood with relentless clinical deterioration, seizures, and intellectual decline. Bulbar symptoms may be prominent. Some adults with a similar disorder, though without megalencephaly, have been described. Characteristically there is widespread Rosenthal fiber formation (Fig. 22) in the subependymal, subpial, and perivas-

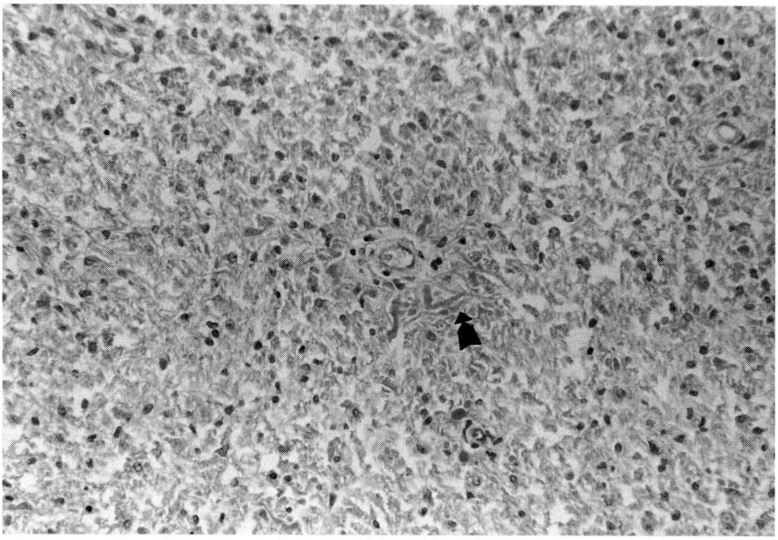

Figure 22 Alexander disease is characterized by intense fibrillary gliosis and Rosenthal fiber (arrowhead) formation, especially within the white matter.

cular locations. Myelin loss may be extensive. Astrocyte numbers are increased and may show atypia. Difficulty may be encountered in trying to separate AD from diffuse gliomatosis cerebri, but in gliomatosis cerebri there is much less Rosenthal fiber formation. Elevated levels of alpha β-crystallin, a heat shock protein, have been reported in AD brains, but the significance of this is unknown. Alpha β-crystallin deposition is typically associated with Rosenthal fiber formation, irrespective of the cause, though alpha β-crystallin is also seen in neuronal cytoplasmic inclusions of several neurodegenerative disorders (see Chap. 8).

C. Wilson Disease (WD)

WD is an autosomal-recessive disorder characterized by widespread copper deposition and reduction in ceruloplasmin levels. The gene for WD, which is located at 13q14-q21, has been cloned and encodes a copper-transporting ATPase protein (ATP7B). The WD gene is remarkably similar to the Menkes disease gene, designated ATP7A. Multiple mutations of the ATP7B gene have been reported in patients with WD. Genotype-phenotype correlations are at a preliminary phase, but some of the mutations reported are associated with early-onset disease, which may occur as a result of interruptions to the reading frame, thereby leading to complete protein deficiency. The basic disease mechanism is still unknown, and the relationship between the copper-binding ATPase protein and ceruloplasmin remains to be determined. Ceruloplasmin, the gene for which is located on chromosome 3, transports copper from the liver and also functions as a copper donor to certain enzymes.

In WD there is widespread copper deposition, especially in liver and brain. When the liver is overloaded, copper diffuses into the blood and is transported to kidney and brain. The brain typically shows bilateral areas of dark-brown discoloration and shrinkage involving the caudate and putamen. Microscopically these areas show vacuolation and astrocytic hyperplasia. Astrocytes are enlarged and of the Alzheimer type II variety. Similar cells may contain yellow-brown granules that stain positively for copper. There may be neuronal loss in the putamen. The globus pallidus is less severely affected. The cortex may show microscopic spongy change. In one case neuropathologic changes were present in the striatum, some 10 days following failed liver transplantation, in spite of improvement in the patient's dystonic posturing. Deposition of copper in Descemet's membrane is responsible for the classic Kayser-Fleischer rings.

D. Menkes Kinky Hair Disease (MKHD)

MKHD is a rare X-linked disorder of copper metabolism which has been shown to be due to mutations in the ATP7A gene at Xq12-q13 which codes for a copper-binding protein. The structure of the ATP7A gene is similar to the Wilson disease ATP7B gene. In MKHD, copper is distributed unevenly, as a result of which it is unavailable for synthesis of cuproenzymes. The typical phenotype includes twisted colorless hair, seizures, hypotonia, and neurological deterioration. The phenotype is variable but results from functional impairment of multiple cuproenzymes. Deficiency of tyrosinase results in the pale hair. Defective elastin and collagen cross-linking occurring as result of lysyl oxidase deficiency, leads to fraying of vascular elastic tissue and vascular dilatation. In the brain there is diffuse atrophy accompanied by patchy foci of neocortical necrosis. The atrophic cerebellum shows swelling of Purkinje cell dendrites and accumulation of numerous mitochondria. The mitochondrial proliferation could possibly arise in response to deficiency of a cuproenzyme such as cytochrome c oxidase.

E. Progressive Neuronal Degeneration of Childhood with Liver Disease (PNDC; Alpers-Huttenlocher syndrome)

This very rare disorder is characterized by intractable seizures including prolonged status epilepticus, progressive neurological deterioration, and terminal hepatic dysfunction. The cause is unknown but a metabolic basis is likely because of liver involvement and rare familial occurrence. Death usually occurs within 2 to 3 years, often after prolonged seizure activity. At autopsy the severity of liver involvement is often greater than anticipated on the basis of liver function tests which themselves may not become abnormal until late in the illness. Fatty change, fibrosis, and even cirrhosis with prominent bile duct proliferation are typical hepatic findings. The brain demonstrates widespread atrophy, but the striatum shows severe involvement. A useful clue is the presence of very severe occipital involvement. Microscopically, there are neuronal loss, gliosis, and spongy change. No genetic or metabolic abnormalities have been reported in this condition, and in particular there is no substantive evidence that the disorder is mitochondrial in origin.

XIII. ALCOHOL-INDUCED NEUROLOGIC DISORDERS

While there may be some controversy about the role of alcohol as a toxic agent in the development of cerebral atrophy, there is general agreement that thiamine deficiency, acute electrolyte shifts, and the direct toxic effects of alcohol, particularly on muscle, combine to produce a constellation of well-recognized clinicopathologic syndromes. The cardinal manifestations of prolonged alcohol dependency include Wernicke-Korsakoff syndrome, central pontine myelinolysis, neuropathy and myopathy, and cerebellar degeneration. The considerable individual variation in susceptibility to the development of these syndromes may in part be determined by genetic factors.

A. Wernicke-Korsakoff Syndrome (WKS)

Thiamine deficiency may occur following chronic starvation from any cause and is a particular feature of chronic alcoholics who favor spirits rather than beer, which is usually fortified with thiamine and other vitamins. Wernicke encephalopathy (WE) includes diplopia with nystagmus, lateral rectus palsy, ataxia, and a global confusional state. Korsakoff psychosis (KP) is characterized by loss of retentive memory with confabulation in an otherwise alert individual and is referred to by some as the psychic manifestation of WE. The clinically distinct syndromes of WE and KP are classified pathologically together under a single term—Wernicke-Korsakoff syndrome (WKS). Thiamine is a cofactor for pyruvate dehydrogenase, which catalyzes the oxidation of pyruvate to acetyl-CoA. It is also required for the metabolism of α-ketoacids and α-ketoglutarate. Deficiency results in impaired energy metabolism.

Many of the neuropathologic features of WE are similar to those seen in mitochondrial disorders, an observation which has led to inappropriate use of the term "Infantile Wernicke's" to describe Leigh disease. The neuropathologic features of WE are dominated by a unique topography which includes mamillary bodies, periaqueductal gray matter, floor of the fourth ventricle, paraventricular regions of the thalamus and hypothalamus, and the cerebellar vermis.

In KP, there is additional involvement of the medial dorsal nucleus of the thalamus. The involved mamillary bodies are recognized by their brown, shrunken appearance. Microscopically, involved areas of brain show capillary proliferation with hemosiderin deposition and varying degrees of neuronal loss depending on the duration of the disorder. Infiltration by macrophages and astrocytic hyperplasia are common. The mortality rate may reach 20% or more if diagnosis and treatment are delayed, and, even in patients who receive treatment in established cases, there may be long-term memory impairment.

B. Central Pontine Myelinolysis and Related White Matter Disorders (see also Chap. 5)

CPM is characterized by an area of demyelination in the basis pontis which is distinguished from an MS plaque by its symmetry and paucity of infiltrating inflammatory cells such as macrophages and lymphocytes (Fig. 23). Extrapontine myelinolysis (EPM) may be present, and in some cases of EPM the pons may show minimal or no involvement. Antemortem MR diagnosis of CPM has resulted in recognition of a wide-ranging clinical presentation which includes altered mental status; pseudobulbar palsy; extrapyramidal symptoms such as dystonia, quadriplegia, and "locked-in syndrome," and seizures. Common to many cases is the overly rapid correction of hyponatremia resulting in osmotic stress which induces brain dehydration and mechanical separation of axons from myelin sheaths. Based on animal experimental evidence it has been sug-

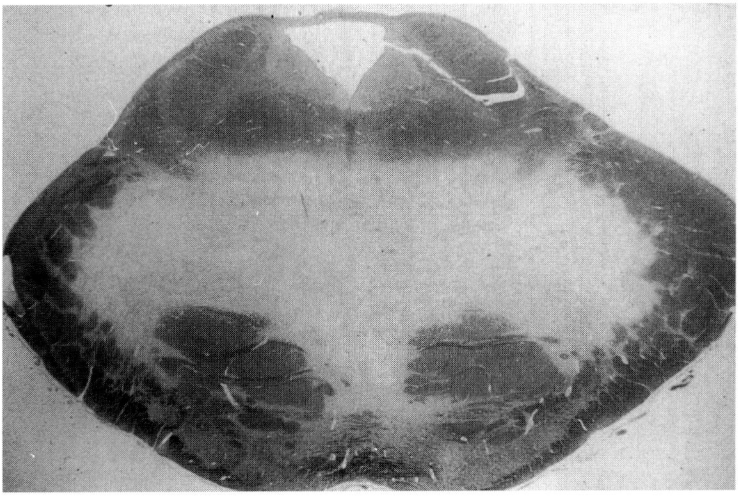

Figure 23 Luxol fast blue-stained section of pons showing large confluent area of demyelination typical of central pontine myelinolysis (CPM). (See also Chap. 5.)

gested that a sodium correction rate of less than 20 mEq/L/24 hours is unlikely to lead to CPM, but this is not supported by clinical experience where CPM has been shown to develop at a correction rate of less than 10 mEq/L/24 hours and may also occur with no or poorly documented electrolyte abnormalities (see Chap. 5). Several case studies describe a patchy demyelinating condition in the corpus callosum in chronic alcoholism under the familiar rubric of Marchiafava-Bignami disease (MBD). Some patients with MBD have presented with symptoms attributable to a callosal lesion including apraxias and disconnection syndromes. However, there are no distinguishing pathologic features that allow MBD to be separated from EPM.

C. Cerebral and Cerebellar Atrophy

Some patients with chronic alcohol abuse develop diffuse cerebrocortical atrophy. Doubts about the significance of cerebral atrophy in chronic alcohol dependency as assessed by postmortem volumetric studies have been resolved, at least in part, by longitudinal MR studies of abstaining and relapsing alcoholics. Documentation of atrophy by MR in chronic alcoholics is followed by improvement in cortical gray matter and in sulcal and lateral ventricular volumes within 3 weeks of abstinence. There is no good evidence that this increased volume is due to increased brain water, and convincing explanations for a return toward normal brain volume are lacking. Development of a progressive cerebellar ataxia with vermian atrophy is well recognized in chronic alcoholics (Fig. 24).

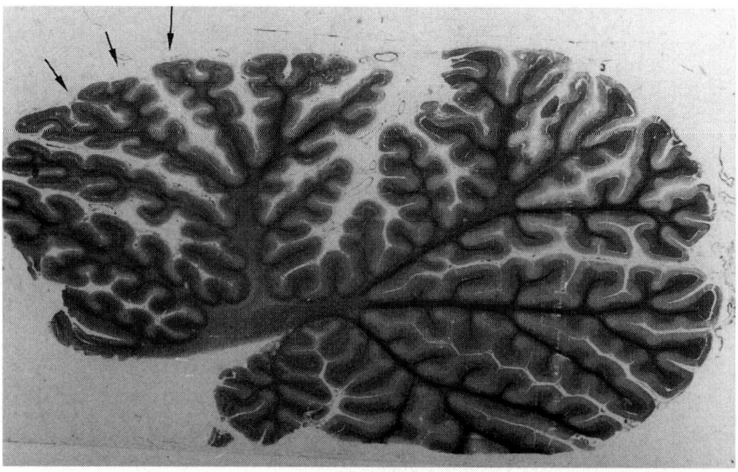

Figure 24 Anterior cerebellar vermian atrophy (arrows) in a patient with history of longstanding alcohol abuse. Note enlarged interfolial spaces. By contrast, note relative preservation of inferior vermis (lower right of micrograph).

Some postmortem studies have shown a loose correlation between the level of alcohol consumption and the severity of Purkinje cell loss, which is independent of age. The cerebellar atrophy is usually independent of cerebrocortical atrophy, but the mechanism of selective Purkinje cell vulnerability has not been determined.

D. Neuropathy and Myopathy (see also Chap. 10)

Leaving aside focal compressive neuropathies induced by prolonged immobilization during alcoholic stupor and disulfiram-induced neuropathy, the typical alcoholic peripheral neuropathy is symmetrical, painful, sensorimotor, and axonal in origin. Autonomic involvement may be present. A toxic effect of alcohol is most likely, given that there is a reasonably good inverse correlation between the neurophysiological indices of neuropathy and the level of alcohol consumption. As many as 50% of a population of chronic alcoholics will have histologic evidence of muscle disease, usually in the form of type II fiber atrophy. Protein synthesis is decreased in such patients. Contributory factors include associated chronic liver disease, acetaldehyde-induced impairment of protein translation, and direct toxic effects of alcohol. Chronic protein malnutrition does not appear to play an important part in the development of muscle fiber atrophy. Acute alcohol-induced rhabdomyolysis is usually associated with binge drinking and a period of prolonged immobilization resulting in muscle compression. Decreased protein intake during binge drinking may be an additional factor in the development of rhabdomyolysis. Additional contributory factors may include coincidental ingestion of nonsteroidal antiinflammatory drugs or cocaine. Hypophosphatemia may also contribute to the development of rhabdomyolysis in chronic alcoholics. It has been suggested that chronic alcoholic myopathy characterised by type II fiber atrophy is associated with deficiencies in the glycolytic pathway and that acute rhabdomyolysis arises as a result of superimposed mitochondrial failure, leading to a severe energy crisis in muscle. Clinically, in acute rhabdomyolysis there is severe muscle pain with cramps, swelling, and weakness. Affected muscles are tender. Creatine kinase levels are high and myoglobinuria is usual. Histologically there is segmental myofiber necrosis followed by acute inflammatory cell infiltration and ultimately by evidence of myofiber regeneration. Most patients show good recovery of muscle function but are prone to develop additional attacks of rhabdomyolysis if drinking is resumed, which is usual. Hypokalemic myopathy may also occur in chronic alcoholics and is recognized by the presence of vacuolated muscle fibers.

E. Fetal Alcohol Syndrome

The association between a particular pattern of facial dysmorphism and alcohol consumption in pregnancy has been recognized since the early 1970s. The toxic

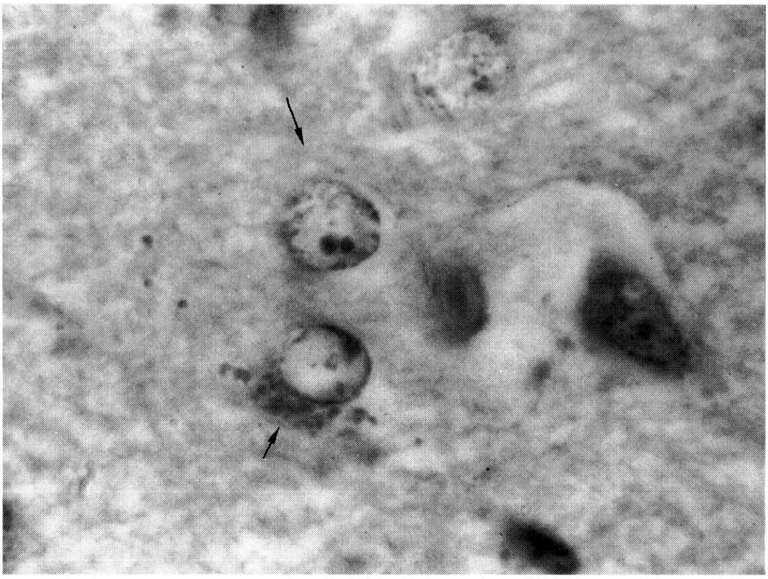

Figure 25 Alzheimer type II astrocytes (arrows) in cortex from a patient with acquired non-Wilsonian hepatocerebral degeneration. Note prominent intranuclear inclusions and minimal cytoplasm.

effects of alcohol on the developing nervous system have been convincingly demonstrated in animal experiments. Clinically, affected children are recognized by the presence of short palpebral fissures, a thin upper lip, incomplete jaw development, growth retardation involving the skeleton and brain, and varying degrees of mental handicap. Less than 10% of the children of alcoholic mothers develop the full syndrome, but a large number of children born to alcoholic mothers will show less severe changes. Neuropathologic examination of small numbers of cases has shown arrested neuronal migration resulting in white matter heterotopias together with more severe changes including agenesis of the corpus callosum.

F. Hepatic Encephalopathy and Acquired Hepatocerebral Degeneration

It is now clear that the development of either acute or chronic hepatic encephalopathy (HE) in patients with portocaval shunting is not solely due to a direct toxic effect of ammonia on neurons, glia, and the blood-brain barrier. Evidence is increasing that ammonia may alter intracerebral levels of neurotransmitters and their receptors and lead to failure of neurotransmission. Alterations in glutamate levels and in the levels of some gamma-aminobutyric acid (GABA) receptors are present in such patients. Blockade of the N-methyl-D-aspartate (NMDA) type of glutamate receptor may, in experimental situations, reduce the mortality from ammonia intoxication. Neuropathologic examination of patients with acute HE may reveal edema. Invariably there is an increased number of swollen astrocytes with large pale nuclei (Alzheimer type II) which are usually located in the deeper cortical layers and in the striatum (Fig. 25). In patients with chronic HE, additional changes including cortical laminar cavitatory necrosis are present. Occasionally this change may be visible on gross examination of the brain. The putamen and globus pallidus may show similar cavitary change which may be detected on MR examination as bilateral symmetric hyperintensities early in the course of chronic HE. However, there is relatively poor correlation between the presence of these signal changes and the degree of hepatic failure.

REFERENCES

1. Agamanolis DP. The pathology of lysosomal storage diseases. Pathol Annu 1995; 30(Pt 1):247–285.
2. Andresen BS, Bross P, Jensen TG, et al. Molecular diagnosis and characterization of medium-chain acyl-CoA dehydrogenase deficiency. Scand J Clin Lab Invest Suppl 1995; 220:9–25.
3. Bachmann C. Ornithine carbamoyl transferase deficiency: findings, models and problems. J Inherit Metab Dis 1992; 15:578–591.
4. Brismar J, Aqeel A, Brismar G, Coates R, Gascon G, Ozand P. Maple syrup urine disease: findings on CT and MR scans of the brain in 10 infants. AJNR 1990; 11:1219–1228.
5. Brismar J, Ozand PT. CT and MR of the brain in glutaric acidemia type I: a review of 59 published cases and a report of 5 new patients. AJNR 1995; 16:675–683.
6. Brockington M, Alsanjari N, Sweeney MG, Morgan Hughes JA, Scaravilli F, Harding AE. Kearns-Sayre syndrome associated with mitochondrial DNA deletion or duplication: a molecular genetic and pathological study. J Neurol Sci 1995; 131:78–87.
7. Brusilow SW, Maestri NE. Urea cycle disorders: diagnosis, pathophysiology, and therapy. Adv Pediatr 1996; 43:127–170.
8. Chuang JL, Fisher CR, Cox RP, Chuang DT. Molecular basis of maple syrup urine disease: novel mutations at the E1 alpha locus that impair E1 (alpha 2 beta 2) assembly or decrease steady-state E1 alpha mRNA levels of branched-chain alpha-keto acid dehydrogenase complex. Am J Hum Genet 1994; 55:297–304.
9. Coates PM. New developments in the diagnosis and investigation of mitochondrial fatty acid oxidation disorders. Eur J Pediatr 1994; 153(7 suppl 1):S49–56.
10. Collier DA, Barrett TG, Curtis D, et al. Linkage of Wolfram syndrome to chromosome 4p16.1 and evidence for heterogeneity. Am J Hum Genet 1996; 59:855–863.
11. De-Gasperi R, Gama Sosa MA, Battistini S, et al. Late-onset GM2 gangliosidosis:

Ashkenazi Jewish family with an exon 5 mutation (Tyr180→His) in the Hex A alpha-chain gene. Neurology 1996; 47:547–552.
12. Favre JP, Becker F, Lorcerie B, Dumas R, David M. Vascular manifestations in homocystinuria. Ann Vasc Surg 1992; 6:294–297.
13. Felice KJ, Schneebaum AB, Jones HR Jr. McArdle's disease with late-onset symptoms: case report and review of the literature. J Neurol Neurosurg Psychiatry 1992; 55:407–408.
14. Fensom AH, Benson PF. Recent advances in the prenatal diagnosis of the mucopolysaccharidoses. Prenat Diagn 1994; 14:1–12.
15. Ferenci P, Gilliam TC, Gitlin JD, et al. An international symposium on Wilson's and Menkes' diseases. Hepatology 1996; 24:952–958.
16. Ferreiro JA, Robert MA, Townsend J, Vinters-HV. Neuropathologic findings after liver transplantation. Acta Neuropathol 1992; 84:1–14.
17. Fournier B, Smeitink JA, Dorland L, Berger R, Saudubray JM, Poll BT. Peroxisomal disorders: a review. J Inherit Metab Dis 1994; 17:470–486.
18. Glasgow JF, Moore R. Current concepts in Reye's syndrome. Br J Hosp Med 1993; 50:599–604.
19. Goebel HH. The neuronal ceroid-lipofuscinoses. J Child Neurol. 1995; 10:424–437.
20. Hamilton RL, Haas RH, Nyhan WL, Powell HC, Grafe MR. Neuropathology of propionic acidemia: a report of two patients with basal ganglia lesions. J Child Neurol 1995; 10:25–30.
21. Harding BN. Progressive neuronal degeneration of childhood with liver disease (Alpers-Huttenlocher syndrome): a personal review. J Child Neurol 1990; 5:273–287.
22. Harding BN, Alsanjari N, Smith SJ, et al. Progressive neuronal degeneration of childhood with liver disease (Alpers' disease) presenting in young adults. J Neurol Neurosurg Psychiatry 1995; 58:320–325.
23. Hirano M, Silvestri G, Blake DM, et al. Mitochondrial neurogastrointestinal encephalomyopathy (MNGIE): clinical, biochemical, and genetic features of an autosomal recessive mitochondrial disorder. Neurology 1994; 44:721–727.
24. Holton JB. Galactosaemia: pathogenesis and treatment. J Inherit Metab Dis 1996; 19:3–7.
25. Iwaki T, Iwaki A, Tateishi J, Sakaki Y, Goldman JE. Alpha beta-crystallin and 27-kd heat shock protein are regulated by stress conditions in the central nervous system and accumulate in Rosenthal fibers. Am J Pathol 1993; 143:487–495.
26. Jog MS, Lang AE. Chronic acquired hepatocerebral degeneration: case reports and new insights. Mov Disord 1995; 10:714–722.
27. Kamiya M, Eimoto T, Kishimoto H, et al. Glutaric aciduria type II: autopsy study of a case with electron-transferring flavoprotein dehydrogenase deficiency. Pediatr Pathol 1990; 10:1007–1019.
28. Kaul R, Gao GP, Matalon R, et al. Identification and expression of eight novel mutations among non-Jewish patients with Canavan disease. Am J Hum Genet 1996; 59:95–102.
29. Kimura S, Hara M, Nezu A, Osaka H, Yamazaki S, Saitoh K. Two cases of glutaric aciduria type 1: clinical and neuropathological findings. J Neurol Sci 1994; 123:38–43.

30. Kohlschutter A, Gardiner RM, Goebel HH. Human forms of neuronal ceroid-lipofuscinosis (Batten disease): consensus on diagnostic criteria, Hamburg 1992. J Inherit Metab Dis 1993; 16:241–244.
31. Kril JJ. Neuropathology of thiamine deficiency disorders. Metab Brain Dis 1996; 11:9–17.
32. Lee PJ, Leonard JV. The hepatic glycogen storage diseases—problems beyond childhood. J Inherit Metab Dis 1995; 18:462–472.
33. Lewis W, Dalakas MC. Mitochondrial toxicity of antiviral drugs. Nat Med 1995; 1:417–422.
34. Mariani P, Coudray, Lucas C, et al. Glutamine metabolism and neuropathological disorders in experimental hepatic encephalopathy: effect of transplanted hepatocytes. Surgery 1996; 120:93–99.
35. Matalon R, Michals K, Kaul R. Canavan disease: from spongy degeneration to molecular analysis. J Pediatr 1995; 127:511–517.
36. Morris AA, Leonard JV, Brown GK, et al. Deficiency of respiratory chain complex I is a common cause of Leigh disease. Ann Neurol 1996; 40:25–30.
37. Moses SW. Muscle glycogenosis. J Inherit Metab Dis 1990; 13:452–465.
38. Nicoll JA, Moss TH, Love S, Campbell MJ, Schut WH. Clinical and autopsy findings in two cases of MELAS presenting with stroke-like episodes but without clinical myopathy. Clin Neuropathol 1993; 12:38–43.
39. Oldfors A, Holme E, Tulinius M, Larsson NG. Tissue distribution and disease manifestations of the tRNA(Lys) A$\rightarrow$G(8344) mitochondrial DNA mutation in a case of myoclonus epilepsy and ragged red fibers. Acta Neuropathol 1995; 90:328–333.
40. O'Neill CA, Eisensmith RC, Croke-DT, Naughten ER, Cahalane SF, Woo SL. Molecular analysis of PKU in Ireland. Acta Paediatr Suppl 1994; 407:43–44.
41. Phaneuf D, Wakamatsu N, Huang JQ, et al. Dramatically different phenotypes in mouse models of human Tay-Sachs and Sandhoff diseases. Hum Mol Genet 1996; 5:1–14.
42. Philippart M, Carrel RE, Landing BH. Tay-Sachs disease with atypical chronic course and limited brain storage: alpha-locus hexosaminidase genetic compound. Neurochem Res 1995; 20:1323–1328.
43. Pons R, De Vivo DC. Primary and secondary carnitine deficiency syndromes. J Child Neurol 1995; 10(suppl 2):S8–24.
44. Powers JM. The pathology of peroxisomal disorders with pathogenetic considerations. J Neuropathol Exp Neurol 1995; 54:710–719.
45. Riordan EP, Sanders MD, Govan GG, Sweeney MG, Da Costa J, Harding-AE. The clinical features of Leber's hereditary optic neuropathy defined by the presence of a pathogenic mitochondrial DNA mutation. Brain 1995; 118:319–337.
46. Rotig A, Bourgeron T, Chretien D, Rustin P, Munnich A. Spectrum of mitochondrial DNA rearrangements in the Pearson marrow-pancreas syndrome. Hum Mol Genet 1995; 4:1327–1330.
47. Ruitenbeek W, Poels PJ, Turnbull DM, et al. Rhabdomyolysis and acute encephalopathy in late onset medium chain acyl-CoA dehydrogenase deficiency. J Neurol Neurosurg Psychiatry 1995; 58:209–214.
48. Schwankhaus JD, Parisi JE, Gulledge WR, Chin L, Currier RD. Hereditary adult-on-

set Alexander's disease with palatal myoclonus, spastic paraparesis, and cerebellar ataxia. Neurology 1995; 45:2266–2271.

49. Seneca S, De Meirleir L, Liebaers I, Lissens W. Importance of sequence analysis in NARP syndrome. J Inherit Metab Dis 1995; 18:97–98.
50. Soupart A, Penninckx R, Stenuit A, Perier O, Decaux G. Reinduction of hyponatremia improves survival in rats with myelinolysis-related neurologic symptoms. J Neuropathol Exp Neurol 1996; 55:594–601.
51. Sparaco M, Bonilla E, DiMauro S, Powers JM. Neuropathology of mitochondrial encephalomyopathies due to mitochondrial DNA defects. J Neuropathol Exp Neurol 1993; 52:1–10.
52. Sum JM, Twiss JL, Horoupian DS. Selective death of immature neurons in methylmalonic acidemia of the neonate: a case report. Acta Neuropathol 1993; 85:217–221.
53. Suzuki K. Neuropathology of late onset gangliosidoses. A review. Dev Neurosci 1991; 13:205–210.
54. Talente GM, Coleman RA, Alter C, et al. Glycogen storage disease in adults. Ann Intern Med 1994; 120:218–226.
55. Tsujino S, Shanske S, DiMauro S. Molecular genetic heterogeneity of phosphoglycerate kinase (PGK) deficiency. Muscle-Nerve 1995; Suppl 3:S45–49.
56. Tsujino S, Shanske S, Sakoda S, Toscano A, DiMauro S. Molecular genetic studies in muscle phosphoglycerate mutase (PGAM-M) deficiency. Muscle-Nerve 1995; Suppl 3:S50–53.
57. Tumer Z, Horn N. Menkes disease: recent advances and new insights into copper metabolism. Ann Med 1996; 28:121–129.
58. Ullrich K, Moller H, Weglage J, et al. White matter abnormalities in phenylketonuria: results of magnetic resonance measurements. Acta Paediatr Suppl 1994; 407:78–82.
59. van de Vlasakker CJ, Gabreels FJ, Wijburg HC, Wevers RA. Clinical features of Niemann-Pick disease type C. An example of the delayed onset, slowly progressive phenotype and an overview of recent literature. Clin Neurol Neurosurg 1994; 96:119–123.
60. Verity MA, Turnbull DM. Assay of acyl-CoA dehydrogenase activity in frozen muscle biopsies: application to medium-chain acyl-CoA dehydrogenase deficiency. Biochem Med Metab Biol 1993; 49:351–362.
61. Wallace DC. Diseases of the mitochondrial DNA. Annu Rev Biochem 1992; 61:1175–212.
62. Weisz B, Spirer Z, Reif S. Niemann-Pick disease: newer classification based on genetic mutations of the disease. Adv Pediatr 1994; 41:415–426.
63. West JR, Chen WJ, Pantazis NJ. Fetal alcohol syndrome: the vulnerability of the developing brain and possible mechanisms of damage. Metab Brain Dis 1994; 9:291–322.
64. Wraith JE. The mucopolysaccharidoses: a clinical review and guide to management. Arch Dis Child 1995; 72:263–267.
65. Yamaguchi K, Hirabayashi K, Honma K. Methylmalonic acidemia: brain lesions in a case of vitamin B12 non-responsive (mut0) type. Clin Neuropathol 1995; 14:216–222.

10

Muscle and Nerve Disease

I. INTRODUCTION

This chapter will focus on the interpretation of muscle biopsy, with less emphasis on nerve biopsy interpretation. Nerve biopsy has declined in popularity due to patient intolerance of a somewhat painful procedure, often having long-term sequelae, and recognition of the relatively low yield of therapeutically useful diagnostic information likely to be obtained. The last few years have witnessed unprecedented advances in understanding the biochemical basis and molecular pathogenesis of muscle disease. The muscular dystrophies, previously associated with a plethora of quasiscientific descriptive clinical terms, can now be subclassified on the basis of immunohistochemical analysis of sarcolemmal membrane proteins. Advances in histochemistry have shown that the mitochondrial myopathies form a larger proportion of myopathies than was previously considered. These advances can now be implemented in the routine diagnostic laboratory.

A. Tissue Preparation

Any laboratory with experience in frozen section technique can easily carry out muscle biopsy preparation, provided a few simple steps are followed. Transportation of muscle to the laboratory wrapped in saline moistened gauze (not soaked and not frozen) with a minimum of delay is essential, although a delay of a few hours can be tolerated without damage to the biopsy. In extreme situations a muscle may be left overnight in a 4°C refrigerator with reasonable enzymatic preservation. Transverse orientation of the specimen is aided by use of a dissecting microscope. Ice crystal artifact is minimized by dusting the muscle biopsy lightly with talcum powder prior to immersion in liquid nitrogen. For good quality electron microscopy it is essential that the specimen be plunged into glutaraldehyde immediately after biopsy, preferably lightly stretched on a clamp, although when biopsies are received from outside institutions this is not always possible. The stored frozen block may be used for subsequent DNA extraction. Dynamic studies of mitochondrial function require optimum preservation of mitochondria. In this situation it is essential that the muscle be frozen immediately on removal from the patient. Such studies are available only through specialized laboratories by prior request. Formalin-fixed paraffin-embedded muscle is of minimal diagnostic use (e.g., for a rapid screen for dystrophic or inflammatory changes before histochemistry has been completed).

B. Biopsy Site

The choice of muscle for biopsy is determined by clinical examination. A clinically involved muscle demonstrating three-fifths power is best. Open biopsy provides the largest tissue sample, although needle biopsy is very useful for sampling several muscles and is particularly suitable in children. It has the added benefit of leaving minimal scarring; however, not all muscles are amenable to needle biopsy. Injection and electromyography sites must be avoided. Many muscle diseases show regional variation in severity, so it is possible to have a normal biopsy in a patient with severe muscle disease.

C. Biopsy Interpretation

It is helpful to adopt a planned anatomical approach to muscle biopsy interpretation. A standard battery of histochemical stains must be carried out on each biopsy and any additional immunohistochemical stains should be requested on the basis of an informed assessment of the preliminary biopsy appearances. Blanket testing of all muscles using all of the available histochemical *and* immunohistochemical stains is wasteful of resources. Very few individual biopsy features are specific for a particular disease; establishment of a diagnosis is based on the summation of individual histologic features. It is wise to remain aloof from the clinical information when initially interpreting the biopsy. However, the ultimate diagnosis of a patient's neuromuscular disorder will depend on the convergence of clinical, electrophysiological, biochemical, and biopsy data. It is very easy to be swayed into making a particular diagnosis by a neurologist confident of his or her clinical diagnostic acumen.

An anatomical approach to biopsy interpretation, in which the sarcolemmal membrane, nuclei, sarcoplasm, endomysium, perimysium, epimysium, and blood vessels are systematically evaluated, is described.

There are very few diagnoses which remain completely undetected after examination of the hematoxylin and eosin- (H&E) stained sections. In practice it is helpful to commence viewing the biopsy from the periphery towards the center.

1. Epimysium, Endomysium, and Perimysium

Inflammatory cell infiltration and fibrosis are the two principal pathological changes that involve these areas. Endomysial fibrosis is a virtually pathognomonic feature of muscular dystrophy (Fig. 1). Complete replacement of endomysium by fat and fibrous tissue confirms the biopsy as end stage and of limited diagnostic usefulness, although rare residual muscle fibers or spindles should be sought to ensure that the specimen is of muscle origin. Epimysial fibrosis may herald the presence of scleroderma.

2. Inflammation

It is essential to decide where the inflammatory process is centered. Angiocentric inflammation is very suggestive of vasculitis and vessel wall necrosis must be sought. Care should be taken to lower the diagnostic threshold for vasculitis, since it is unusual in muscle to observe the full-blown picture of vessel wall

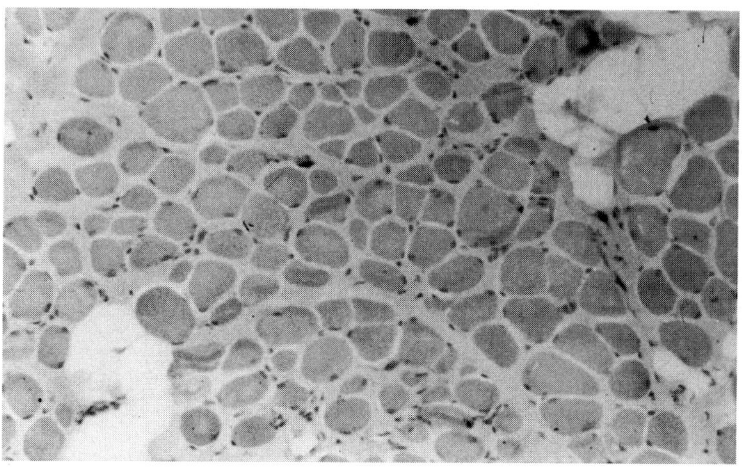

Figure 1 Endomysial fibrosis. Replacement of endomysium by fibrous tissue resulting in separation of individual fibers. A Van-Gieson stain may help to accentuate endomysial fibrosis.

necrosis, eosinophils, lymphocytes, and so on typical of polyarteritis nodosa (PAN) (Fig. 2). Multiple levels may reveal more severe vessel change. Irregular fibrous thickening may suggest previous or healed vessel wall injury. A purely lymphocytic vasculitis may be observed in systemic lupus erythematosus (SLE). Immunofluorescent detection of immunoglobulins and complement together with complement components should be carried out on all muscle biopsies with vasculitis. An epimysial inflammatory infiltrate with sparing of the endomysium and perimysium suggests fasciitis, in which eosinophils may be prominent. A skin biopsy with subcutaneous fat will complement the muscle biopsy when one is trying to make a diagnosis of fasciitis.

3. *Endomysial Inflammation*

Endomysial lymphocytic inflammation is present in polymyositis (PM), dermatomyositis (DM), inclusion body myositis (IBM), and mixed connective tissue disease (MCTD). The intensity of the inflammatory infiltrate in these four conditions may vary enormously (Fig. 3). Previous treatment and long-standing disease may diminish the extent of the inflammatory infiltrate. PM may be very focal. PM and IBM are suggested when the infiltrate targets muscle fibers, whereas in DM the infiltrate tends to be located around the small capillaries. Necrosis of muscle fibers, with or without surrounding macrophages, is promi-

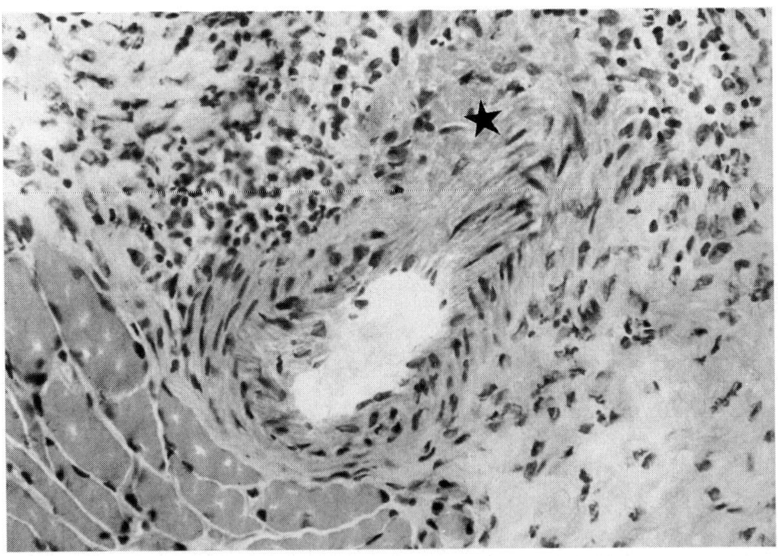

Figure 2 Polyarteritis nodosa. A perimysial blood vessel demonstrates a patchy mixed cellular infiltrate together with focal vessel wall destruction and fibrin deposition (star).

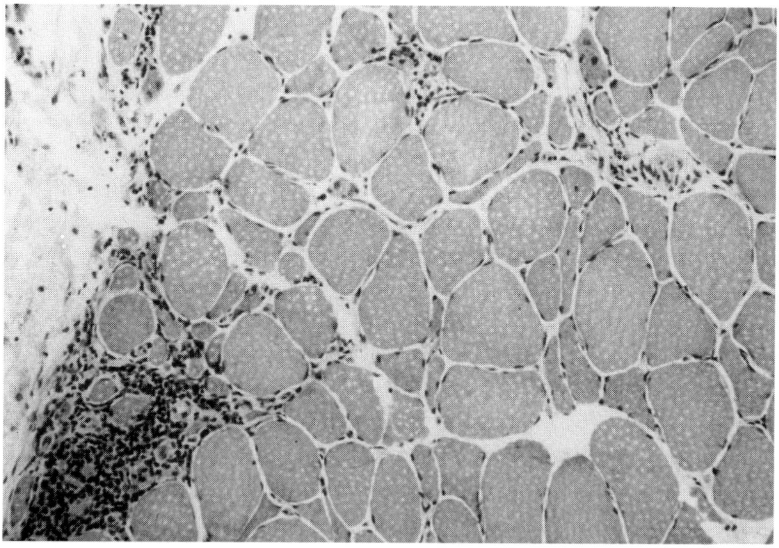

Figure 3 Polymyositis. Muscle demonstrates a patchy but well-defined endomysial lymphocytic infiltrate. Biopsy also shows fiber atrophy that may be due to involvement of the intramuscular nerve twigs by inflammatory process or due to steroid therapy (type 2 fiber atrophy only).

nent in PM especially when the disease is acute, but there is no clear relationship between the degree of inflammatory cell infiltration and extent of necrosis (Fig. 4). Necrosis of muscle fibers is less pronounced in DM. Capillary loss in DM is best seen in plastic-embedded semithin sections and is usually associated with atrophy of the perifascicular fibers, particularly in juvenile DM. The membrane attack complex (MAC) of complement is more likely to be found in the vessels of DM than in PM. Differential expression of the major histocompatibility complexes (MHC I and II) has been suggested as a means to differentiate DM and PM, but supportive evidence from the literature is scanty. The presence of rimmed vacuoles (Figs. 5, 6) in muscle sarcoplasm suggests IBM; the inclusion bodies of IBM may be difficult to detect by light microscopy but electron microscopy should reveal the typical tubulofilamentous structures (Fig. 7). IBM biopsies may show evidence of mitochondrial dysfunction in the form of ragged red fibers and interfiber mosaicism for cytochrome oxidase and succinic dehydrogenase (see below). Atrophic fibers may be present in both IBM and PM, suggesting the presence of denervation. Any of the connective tissue diseases may show focal endomysial chronic inflammation but there is usually little associated muscle fiber necrosis. A diagnosis of MCTD can only be sug-

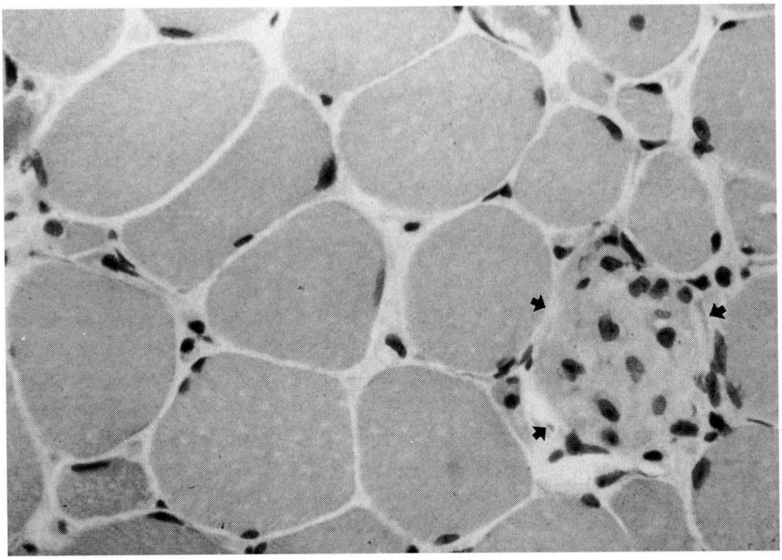

Figure 4 Polymyositis. A single necrotic fiber (arrows) is engulfed by macrophages; note absence of lymphocytes.

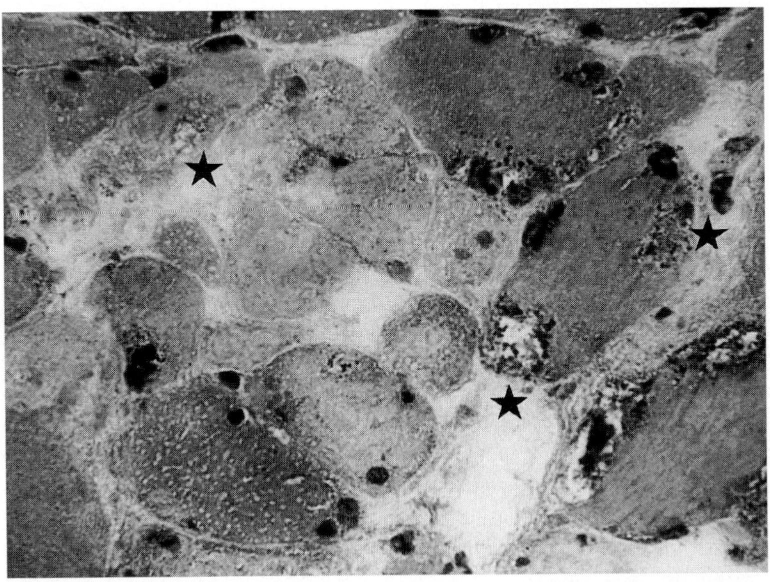

Figure 5 Inclusion body myositis. Numerous rimmed vacuoles, some indicated by stars.

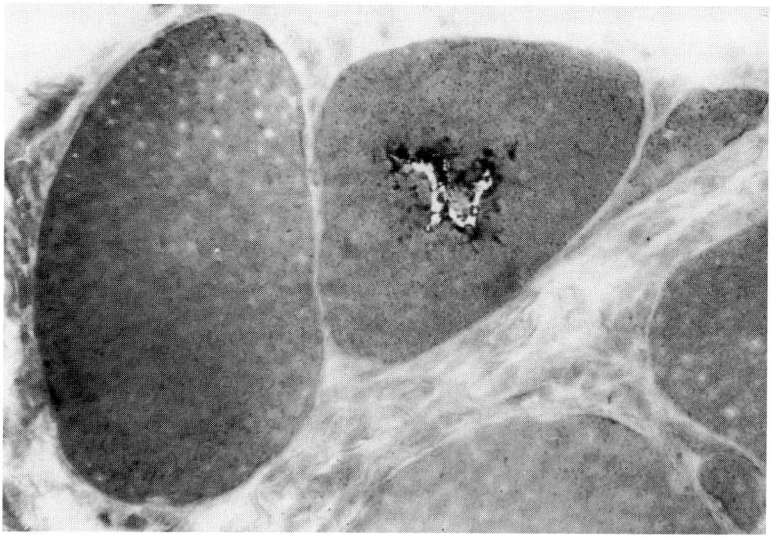

Figure 6 Rimmed vacuole in IBM muscle biopsy.

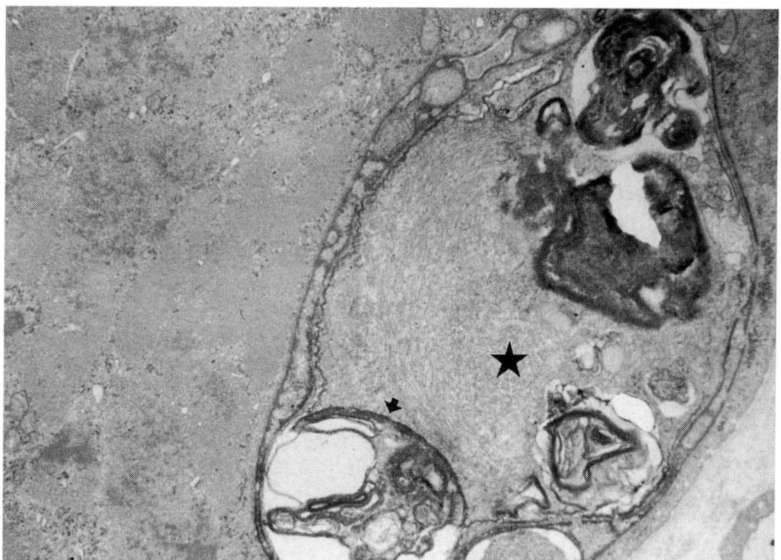

Figure 7 IBM (electron micrograph) showing inclusion body with filamentous aggregates (star) together with granular membranous profiles (arrow).

gested based on examination of muscle biopsy, since there are no defining histological features. An eosinophilic endomysial infiltrate should raise the possibility of a parasitic infestation and the larvae of trichinosis and cysticercosis should be sought. The presence of granulomas is suggestive of sarcoidosis (Fig. 8), but tuberculosis and *Mycobacterium avium intracellulare* (MAI) infection (in patients with human immunovirus (HIV) infection) should be considered.

4. Fiber Size Variation

A biopsy showing uniform fiber size is unlikely to be abnormal unless all fibers are uniformly small, which may occur in spinal muscular atrophy (SMA). Transversely oriented fibers are essential in making this interpretation to avoid artifact-induced fiber size vbariation due to oblique sectioning. Avoid the interpretation of fibers located close to fascia, where variation in size is normal. Fiber splitting, a feature of muscular dystrophy and other myopathies, will also cause apparent size variation. The presence of randomly distributed atrophic angulated fibers is suggestive of denervation, but histochemical fiber typing is essential to show that the process is nonselective. Groups of angulated atrophic fibers on the H&E section are diagnostic of denervation (Fig. 9). The diagnosis of denervation in early infancy is difficult since the denervated fibers have a

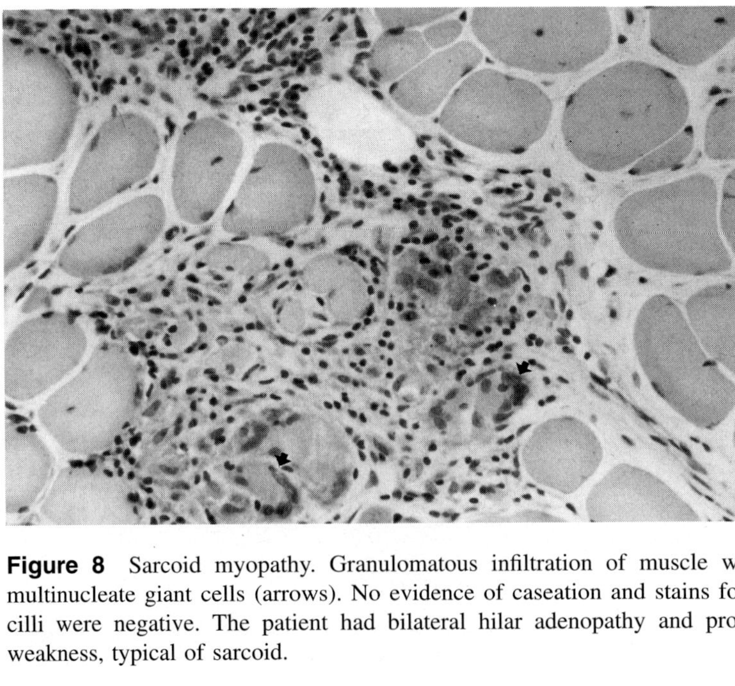

Figure 8 Sarcoid myopathy. Granulomatous infiltration of muscle with numerous multinucleate giant cells (arrows). No evidence of caseation and stains for tubercle bacilli were negative. The patient had bilateral hilar adenopathy and proximal muscle weakness, typical of sarcoid.

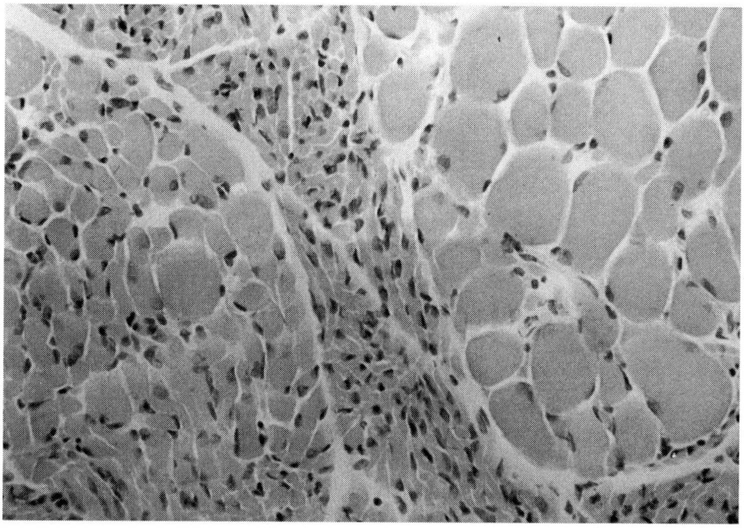

Figure 9 Grouped atrophy. Group of small angulated atrophic fibers (at center) contrasts with another group of normal-sized fibers (at right). A diagnosis of denervation can be made without recourse to histochemistry when this pattern of atrophy is present.

rounded configuration and grouping of fibers (see below) according to histochemical type is invariably absent (Fig. 10). In this situation, it may be helpful to assess the mean lesser fiber diameter of at least 100 fibers using an eyepiece graticule with a vernier scale. Genetic testing for SMA, the most common cause of denervation in the newborn, is now widely available. Perifascicular fiber atrophy is a feature of dermatomyositis, especially juvenile DM (Figs. 11, 12). An increase in fiber size may occur as a physiological response to slowly evolving, long-standing denervation. Large rounded fibers are typical of muscular dystrophy.

5. *Sarcolemmal Nuclei*

As fetal muscle undergoes maturation, nuclei adopt a peripheral position under the sarcolemmal membrane. Persistence of central nuclei in a majority of fibers is typical of centronuclear myopathy (Fig. 13). Central nuclei are also a feature of myotonic dystrophy (MyD), although the availability of [CTG] triplet repeat testing to confirm the diagnosis of MyD means that muscle biopsy is now rarely carried out in this condition. Central nuclei are normally found in fibers at tendon insertion sites. Chronic denervation and some myopathies may also show central nuclei. Central nucleation in less than 4% of fibers is not considered pathological. Proliferation of subsarcolemmal nuclei is typical of denerva-

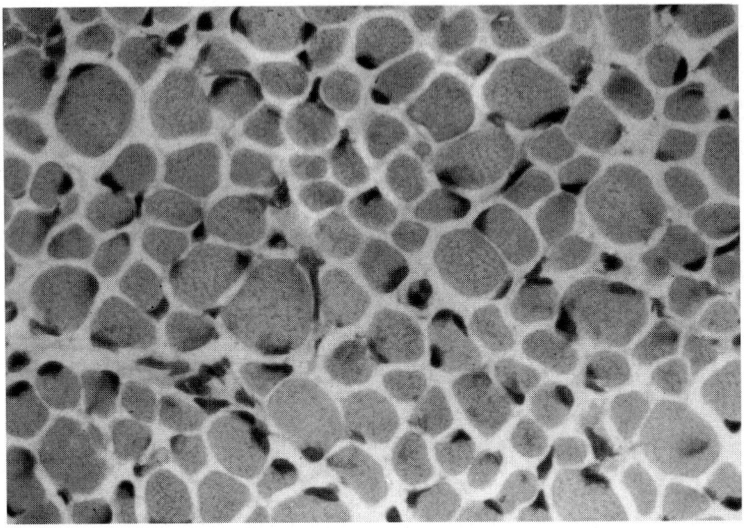

Figure 10 Spinal muscular atrophy. Muscle biopsy from newborn infant with profound hypotonia shows marked variation in fiber size with a rounded profile present in a majority of fibers. No evidence of fiber type grouping on histochemistry; nevertheless appearances are typical of denervation in this age group.

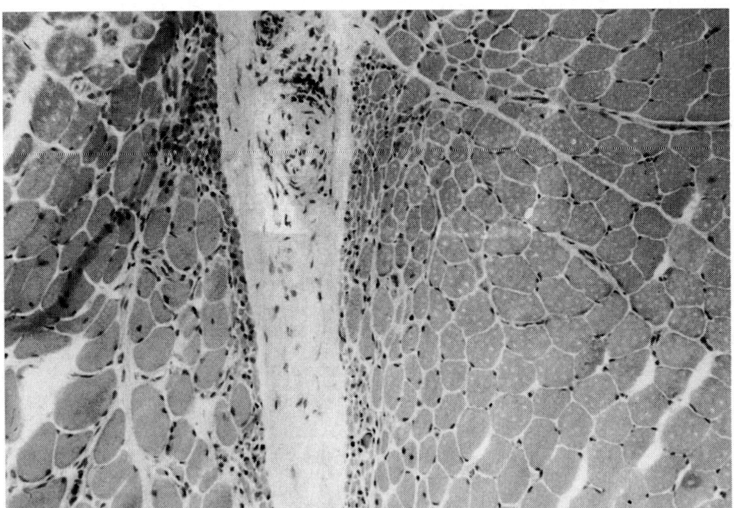

Figure 11 Dermatomyositis. Profound perifascicular atrophy with central areas of muscle fascicles showing little or no fiber size variation.

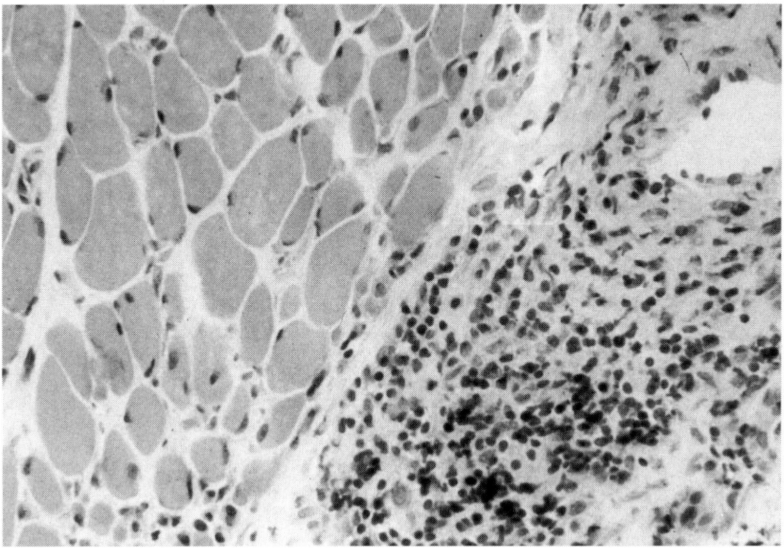

Figure 12 Dermatomyositis. Same biopsy as in Figure 11 shows perivascular lymphocytic infiltrate in perimysium and associated perifascicular muscle fiber atrophy typical of dermatomyositis.

tion. Proliferating subsarcolemmal nuclei may be mistaken for lymphocytes but immunostaining with a lymphocyte marker will resolve the issue. Regenerating fibers are characterized by large vesicular subsarcolemmal nuclei.

6. Sarcoplasm

Poor tissue preparation and contraction artifact may cause alteration in sarcoplasmic staining intensity and such changes may be mistaken for necrosis. Pale sarcoplasm is suggestive of fiber necrosis and need not be accompanied by any inflammatory reaction adjacent to or within the necrotic fiber (Fig. 14). As fiber necrosis advances, macrophages infiltrate the fiber. This feature should not necessarily be construed as evidence for an inflammatory myopathy. Rhabdomyolysis with widespread myofiber necrosis may result from a toxic, metabolic, or septic/infectious cause. Myofiber necrosis is a typical feature of the muscular dystrophies and inflammatory myopathies. Regional limb ischemia will invariably lead to extensive myofiber necrosis. Fiber necrosis may be accompanied by regeneration, in which the regenerating fibers are characterized by basophilic sarcoplasm with a reduction in sarcoplasmic volume, an increase in nuclear size, and the presence of prominent nucleoli. Immunohistochemical staining with antibodies to fetal myosin highlights the regenerating fibers, which are

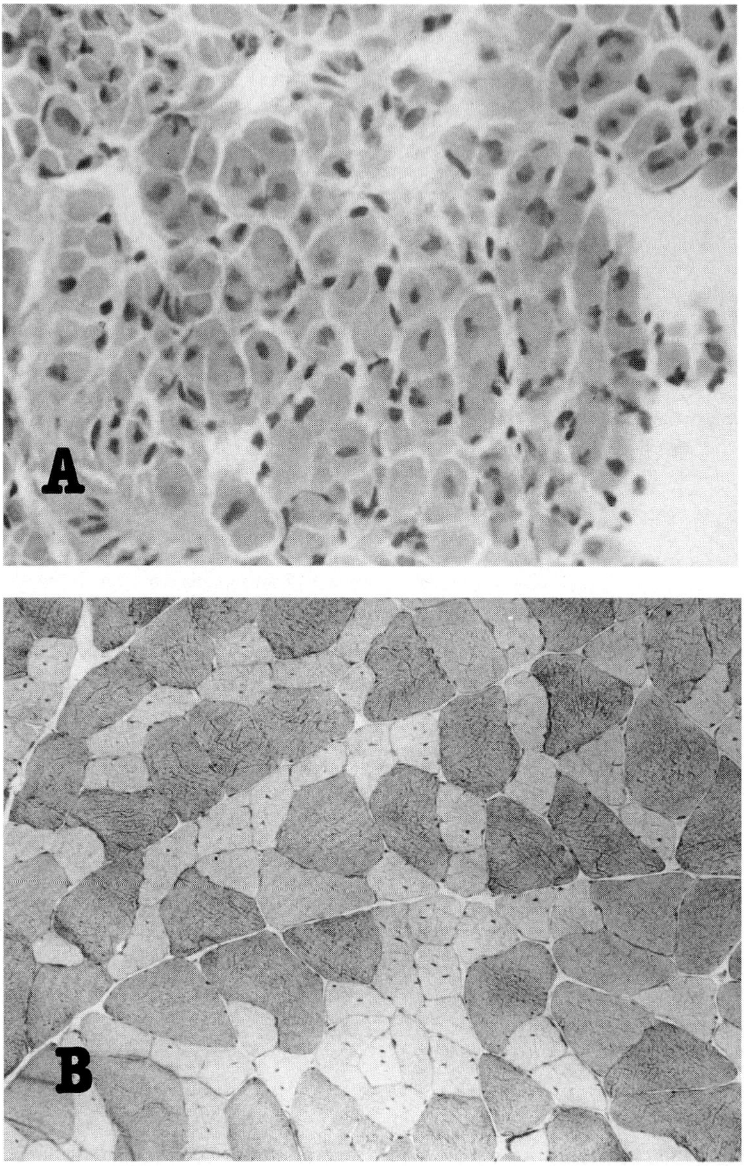

Figure 13 Central nucleation. A. Muscle biopsy demonstrates that virtually all fibers have centrally located nuclei typical of myotubular myopathy. B. Type 1 fiber hypotrophy with central nucleation (routine ATPase stain). This patient had elevated [CTG] repeats diagnostic of myotonic dystrophy.

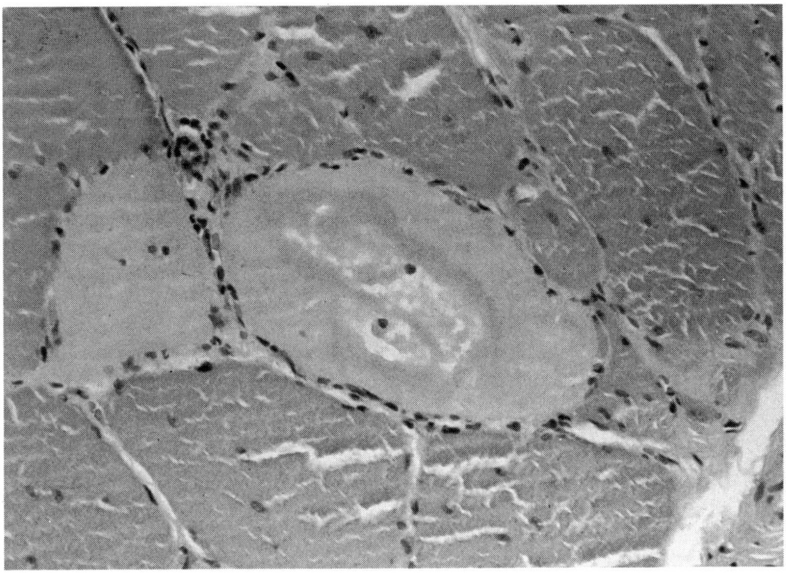

Figure 14 Myofiber necrosis. Centrally located pale muscle fibers with lack of fine sarcoplasmic details, typical of early necrosis; note absence of inflammatory cell infiltrate.

always considered pathological. There is often little or no concordance between the prevalence of necrotic and regenerating fibers in a particular biopsy.

Sarcoplasmic vacuoles are present in a variety of conditions. Sometimes ice-crystal artifact may simulate vacuolar change, but in general ice crystallization produces large non-membrane-bound holes affecting all fibers (Fig. 15). With the exception of lipid vacuoles, which are usually small and evenly dispersed throughout the muscle fiber, most pathological vacuoles are sparse, large, single, and centrally located. A rim of basophilic granular staining may be visible around the edge of the vacuole on the H&E stain: so-called rimmed vacuoles (Fig. 5). These may be present in inclusion body myositis, distal myopathy with rimmed vacuole formation (DMRV), Marinesco-Sjögren syndrome, and oculopharyngeal muscular dystrophy (OPMD). In the assessment of vacuoles the Oil-red O, PAS, and acid phosphatase stains are helpful. PAS positive glycogen-containing vacuoles are typical of acid maltase deficiency (Fig. 16) and may also be present in partial phosphofructokinase deficiency. The Oil-red O positive vacuoles of lipid myopathy are typically tiny and multiple. The acid phosphatase stain is intensely positive in the vacuoles seen in lysosomal storage disorders affecting muscle. Vacuole formation may be present in hypokalemic

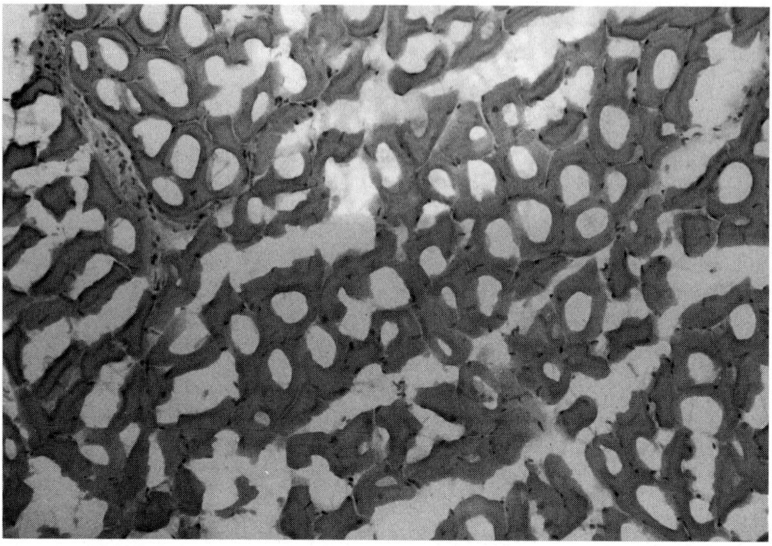

Figure 15 Ice crystal artifact. Large regular vacuoles induced by ice crystal formation. Occasionally, deeper sections of muscle may show a diminution in the severity of ice crystal artifact.

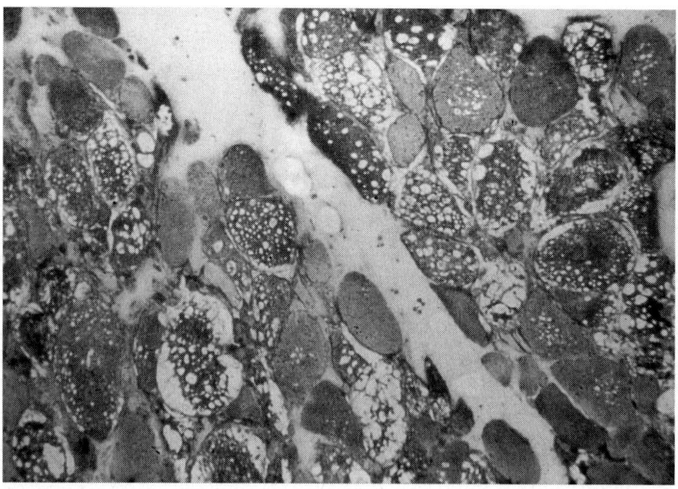

Figure 16 Acid maltase deficiency. Extensive subsarcolemmal and sarcoplasmic vacuolar change. PAS stain was positive for glycogen.

periodic paralysis (Fig. 17). An X-linked myopathy characterized by the presence of vacuolated muscle fibers has also been described. In general, however, most sarcoplasmic vacuoles are autophagic and are best seen with the acid phosphatase stain.

The other major sarcoplasmic pathological finding is fiber splitting, which is a feature of muscular dystrophy. However, any large hypertrophied fiber may undergo splitting. The small fiber fragments that have split from the parent fiber may simulate groups of atrophic fibers and result in an erroneous diagnosis of denervation. Fiber splitting is a normal feature close to the myotendinous insertion.

D. Special Stains and Interpretation

The routine special stains used in the assessment of a muscle biopsy include the following:

Hematoxylin & eosin
Gomori trichrome
Oil-red O
Periodic acid schiff with or without diastase
Acid phosphatase
Adenosine triphosphatase at pH 10.2, 4.6, and 4.3

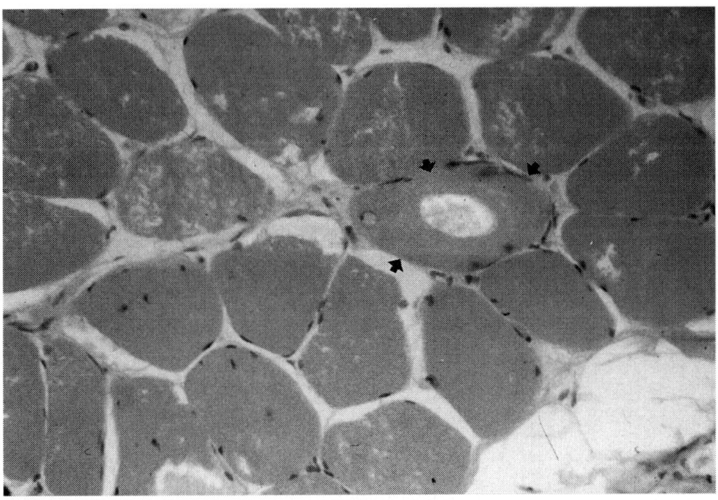

Figure 17 Hypokalaemic periodic paralysis. Large centrally located vacuole in one fiber (arrows).

Nicotinamide adenine dinucleotide dehydrogenase
Combined cytochrome oxidase–succinic dehydrogenase (COX-SDH)
Myophosphorylase

Considerable technical expertise is required to ensure minimal day to day variability in the quality of staining.

1. Gomori Modified Trichrome

Normally the sarcoplasm displays a fine granular staining pattern denoting the presence of intermyofibrillar mitochondria. Mitochondria-rich type 1 fibers may be distinguishable from type II fibers. This is probably the most useful of all muscle stains. Ragged red fibers (RRFs), the cardinal histological feature of mitochondrial myopathy, have a dark red/brown appearance in the subsarcolemmal region (Fig. 18) with the use of this stain. Electron microscopy of the RRFs reveals clusters of normal or morphologically abnormal mitochondria. The abnormal forms may have a paracrystalline appearance in place of normal cristae. There is controversy about the pathological significance of rare isolated RRFs, especially in elderly patients in whom they are frequently regarded as a normal phenomenon of aging without any associated defect in mitochondrial function. Assessment of cytochrome oxidase (COX) activity complements the Gomori trichrome. COX activity will be reduced or lost when mutations/deletions involve the COX genes in mitochondrial DNA (mtDNA). In response, nuclear-encoded succinic dehydrogenase (SDH) activity will increase. This enhanced compensatory SDH activity is demonstrable in tissue sections and is

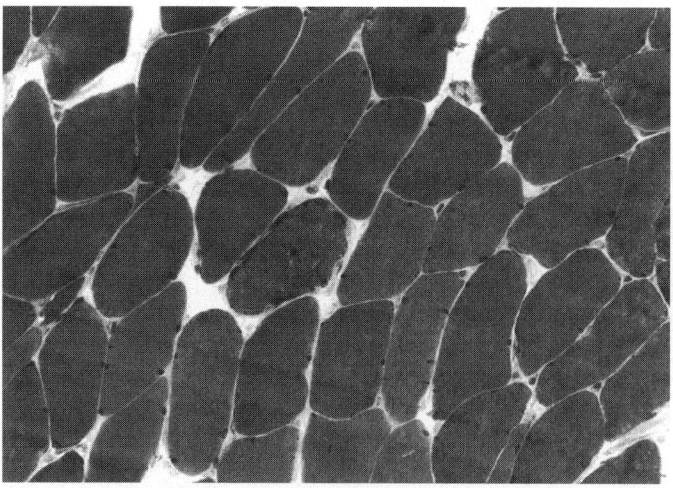

Figure 18 Mitochondrial myopathy. Gomori trichrome stain shows increased subsarcolemmal staining characteristic of ragged red fiber formation.

best seen in the combined COX-SDH stain. Using this technique, our laboratories always regard RRFs as significant, at least in the sense of having an associated biochemical defect. Ragged red fibers must be differentiated from tubular aggregates, which also accumulate in a subsarcolemmal location and stain red with the Gomori trichrome technique. Tubular aggregates do not have the ragged appearance of RRFs, and their tubular structure is readily evident on ultrastructural examination. They are not specific for any disease process. Nemaline (from the Greek *nema,* meaning thread) rods stain dark green to brown–black with the Gomori trichrome stain and are located beneath the sarcolemmal membrane and close to the nucleus (Fig. 19). Electron microscopy may demonstrate continuity between the rods and Z-lines or Z-disks. Nemaline rods are a diagnostic feature of nemaline myopathy, a clinically heterogeneous condition varying from a congenital rapidly fatal form to a nonprogressive form with minimal disability. Nemaline rods have also been reported in patients with HIV infection, and rare rod bodies may be seen in otherwise normal or minimally abnormal muscle. The rods may be immunostained with antibodies to actin or alpha-actinin.

2. *Periodic Acid–Schiff*

Assessment of muscle glycogen content by direct visual inspection of the periodic acid–Schiff (PAS) stain is next to impossible except when there is massive glycogen accumulation. Electron microscopy should always be carried out to confirm the presence of excess intermyofibrillar glycogen (Fig. 20). Techniques

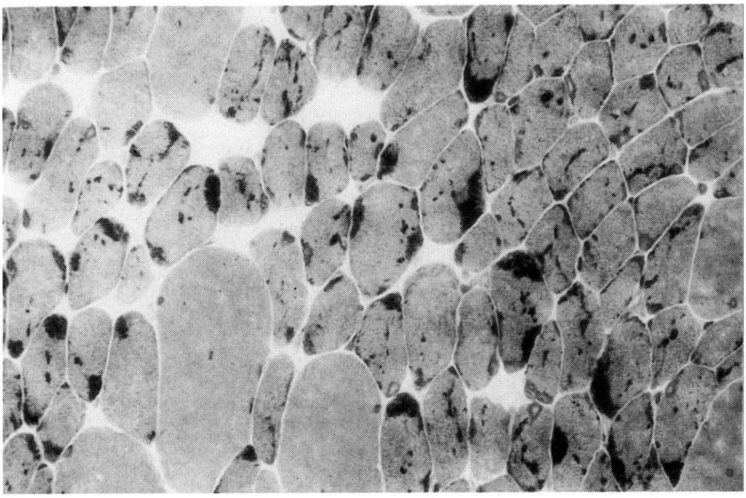

Figure 19 Nemaline myopathy. Gomori trichrome demonstrates rodlike subsarcolemmal structures typical of nemaline myopathy in most fibers. Also note fiber size variation.

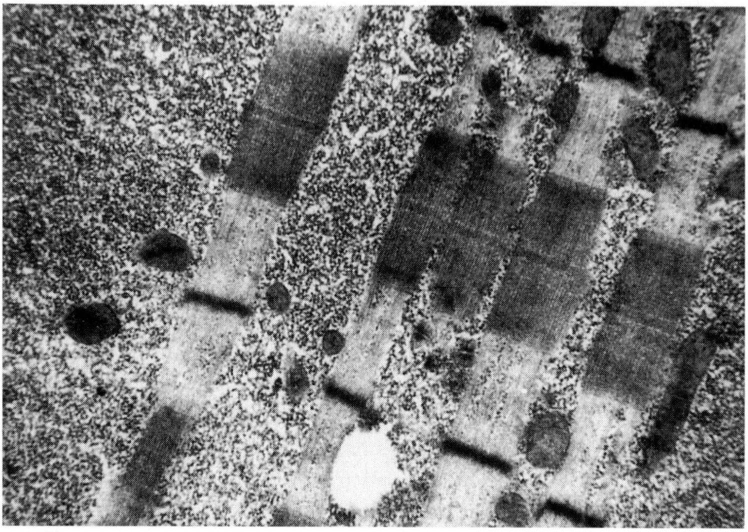

Figure 20 McArdle disease. Extensive intermyofibrillar glycogen deposition seen on electron microscopy.

to assess glycogen content, such as measurement of the optical intensity of the PAS-stained sections, are not routinely available. A myophosphorylase stain should always be routinely carried out because glycogen excess may be absent in some patients with McArdle disease. Blood vessels serve as an internal control in McArdle disease and will show normal reactivity that contrasts with the depleted sarcoplasm. The presence of diastase-resistant material suggests the presence of one of the other glycogenoses, particularly type IV.

3. Oil-red O

Large fat droplets overlying muscle fibers are frequently encountered in technically suboptimal preparations and should be disregarded. A well-prepared lipid stain should demonstrate fine red sarcoplasmic droplets and it should be possible to discern two distinct fiber types: type I fibers normally contain more lipid than type II fibers (Fig. 21). However considerable experience is required when trying to assess the amount of lipid present and in all suspected cases of lipid storage myopathy it is essential to have electron microscopic verification of the excess lipid. Confirmation of lipid excess should stimulate a search for fatty acid oxidation defects as well as deficiency of carnitine, carnitine palmitoyltransferases I and II, carnitine-acylcarnitine translocase, very long chain acyl-CoA dehydrogenase, and the mitochondrial trifunctional protein. The frozen

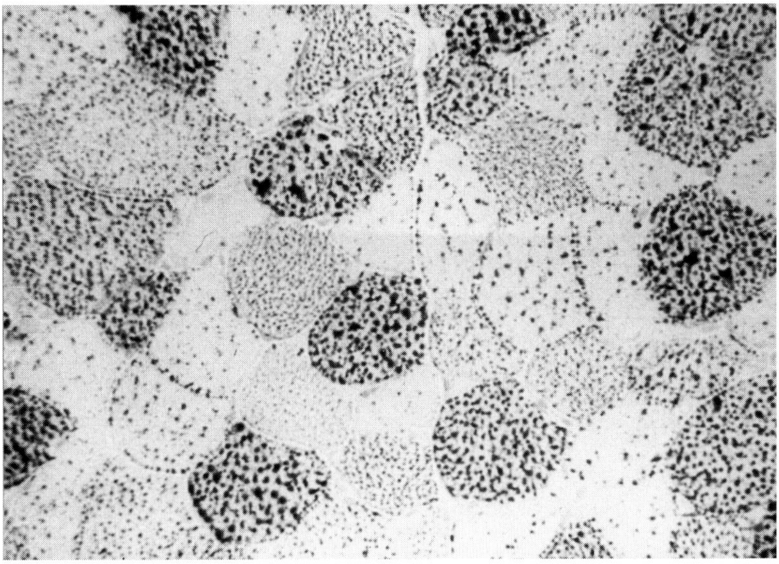

Figure 21 Lipid storage myopathy. Oil-red-O stain reveals extensive sarcoplasmic lipid deposition. Type 1 fibers contain more lipid than type 2 fibers.

muscle should be retained for direct measurements of these enzymes in cases of suspected lipid storage myopathy.

4. Adenosine Triphosphatase; Myofibrillar ATPase

Differentiation of muscle fibers into types I and II is best accomplished with the ATPase reaction. Further subclassification of type II fibers is achieved by preincubation at pH 4.3 and pH 4.6. Individual muscles vary according to the relative proportions of type I and type II fibers and care should be taken in the interpretation of fiber type distributions in biopsies obtained from unfamiliar sites. The differing histochemical fiber types are normally randomly distributed, giving rise to the classic "checkerboard" or mosaic pattern (Fig. 22). In evaluating ATPase reactions, the first step is determine whether the mosaic pattern is preserved or lost. If the pattern is lost, is it because there is poor fiber type differentiation; or because one fiber type is predominant; or because the fibres, although present in more or less equal numbers, are unevenly distributed due to fiber type grouping (Fig. 23)? Poor fiber type differentiation may be due to poor technique but may also be present in some cases of muscular dystrophy. Type I fiber type predominance is present in some myopathies and may, in certain circumstances, be present in denervation (see below).

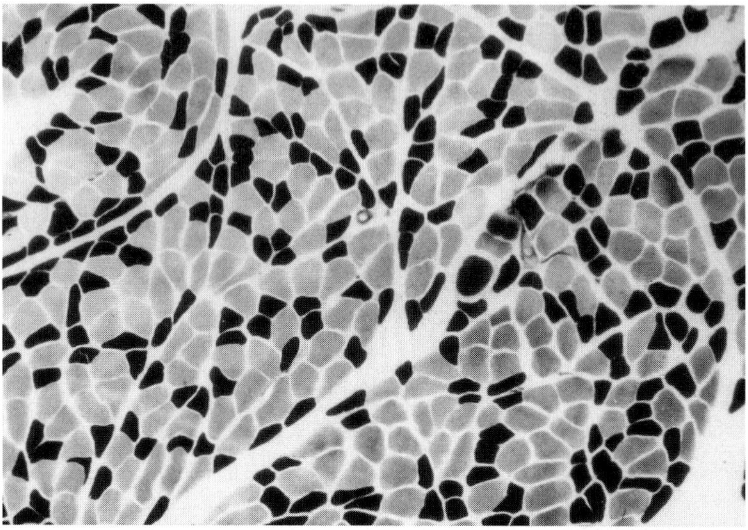

Figure 22 Mosaic fiber type pattern. Typical checkerboard or mosaic pattern of fiber type distribution. In this case the type 2 fibers (dark) are considerably smaller than the type 1 fibers. (ATPase pH 10.2.)

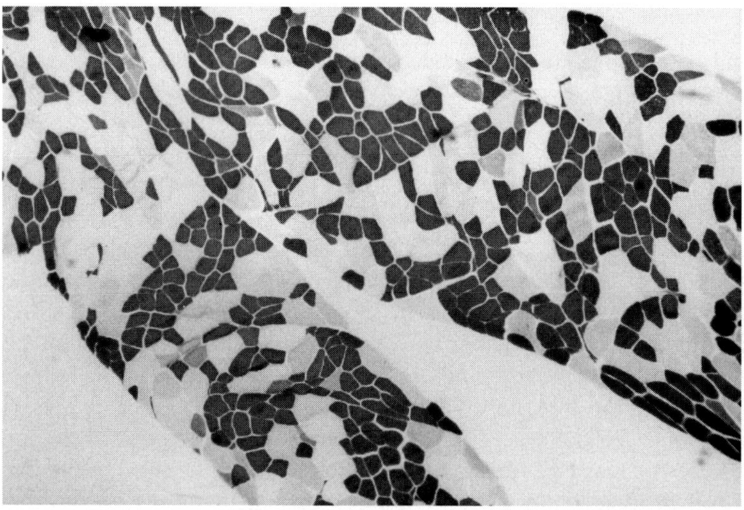

Figure 23 Fiber type predominance. Type 2 fiber predominance causes difficulty in interpretation: there is apparent grouping of the type 2 fibers. However, there is no evidence of any grouping involving type 1 fibers. A diagnosis of denervation cannot be based on grouping that involves one fiber type alone.

5. *Fiber Type Grouping*

Mathematical models constructed to assist in the assessment of fiber type grouping are not useful in daily practice. Arbitrary assessment, including the detection of a minimum of 16 fibers of identical type to constitute a group, or determination of grouping when three fibers of the same histochemical type touch each other and are completely surrounded on all sides by fibers of the same histochemical type, is a good practical approach. Groups of both type I and type II fibers must be present for a diagnosis of fiber type grouping. When the groups are very large, occasionally the biopsy may consist only of a large fascicle composed of fibers all of one histochemical type (Fig. 24). This is difficult to resolve but as long as the histochemical technique is above reproach one can suggest denervation as the most likely diagnosis. Denervation may be diagnosed without fiber type grouping when there is random atrophy of fibres: nonselective atrophy of type I and type II fibres. In equivocal cases, knowledge of the electromyographic and clinical findings may be helpful. Denervation is a dynamic evolving process in which a biopsy captures only a tiny area of one muscle at a particular time. Figure 25 is an attempt to show how the process may evolve over time.

6. *NADH–Tetrazolium Reductase*

A number of features may be seen with this stain. Disruption of the central myofibrillar pattern is a nonspecific feature and may be seen in both myopathies and denervation (Fig. 26). Targetoid change is a feature of denervation. Other features

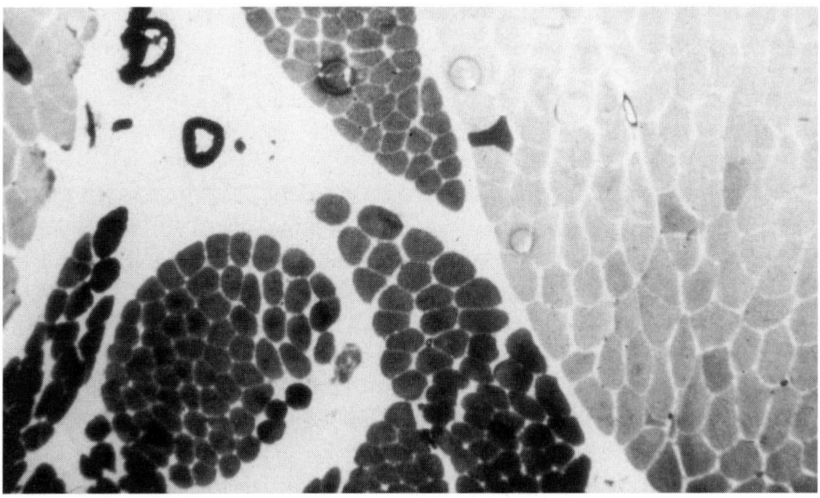

Figure 24 Panfascicular fiber type grouping. This pattern may be extremely difficult to interpret if the biopsy is nonrepresentative (i.e. only one fascicle of a single fiber type may be biopsied); in that context a diagnosis of denervation cannot be established.

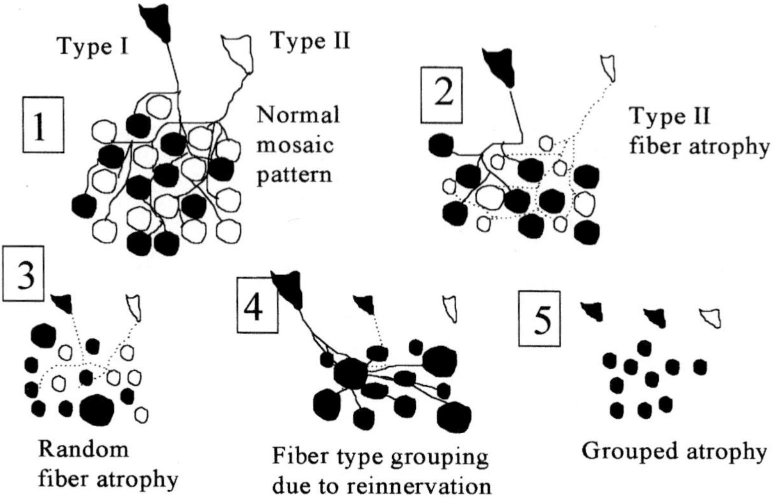

Figure 25 Evolution of denervation atrophy with reinnervation. The motor unit consists of a variable number of fibers together with the parent neuron, its axon, and intramuscular nerve branches. The parent neuron determines the histochemical profile of the muscle, all fibers within a unit having the same histochemical type (panel 1). The denervating process may begin anywhere from anterior horn cell distally, and in this instance (panel 2) atrophy of all type II fibers is depicted. As the disease process progresses (panel 3), other neurons are affected and further muscle fibers undergo atrophy, resulting in random fiber atrophy. Axons of surviving neurons (panel 4) sprout and reinnervate the atrophic fibers which then take on the histochemical profile of the new parent neuron, resulting in fiber type grouping. Finally, when the denervating process spreads further and there are no residual neurons capable of sprouting, all of the muscle fibers undergo atrophy: so-called group atrophy.

of denervation that may be observed with this stain include fiber type grouping and the presence of small, atrophic, intensely stained type 1 fibers. However the relatively poor fiber type differentiation seen with this stain makes it unreliable for assessment of fiber types in comparison to ATPase preparations. Central core disease, as the name implies, is characterized by central pale staining areas in individual muscle fibers (Fig. 27). Increased subsarcolemmal staining due to increased numbers of mitochondria is typical of mitochondrial myopathies.

E. Other Histochemical Stains

The variability of glycogen accumulation in myophosphorylase deficiency is such that a myophosphorylase stain should be performed on all muscle biopsies. Acid phosphatase is a very useful marker of increased lysosomal activity.

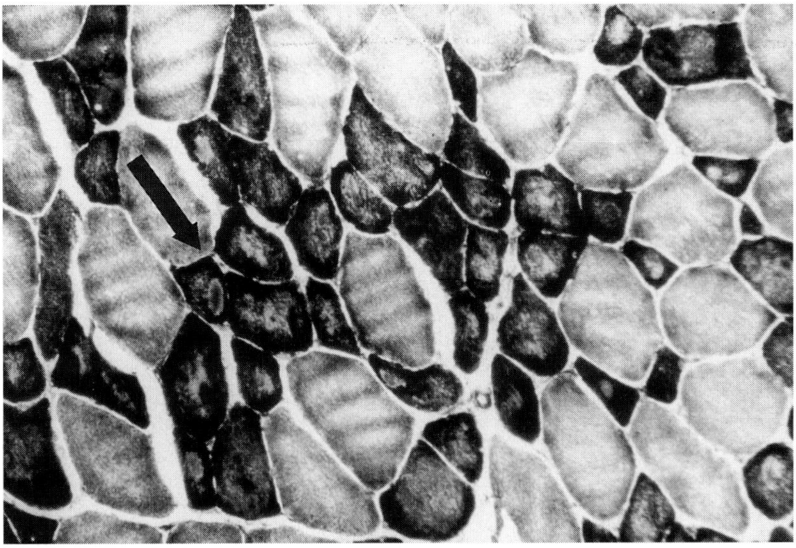

Figure 26 Myofibrillar disruption. The NADH stain shows central myofibrillar pallor with targetoid change (arrow). Note small angulated intensely stained fibers. Overall appearances are those of denervation.

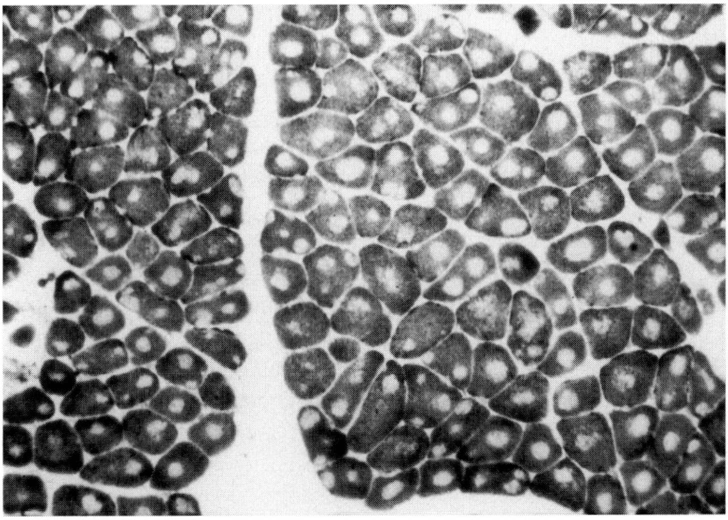

Figure 27 Central core disease. NADH-stained section demonstrates numerous central cores typical of central core myopathy.

Increased reactivity is present in most of the lysosomal storage disorders but also in conditions in which there is increased muscle fiber degradation from whatever cause. Cytochrome oxidase (COX) is an essential stain for the investigation of mitochondrial disease in which the COX activity is depleted or absent. The histological assessment of COX depletion is difficult and is compounded by day-to-day variability in staining intensity. The activity of COX, which is encoded by mitochondrial DNA, will be reduced or lost when mutations/deletions involve the COX genes. In response, nuclear-encoded succinic dehydrogenase (SDH) activity will increase. This enhanced compensatory SDH activity is demonstrable in tissue sections, but correlation of the diminished COX activity with enhanced SDH activity in parallel sections is laborious and time-consuming. These problems are easily overcome by combining the COX and SDH stains. COX depletion will be instantly apparent by the blue appearance of the compensatory increased SDH activity.

F. Immunohistochemistry

Muscle biopsy interpretation has been revolutionized by immunohistochemistry (IHC). Advances in the characterization of sarcolemmal proteins and recognition that defects in the genes encoding such proteins may lie at the heart of the multiple differing forms of muscular dystrophy have been among the most important recent developments in muscle pathology. The individual proteins and related diseases will be reviewed below. Interpretation of the immunohistochemical reactions using antibodies to the individual proteins differs from conventional IHC in that frozen sections are usually required. Extreme care is needed to ensure that only 6μm thick sections of muscle are used; thick sections will give false-positive reactions. In the early stages of acquiring experience with these antibodies it is crucial that biochemical confirmation of any alterations, reductions, or absences of particular proteins be obtained with Western blotting. This is only available in a few specialized centers and it is helpful if the antibodies used in the IHC are the same as those used in the Western blot. Some antigens, particularly merosin-associated epitopes, may survive prolonged storage (periods of up to 10 years). Therefore, it is possible to take archival frozen sections of muscle, remove the cover slip, destain the sections, and incubate the decolorized sections with merosin antibodies, thereby allowing reassessment of old biopsies previously classified as "dystrophy, type unspecified" (Fig. 28). Either peroxidase- or fluorescein-labeled antibodies may be used. Desmin IHC is worth considering in any undiagnosed myopathy, since the accumulation of sarcoplasmic desmin-positive material is common to a number of myopathies. In the past these were variously termed "myopathy with myofibrillar inclusions," "spheroid body myopathy," "cytoplasmic body myopathy,"

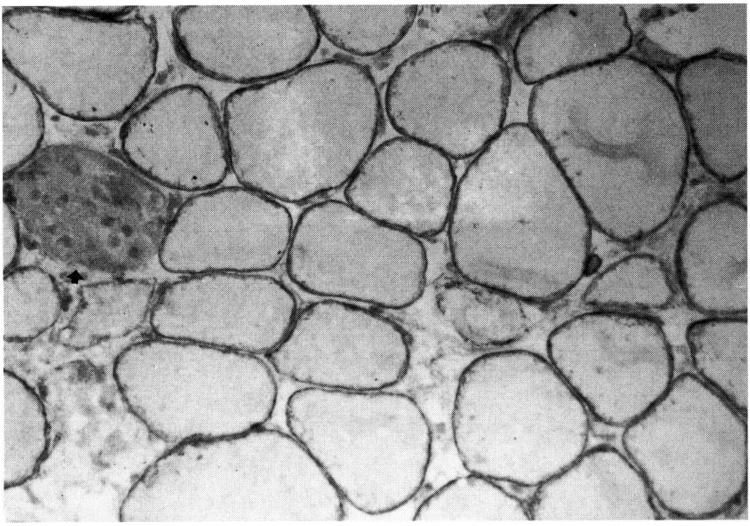

Figure 28 Immunohistochemistry. Archival frozen section of skeletal muscle destained and immunoreacted with an antibody to merosin. Note fine sarcolemmal membranous staining and absence of staining from necrotic fiber. Spectrin is used as an internal control for membrane integrity (not demonstrated in this panel).

and so on. These have now been collected under the umbrella term "myofibrillar myopathy with abnormal foci of desmin positivity." So far, there is little clinical application for antibodies directed against myosin, actin, or actinin epitopes, although it is likely that this situation will change as the emphasis in muscle research shifts from sarcolemmal to sarcoplasmic proteins. In addition, antibodies directed against the various mitochondrial protein subunits have not yet come into widespread usage. Antibodies directed against T cells and T-cell subsets, activated T cells, B cells, macrophages, proliferating cells, natural killer cells, class I and II molecules from the major histocompatibility complex (MHC), and various cytokines may be of limited usefulness in trying to differentiate the various inflammatory myopathies. MHC class I molecules are located in perifascicular fibers in DM. In PM, MHC expression is more intense and is located mainly in non-necrotic partially invaded cells. MHC class II molecule expression is present in endothelial cells in a variable fashion in both DM and PM. In summary the repertoire of immunohistochemical stains that may aid in the diagnosis of muscle disease is increasing quickly and their interpretation requires considerable expertise.

II. SPECIFIC CATEGORIES OF MUSCLE DISEASE

A. Muscular Dystrophy

Advances in unravelling the pathophysiological basis of the muscular dystrophies have been spectacular. Within the past 10 years at least three protein families together with several individual proteins have been discovered within or adjacent to the sarcolemmal membrane. Although much is still to be learned about the role of these proteins in maintaining muscle function and structure, it is clear that deficiencies in these proteins result in severe progressive muscle disease. This progress is best illustrated by our current understanding of Duchenne's muscular dystrophy (DMD), in which the absence of dystrophin, a huge sarcolemmal membrane protein, results in severe irreversible muscle fiber destruction. This chapter does not propose to review in detail the genetic and molecular basis of all of the muscular dystrophies, but will concentrate on illustrating how several of the muscular dystrophies can now be diagnosed using antibodies directed against the various sarcolemmal proteins.

Several diagrams have been published to illustrate the position of protein molecules in the sarcolemmal membrane, but it must be remembered that much of this positioning is still conjectural. With the possible exception of DMD and Becker's muscular dystrophy (BMD), none of the muscular dystrophies have distinguishing histopathologic features. All share the following features: fiber size variation with fiber splitting, central nucleation, fiber necrosis with regenerating fibers, and variable endomysial fibrosis. The extent to which any or all of these individual features are present in a particular biopsy depends on the duration of the disease process and the severity of involvement of a particular muscle. Once a dystrophic process is suspected in a muscle biopsy it is necessary to examine the muscle using a panel of antibodies directed against the various muscle membrane-associated proteins.

From the schematic illustration in Figure 29 and table below it is apparent that the association of a particular protein with a specific dystrophy, together with the commercial availability of an antibody to that protein, is currently fulfilled in only a few instances. The dystrophin, merosin, and some of the sarcoglycan-related dystrophies can be easily diagnosed using this approach. It is certain that muscular dystrophies resulting from altered expression of the dystroglycan and syntrophin complexes will be described in the very near future. Rather than have to carry out multiple immunohistochemical analyses with an increasingly large panel of antibodies, it may be more practical to decorate a Western blot prepared from a dystrophic muscle homogenate with multiple antibodies. A Western blot is more sensitive than tissue immunohistochemistry and has the added advantage of allowing a degree of quantification. In several muscular dystrophies a genetic locus has been established but the

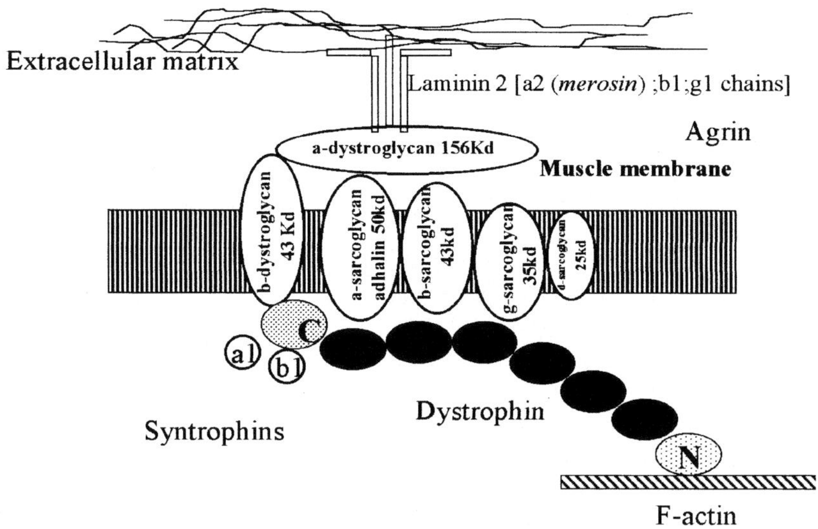

Figure 29 The skeletal muscle cell membrane and its components. The laminin component of the extracellular matrix is a heterotrimer linked to glycoproteins on and within the muscle cell membrane. These glycoproteins or dystroglycans link laminin to the dystrophin molecule located on the cytoplasmic face of the sarcolemmal membrane. The dystrophin molecule is linked to the cytoskeletal filaments through binding of its N-terminal to F-actin. It is easy to appreciate that loss of one of the links in this complex could lead to muscle fiber disruption. Other proteins, namely the sarcoglycans, also span the muscle cell membrane and form links with the dystrophin molecule. The syntrophins, which are attached to the C-terminal end of the dystrophin molecule, are located entirely within the sarcoplasm and do not span the sarcolemmal membrane. Their structural role is not well understood. There are minor alterations in the arrangement of these proteins at the neuromuscular junction. Agrin, which is involved in the organization of the acetylcholine receptors, and utrophin (a dystrophin homologue) are both present at the neuromuscular junction.

relevant protein has yet to be determined. As might be expected, the majority of this group show autosomal dominant inheritance. Included are the limb girdle (types 1A & 1B), facioscapulohumeral, distal and oculopharyngeal muscular dystrophies. It is not possible to make a specific histological diagnosis in these dystrophies.

The location and putative interrelationships of the various membrane proteins are illustrated in Figure 29.

B. Dystrophinopathies (Duchenne's and Becker's Muscular Dystrophy)

DMD has an incidence of approximately 1:3500 and is inherited in an X-linked recessive manner. The DMD gene, one of the lagest known, spans 2400 kb and is located on the X chromosome (Xp21.1) where it has 79 exons that encode a 14kb mRNA transcript. This mRNA encodes a 3685 amino acid, 427kDa protein termed dystrophin. Two-thirds of DMD patients have large scale deletions clustered in a hot-spot in the center of the gene. DMD differs from BMD in that the deletions usually result in an interruption of the reading frame and consequent complete loss of dystrophin. In BMD the reading frame is maintained and protein is produced, although in insufficient amounts to maintain the structural integrity of the muscle. This genetic difference is reflected in the complete absence of any histochemically detectable dystrophin from the DMD biopsies, whereas BMD biopsies usually exhibit definite but patchy staining for dystrophin (Table 1, Fig. 30). New point mutations and small deletions may also interrupt the reading frame and result in the DMD phenotype. The difficulty in detecting small deletions and point mutations in such a large gene is self-evident and presents particular problems in carrier detection among

Table 1 Muscular Dystrophies: Genetic and Immunohistochemical Features

Protein	Disease	Size (kDa)	Locus	Commercial antibodies available
Dystrophin	Duchenne's Becker's	427	Xp21	Yes (antibodies to amino, carboxy, and rod portions of the molecule must be used)
Calpain 3	LGMD2A	95	15q15.1	No
α-sarcoglycan (Adhalin)	LGMD2D	50	17q12	Yes
β-sarcoglycan	LGMD2E	43	4q12	Yes
γ-sarcoglycan	LGMD2C	35	13q12	Yes
δ-sarcoglycan	LGMD2F	25	5q33	No
Merosin	Merosin deficient congenital muscular dystrophy	90	6q22	Yes
Emerin	Emery-Dreifuss	34	Xq28	No
Myotonin-protein kinase	Myotonic Dystrophy	72	19q	No

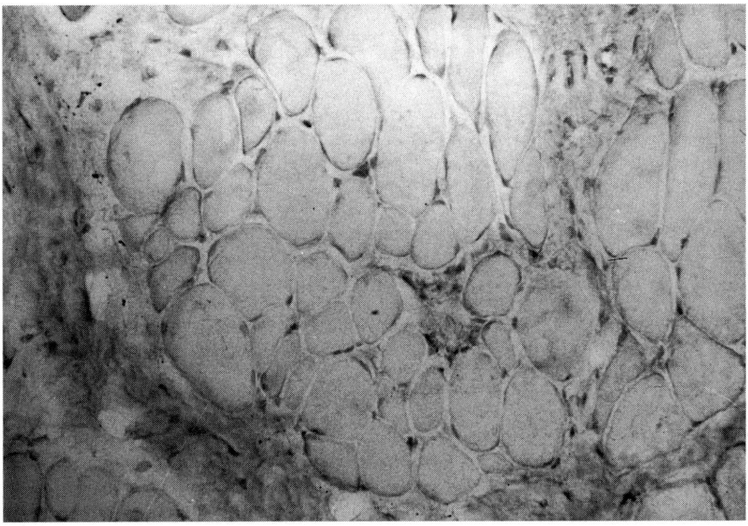

Figure 30 Becker muscular dystrophy. Muscle immunoreacted with antibody to carboxy-terminal portion of dystrophin molecule to show patchy membranous immunostaining. Individual fibers demonstrate variability in the intensity of staining. Virtually all fibers show some staining. In DMD there is complete absence of immunoreactivity.

mothers of isolated cases of DMD. Considerable care has to be taken before concluding that a given patient represents a new spontaneous mutation. Loss of dystrophin in DMD is sometimes accompanied by a reduction in the staining intensity of the other dystrophin-associated molecules, presumably due to loss of anchorage rather than to any defect in the gene(s) encoding these proteins.

C. Limb-Girdle Muscular Dystrophy

The limb-girdle muscular dystrophies (LGMDs) (Table 2) have emerged from the "waste basket" of undiagnosed muscular dystrophies. Advances in protein chemistry applied to muscle have yielded important new information about the composition of the sarcolemmal membrane. In the LGMDs these new discoveries have proved most helpful. The LGMDs are a heterogeneous group of muscular dystrophies that have in common clinical involvement of the pelvis and shoulder musculature and show variable clinical progression and severity. There may also be cardiac involvement. Onset may be at any age but is most common in the teenage years. Involvement of face or distal musculature, at least in the early stages of the disease, is unusual. Creatine kinase is usually elevated, although variably so. The recessive forms due to sarcoglycan deficiency are usually most severe whereas the dominant and nonsarcoglycan-related forms have

Table 2 Limb-girdle Muscular Dystrophies

LGMD subtype	Inheritance	Locus	Protein	Possible identifying features
1A	Dominant	5q31		Young adults, slow progression
1B	Dominant	1q11-21		Cardiac abnormalities
2A	Recessive	15q15	Muscle specific calpain	Isolated community on Reunion Island and Amish families: variable phenotype
2B	Recessive	2p13-p16		Onset 15+ and slow progression. Miyoshi myopathy linked to same locus
2C	Recessive	13q12	γ-sarcoglycan	Severe phenotype; G-A mutation in codon 283 replacing a conserved cysteine in the extra-cellular domain of γ-sarcoglycan by a tyrosine.
2D	Recessive	17q12-21	α-sarcoglycan (adhalin)	Variable phenotype; no relation between disease severity and amount of adhalin expressed. Secondary adhalin deficiency may result from mutations in γ-sarcoglycan gene on chromosome 13.
2E	Recessive	4q12	β-sarcoglycan	A Thr-to-Arg missense mutation within the β-sarcoglycan gene leads to reduced expression of β-sarcoglycan. Secondary loss of adhalin and γ-sarcoglycan may occur.
2F	Recessive	5q33	δ-sarcoglycan	Single nucleotide deletion that alters reading frame and leads to complete protein loss.

a milder clinical course. However, there is considerable overlap in the clinical features of the different subtypes of LGMD. The relative proportions of each of the subtypes in any community remain to be determined but it has been estimated that approximately 11% of all nondystrophin dystrophies are related to sarcoglycan abnormalities. Reports to date are biased because of necessity they contain data on large informative kindreds with little information on sporadic cases. From the viewpoint of biopsy, the diagnosis of LGMD should be suspected when the biopsy is clearly dystrophic but when immunostaining for dystrophin is normal or near normal. Again it is important to stress that an immunohistochemical reduction in one sarcoglycan protein may be associated with secondary reductions of other sarcoglycans or indeed of the dystrophins. Thus it is essential that a Western blot be carried out, particularly when identifying the index case in a particular family. Correlations between the severity of the clinical phenotype and the degree of protein deficiency as assessed by Western blot remain to be established. As more data emerge concerning the mutations that give rise to the sarcoglycan deficiencies it is likely that a genetic diagnosis for the LGMDs will become available in the near future. Very little is known about the non-sarcoglycan-related LGMDs at this time other than a suspected role for muscle-specific calpain in LGMD2A.

D. Other Dystrophies

1. Emery–Dreifuss Muscular Dystrophy

Emery–Dreifuss muscular dystrophy (EMD) is an X-linked dystrophy characterized by muscle weakness, contractures, and cardiac involvement with arrhythmias and a risk of sudden death. Onset is usually in the first two decades. The biopsy does not show identifying diagnostic features. The EMD gene is located at Xq28 and the gene product, emerin, is a widely distributed 34kD nuclear membrane protein that shows homology with thymopoietins and the nuclear parminin-associated protein, LAP2, both members of a family of inner nuclear membrane proteins. Emerin expression is absent from skeletal muscle in patients with EMD. However, antibodies to emerin are not yet commercially available. The widespread expression of emerin means that skin or leukocytes may be used as an alternative to muscle for diagnosis and female carriers may be detected by demonstration of reduced but not absent levels of emerin. A variety of different mutations in the emerin gene have been described including several different mutations from the same EMD family.

2. Facioscapulohumeral Muscular Dystrophy

Facioscapulohumeral muscular dystrophy (FSHD) is an autosomal dominant dystrophy characterized by progressive weakness and atrophy of the facial, shoulder girdle, and upper arm muscles. Onset is variable, with some patients not manifesting the disease until midlife. Other features that may be present include hypertrophic cardiomyopathy, sensorineural deafness, and retinal telangiectasia. Disease progression is slow and life expectancy may be normal. FSHD is one of the more common dystrophies and is recognized as the great mimicker on biopsy with chronic inflammation, denervation, and dystrophic features all likely to be encountered. The gene responsible for FSHD has been localized to chromosome 4q35. A number of tandem repeats are located at this site. The functional role of these repeats (if any) is unknown. Deletion of a number of these nonexpressed repeats results in the generation of fragments that are considerably smaller than those encountered in normal muscle.

Their detection is the basis for diagnostic genetic testing for FSHD. There is a reasonable correlation between the deletion size at this locus and the age at onset of FSHD. How these deletions of nonexpressed regions result in disease is as yet undetermined. Some FSHD families do not show linkage to this locus.

3. Myotonic Dystrophy

Myotonic dystrophy (MyD) is one of the most common of all muscular dystrophies with an incidence of up to 13:100,000 live births. It is particularly common in French Canada. Myotonia or delayed muscle relaxation after contraction or following percussion is present in a variety of muscle disorders classified into dystrophic and nondystrophic types. The nondystrophic myotonias include hypokalemic periodic paralysis, paramyotonia congenita, and myotonia congenita. All the myotonias have in common a disorder of muscle membrane involving either ion channels (sodium or potassium) or a protein kinase involved in regulation of the membrane channels. MyD is differentiated from the other myotonias by the presence of systemic disease and muscle wasting and shows autosomal dominant inheritance. The disorder is caused by expansion of an unstable [CTG] trinucleotide repeat in the 3′ untranslated region of the myotonin proteinase (MtPK) gene on chromosome 19q13.31. As with most triplet repeat diseases, the manner in which this abnormal unstable expansion results in disease is still poorly understood. Severely affected individuals may have as many as 2000 copies of the [CTG] triplet in comparison to less than 100 copies in mildly affected individuals and less than 30 copies in normals. Antibody studies have localized MtPK mainly to the I-band and in the terminal cisternae of the sarcoplasmic reticulum. Systemic features of MyD include cardiac conduction defects with risk of sudden death, variable mental retardation, hypogonadism, and the easily recognized frontal balding, temporal wasting, and cataracts. Disease may onset at any age and in general an earlier onset is associated with a greater number of repeats. A congenital form occurs and may easily be mistaken for another neuromuscular disease if the mother is not examined. Prominent features of the congenital form include decreased fetal movements, hydramnios with hypotonia, and arthrogryposis at birth. Muscle biopsy is rarely performed for MyD since the diagnosis is easily made on the basis of the number of triple repeats present in blood. Classic biopsy feature included ring fibers, type I fiber hypotrophy, central nuclei, and sarcoplasmic masses.

4. Regional Dystrophies

Occasionally a biopsy will be accompanied by a request to confirm the diagnosis of distal myopathy or scapuloperoneal or scalpulohumeral dystrophy. There is still much confusion about whether these are distinct clinicopathological entities. Both neurogenic and myopathic disorders may present with this pattern of muscle involvement. Thus interpretation of the muscle biopsy in this context should be directed towards the establishment of a primary pathologic process (i.e., denervation vs. myopathy/dystrophy) rather than at futile attempts to make an eponymic diagnosis. These biopsies are particularly difficult to interpret since virtually all of the biopsy features of a myopathic or dystrophic process may be present in long-standing denervation. The best approach is to look for evidence of denervation in the form of fiber type grouping while at the same time remembering that large hypertrophied fibers that have undergone splitting may simulate grouped atrophy. However these split fibers are usually rounded rather than angular and atrophic. Small fibers intensely stained with NADH also suggest denervation. If neither of these fatures are present it is difficult to support a diagnosis of denervation. Rimmed vacuoles or hyaline bodies may point to one of the syndromes listed below. Ultimately one may have to rely on the electromyogram (EMG) and nerve conduction studies to resolve the issue.

E. Inflammatory Myopathy

The inflammatory myopathies (IM) include inclusion body myositis (IBM), polymyositis (PM), and dermatomyositis (DM). Occasionally other myopathies or dystrophies such as FSH may be associated with an intense inflammatory cell infiltrate and simulate one of these three conditions on biopsy. There is a ten-

Table 3 Histologically Verifiable Distal Neuromuscular Disorders Likely To Cause Diagnostic Difficulty

Distal myopathy with	
Rimmed vacuoles	Adult-onset sporadic
Rimmed vacuoles and cytoplasmic inclusions	Autosomal dominant
Rimmed vacuoles	Autosomal recessive; chromosome 9
Scapuloperoneal syndrome with	
Hyaline (myosin heavy-chain-positive) cytoplasmic bodies	Autosomal dominant
Hyaline desmin-containing cytoplasmic inclusions,	Autosomal dominant; chromosome 12q24.1-q.24.3
Various other late-onset spinal muscular atrophies	SMA type III
GM2 gangliosidosis	(Kugelberg-Welander disease)

dency at some institutions to make a clinical diagnosis of IM without recourse to biopsy. This is regrettable because subsequent biopsies taken after the patient has failed to show the expected response to steroids are likely to be very difficult to interpret because of a reduction in the inflammatory component together with possible steroid-induced atrophy. Although the three IMs are distinct pathological entities with different causes, they do not show major clinical differences. All usually have their onset after the age of 50, although childhood forms of DM and PM are described. A weak association with cancer is present with DM. Muscle weakness is as likely to be distal as proximal in IBM. A skin rash is absent in IBM and PM.

1. Inclusion Body Myositis

IBM is possibly the most common inflammatory myopathy in adults, with men more likely to be affected than females. Hereditary forms have been described but most cases are sporadic. IBM begins slowly, often in the distal muscles, particularly with finger–wrist involvement. In contrast to PM and DM, IBM is typically not associated with other disorders. Great care must be taken with interpretation of suspected IBM biopsies since the appearances are highly variable. The most characteristic finding is rimmed vacuoles with basophilic granules located at the edge of centrally placed sarcoplasmic vacuoles (Figs. 5, 6). Their number varies enormously, with some IBM biopsies showing few if any vacuoles. Groups of atrophic fibers may be present and simulate denervation. Fiber hypertrophy may be present. The presence of ragged red fibers (RRFs) and interfiber mosaicism on the COX-SDH stain has led to speculation about a mitochondrial basis for IBM, and indeed mtDNA deletions have been reported in some patients. Lymphocytic infiltrates surround and invade muscle fibers with the partially invaded fibers, but not others, likely to show MHC-class I expression. The infiltrating cells are usually cytotoxic T lymphocytes and macrophages. The characteristic filaments of IBM require ultrastructural demonstration (Fig. 7) and may be seen in either the nucleus or cytoplasm. In the cytoplasm they may lie adjacent to membranous whorls. Filaments may measure up to 20 nm in diameter and should not be confused with normal sarcoplasmic filaments, such as myosin and actin. IBM-like filaments and rimmed vacuoles may be observed, although not simultaneously, in other muscle diseases. When a biopsy shows invasion of nonnecrotic fibers by lymphocytes and contains both vacuoles and typical filaments, a definitive diagnosis of IBM can be made irrespective of the clinical history. A diagnosis of possible IBM is made when the biopsy only shows invasion of nonnecrotic fibers by lymphocytes with no vacuoles or filaments detected. Familial IBM must not be confused with hereditary inclusion body myopathy without inflammation. The presence of beta/A4 amyloid and other proteins associated with Alzheimer's disease in myofibers of IBM has raised many questions about its causes. Demonstration of congo red-positive amyloid is not essential for the diagnosis of IBM. Sequences of the amyloid precursor protein (APP) and ubiquitin have been demonstrated in IBM muscle, as have paired helical filaments and apolipoprotein-E. It has been suggested that production of these proteins in muscle might represent an induced response to a virus-derived transcription factor and that the inflammatory response is directed against such proteins. However, the fact that fibers partially invaded by lymphocytes are overwhelmingly more common than fibers containing amyloid or other proteins would seem to offer little support for this hypothesis, as does the apparent failure of IBM to show much improvement in response to immune suppression. There is evidence that the vacuoles may arise as a result of nuclear damage, the remnants of which can be recognized as the membranous whorls in the sarcoplasm. How the nuclear damage is brought about remains unknown. It is also possible that nuclear injury results in mitochondrial dysfunction, as evidenced by RRFs and COX depletion. Currently there are new data emerging on the significant role played by the nucleus in regulating the expression of mitochondrial proteins. Disruption of the nuclear regulatory mechanisms could conceivably also induce secondary mitochondrial injury in the form of RRFs, COX depletion, and mtDNA deletions, similar to that seen in IBM. As yet there are no genetic clues available from linkage studies of hereditary forms of IBM to provide insights into possible disease mechanisms in this disorder. The natural history of IBM is one of relentless but slow progression over many years, although this may be hastened by futile persistence in treating affected patients with high doses of steroids.

2. *Polymyositis*

More common in women, polymyositis (PM) typically presents with subacute proximal muscle weakness with pain and tenderness present in as many as 50% of patients. Distal weakness is frequently present but only usually detected on examination. Involvement of pharyngeal and neck muscles as well as the diaphragm may lead to dysphagia, weakness of head flexion, and respiratory insufficiency. Cardiac involvement is well documented in PM, although its prevalence is disputed. It is important to exclude coexistent ischemic heart disease. Creatine kinase (CK) level elevation in PM may reach 30–40 times normal but the CK may also be normal, depending on the stage of disease.

Having decided that a biopsy essentially shows inflammatory change, it is best initially to look for the characteristic features of IBM and DM. Having assured oneself that these are absent, it is then usually easier to make the diagnosis of PM, with only a mixed connective tissue disease (MCTD) likely to cause any difficulty. The inflammatory infiltrate in PM (Fig. 3) is usually centered on individual muscle fibers, whereas in DM the infiltrate is located around the small capillary vessels. In some cases of PM the inflammatory infiltrate may be very sparse. CD8-positive lymphocytes together with macrophages are prominent. Necrosis of muscle fibers (Fig. 4), with or without surrounding macrophages, is prominent in PM, especially when the disease is acute. Muscle fiber necrosis is less evident in DM, in which the capillary bed bears the brunt of the immune attack. Muscle fiber injury is initiated by sensitized CD8+ cytotoxic T cells that recognize as yet uncharacterized antigens in the context of major histocompatibility complex (MHC) class I expression. A restricted (oligoclonal) pattern of T-cell receptor genes in the inflammatory infiltrate suggests that the T-cell response is antigen driven. Previous treatment and disease chronicity can diminish the intensity of the inflammatory infiltrate and in some biopsies there may be little or no inflammation. PM may be very focal. Sometimes the inflammatory infiltrate may impinge on intramuscular nerve terminals and give rise to a picture of denervation (in addition to the inflammatory myopathic changes). This type of secondary denervation is not usually seen in DM and IBM. In attempting to differentiate between PM and the MCTDs it is usually necessary to determine the patient's serological status.

A variety of "myositis-specific antibodies" have been described in PM/DM patients. These antibodies are directed against tRNA synthetases and a translation protein termed signal recognition particle (SRP). Anti-Jo-1, which recognizes a histidyl-t-RNA synthetase, is present in about 20% patients with PM, while elevated antinuclear antibodies are present in up to 40%. Correlations between antibody profile and disease behavior, including response to treatment and association with other organ involvement, are being undertaken. Much has been written about the patterns of cytokine expression in PM and other inflammatory myopathies but it is difficult to discern consistent patterns of expression in the various publications. In particular it is difficult to draw any correlation between disease severity and cytokine expression. Cytokine expression is also present in some *non*inflammatory muscle diseases such as Duchenne's muscular dystrophy. Clinicians must be aware that a diagnosis of PM or indeed DM is based on a triad of clinical, histological, and biochemical indices, and that an absence of inflammation from the muscle biopsy does not preclude a diagnosis of PM. A particular problem for both clinician and pathologist is the development of symptom recurrence and increasing weakness in a patient with established PM who is already taking steroids. Does the patient require more steroids for persistently active disease or is the increasing weakness due to steroid excess? A normal or near-normal CK favors a steroid effect, but in some instances it may be necessary to carry out a repeat biopsy.

3. *Dermatomyositis*

Dermatomyositis (DM) differs from IBM and PM in the presence of a rash and an increased propensity to occur in children as well as adults, in whom it is more common in women. The classic red–purple rash involves the periorbital and malar regions as well as the arms and legs. Elevated red scaly lesions may be present over the knuckles. An accompanying vasculitis may involve other organs but particularly the subcutaneous tissues, where the lesions may ulcerate and undergo calcification. DM is best regarded as an inflammatory vasculopathy in which the muscle capillaries bear the brunt of the disease. This is reflected in the muscle biopsy appearance, where careful examination of plastic embedded 1 μm thick sections (or alkaline phosphatase histochemistry) will demonstrate a reduction in the number of capillary vessels. Important though this finding is for understanding the disease, it is difficult for the inexperienced pathologist to come to terms with assessment of capillary density in skeletal muscle. However, the effects of the capillary involvement may be seen in the form of perifascicular atrophy with relative sparing of the fascicular center. This atrophy is readily apparent on ATPase stains. The perifascicular region is thought to represent a watershed zone that is most vulnerable to ischemia (Fig. 11). In children the ischemic process may be more severe and result in infarction of muscle. The inflammatory cell infiltrate is different from that seen in PM: it surrounds blood vessels rather than muscle fibers and contains more B cells and CD4+ T-cells. The C5b-9 membrane attack complex as well as C3 and other immunoglobulins may be located in the muscle vasculature. Frank necrosis of blood vessels (Fig. 31) may be accompanied by thrombosis and in this situation it may be very difficult to exclude a systemic vasculitis. Intact endothelial cells may show characteristic (although *not* specific to this disorder) tubuloreticular inclusions on electron microscopy. As with PM, the inflammatory process may be very patchy, but some experienced pathologists are happy to make a diagnosis of DM in the presence of capillary depletion alone.

F. Congenital "Structural" Myopathies

This group is rather loosely defined but includes those myopathies in which onset is early in childhood (usually the neonatal period) and in which there is a recognizable histological abnormality by which the myopathy is designated. Mitochondrial myopathies, dystrophies, and metabolic disorders are not included in this group, for obvious reasons. These disorders are rare in comparison to other myopathies and in many instances only a handful of cases have been reported. Only the more common congenital structural myopathies will be considered. All show early onset, usually in the neonatal period, with relatively slow progression, although there are exceptions. All require biopsy for a specific diagnosis; indeed, the biopsy appearances have given rise to the names of most of the congenital myopathies. In considering these myopathies it is helpful to classify them on the basis of the site of abnormality:

Site of involvement	Myopathy
Sarcomere	Core diseases
Z-disc	Nemaline rod
Nucleus	Centronuclear
Fibre size	Congenital fiber type disproportion
Myofibrils	Desmin associated
	Cytoplasmic body
	Spheroid body
	Mallory body
	Myopathy with granulofilamentous inclusions
	Intermediate filament
Unusual inclusions	Fingerprint body
	Reducing body
	Tubulomembranous body

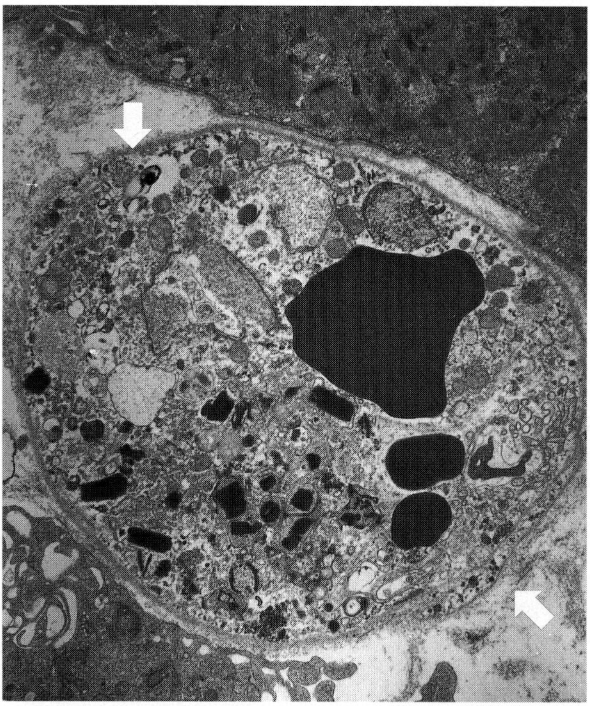

Figure 31 Dermatomyositis. Electron micrograph shows a necrotic capillary (arrows). Endothelial cytoplasmic tubuloreticular inclusions may also be seen in intact microvessels, though not in this case.

1. *Core Diseases*

Although there are many types of core, all have in common a circular area in which myofibrils are lost. This is best detected by loss of NADH staining and a relative absence of mitochondria on electron microscopic examination. Differentiation of structured cores, which show some preservation of myofibrillar architecture, from unstructured cores in which the architecture is completely lost, is not particularly helpful from a diagnostic viewpoint since both types of cores may be found in the same muscle. The basis on which cores form is debated, but mechanical factors such as tenotomy and immobilization as well as neural factors are important in their development, at least in the experimental situation. Cores are generally more common in type 1 fibers and may extend the entire length of a muscle fiber. In longitudinal sections there is Z-band streaming. The mechanisms by which the cores lead to muscle weakness are not well described, but we assume that muscle contractility is diminished by core formation.

Central core disease (CCD) is the prototype of this group of disorders. Early onset hypotonia with delayed motor milestones, proximal weakness, occasional cramps, and relative sparing of facial muscles is typical. The frequent coexistence of skeletal abnormalities including pes cavus and scoliosis occasionally leads to an erroneous diagnosis of peripheral neuropathy. As well as cores and type I fiber predominance, biopsies may show central nuclei and fiber size variation.

CCD often shows autosomal dominant inheritance, the gene having been mapped to a locus at chromosome 19q13.1 close to the gene for malignant hyperthermia susceptibility (MHS). MHS is caused by dysfunction of the ryanodine receptor calcium-sensitive, calcium-release channel of skeletal muscle sarcoplasmic reticulum. The ryanodine receptor gene (RYR1) that encodes the human skeletal muscle ryanodine receptor has been localized to chromosome 19q13.1–13.2. Several different single point mutations have been identified in the human skeletal muscle RYR gene in families with a predisposition to MH. A cluster of mutations has also been described in patients with combined CCD and MHS. Nearly all patients with CCD are susceptible to MH but not all patients with MHS have underlying CCD. Thus the biopsy appearances alone cannot be used to screen for MHS.

Biopsies for MHS should undergo *in vitro* contractility testing in response to various agents known to precipitate MH in susceptible individuals and this can only be done in specialized laboratories. Why some individuals develop CCD and others MHS in response to similar mutations is as yet unknown. The clinical heterogeneity of CCD must be stressed, with some patients not presenting until adulthood and some having a more rapidly progressive course than others. Multicore/minicore disease, in which there are tiny circular foci of degenerative change (on transverse section) in muscle fibers, shares many clinical features with CCD but as yet has failed to display sufficient identifying features to warrant a separate description. There is no evidence yet of genetic linkage to a particular locus. Core-targetoid fibers are also often encountered in denervation atrophy of muscle.

2. *Nemaline Rod Myopathy*

Nemaline rod myopathy (NRM; also known as rod body myopathy) is characterized by the presence of dark green to bluish black (Gomori trichrome stain) subsarcolemmal deposits (Fig. 19) composed of Z-band derived proteins showing immunopositivity for alpha-actinin. Two major clinical types are described: a severe neonatal-onset form and a more slowly progressive mild form that may begin in later childhood or adulthood. Most infants with the neonatal form have severe respiratory and feeding difficulties as well as profound hypotonia. Involvement of heart muscle may be present. In the later-onset form weakness may be very mild. A dysmorphic facies is often accompanied by scoliosis and pes cavus. Cardiac involvement may be present in this form as well. Diagnosis can only be made on biopsy, on which the rods (which measure 3–6 μm in length and up to 3 μm in width) are located beneath the sarcolemmal membrane on the Gomori trichrome stain. Rods may be present in virtually all or few muscle fibers but are more common in type 1 fibers. Type I fibers are also predominant and are usually smaller than type 2 fibers. The rods are electron dense and lie in continuity with streaming z-bands. Any clinically affected muscle including heart muscle may contain rods.

Immunolabeling of NRM sections shows that alpha-actinin is present in the rods. There may also be variable immunostaining with tropomyosin antibodies. These two proteins are likely to be of causative importance in the disease; mutations in the tropomyosin gene (TPM3) on chromosome 1q22-23 have been reported in a family with autosomal dominant nemaline myopathy. However, linkage to the genes for human muscle-specific alpha-actinin, (ACTN2 on chromosome 1q and ACTN3 on chromosome 11) remains to be demonstrated. Nemaline rods (usually in small numbers) may also be observed in many other muscle disorders but NRM is characterized by an absence of other muscle pathology, excluding that described above.

3. *Centronuclear Myopathy*

Centronuclear myopathy (CNM) is diagnosed on the basis of at least 30% of muscle fibers having centrally located nuclei in both fiber types (Fig. 13A), together with a predominance of type I fibers that are generally smaller than the type 2 fibers, and an absence of other major histopathological alterations. The diagnosis can be made on a hematoxylin and eosin-stained transverse section of muscle. The resemblance of these centrally nucleated fibers to fetal myotubes has given rise to the term "myotubular myopathy." However, some have reserved this eponym for those patients in whom the disease is X linked and in whom the centrally nucleated fibers are extremely small and closely resemble fetal muscle. This X-linked form results in severe weakness and hypotonia and is usually fatal. An arrest of the normal maturational migration of sarcolemmal nuclei or a failure of normal sarcoplasmic development is a possible explanation for persistence of this immature muscle appearance. Early- and late-onset forms of CNM are described but neither has any clinical features that allow differentiation from other forms of congenital myopathy. In both forms, clinical progression is slow with skeletal deformities commonly encountered. Central nuclei in isolation are not specific for CNM or myotubular myopathy. CNM is often familial, with autosomal dominant inheritance present in many cases. Adult and neonatal forms of myotonic dystrophy (MyD) may show extensive central nucleation (Fig. 13B). The adult form of MyD usually is easily recognizable by the presence of ring and hypertrophied fibers, but it is not possible to make a confident differentiation between neonatal MyD and CNM; thus expanded [CTG] repeats should be sought in blood from patients with suspected MyD (see above).

4. Congenital Fiber Type Disproportion

Congenital fiber type disproportion (CFTD) is suggested when a child with neonatal weakness and hypotonia is found to display type 1 fibers uniformly more than 15% smaller than type 2 fibers. There is considerable clinical heterogeneity, with some children dying as a result of respiratory failure and others showing near-normal attainment of motor milestones, suggesting perhaps that CFTD is not yet a clearly defined clinicopathological entity. Familial cases of CFTD are rare and there are no published linkage studies. It is not possible to predict the clinical outcome on the basis of the biopsy appearances.

5. Desmin-Related Myopathies

A number of congenital myopathies characterized by dissolution of myofibrils and accumulation of Z-disk material resulting in the formation of globular masses comprising myofibrils and altered Z-disk material have been labeled with a confusing variety of terms. The sarcoplasmic masses show variable desmin immunoreactivity and this has led to a proposal that these myopathies be termed "desminopathies." However, it has recently been shown that the sarcoplasmic masses comprise two types. In one, components of degenerate myofibrils accumulate as hyaline structures. These hyaline lesions show variable desmin immunoreactivity and also increased expression of actin, alpha-actinin, and various myosins. In the other, there is myofibril destruction associated with Z-disc remnants. These nonhyaline lesions are depleted of actin, alpha-actinin, and myosin but show strong immunoreactivity for desmin. Myofibrillar myopathy with abnormal foci of desmin positivity is a more satisfactory term, use of which avoids much of the confusion in this category of congenital myopathy. The gene for human desmin has been assigned to chromosome 2q35. Knockout of the desmin gene in a mouse model results in a myopathic syndrome in these animals. However, to date there is no evidence for linkage of any of the myofibrillar myopathies to defects in the desmin gene. It is likely that desmin accumulation is a secondary event precipitated by a primary myofibrillar disease process, the nature of which is as yet undetermined. Involvement of distal musculature and cardiac muscle may be present in some of the myofibrillar myopathies and intestinal smooth muscle involvement has also been described.

6. Myopathy with Unusual Inclusions

A variety of congenital myopathies, in which electron microscopy demonstrates unusual inclusions, have been described. These must not be confused with inclusion body myositis (IBM), hence the term "myopathy with unusual inclusions." Little is known of the cause(s) of this group of muscle diseases. Nearly all descriptions are based on isolated case reports with no large series published. Fingerprint bodies are located beneath the sarcolemmal membranes and although these may also be observed in MyD and in some inflammatory myopathies, they have been reported in association with a slowly progressive myopathy characterized by type 1 fiber hypotrophy. In reducing body myopathy, the diagnostic inclusions may be seen as pink sarcoplasmic masses on the H&E stain with strong positive reactions for menadione-linked α-glycerophosphate-dehydrogenase. On ultrastructural examination the bodies consist of dense granules and filaments with variable amounts of glycogen and may be immunopositive for desmin. In some reports it is difficult to differentiate between these inclusions and the myofibrillar inclusions described above. A fatal familial myopathy with reducing bodies has been described. Tubular aggregates are dense basophilic subsarcolemmal areas that stain positively for NADH and consist of double-walled parallel strictures sharply demarcated from adjacent myofibrils. They originate in the sarcoplasmic reticulum. Heat shock protein may be expressed in the tubular aggregates. They are not specific and have been described in partial cytochrome-c-oxidase deficiency, chronic progressive external ophthalmoplegia and myalgia, hypokalemic periodic paralysis, and in a familial limb-girdle myasthenic syndrome. However, three relatively well-characterized neuromuscular syndromes are described in which tubular aggregates are a dominant histological feature and include a congenital myasthenic syndrome, exertional myalgia with cramps, and a slowly progressive myopathy that may have a limb-girdle distribution and may show dominant inheritance.

G. Mitochondrial Myopathies

Many of the theoretical and practical aspects of mitochondrial disease have been reviewed in detail in Chapter 9. This brief section serves to illustrate the various investigations that should be carried out on a muscle biopsy in which mitochondrial disease is suspected. The biopsy may be obtained from a patient with a systemic metabolic disorder of possible mitochondrial origin or from a patient with obvious muscle disease. In either case it is necessary to carry out the full range of mitochondrial investigations, including DNA analysis. Frozen muscle tissue should always be retained on such patients. Preliminary investigations are directed at demonstrating mitochondrial proliferation using the Gomori trichrome stain and electron microscopy (EM). This must be supplemented with cytochrome oxidase (COX) and succinic dehydrogenase (SDH) histochemistry. Ragged red fibers (RRFs) (Fig. 18) are focal in their distribution and do not extend the entire length of any individual muscle fiber. Absence of RRFs or of EM demonstration of mitochondrial proliferation or abnormal mitochondrial morphology (Fig. 32) does not preclude mitochondrial disease. Muscle may not be clinically or morphologically affected, but may harbor mitochondrial DNA mutations or deletions. The most sensitive method for detection of mitochondrial disease in muscle is the combined COX-SDH stain. A mosaic pattern clearly indicates COX deficiency supplemented by increased SDH activity. COX is largely encoded by mtDNA whereas SDH is encoded by nuclear DNA. The nucleus attempts to compensate for COX depletion by increasing SDH transcription. There is a poor correlation between the number of COX-deficient fibers and RRFs. In general the COX^-/SDH^+ fibers outnumber the RRFs. Both mutations and deletions can cause COX deficiency. If the deletion/mutation affects COX genes, then COX depletion will be severe; less severe COX deficiency may result from mutations involving the mitochondrial tRNA genes. Normal COX activity is usual in biopsies from patients with point mutations, such as those in Leber hereditary optic neuropathy. Antibodies directed against various mtDNA encoded polypeptides are not yet available for routine diagnostic use.

In the evaluation of mitochondrial myopathies, the principal objectives are to establish the relationships between functional disturbances of mitochondria in the form of altered oxidative phosphorylation and mitochondrial respiratory chain complexes, and to establish the site of any underlying mutation in mtDNA or nuclear DNA. In the case of nuclear-encoded mutations, it may be next to impossible to determine their site at this time. Finally, the relative proportions of mutant and wild type DNA in the affected muscle or indeed in affected individual muscle fibers should be determined. All of this is difficult to achieve in most routine laboratories. In practice, the muscle biopsy as assessed in a routine laboratory provides supportive evidence for mitochondrial dysfunction in the form of a) mitochondrial proliferation as demonstrated by the Gomori trichrome stain and EM and b) mitochondrial dysfunction (COX depletion with or without increased SDH activity). Other studies such as *in situ* hybridization analysis with mtDNA probes and immunohistochemistry using

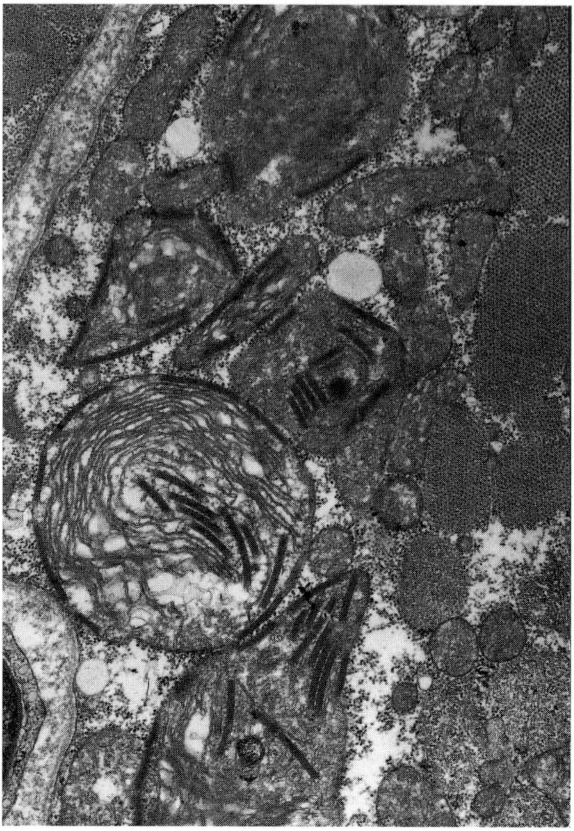

(A)

Figure 32 Mitochondrial myopathy. Various types of dysmorphic features may be seen within and among mitochondria, as illustrated in these electron micrographs. Mitochondria, often in a subsarcolemmal location, may be massively enlarged and increased in number (panel A), with curvilinear or circular cristae and electron dense rodlike structures within the mitochondria. The normal crystal pattern (panel B) may be replaced by stacks of paracrystalline electron dense structures. Rare mitochondrial abnormalities of this type may occur in otherwise "healthy" muscle, and absence of these ultrastructural changes does *not* rule out a mitochondrial myopathy.

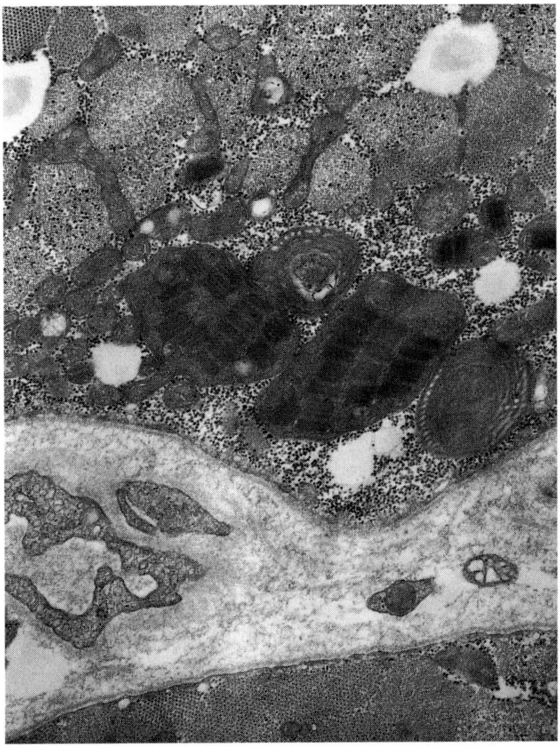

(B)

antibodies directed against mitochondrial encoded polypeptides are unlikely to be carried out in a routine laboratory. Measurements of individual respiratory chain complexes are usually performed in specialized mitochondrial or biochemistry laboratories.

H. Toxic Myopathies

From the pathologist's perspective, toxic myopathies provide diagnostic challenges mainly because so few have specific biopsy findings. The dramatic clinical features of acute rhabdomyolysis or myoglobinuria are rarely matched by the muscle biopsy appearances, which are often surprisingly bland. Correlation between elevated creatine kinase and muscle fiber necrosis is often poor. It is also surprising how frequently clinicians fail to consider a toxic or drug-related cause in patients with otherwise unexplained myopathies. Toxic or drug-induced muscle disease frequently manifests on biopsy as one of the major and relatively stereotyped patterns of muscle injury. In this section, attention will be drawn only to the more common toxic or drug-induced causes of differing patterns of muscle injury. Mechanisms of injury include a direct toxic effect on muscle; prolonged and sustained muscle fiber contraction with resultant energy deprivation; indirect injury induced by ischemia as a result of drug-induced hypotension; immobilization with resultant crush injury; or interference with the sarcoplasmic tubule system.

1. Necrosis

Widespread necrosis will lead to release of myoglobin into the serum (myoglobinemia) and ultimately, if the necrosis is sufficiently severe, into urine (myoglobinuria). The causes of myoglobinuria are numerous but the list can be narrowed to the following: sustained muscle fiber contraction, either voluntary (e.g., severe exercise) or involuntary (e.g., tetanus, status epilepticus, neuroleptic malignant syndrome, hyperpyrexia, etc.); muscle ischemia; crush injury; metabolic disorders including those of fatty acid metabolism and mitochondrial dysfunction (see Chap. 9); septicemia; and drugs or toxins. The clinical scenario will eliminate many of these conditions and a biopsy will not necessarily be carried out. In the remainder the pathologist must look carefully for evidence of lipid excess or features of mitochondrial disease. All the pathologist can do subsequently is to suggest the possibility of drug or toxic myopathy if there are no other histological pointers to the cause of the necrosis. Histological verification of myofiber necrosis in the absence of a macrophage infiltrate around the necrotic fibers is difficult to detect on H&E-stained sections, but fiber pallor is an important clue, as is loss of granular staining on the Gomori trichrome.

Alcohol toxicity is an important cause of muscle fiber necrosis. A variety of muscle changes may be seen in chronic alcohol toxicity, the most common of which is an acute necrotizing myopathy that usually first occurs during a period of particularly heavy drinking or paradoxically, following cessation of heavy alcohol intake. Muscle pain and tenderness are followed by muscle swelling and, if severe, by myoglobinuria and renal failure. The biopsy appearances depend on the stage of the disease. Pale necrotic fibers are gradually replaced by a macrophage infiltrate together with regenerative change in the form of basophilic fibers. Provided the renal complications of myoglobinuria are overcome, prospects for full functional recovery are excellent but unfortunately most patients continue to drink and experience further episodes of muscle necrosis. Electrolyte depletion, especially of potassium, may lead to a vacuolar myopathy (see below). There is no good evidence that chronic alcohol excess produces a stereotyped myopathy; most alcoholics with chronic muscle weakness have a neuropathy.

The cholesterol lowering agents, especially the fibric acid derivatives and the 3-hydroxy-3-methylglutaryl coenzyme A (HMG-CoA) inhibitors, are especially prone to induce a necrotizing myopathy (CLAM) that is considerably more likely to occur with combination therapy. Some patients taking these drugs may develop a myotonic syndrome in addition to necrotizing myopathy. The likelihood of developing a myopathy is greatly increased if there is concomitant usage of cyclosporine, for example, in heart transplant recipients. Lysosomal accumulation and muscle fiber necrosis may be present on biopsy. It is thought that some of the cholesterol-lowering agents may lead to decreased synthesis of some of the essential metabolites in the respiratory chain, especially ubiquinone.

Prolonged muscle overactivity, a result of voluntary sustained muscle contraction during vigorous exercise, may result in muscle fiber necrosis although this is usually limited to the exercised muscle. Prolonged involuntary and generalized muscle fiber contraction may occur in status epilepticus, in tetanus, and with strychnine poisoning. Drug-induced neuroleptic malignant syndrome may also lead to similar prolonged muscle contraction.

When myofiber necrosis is accompanied by an intense mixed inflammatory cell infiltrate that appears to originate from muscle fascia, one should consider the possibility of a necrotizing fascitis. Infection with group A streptococcal strains (especially M types 1 and 3) that produce a pyrogenic exotoxin may lead to a widespread toxic streptococcal shock syndrome.

2. *Lysosomal Accumulation*

In addition to suggesting the presence of an underlying inherited storage disorder, the presence of a large number of lysosomes should also lead to consideration of toxicity from one of the amphiphilic drugs. These drugs, because of their charge status, are able to interact with membrane lipids and form complexes resistant to lysosomal degradation. This category of drugs is very large but myopathy is encountered most frequently with administration of the chloroquine-based antimalarials and amiodarone and perhexiline used in the treatment of cardiac arrhythmias and angina. In addition to widespread fiber necrosis and vacuolar change, muscle biopsy will show increased acid-phosphatase reactivity combined with accumulation of large numbers of myeloid bodies and other cytoplasmic degradation products on electron microscopy. Many patients will have an associated neuropathy with consequent denervation changes on biopsy.

3. *Fiber Atrophy*

Atrophy of type 2 fibers (Fig. 23) is a characteristic feature of corticosteroid excess. Development of this steroid myopathy is dose dependent, although some patients have developed an acute quadriplegic myopathy days after administration of high doses of steroid. Virtually all patients on long-term steroid treatment will gradually develop muscle weakness. It may be very difficult to determine if increasing weakness in a patient with an inflammatory myopathy is due to acceleration of the disease process or to steroid excess. An absence of inflammatory change on biopsy does not preclude active inflammatory myopathy, but the presence of type 2 fiber atrophy is very suggestive of steroid excess, provided there was no prolonged disuse prior to biopsy. Muscle protein breakdown is greatly enhanced by steroids.

4. *Inflammation*

It is always important to consider a drug-induced cause in the evaluation of an inflammatory muscle biopsy. An endomysial chronic inflammatory cell infiltrate may be seen with a variety of drugs, including D-penicillamine, penicillin, sulfonamides, cimetidine, and procaineamide. Eosinophils may be present. When eosinophils are dominant, the eosinophilia–myalgia syndrome (EMS) should be considered. This unusual disorder, which was initially thought to be a variant of eosinophilic fasciitis, was subsequently considered to have arisen as a result of ingestion of a contaminant of L-tryptophan (LT) found in certain health foods. More recently, doubt has been cast on the validity of the epidemiological studies that linked EMS and LT. Nevertheless there is a distinct clinicopathological syndrome characterized by muscle pain, weakness, and scleroderma-like changes in skin and soft tissues with an inflammatory infiltrate in fascia and adjacent muscle in which a history of exposure to LT should be sought. A peripheral and tissue eosinophilia is usually present. A sensorimotor neuropathy may also occur. None of the immunological features of Churg-Strauss syndrome or polyarteritis nodosa are present.

5. *Mitochondrial Proliferation*

Long-term zidovudine (AZT) therapy in patients with AIDS has been shown to be associated with a variety of neuromuscular symptoms, but particularly with painful proximal weakness, wasting, and elevated creatine kinase levels. The condition usually improves after withdrawal of the drug. Muscle biopsy demonstrates ragged red fibers, proliferation and abnormal enlargement of mitochondria (often with abnormal cristae), and the appearance of electrondense structures in the mitochondrial matrix. In severe cases there may be myofiber necrosis. Depletion of mitochondrial DNA may be present and there is usually a reduction in the activity of several mitochondrial respiratory chain enzymes. As a result of respiratory chain inhibition there may be an accumulation of fat in the muscle. As many as 20% of patients taking AZT for 6 months (or more) will have symptomatic muscle disease. AZT is one of a group of antiviral nucleoside analogues that should show selective interference with viral DNA replication but which, in high doses over an extended period of time, may inhibit cellular and mitochondrial DNA polymerase. Involvement of peripheral nerve as well as other organs including heart and liver has been reported.

6. *Myosin-Deficient Myopathy with Z-Band Disruption.*

It is becoming increasingly common to receive muscle biopsies from patients who experience weakness in the critical care setting. Many of these patients will have prior subclinical neuromuscular disease that manifests itself when the extra demands of independent respiration are placed on them. Critical care polyneuropathy is well characterized and relatively easy to differentiate from Guillain-Barré syndrome. The recognition of persistent neuromuscular blockade secondary to pancuronium and vancuronium is usually obvious. Some patients with weakness in the critical care setting have a myopathy that may be severe and necrotizing. Muscle fiber necrosis may occur in up to 50% of patients in a critical care unit. A multiplicity of factors may be responsible for the widespread muscle fiber necrosis including steroids, infection, and antibiotics. In this respect the myopathy does not differ from the "neuropathy of critical care." Type 2 fiber atrophy coupled with loss of myosin ATP-ase staining as well as electron microscopic demonstration of loss of myosin thick filaments is said to be characteristic.

7. *Vacuoles*

The presence of centrally located nonrimmed vacuoles containing variable amounts of pale staining material always raises the possibility of hypokalemia. In addition to the hypokalemia associated with various forms of familial periodic paralysis, hypokalemia of sufficient severity to cause muscle weakness and myopathic changes may occur following treatment with or ingestion of licorice-containing drugs, thiazide diuretics, alcohol excess, and barium or lithium. Weakness in the nonperiodic forms is usually proximal and painless. Occasionally, the ingestion of licorice may lead to a secondary myoadenylate deaminase deficiency. Some of the amphiphilic drugs may induce vacuolar change as well the more usual necrotizing myopathy.

8. *Fibrosis*

Focal endomysial fibrosis may result from repeated intramuscular injections, but this is usually accompanied by hemosiderin deposition.

III. DENERVATION ATROPHY INCLUDING MOTOR NEURON DISEASE AND SPINAL MUSCULAR ATROPHY

A. Spinal Muscular Atrophy

This section will deal with general aspects of the more common denervating diseases affecting children and adults. A review of the causes of the "floppy baby" is well beyond the scope of this section and chapter. As already indicated, it may be exceptionally difficult to make a definitive diagnosis of denervation on biopsy, particularly in early childhood. Considerable experience is required. One of the most challenging tasks in muscle histology is to make a diagnosis of denervation in a ventilator-dependent neonate suspected of having spinal muscular atrophy (SMA), with the obvious implication for discontinuance of ventilatory support once the biopsy is considered positive for denervation. The unraveling of SMA genetics and the ability to search for mutations in the SMA gene have helped enormously to resolve the issue of accurate diagnosis in this age group.

SMA is the second most common autosomal recessive (AR) disease of childhood. Loss of anterior horn cells, through poorly understood mechanisms, leads to muscular atrophy with resultant weakness and inevitably to involvement of respiratory muscles and death. Three clinically well-characterized forms of AR-SMA have been described and all are caused by defects (usually deletions) in the survival motor neuron (SMN) gene on chromosome 5q13. Clinical types of SMA are defined by age of onset and rapidity of disease progression, with SMA-I beginning *in utero* and usually resulting in death in infancy. SMA-II has its onset between 3 and 15 months and patients survive into adolescence, while SMA-III begins from 3 to 17 years and usually has a much slower course.

The genetics of SMA is complicated. THE SMN gene resides in a duplicated area of chromosome 5, with the result that there are two copies of the SMN gene on each chromosome. These are designated as telomeric or centromeric depending on their position. Recently, a second candidate gene, termed the neuronal apoptosis inhibitory protein (NAIP) gene, was located in the same general region as the SMN gene. It is postulated that mutations in this gene lead to a failure of the normal inhibition of neuronal apoptosis. Virtually all SMA patients lack both copies of exons 7 and 8 of the $SMN_{telomeric}$ gene and as many as 50% of type I SMA patients lack both copies of the NAIP of exons 4 and 5 of the NAIP gene. The problem in attempting to make a genetic diagnosis is that normal healthy carriers may be missing part of the SMN or NAIP genes. A variety of genotypes for the SMN and NAIP genes have been used to generate probabilities for the presence of SMA when deletions are present or absent. When exon 7 of the $SMN_{telomeric}$ is deleted, the probability of SMA being present is greater than 98% but care should be taken to establish norms for individual populations. When the $SMN_{telomeric}$ gene is intact, the probability of SMA is approximately 17 times less than the population risk.

At this time it is probably wise to carry out a muscle biopsy that can be used to support the genetic diagnosis and vice versa. The SMN gene product is as yet unknown but clearly its structure and function will be of enormous interest in trying to understand the nature of the highly selective anterior horn cell loss and formation of spinal grey matter spheroids that typify the spinal cord pathology of this condition. Dominant and X-linked forms may occur, although the X-linked form (Kennedy's syndrome) is clinically and genetically different, being late in onset and due to [CAG] expansion in the androgen receptor gene.

B. Motor Neuron Disease (Amyotrophic Lateral Sclerosis)

Both motor neuron disease (MND) and amyotrophic lateral sclerosis (ALS) are used synonymously to describe a relentlessly progressive and invariably fatal degenerative disorder of motor systems, both upper and lower (see also Chap. 8). Typically the spinal cord, brainstem, and motor cortex are involved to varying degrees in individual cases. Over 90% of cases are sporadic, with familial cases making up an increasingly larger percentage as ascertainment increases. Geographic clustering on the island of Guam and in the Kii peninsula of Japan has provided useful natural experiments to help unravel the environmental and genetic factors involved in ALS. Median age of onset is 55 years. More than 50% of patients are dead within 3 years. Clinical variants characterized by involvement of cortex, substantia nigra, cerebellum, or other systems are recognized but form a tiny minority. Diagnostic criteria have been established. The diagnosis is exclusively clinical and is based on the pattern of motor system involvement and on the exclusion of ALS/MND-like syndromes such as a compressive myelopathy (excluded using magnetic resonance imaging [MRI]); multifocal motor neuropathy with conduction block (nerve conduction studies exclude this entity); paraproteinemic motor neuropathies (serum protein electrophoresis excludes); and benign fasciculations (clinical experience excludes).

The autopsy examination in fatal cases should be thorough and include examination of upper and lower extremity proximal and distal muscles as well as intercostal and diaphragm muscles. Motor nerves should be sampled; the nerve to peroneus brevis and or the deep peroneal nerves are both easily accessible. The spinal cord together with all of the roots should be removed en bloc. It is always useful to harvest fresh frozen spinal grey matter for immunohistochemical or research studies.

The neuropathological findings at autopsy are those of profound muscle wasting with shrinkage of the ventral roots. Gross changes in the motor cortex are usually minimal. On microscopic examination there is anterior horn cell loss with gliosis and corticospinal tract wallerian degeneration in those cases with upper motor neuron involvement. Anterior horn cell loss may be very patchy and it may be useful to make longitudinal sections of the spinal grey matter to demonstrate the full extent of this loss. Residual neurons are pyknotic or, alternatively, large with pale cytoplasm. Neuronophagic neurons may be present, especially in rapidly progressive cases and in some there may be a lymphocytic inflammatory infiltrate. The rostral extent of the corticospinal tract degeneration is highly variable but may extend proximally to the cerebral peduncles and into the internal capsules. In some patients the disease may preferentially affect the cervical cord and muscles of respiration, resulting in earlier death and minimal changes outside the cervical spinal cord region. The motor cortex may show loss of large Betz cells and other large neurons. Although clinical sensory findings tend to exclude the diagnosis of ALS, it is not unusual to find involvement of the spinocerebellar tracts as well as neuronal loss in dorsal root ganglia at autopsy. Other areas of brain not typically involved in ALS should be examined very carefully in view of the established associations of MND with dementia, parkinsonism, and other conditions.

More detailed studies of the ventral horn pathology reveal striking findings including the presence of spheroids in the proximal axon. The spheroids contain phosphorylated neurofilaments and ubiquitin. Similar accumulation of axonal spheroids may be seen in the ventral grey matter of SMA patients (Fig. 33). Thus it would seem likely that cytoskeletal neurofilamentous alterations play some role in the degeneration of motor neurons. This has prompted speculation about possible alterations in one of the three neurofilament polypeptide subunits in ALS. The C-terminal region of human neurofilament heavy chain (NEFH) contains a large cluster of three repeating amino acids Lys-Ser-Pro (KSP). This is a key site for the formation of cross-links in the neurofilament

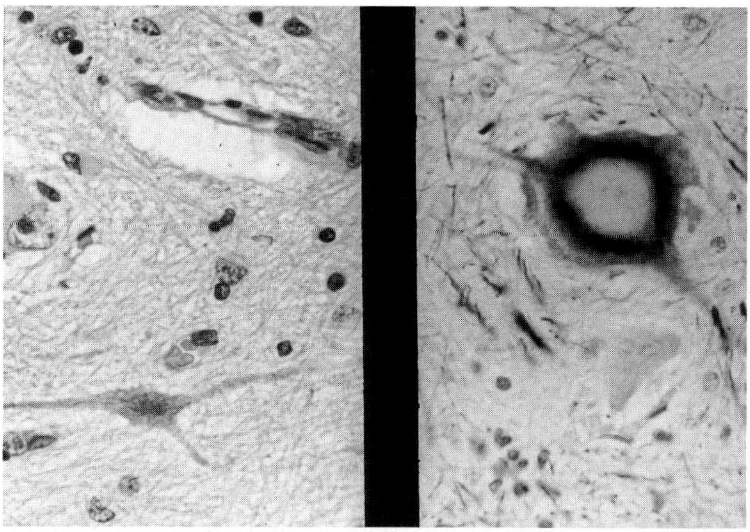

Figure 33 Spinal muscular atrophy. Spinal cord from newborn infant with spinal muscular atrophy shows small shrunken anterior horn cell (left panel) with surviving ventral motor neuron (right panel) demonstrating marked somatic distention and extensive neurofilament immunopositivity.

proteins and also for phosphorylation. Defects in either process could result in spheroid formation. There is considerable polymorphism in the encoding site for NEFH. As a first step in unraveling this process it was hypothesized that familial ALS (FALS) might be linked to mutations in the NEFH gene. However, screening of the KSP repeat region of the NEFH gene in a large number of patients with FALS, who did not have any of the other known FALS-associated gene defects (see below), failed to reveal any disease-linked mutations in the NEFH gene. It has also not been possible to demonstrate any mutations in the genes encoding the medium and light chains of neurofilament.

Research in another direction has also been of limited value in explaining the distinctive neuropathology of human ALS. About 20% of patients with FALS have mutations in the gene that encodes superoxide dismutase 1 (SOD1). The SODs, of which there are three, are a group of metalloenzymes that act as free radical scavengers by promoting the conversion (dismutation) of superoxide ions into hydrogen peroxide and oxygen. SOD1 is widely distributed in the nervous system and especially in neurons. The gene for SOD1 is located on chromosome 21q22.1. It was initially thought that the FALS-associated mutations in SOD1 caused a reduction in the SOD1 activity with consequent reduced neuronal protection. However, it was later discovered that transgenic mice expressing many of the more than 45 FALS linked mutations in the SOD1 gene demonstrate normal or increased levels of SOD1. Some transgenic mice known to express very high levels of SOD1 fail to display any of the neuropathological findings typical of ALS. Nevertheless, several lines of transgenic mice harboring certain SOD1 mutations develop ALS-like neuropathologic changes in spite of normal or elevated levels of SOD1. It seems that the mutant SOD1 is associated with gain of an adverse or toxic property, but how this gain of adverse function results in spheroid formation or indeed how it accounts for the selective vulnerability of motor neurons is as yet unknown.

In search of environmental cause(s) that can reasonably account for the observed pathology, most interest has focused on the role of excitatory amino acids (EAA) as possible mediators of neuronal injury. The Guamanian form of ALS has been linked to the ingestion of an excitatory neurotoxin present in the seeds of the *Cycas circinalis* plant. Ingestion of this toxin (β-N-methylamino-L-alanine [BMAA]) can induce spinal motor neuron degeneration in experimental primates. Application of other excitotoxic agonists with specificity for the main glutamate receptors to spinal cord in vivo results in histological changes similar to those observed in transgenic mice expressing mutant SOD1. The changes include formation of axonal swellings. As a result of this work, specific glutamate-release-blocking drugs have been introduced as a treatment for ALS, although so far with limited effect. The EAA-induced injury is probably mediated through selective glutamate receptors and new selective glutamate receptor blocking drugs seem likely to be designed and introduced for the treatment of ALS in the near future. In summary, any proposed new cause for ALS should, in part at least, explain the distinctive and highly selective neuropathology.

IV. MYASTHENIA GRAVIS AND MYASTHENIC SYNDROMES

The neuromuscular junction (NMJ) consists of the presynaptic nerve terminal, a synaptic space, and a postsynaptic receptor. Acetylcholine (ACh) is stored in synaptic vesicles located in the presynaptic nerve terminal. The synaptic space is lined by a basal lamina in which acetylcholinesterase is stored. The postsynaptic acetylcholine receptor (AChR) molecules packed into junctional folds in the muscle membrane consist of two α, one β, one δ, and one ϵ subunits. These protein subunits surround an ion channel and are arranged in a perpendicular manner in the junctional fold membrane. Released ACh crosses the synaptic space to bind with the AChR receptor complex, as a result of which there is a structural change in the AChR and the pore opens. Later the ion channel closes, the ACh is released and undergoes breakdown to choline and acetate, with the former taken up again by the presynaptic nerve terminal for resynthesis into more ACh under the influence of acetylcholinesterase. Myasthenia, characterized by weakness on exertion with fatigability, may result from disturbances in any of these steps and the various myasthenic disorders are described in the following sections.

A. Autoimmune Myasthenia Gravis

Classic myasthenia gravis fulfills all of the criteria for an autoimmune disorder: AChR antibodies are present in over 90% of patients. These complement-binding antibodies may be located at the NMJ, where ultrastructural studies demonstrate simplification of the receptor folds. AChR antibodies are the cause of passively transferred MG in neonates born to MG mothers. Removal of the AChR antibodies is associated with clinical improvement. The main immunogenic region of the AChR has been localized between residues 67 and 76 of the AChR α-subunit. That is not to say, however, that the (polyclonal) AChR antibodies are only targeted to this region of the α-subunit. In fact the AChR assay utilizes detergent-solubilized human muscle receptors that are radiolabeled with iodinated α-bungarotoxin; addition of patient serum containing AChR antibodies results in IgG-mediated immunoprecipitation that is then measured. As with most autoimmune diseases, the nature of the initial trigger for the formation of AChR antibodies is unknown. There is no convincing evidence to implicate the usual suspects such as viruses, which might share antigenic determinants with the α-subunit, in disease pathogenesis. The association between MG and thymic hyperplasia and thymoma obviously raises interesting questions about shared thymic and AChR immunogenic determinants. There is intrathymic expression of AChR (specifically the α-subunit) in thymic epithelial cells, but the level of expression is similar in normal thymuses and those removed from patients with MG. More recently two isoforms of the α-subunit have been described. They differ by the presence of a 25 amino-acid insert encoded by the P3A exon. It is possible that the differential expression of alpha subunit isoforms in MG-associated thymic tissues and normal thymus might contribute to disease pathogenesis. On the efferent side of the immune response, it has been shown that cultured thymic lymphocytes from MG patients spontaneously produce AChR antibodies and that AChR-specific T cells are present in large numbers in MG-associated thymic tissue. The interdigitating reticulum cells of the thymus are capable of antigen presentation. It thus appears that all of the components required to initiate and propagate the immune response in MG are resident in the thymus, although the initial trigger remains elusive.

B. Inherited Defects in Receptor Proteins

A variety of inherited congenital myasthenic syndromes have been reported. All are rare but have in common mutations involving the genes encoding the protein subunits in the AChR. The protein defects lead to abnormal, usually prolonged, channel opening times. These patients are often misdiagnosed as harboring a myopathy or neuropathy; the muscle biopsy may show minimal myopathic features.

C. Drugs

Existing MG can be made worse by certain drugs, while other drugs can induce an autoimmune myasthenic syndrome. Drugs such as the aminoglycosides decrease ACh release and should be avoided in MG patients. Other drugs such as quinidine and procainamide have less well-characterized deleterious effects on MG and should also be avoided. Chloroquine and penicillamine may induce an autoimmune MG syndrome with anti-AChR antibody formation.

D. Lambert–Eaton Myasthenic Syndrome

Lambert–Eaton myasthenic syndrome (LEMS) is an autoimmune presynaptic myasthenic syndrome in which antibodies are targeted against the voltage-sensitive calcium channels (VSCC) on the presynaptic nerve terminal. LEMS IgG antibodies can be demonstrated by immunoelectron microscopy bound to the VSCC channels on presynaptic nerve terminal. The antibody binding causes depletion of the VSCCs with a consequent reduction in calcium entry to the nerve terminal during activity. This in turn leads to a reduction in ACh release. About 60% of LEMS cases are paraneoplastic, with small cell carcinoma of lung the most frequent associated tumor. LEMS-associated tumors may express VSCCs. Nonparaneoplastic LEMS may be associated with other autoimmune disorders.

Muscle biopsy on a patient with MG may be relatively unrevealing or may show collections of lymphocytes only. From the pathologist's viewpoint the handling of nerve and muscle biopsies taken to include the NMJ requires considerable skill, but with a plethora of available techniques including immunoelectron, freeze fracture, transmission and confocal electron microscopy, a vast amount of information can be obtained. In reality, however, autoimmune MG and LEMS constitute over 95% of all myasthenic disorders in all ages, whereas the congenital myasthenic disorders are exceptionally rare.

V. PERIPHERAL NERVE DISEASE

Evaluation of peripheral nerve disease is complex and in general should only be undertaken by an experienced neurologist. Unfortunately, many physicians are of the belief that the simplest and most effective way to evaluate a patient with peripheral neuropathy is to obtain a nerve biopsy. Nerve biopsy in this situation may or may not yield useful diagnostic information and almost certainly will give rise to long-term discomfort for the patient. The specific indications for nerve biopsy are relatively few. Developments in molecular genetics have meant that many diagnoses can be obtained without recourse to biopsy, which is a reflection of the excellent work in peripheral neuropathy carried out by a small number of superb researchers.

It is no longer acceptable, at least in terms of patient benefit, to carry out nerve biopsy simply to confirm the presence of a neuropathy. Nerve conduction (NC) can readily provide this information. Detailed NC studies can, in most cases, indicate the fiber population affected by the disease process. NC studies will also indicate the distribution of the disease process, something a single nerve biopsy cannot achieve. NC studies, which must include measurements of the compound muscle action potential (CMAP) and the sensory nerve action potential (SNAP), provide consistent and reproducible measures of assessing peripheral nerve function over time and can be used to monitor response to treatment, something that peripheral nerve biopsy clearly cannot do.

Most physicians who are inexperienced in the evaluation of peripheral nerve disease favour an approach by which a vast number of frequently unhelpful investigations are carried out, sometimes including inappropriate nerve biopsy. In the evaluation of a patient with peripheral nerve disease, several key features of the disease process must be determined, including level of functional involvement, (motor, sensory, autonomic, or combined features); anatomical distribution (symmetrical or asymmetrical distribution; cranial nerve involvement; stocking and glove pattern or isolated individual nerve); time course (acute, subacute, relapsing–remitting, and age of onset); presence or absence of family history; other organ involvement (e.g., associated carcinoma, end organ failure, or central nervous system involvement); laboratory support (measurement of cerebrospinal fluid protein, serum antibodies, mutation detection, and possibly nerve biopsy). Having determined these features one should be in a position to tailor the investigations to those most likely to yield a pathological diagnosis. It may not be necessary to include a nerve biopsy in the patient evaluation. In many cases, it may be as important to evaluate other family members clinically.

As an alternative to nerve biopsy, skin biopsies have been used to evaluate the density of small sensory nerve fibers. In patients with purely sensory symptoms and minimal signs, it can be difficult to determine if organic disease is present (even with sensory nerve action potentials). A small full-thickness punch skin biopsy from a symptomatic area can be used to evaluate loss of intraepidermal nerve fibers. A 50 μm thick free-floating section of formalin-fixed skin is evaluated with a neuron-specific ubiquitin hydrolase (PGP 9.5) antibody and the number of immunopositive nerve terminals compared with age-matched controls. Each laboratory should establish its own panel of age-related controls.

A. Peripheral Nerve Biopsy

The threshold for nerve biopsy varies from center to center, but in general clinicians should be advised that a biopsy not be undertaken unless the laboratory is willing to use a combination of semithin (Fig. 34) 1 μm thick plastic embedded sections, electron microscopy, immunofluorescence, and (osmicated) teased fibers (Fig. 35). The use of these techniques in the evaluation of peripheral nerve requires considerable experience. The biopsy is more likely to yield a specific pathological diagnosis if the process is asymmetrical (mononeuritis multiplex) and if there is sensory loss. Nerve biopsy is also more likely to yield diagnostic information in the elderly, in whom an occult vasculitis or plasma cell dyscrasia is frequently encountered for the first time. It is extraordinary how frequently sensory nerves are biopsied in patients with purely motor symptoms and signs. Nerve biopsies should only be undertaken by surgeons experienced in the technique, willing to take the care and time required to locate the appropriate nerve, and handle it in a sensitive manner so as to reduce iatrogenic artifact. It is essential that the whole nerve be biopsied and that the biopsy include epineurium and blood vessels. Pure motor nerve biopsies can also be obtained where it is obviously advisable to take only a single fascicle. In general it is useful to have a muscle biopsy obtained coincidentally with each nerve biopsy.

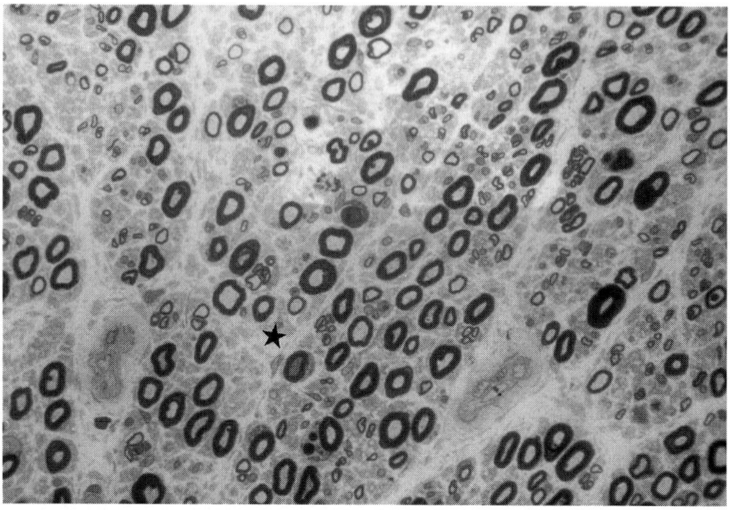

Figure 34 Sural nerve showing patchy axonal loss. Semithin plastic-embedded section of sural nerve stained with toluidine blue to demonstrate large and small myelinated fibers and patchy replacement of endoneurium by collagen (star).

The choice of nerve for biopsy is dictated by the disease distribution. The sural and superficial peroneal nerves are the two sensory nerves most frequently biopsied. Nearly all morphometric data on age-related patterns of fiber size density and distribution relates to these nerves. For motor biopsy, either the nerve to peroneus brevis or a fascicle of the deep peroneal nerve may be obtained.

The biopsied nerve is gently laid across moistened gauze and transported to the laboratory, where a 4 mm section is removed for immunofluorescence. The remainder is suspended in glutaraldehyde and used for preparation of semithin (1 μm thick) plastic sections and electron microscopy, teased fiber preparation, conventional paraffin embedding; paraffin sections can be used to screen for amyloid or inflammation. In evaluating a nerve biopsy the plastic embedded semithin sections provide most diagnostic information. Objectives in examining the plastic sections are as follows: determination of disease presence or disease processes that may contribute to neuropathy (vasculitis, amyloidosis); assessment of fiber density, with specific reference to normal age-related controls using morphometry; characterization of the basic pathological process (i.e., primary axonal or primary demyelination); and determination of the cause of the pathological process.

To determine fiber density, an image is projected onto a digitizing tablet. Individual fibers are counted and the density expressed per mm^2. Individual

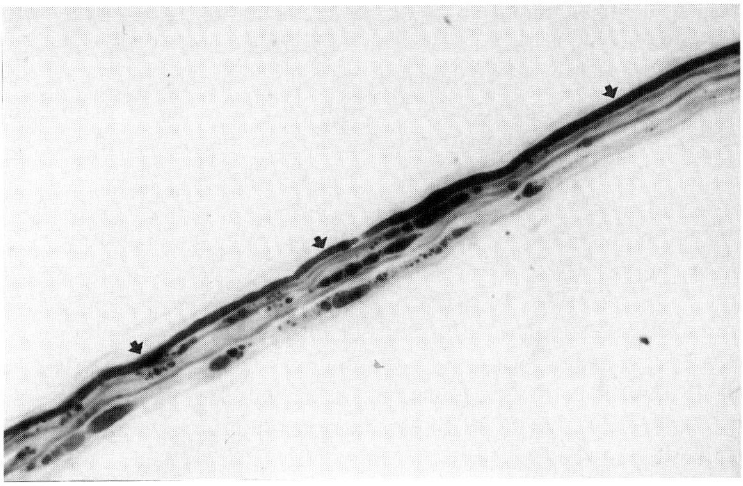

(A)

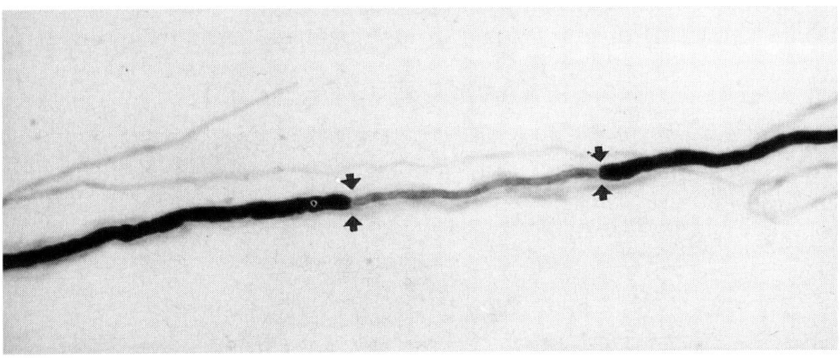

(B)

Figure 35 Osmicated teased nerve fiber preparations are useful in differentiating a neuropathy characterized by axonal damage/Wallerian degeneration from one due primarily to segmental demyelination. Panel A shows several parallel fibers demonstrating osmiophilic ovoids and loss of continuity, characteristic of Wallerian/axonal degeneration (uppermost fiber, indicated by arrows, is relatively intact). Panel B shows features of segmental demyelination. A myelinated fiber is intact but shows marked thinning of its myelin sheath between two internodes, indicated by arrows. From this static image, it is impossible to ascertain whether this "internode" is undergoing demyelination or remyelination; it is thus most accurately described in a biopsy report as representing a "hypomyelinated segment."

fiber size is traced using a cursor so as to allow calculation of fiber diameter. Myelin sheath thickness is also assessed. The data are entered into a computer. A number of imaging software programs are available and are relatively easy to operate. It is imperative that results be expressed in terms of age-related control populations established for the nerve under examination. Without controls it is easy to overcall age-related fiber loss in the elderly.

Demyelination, depending on the stage of the disease process, is characterized in the early phase by an accumulation of myelin-filled macrophages, some of which may be observed insinuating themselves between the myelin lamellae (Fig. 36). As myelin is stripped from the axon, there is a gradual appearance of naked axons devoid of myelin sheaths. As the disease progresses, axons surrounded by disproportionally thin myelin sheaths are observed. If there are repeated episodes of demyelination, onion bulb formation will be observed (Fig. 37). Ideally, teased fiber preparations must be examined for an adequate assessment of the myelination status (Fig. 35). At least 100 fibers must be assessed and data on the internode length, myelin sheath thickness, and presence or absence of myelin ovoids should optimally be obtained. These data are also analyzed using an appropriate software program. Endoneurial deposition of immunoglobulin may be detected using immunofluorescence and can be further localized to the myelin lamellae using immunoelectron microscopy.

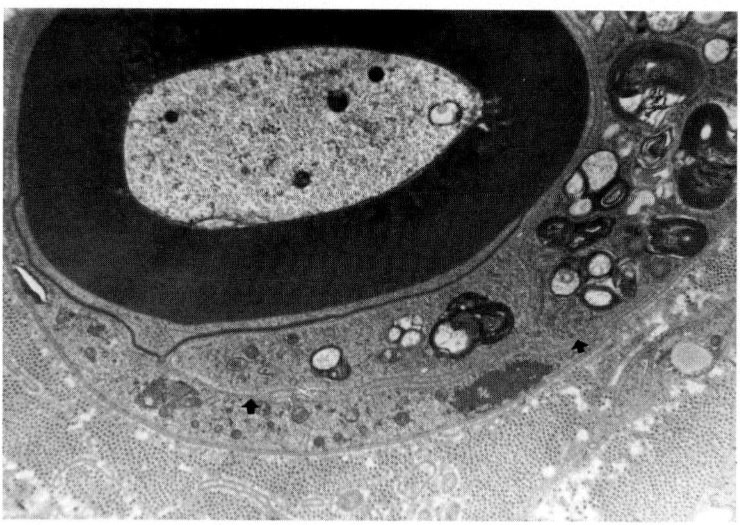

Figure 36 Inflammatory demyelinating neuropathy. Macrophage cytoplasm (arrows) extends between myelin layers with myelin degradation products present in macrophage cytoplasm in this electron micrograph.

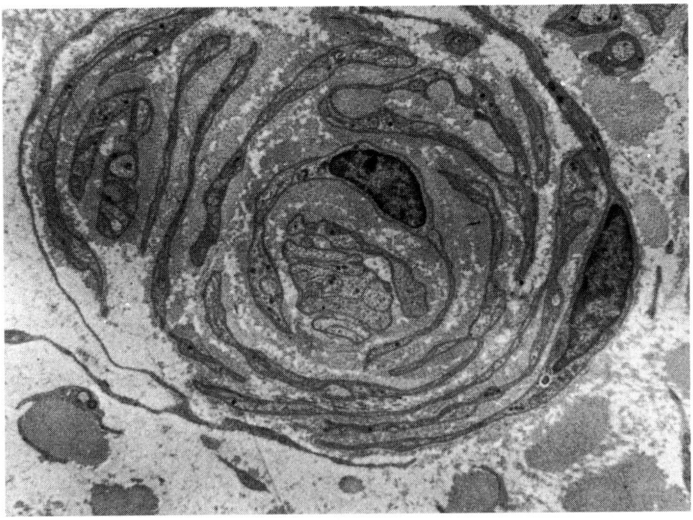

Figure 37 Chronic inflammatory demyelinating neuropathy. Electron micrograph shows extensive onion bulb formation with reduplication of Schwann cell processes, presumably a result of cycles of axonal demyelination/remyelination.

The histological appearances of an axonal neuropathy obviously depend on the timing of biopsy in relation to the evolution of the disease. A variety of changes ranging from acute Wallerian degeneration (Fig. 38) through to an end-stage nerve virtually devoid of axons and showing extensive endoneurial fibrosis may be observed. In the acute phase of an axonal neuropathy there is axonal swelling and condensation of neurofilaments and other axonal organelles. Axonal spheroid formation may be present. Secondary myelin degradation is usually conspicuous. Regeneration is characterized by clusters of small thinly myelinated axons.

B. Specific Pathological Diagnoses

The number of specific diagnoses that can be made on biopsy is small in comparison with the vast number of differing causes of peripheral neuropathy. As knowledge of the molecular biology and genetics of peripheral nerve disease increases it is possible that newly developed antibodies targeted against myelin and axonal components will become available. However, it is difficult to see a revolution in diagnostic peripheral nerve work developing on a similar scale to that occurring in muscle disease, given all of the reasons outlined above.

As with muscle biopsy interpretation, a systematic approach is advised. The epineurium is carefully evaluated for evidence of vasculitis. In peripheral

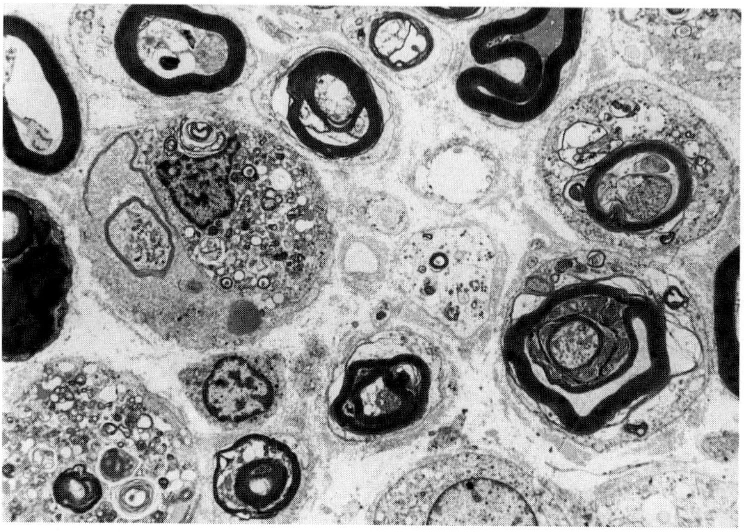

Figure 38 Wallerian degeneration. Varying degrees of axonal disintegration with accumulation of myelin debris (electron micrograph).

nerve, vasculitis may be extremely patchy and range from a few perivascular lymphocytes to frank fibrinoid necrosis of a vessel wall, although it is rare to see the latter. Rarely can a conclusion be drawn about the presence or absence of a vasculitis if the biopsy does not include epineurium. Once vasculitis is detected, immunofluorescence is essential to characterize any antibodies or immune complexes present. An extensive eosinophilic infiltrate should raise the possibility of Churg-Strauss disease. Other vascular changes include those seen in cerebral/autosomal dominant arteriopathy with subcortical infarcts and leukoencephalopathy (CADASIL), where the epineural vessel wall cells are swollen and contain granular osmiophilic material. Hyaline thickening may be seen in diabetes but biopsy is obviously not required to make a diagnosis of diabetic neuropathy. Amyloid deposits may be located either in vessels or within the perineurium or endoneurium. Multiple sections should be examined since amyloid deposition is typically focal. In some patients with genetically proven hereditary amyloid neuropathy, there may be no visible amyloid (Fig. 39) in the nerve biopsy. Immunohistochemistry is required to subtype the various amyloids (Table 4). Inflammation may be present in the epineurium without involvement of blood vessels. A granulomatous epineural inflammatory process should raise the possibility of sarcoidosis or (in the appropriate geographic region) leprosy. Lymphomatous infiltration may also be seen on nerve biopsy.

The perineurium functions to provide mechanical support to the nerve and to prevent unwanted diffusion into or out of the endoneurial compartment. It may show inflammatory cell infiltration in a necrotizing vasculitis or when involved by sarcoidosis. Isolated perineuritis may occur in the absence of any other pathology and specifically in the absence of vasculitis, and has been reported in association with a mononeuritis multiplex. The most common pathological response of the perineurium is thickening due to increased connective tissue, a common finding in most long-standing axonal neuropathies. Perineural thickening is also a feature of neurofibromatosis.

The endoneurium comprises the connective tissue elements within the fascicle in which the individual axons are located. Both collagen and poorly staining granular material are present. Fibroblasts are the dominant cell type, although rare macrophages may occasionally be present without any associated pathology. Endoneurial edema is a common response to a breakdown in the blood–nerve barrier or when there is increased deposition of large molecules such as galactose within the endoneurium. A hyperosmolar state is induced and water flows along the osmotic gradient, causing nerve swelling. The easiest way to recognize endoneurial edema is by a widening of the subperineurial space. Endoneurial edema increases the endoneurial fluid pressure and may, if prolonged, lead to further nerve injury by compression. Accumulation of endoneurial macrophages may be present in acute Wallerian degeneration and in demyelination. Lymphocytes may be present in inflammatory demyelinating neuropathies. Endoneurial fibrosis is a nonspecific finding in most long-standing neuropathies.

Schwann cells have a limited repertoire of reactions to injury, the most characteristic of which is proliferation and the production of cytoplasmic extensions in an attempt to form new myelin. Both axonal injury and primary demyelination will stimulate Schwann cell proliferation. Repeated episodes of demyelination lead to layers of Schwann cell cytoplasm wrapping themselves around naked axons to form onion bulbs (Fig. 37). Lysosomal storage products may accumulate within Schwann cell cytoplasm (see Chap. 9) but should not be confused with the π or μ granules of Reich (Fig. 40). Rare neuropathies may be attributed to mitochondrial disease, although it is very unusual to find Schwann's cell mitochondrial proliferation in this situation. Toxic drug-related inclusions similar to those seen in the drug-induced toxic myopathies may also be present in Schwann's cells. Having assessed axonal density and degree of myelination, it is useful to check for axonal swelling or spheroid formation. Axonal spheroids may be found in some toxic neuropathies (iminodipropionitrile and n-hexane), in vitamin E and alpha-N-acetylgalactosaminidase deficiency, and in Niemann-Pick disease type II. Widening of the myelin lamellae (Fig. 41) was originally thought to be a diagnostic feature of paraproteinemic neuropathies, but has also been described in Guillain-Barré syndrome.

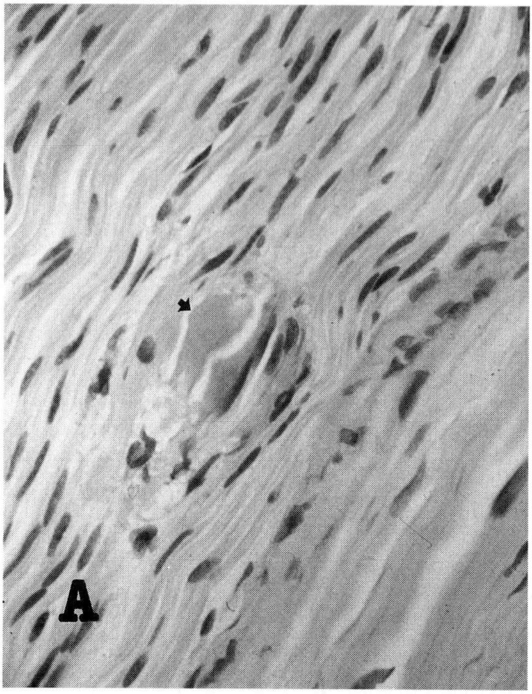

Figure 39 Amyloid neuropathy. A. Longitudinal section of peripheral nerve stained with Congo red to reveal globular mass of amyloid (arrow) that exhibits apple green birefringence on examination with polarized light (B).

"Sausage-like" swellings of myelin referred to by the term "tomaculous neuropathy" are characteristic of hereditary neuropathy with propensity for pressure palsies (HNPP). These can only be properly assessed on teased fiber preparations.

Three areas of peripheral nerve pathology have been selected for particular mention: amyloid neuropathy, hereditary sensorimotor neuropathies, and immune-mediated neuropathies, on the basis that there has been significant progress in characterizing these neuropathies over the last 3-5 years.

1. Amyloid Neuropathy

The amyloid neuropathies have benefited enormously from the explosion of knowledge in neurogenetics. Over 30 different genetic forms of amyloid neuropathy have been described. Although we still have a poor understanding of the mechanisms of amyloid-induced nerve injury, it is only a matter of time

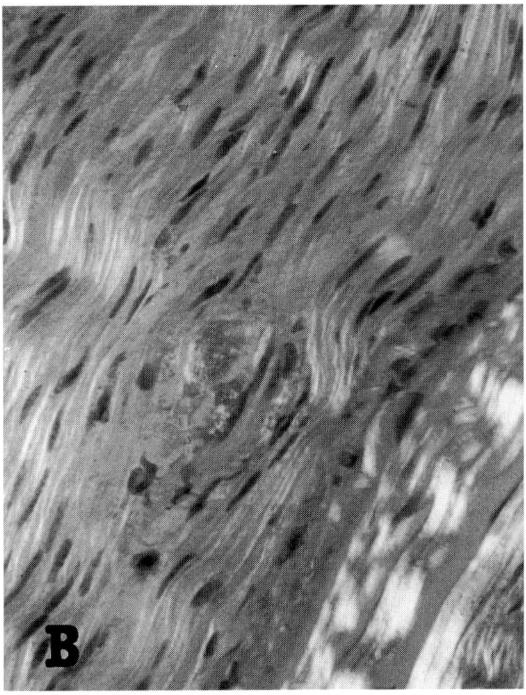

before transgenic animal models provide the answers to this question as they are now so eloquently doing in the "amyloid dementias." Table 4 lists the salient features of the amyloid neuropathies.

2. *Hereditary Motor and Sensory Neuropathies*

The complexity of the nodes of Ranvier and paranodal regions is evidenced by the discovery of an increasing number of molecules that appear to be selectively localized to different parts of the nodes and that are essential for the proper functioning and stability of nodes. There are also important biochemical differences between peripheral and central myelin. Abnormalities in some of these molecules may play a role in two major categories of peripheral nerve disease: the hereditary–sensorimotor neuropathies and the dysimmune neuropathies. The confusing terminology used in the descriptions of the hereditary–sensorimotor neuropathies (HMSN) is at last being replaced by a terminology firmly grounded in the molecular genetics and biochemistry of peripheral nerve myelin and axonal components. Both HMSN and Charcot-Marie-Tooth eponyms are in current use but the subsequent numerical designation into types I or II is the same. The various hereditary neuropathies classified according to protein abnormality are summarized in Table 5.

Table 4 Amyloid Neuropathies

Protein	Gene	Mutations	Phenotype	Pathology	Other aspects
Familial					
Transthyretin (TTR) 127 amino acid; β-pleated structure, produced mainly in liver	Single copy gene 18q11.2–q12.1 four exons	At least 30 point mutations described, mainly in exons 2 & 3. Autosomal/dominant inheritance with variable penetrance	Portuguese form (Met 30 substitution) and Irish–Appalachian form (Ala 60 substitution) plus multiple other ethnic types	Progressive loss of small fibers and later loss of large fibers; amyloid deposited in any area of nerve; amyloid subtype confirmed in tissue with immunohistochemistry	Liver transplant may arrest progress. Mechanism of nerve injury not determined. Cardiomyopathy often fatal. Severe autonomic involvement. Various TTR assays available
Apolipoprotein A-1	Chromosome 11	Gly→Arg 26	Iowa form	No specific features	
Gelsolin, an actin-modulating protein that exists in both secretory and intracellular forms	Single gene on chromosome 9 encodes both forms	G-to-A mutation at codon 187 resulting in substitution of asparagine for aspartic acid at position 15	Mainly Finnish but Dutch, Irish–American families also. Lattice corneal dystrophy and progressive cranial neuropathy		

Acquired				May have plasma cell dyscrasia with malignant paraproteinemia or "monoclonal gammopathy of undetermined significance (MGUS)" especially IgM kappa. Liver transplant attempted for patient with MGUS and severe neuropathy
Light chains	Either a compression neuropathy (e.g., carpal tunnel) or generalized neuropathy		Immunohistochemistry demonstrates light-chain origin of amyloid	
β_2Microglobulin	Compressive neuropathy (e.g., carpal tunnel) in patients on long-term dialysis			

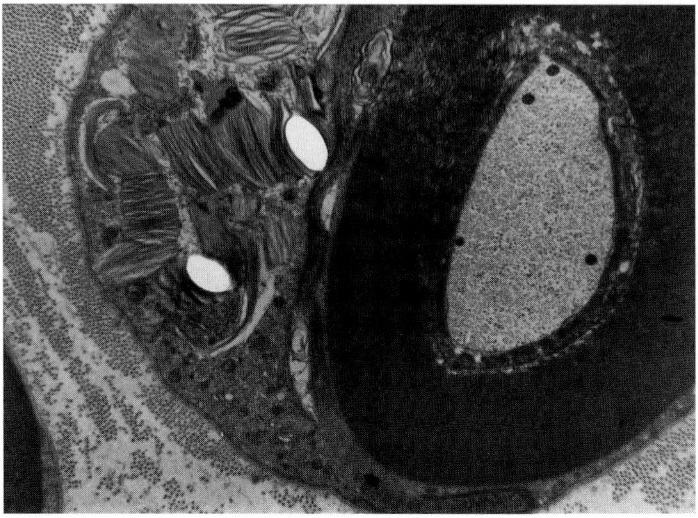

Figure 40 Sural nerve. Electron micrograph shows Reich granules, with parallel stacks of membranes, in Schwann cell cytoplasm.

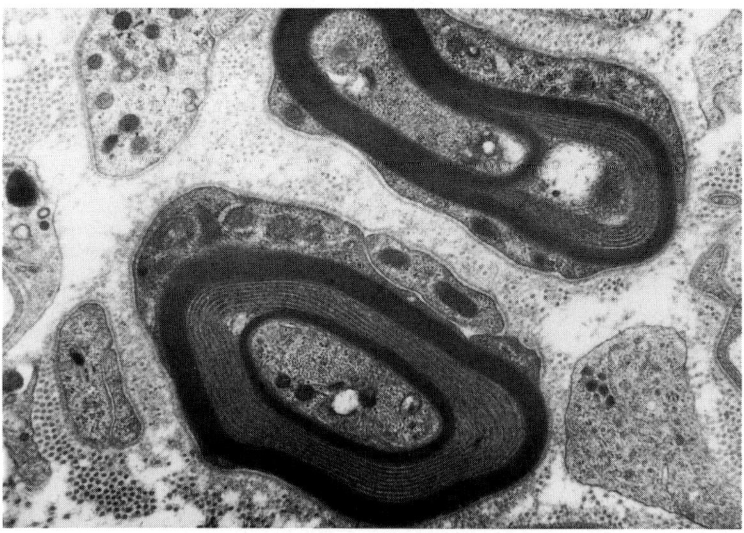

Figure 41 Dysimmune neuropathy. Splitting of myelin lamellae characteristic of immune-mediated neuropathy.

3. Dysimmune Antibody-Mediated Neuropathy

Many nodal and paranodal molecules are capable of serving as antigens for the initiation and maintenance of immune-mediated peripheral nerve injury. A number of neuropathies have been linked to the presence of circulating antibodies with varying degrees of reactivity against these myelin and neuronal/axonal antigens. The hope that these antibodies might provide insights into mechanisms of peripheral nerve disease has yet to be fulfilled. Furthermore, with one exception, most of the antibodies may be present in the absence of peripheral nerve disease. There is at present little justification for mass screening of peripheral neuropathy patients for the presence of these antibodies. Nevertheless, it is likely that current research into the role of these antibodies in peripheral nerve injury will yield important results over the next few years. Also, the demonstration of possible immune mechanisms of nerve injury opens opportunities for treatment. Salient features of these dysimmune neuropathies are summarized in Table 6.

From this brief account of peripheral nerve pathology it is apparent that few of the many diagnoses in peripheral nerve disease can be made based on biopsy. However, a genetic and immunological approach is now at least as likely as biopsy to provide important diagnostic information.

Table 5 Hereditary Motor and Sensory Neuropathies[a]

Neuropathy	Protein	Gene & locus	Mutation	Pathology
HMSN Ia (Type 1 HMSN is demyelinating with slowed nerve conduction velocities)	PMP-22: 170 kDa glycoprotein associated with PNS myelin and Schwann cells. Forms <5% of peripheral myelin protein and probably functions to regulate cell proliferation and Schwann cell–axonal adhesion	Chromosome 17p11.2-p12; dominant; A 1.7-kb recombination hotspot region lying within misaligned flanking repeats	Most patients have duplication (three copies) Rare point mutation G368→T in exon 5 of PMP22	Nodal widening or paranodal demyelination with PMP-22 immunopositive onion bulbs present. Duplication probably alters amount and distribution of PM-22 in Schwann cells
HMSN Ib (Type 1 HMSN is demyelinating with slowed nerve conduction velocities)	PO: 20 kDa protein member of immunoglobulin superfamily with extracellular, transmembrane, and cytoplasmic domains. Most abundant protein in peripheral nerve myelin (50%) and functions to maintain tight compaction of myelin.	Chromosome 1q22–q23; dominant	Point mutations in exons 2 or 3 coding for extracellular and transmembrane domains. Mutations in cytoplasmic domain cause severe disease	Demyelination with focally folded or uncompacted myelin
X-linked form of type 1	Connexin-32 functions as a gap junction protein. The gap junctions are aqueous channels that connect the cytoplasmic compartments of coupled cells to allow free movement of ions	Chromosome Xq13.1	Mutations include nonsense, missense mutations, deletions, and insertions. Missense mutations show a mild clinical phenotype whereas all nonsense mutations and deletions show severe phenotypes	

Hereditary liability to pressure palsies (HNPP)	PMP-22	Chromosome 17p11.2-p12	Deletion involving the identical 1.5Mb region to that duplicated in HMSN IA	Tomaculous neuropathy with underexpression of PMP-22-mRNA in sural nerve and rare tomaculous fibers show patchy staining of the compact myelin with monoclonal antibody against PMP-22
HMSN III (Déjerine-Sottas):	PMP-22 and PO	Genetically heterogeneous	Mutations in PMP-22 (Ser72Trp, Ser76lle and Leu80Pro) and P0 genes (Ile134Thr in exon 3, and a complex rearrangement in exon 4 genes)	Grossly enlarged nerves; very thin or no myelin sheaths, Schwann cell hyperplasia and onion bulb formation, extensive endoneurial fibrosis, and later axon loss
HMSN IVA	Not yet determined	8q11-21.1		Slow motor nerve conduction velocity (MCV). Nerve biopsy shows severe hypomyelination with basal lamina onion bulbs and no myelin outfolding
HMSN IIa (Primary axonal neuropathy with probable neuronal involvement). Normal conduction velocities	Not yet determined	Heterogeneous with chromosome 1p35p36 designated as minor locus only. Dominant		No onion bulbs, loss of large myelinated fibers; axonal atrophy and degeneration. Depletion of spinal motor and dorsal ganglia sensory neurons at autopsy
IIB (as in IIa)	Not yet determined	Chromosome 3q; dominant		

[a]Listing includes only those for which a gene locus is known.

Table 6 Dysimmune Neuropathies

Antigen	Antibody	Disease	Pathology
GM1 Ganglioside located at node of Ranvier	Low-affinity polyclonal IgM; monoclonal in 10–15%. IgG antibodies in <1% but frequency dictated by assay type. Antibody binding is strongly influenced by the lipid environment of GM1 ganglioside	Multifocal motor neuropathy (MMN) MMN accounts for approx. 3% of all motor syndromes	Motor conduction block. Minimal demyelination on sural nerve biopsy. Antibodies may alter potassium channel status at node of Ranvier. Focal demyelination at site of block (few morphological studies)
GM1, GD1a Ganglioside. *Campylobacter jejuni* shares saccharides with GM1 and GD1a. GD1a is present in the axolemma and exposed at the node of Ranvier	Polyclonal IgG or IgM antibody but of doubtful significance in Guillain-Barré syndrome (GBS), with only about 12% of GBS patients having high anti-GD1A antibodies	Guillain-Barré syndrome	Motor axonal form of GBS rather than usual mixed form. Antibodies deposited at axolemma
GQ1b Ganglioside (sphingoglycolipid). GQ1b epitopes are found on *Campylobacter jejuni*	Polyclonal IgG present in all MFS patients. Antibodies localize to cranial nerves 3, 4, 6	Miller-Fisher syndrome (MFS)	Triad of ophthalmoplegia, ataxia, and areflexia. Autopsy study demonstrated areas of subacute inflammatory necrosis, rostral brainstem tectum and tegmentum

MAG Glycoprotein that makes up <1% all PNS proteins and functions to maintain compaction of myelin. Role in Schwann cell–axonal interactions	IgMk *m*onoclonal *g*ammopathy of *u*ndetermined *s*ignificance (MGUS) Other MGUS of IgG or IgA type do not show anti-MAG reactivity. Role of antibody in causing progression of demyelination unknown	Slowly progressive, distal, symmetrical, sensorimotor neuropathy	Deposits of anti-MAG IgM in the periaxonal regions of the fibers; myelin lamellae split with IgM localized between lamellae
Hu 35–40 kDa RNA-binding proteins	Polyclonal IgG anti-neuronal nuclear antibody (ANNA type 1)	Paraneoplastic sensory neuronopathy	Small cell carcinoma of bronchus, dorsal ganglionitis; involvement of myenteric plexus and encephalomyelitis
Sulfatide Sphingolipid; major acidic glycosphingolipid in peripheral nerve myelin	IgG or IgM class	Chronic sensory neuropathy, very rare cause. 8% of chronic inflammatory demyelinating neuropathy patients have antisulfatide antibodies	

REFERENCES

1. Anderson LVB. Optimized protein diagnosis in the autosomal recessive limb-girdle muscular dystrophies. Neuromusc Disord 1996; 6:443–446.
2. Andreetta F, Tritschler H-J, Schon EA, DiMauro S, Bonilla E. Localization of mitochondrial DNA in normal and pathological muscle using immunological probes: a new approach to the study of mitochondrial myopathies. J Neurol Sci. 1991; 105:88–92.
3. Baeta AM, Figarella-Branger D, Bille-Turc F, Lepidi H, Pellissier JF. Familial desmin myopathies and cytoplasmic body myopathies. Acta Neuropathol 1996; 92:499–510.
4. Bodensteiner JB. Congenital myopathies. Muscle Nerve 1994; 17:131–144.
5. Bushby KMD, Beckmann JS. The limb-girdle muscular dystrophies—proposal for a new nomenclature. 30th and 31st ENMC International Workshops, Naarden, The Netherlands. Neuromusc Disord 1995; 5:337–343.
6. Campbell KP. Adhalin gene mutations and autosomal recessive limb-girdle muscular dystrophy. Ann Neurol 1995; 38:353–4.
7. Carpenter S. Inclusion body myositis, a review. J Neuropathol Exp Neurol 1996; 55:1105–1114.
8. Carpenter S, Karpati G. The pathological diagnosis of specific inflammatory myopathies. Brain Pathol 1992; 2:13–19.
9. Ceuterick C, Martin J-J. Sporadic early adult-onset distal myopathy with rimmed vacuoles: immunohistochemistry and electron microscopy. J Neurol Sci 1996; 139:190–196.
10. Comi GP, Prelle A, Bresolin N, Moggio M, Bardoni A, Gallanti A, et al. Clinical variability in Becker muscular dystrophy. Genetic, biochemical and immunohistochemical correlates. Brain 1994; 117:1–14.
11. Dalakas MC. Polymyositis, dermatomyositis and inclusion-body myositis. N Engl J Med 1991;325:1487–1498.
12. Dalakas MC, Sivakumar K. The immunopathologic and inflammatory differences between dermatomyositis, polymyositis and sporadic inclusion body myositis. Curr Opin Neurol 1996; 9:235–239.
13. De-Bleecker JL, Engel AG, Ertl BB. Myofibrillar myopathy with abnormal foci of desmin positivity. II. Immunocytochemical analysis reveals accumulation of multiple other proteins. J Neuropathol Exp Neurol 1996; 55:563–577.
14. Deisenhammer F, Keir G, Pfausler B, Thompson EJ. Affinity of anti-GM antibodies in Guillain-Barre syndrome patients. J Neuroimmunol. 1996; 66:85–93.
15. De Pinieux G, Chariot P, Ammi-Said M, Louarn F, Lejonc JL, Astier A, et al. Lipid-lowering drugs and mitochondrial function: effects of HMG-CoA reductase inhibitors on serum ubiquinone and blood lactate/pyruvate ratio. Br J Clin Pharmacol 1996; 42:333–337.
16. Devriendt K, Lammens M, Schollen E, Van-Hole C, Dom R, Devlieger H, et al. Clinical and molecular genetic features of congenital spinal muscular atrophy. Ann Neurol 1996; 40:731–738.

17. Dubowitz V. 22nd ENMC sponsored workshop on congenital muscular dystrophy, Baarn, The Netherlands. Neuromusc Disord 1994; 4:75–81.
18. Durham HD, Roy J, Dong L, Figlewicz DA. Aggregation of mutant Cu/Zn superoxide dismutase proteins in a culture model of ALS. J Neuropathol Exp Neurol 1997; 56:523–530.
19. Dyck PJ, Giannini C. Pathologic alterations in the diabetic neuropathies of humans: a review. J Neuropathol Exp Neurol 1996; 55:1181–1193.
20. Dyck PJ, Thomas PK. Peripheral Neuropathy. 3rd ed. Philadelphia: W B Saunders, 1993.
21. Engel AG, Franzini-Armstrong C. Myology. 2nd ed. Vols. I, II. New York: McGraw-Hill, 1994.
22. Farrell M, O'Connell S, Burke M, Droogan O, Brett F. Combined cytochrome oxidase (cox) and succinic dehydrogenase (sdh) muscle histochemistry in the evaluation of suspected mitochondrial disease. J Neuropathol Exp Neurol 1997; 56:619.
23. Feldman BM, Reichlin M, Laxer RM, Targott IN, Stein LD, Silverman ED. Clinical significance of specific autoantibodies in juvenile dermatomyositis. J Rheumatol 1996; 23:1794–1797.
24. Goebel HH. Congenital myopathies. Semin Pediatr Neurol. 1996; 3:152–161.
25. Gregson NA, Rees JH, Hughes RAC. Reactivity of serum IgG anti-GM1 ganglioside antibodies with the lipopolysaccharide fractions of *Campylobacter jejuni* isolates from patients with Guillain-Barré syndrome (GBS). J Neuroimmunol 1997; 73:28–36.
26. Harding AE. From the syndrome of Charcot, Marie and Tooth to disorders of peripheral myelin proteins. Brain 1995; 118:809–818.
27. Hawke SH, Davies L, Pamphlett R, Guo Y-P, Pollard JD, McLeod JG, Vasculitic neuropathy. A clinical and pathological study. Brain 1991; 114:2175–2190.
28. Heffner RR Jr. Inflammatory myopathies. A review. J Neuropathol Exp Neurol 1993; 52:339–350.
29. Hoffman EP. Clinical and histopathological features of abnormalities of the dystrophin-based membrane cytoskeleton. Brain Pathol 1996; 6:49–61.
30. Holland NR, Stocks A, Hauer P, Cornblath DR, Griffin JW, McArthur JC. Intraepidermal nerve fiber density in patients with painful sensory neuropathy. Neurology 1997; 48:708–711.
31. Ikeuchi T, Asaka T, Saito M, Tanaka H, Higuchi S, Tanaka K, et al. Gene locus for autosomal recessive distal myopathy with rimmed vacuoles maps to choromosome 9. Ann Neurol 1997; 1:432–437.
32. Ikonomidou C, Qin YQ, Labruyere J, Olney JW. Motor neuron degeneration induced by excitotoxin agonists has features in common with those seen in the SOD-1 transgenic mouse model of amyotrophic lateral sclerosis. J Neuropathol Exp Neurol 1996; 55:211–224.
33. Jacobs JM. Morphological changes at paranodes in IgM paraproteinaemic neuropathy. Microsc Res Tech 1996; 15; 34:544–553.
34. Latov N. Pathogenesis and therapy of neuropathies associated with monoclonal gammopathies. Ann Neurol 1995; 37 Suppl 1:S32–S42.

35. Le Quintrec JS, Le Quintrec JL. Drug-induced myopathies. Baillieres Clin Rheumatol 1991; 5:21–38.
36. Leys K, Lang B, Johnston I, Newsom-Davis J. Calcium channel autoantibodies in the Lambert-Eaton myasthenic syndrome. Ann Neurol 1991; 29:307–314.
37. Ljunggren A, Duggan D, McNally E, Boylan KB, Gama CH, Kunkel LM, Hoffman EP. Primary adhalin deficiency as a cause of muscular dystrophy in patients with normal dystrophin. Ann Neurol 1995; 38:367–372.
38. Loughlin M. Muscle Biopsy, A Laboratory Investigation. 1st ed Oxford: Butterworth Heinemann, 1993.
39. MacLennan C, Beeson D, Buijs A-M, Vincent A, Newsom-Davis J. Acetylcholine receptor expression in human extraocular muscles and their susceptibility to myasthenia gravis. Ann Neurol 1997; 41:423–431.
40. Manilal S, Man Nt, Sewry CA, Morris GE. The Emery-Dreifuss muscular dystrophy protein, emerin, is a nuclear membrane protein. Hum Mol Genet 1996; 5:801–808.
41. Manley GT, Smitt PS, Dalmau J, Posner JB. Hu antigens: reactivity with Hu antibodies, tumor expression, and major immunogenic sites. Ann Neurol 1995; 38:102–110.
42. Meléndez-Vasquez C, Redford J, Choudhary PP, Gray IA, Maitland P, Gregson NA et al. Immunological investigation of chronic inflammatory demyelinating polyradiculoneuropathy. J Neuroimmunol 1997; 73:124–134.
43. Mercuri E, Pennock J, Goodwin F, Sewry C, Cowan F, Dubowitz L, et al. Sequential study of central and peripheral nervous system involvement in an infant with merosin-deficient congenital muscular dystrophy. Neuromusc Disord 1996; 6:425–429.
44. Mhiri C, Baudrimont M, Bonne G, Geny C, Degoul F, Marsac C, et al. Zidovudine myopathy: a distinctive disorder associated with mitochondrial dysfunction. Ann Neurol 1991; 29:606–614.
45. Mirabella M, Alvarez RB, Bilak M, Engel WK, Askanas V. Difference in expression of phosphorylated tau epitopes between sporadic inclusion-body myositis and hereditary inclusion-body myopathies. J Neuropathol Exp Neurol 1996; 55:774–786.
46. Mora M, Cartegni L, Di Blasi C, Barresi R, Bione S, di Barletta MR, et al. X-linked Emery-Dreifuss muscular dystrophy can be diagnosed from skin biopsy or blood sample. Ann Neurol 1997; 42:249–253.
47. Morrison KE. Advances in SMA research: review of gene deletions. Neuromusc Disord 1996; 6:397–408.
48. Nakano S, Engel AG, Waclawik AJ, Emslie-Smith AM, Busis NA. Myofibrillar myopathy with abnormal foci of desmin positivity. I. Light and electron microscopy analysis of 10 cases. J Neuropathol Exp Neurol 1996; 55:549–562.
49. Naom I, D'Alessandro M, Sewry C, Ferlini A, Topaloglu H, et al. The role of immunocytochemistry and linkage analysis in the prenatal diagnosis of merosin-deficient congenital muscular dystrophy. Hum Genet 1997; 99:535–540.
50. Naom IS, D'Alessandro M, Topaloglu H, Sewry C, Ferlini A, Helbling-Leclerc A, Guicheney P, et al. Refinement of the laminin alpha2 chain locus to human chro-

mosome 6q2 in severe and mild merosin deficient congenital muscular dystrophy. J Med Genet 1997; 34:99–104.

51. Nemni R, Fazio R, Quattrini A, Lorenzetti I, Mamoli D, Canal N. Antibodies to sulfatide and to chondroitin sulfate C in patients with chronic sensory neuropathy. J Neuroimmunol. 1993; 43:79–85.
52. O'Donovan CA, Keogan M, Staunton H, Browne O, Farrell MA. Peripheral neuropathy in Churg-Strauss syndrome associated with IgA-C3 deposits. Ann Neurol 1992; 32:411.
53. Phillips MS, Fujii J, Khanna VK, DeLeon S, Yokobata K, de Jong PJ, MacLennan DH. The structural organization of the human skeletal muscle ryanodine receptor (*RYR1*) gene. Genomics 1996; 34:24–41.
54. Quane KA, Keating KE, Healy JM, Manning BM, Krivosic-Horber R, Krivosic I. Mutation screening of the RYR1 gene in malignant hyperthermia: detection of a novel Tyr to Ser mutation in a pedigree with associated central cores. Genomics 1994; 23:236–239.
55. Ramsay DA, Zochodne DW, Robertson DM, Nag S, Ludwin SK. A syndrome of acute severe muscle necrosis in intensive care unit patients. J Neuropathol Exp Neurol 1993; 52:387–398.
56. Rappaport WD, Valente J, Hunter GC, Rance NE, Lick S, Lewis T, Neal D. Clinical utilization and complications of sural nerve biopsy. Am J Surg 1993; 166:252–256.
57. Reilly MM, Staunton H. Peripheral nerve amyloidosis. Brain Pathol 1996; 6:163–177.
58. Rouleau GA, Clark AW, Rooke K, Pramatarova A, Krizus A, Suchowersky O, et al. SOD1 mutation is associated with accumulation of neurofilaments in amyotrophic lateral sclerosis. Ann Neurol 1996; 39:128–131.
59. Ruchoux M-M, Maurage C-A. CADASIL: Cerebral autosomal dominant arteriopathy with subcortical infarcts and leukoencephalopathy. J Neuropathol Exp Neurol 1997; 56:947–964.
60. Sacanella E, Fernandez-Sola J, Cofan M, Nicolas JM, Estruch R, Antunez E, Urbano-Marquez A. Chronic alcoholic myopathy: diagnostic clues and relationship with other ethanol-related diseases. Q J Med 1995; 88:811–817.
61. Sanders DB. Lambert-Eaton myasthenic syndrome: clinical diagnosis, immune-mediated mechanisms, and update on therapies. Ann Neurol 1995; 37 Suppl 1:S63–S73.
62. Sarnat HB. Vimentin and desmin in maturing skeletal muscle and developmental myopathies. Neurology 1992; 42:1616–1624.
63. Schon EA, Hirano M, DiMauro S. Mitochondrial encephalomyopathies: clinical and molecular analysis. J Bioenerg Biomembr 1994; 26:291–299.
64. Sewry CA, Naom I, D'Alessandro M, Ferlini A, Philpot J, Mercuri E, et al. The protein defect in congenital muscular dystrophy. Biochem Soc Trans 1996; 24:281S.
65. Shimokawa M, Ishiura S, Kameda N, Yamamoto M, Sasagawa N, Saitoh N, et al. Novel isoform of myotonin protein kinase: gene product of myotonic dystrophy is localized in the sarcoplasmic reticulum of skeletal muscle. Am J Pathol 1997; 150:1285–1295.

66. Smolenicka Z, Laporte J, Hu L, Dahl N, Fitzpatrick J, Kress W, Liechti-Gallati S. X-linked myotubular myopathy: refinement of the critical gene region. Neuromusc Disord 1996; 6:275–281.
67. Somerville MJ, Hunter AG, Aubry HL, Korneluk RG, MacKenzie A, Surh LC. Clinical application of the molecular diagnosis of spinal muscular atrophy: deletions of neuronal apoptosis inhibitor protein and survival motor neuron genes. Am J Med Genet 1997; 69:159–165.
68. Spencer MJ, Tidball JG, Anderson LVB, Bushby KMD, Harris JB, Passos-Bueno MR, et al. Absence of calpain 3 in a form of limb-girdle muscular dystrophy (LGMD2A). J Neurol Sci 1997; 146:173–178.
69. Tachi N, Kozuka N, Ohya K, Chiba S, Kikuchi K. CTG repeat size and histologic findings of skeletal muscle from patients with congenital myotonic dystrophy. J Child Neurol 1996; 11:430–432.
70. Targoff IN. Autoantibodies in polymyositis. Rheum Dis Clin North Am 1992; 18:455–482.
71. Tawil R, Forrester J, Griggs RC, Mendell J, Kissel J, McDermott M. Evidence for anticipation and association of deletion size with severity in facioscapulohumeral muscular dystrophy. The FSH-DY Group. Ann Neurol 1996; 39:744–748.
72. Thomas PK, Marques W Jr, Davis MB, Sweeney MG, King RH, Bradley JL, et al. The phenotypic manifestations of chromosome 17p11.2 duplication. Brain 1997; 120:465–478.
73. Topaloglu H, Muntoni F, Dubowitz V, Sewry CJ. Expression of HLA class I antigens in skeletal muscle is a diagnostic marker in juvenile dermatomyositis. J Child Neurol 1997; 12:60–63.
74. Vainzof M, Passos-Bueno MR, Canovas M, Moreira ES, Pavanello RC, Marie SK, et al. The sarcoglycan complex in the six autosomal recessive limb-girdle muscular dystrophies. Hum Mol Genet 1996; 5:1963–1969.
75. Wallgren-Pettersson C, Laing N. 40th ENMC Sponsored International Workshop: nemaline myopathy, Naarden, The Netherlands. Neuromusc Disord 1996; 6:389–391.
76. Wallgren-Pettersson C, Thomas NST. Report on the 20th ENMC sponsored International Workshop: myotubular/centronuclear myopathy. Neuromusc Disord 1994; 4:71–74.
77. Wilhelmsen KC, Blake DM, Lynch T, Mabutas J, DeVera M, Neystat M, Bernstein M, et al. Chromosome 12-linked autosomal dominant scapuloperoneal muscular dystrophy. Ann Neurol 1996; 39:507–520.

Index

Abeta (β/A4) peptide/protein, 125, 130, 464–465, 472–473
Abscess, brain, 109, 177, 187
 causal micro-organisms, 188
 extradural, 188
 neuropathologic features, 188–193
 predisposing factors for, 187, 188
Acceleration/deceleration injury, 151, 159
Acetyl CoA, 542, 560
Acetylcholine receptors, 623
Acid maltase deficiency, 525–527
Acid phosphatase, 590, 616
Acoustic neuroma (*see* Neurilemoma)
Acquired immunodeficiency syndrome (AIDS), 173, 186
 dementia/encephalopathy, 207–208
  neuropathologic features, 210–214
Acquired lesions in developing brain, 431–449
 hemorrhages, 435–439
 infarcts, 439–446
 infections, 446–448
[Acquired lesions, in developing brain]
 toxic exposures, 448–449
Actin, 593
Actinin, 593, 608–609
Activator protein
 for GM2, 521
 for lysosomal enzymes, 513
 Sap-1, 519
Acyl-CoA dehydrogenases, 543, 550
Adenosine triphosphatase, 588–589
Adhalin, 597
Adrenal glands, in adrenoleukodystrophy (ALD), 510
Adrenoleukodystrophy (ALD), 510–512
Adrenomyeloneuropathy (AMN), 510, 512
Agenesis of the corpus callosum, 400, 564
Aging, CNS, 453–457
Aicardi syndrome, 400
Alcohol, and myopathy, 615
Alcohol-induced neurologic disorders, 560–565
Alexander disease, 557–558

Alpers-Huttenlocher syndrome, 559–560
Alpha-N-acetylgalactosaminidase, 631
Alzheimer's disease (senile dementia of Alzheimer type)
  apolipoprotein E and, 473–474
  clinicopathologic features, 458–459, 469–471
  familial (FAD), 473
  historical considerations, 458
  molecular pathogenesis, 471–474
  neuropathologic features, 459–471 (*see also* Amyloid angiopathy, cerebral)
    granulovacuolar degeneration, 461–462
    neurofibrillary tangles, 462–464
      paired helical filaments (PHFs) in, 463, 465
      tau, 463
    neuropil threads, 469
    rodlike bodies of Hirano, 468–469
    senile "neuritic" plaques, 464–466, 467
Amino acidopathies (amino acid disorders)
  galactosemia, 551–552
  homocystinuria, 552
  phenylketonuria (PKU), 551
Aminoglycosides, 624
Amiodarone, 616
Ammonia, 546, 564–565
Amphiphilic drugs, 616
Amyelia, 398 (*see also* Neural tube, defects of)
Amyloid angiopathy, cerebral (CAA) (see *also* Congophilic angiopathy, cerebral)
  and brain ischemia, 128
  angiitis with, 78
  cerebral hemorrhage with, 121, 125
  Dutch familial (HCHWA–D), 125, 472
  Icelandic familial (HCHWA-I; cystatin C amyloid angiopathy, HCCAA), 125
  pathologic features, 129
[Amyloid angiopathy, cerebral]
    evolution/progression of, 468
    immunohistochemistry, 130, 470, 471
  relationship to Alzheimer's disease (SDAT), 125, 466, 468
Amyloid, CNS
  in boxers, 164
  in inclusion body myositis, 603
Amyloid neuropathy, 631, 634–637
Amyloid precursor protein (APP), 125, 472, 473
  in inclusion body myositis, 603
Amyotrophic lateral sclerosis (ALS) (*see also* Motor neuron disease)
  familial, 621
Anencephaly, 395–398 (*see also* Neural tube, defects of)
Aneurysms
  berry/saccular, 103, 105, 106
    association with arteriovenous malformations, 128
    giant, 105, 118
    locations, 114
    pathologic features, 107, 110–113, 115, 117
    risk factors for/associated diseases, 104
  Charcot-Bouchard type, 121, 124, 128
  fusiform/atherosclerotic, 109, 110, 111
  infectious/"mycotic," 107, 109, 119
  traumatic, 111
  vein of Galen, 133, 139
Angiitis (*see also* Arteritis)
  allergic, of Churg-Strauss, 75
  hypersensitivity, 75
  primary, of CNS, 73
  small vessel, 73
  Wegener's granulomatosis, 75, 79
Angioma, venous, 130, 137
Anoxic (hypoxic)-ischemic encephalopathy
  acute, 52, 59
  chronic, 53, 56, 57

[Anoxic (hypoxic)-ischemic encephalopathy]
microscopic features, 53, 55, 58, 59
white matter ("anoxic leukoencephalopathy"), 60, 285
Anterior horn cells
involvement in Tay-Sachs disease, 521
in spinal muscular atrophy, 618
Anti-Hu antibody, 504
Anti-Jo-1, 605
Anti-Ri antibody, 504
Anti-Yo antibody, 504
Antiphospholipid antibodies, 70
Apolipoprotein A-1, 634
Apoptosis (programmed cell death, PCD), 6, 457
in Huntington's disease, 491
in spinal muscular atrophy, 619
Arachnoiditis, post-traumatic, 169
Arginase, deficiency, 549
Arginine, 546
Argininosuccinate lysate (ASL), 547
deficiency, 548
Argininosuccinate synthase (ASS), 547
deficiency, 548
Arnold-Chiari malformations, 413–417
Type I, 413–414
Type II, 414–417
Arrhinencephaly, 400
Arterial injury, 153
dissection, 166
Arterial spasm
in craniocerebral trauma, 163
in spinal cord injury, 168
Arterial territories, watershed/borderzone in, 162
Arteriopathy, HIV-associated, 69, 70, 76
Arteriosclerosis/arteriolosclerosis, cerebral, 116, 123, 124
Arteriovenous malformation (AVM), 105, 128, 130–132, 134–135
Arteritis
giant cell, 71, 73, 77
with amyloid angiopathy (CAA), 78
[Arteritis]
Takayasu's, 71, 73
temporal, 71, 73, 77
temporal artery biopsy in, 73
Arthrogryposis, 601
Arylsulfatase, 517
Aspartoacyclase, 557
Aspergillosis, 240–241
Aspirin, and Reye's syndrome, 544
Astroblastoma (*see* Astrocytomas)
Astrocytes, 3, 19–24, 434
Alzheimer type II, 23, 547, 559, 565
Bergmann type, 19
fibrillary, 19
functions of, 19
gemistocytic, 19, 100
glial fibrillary acidic protein (GFAP) in, 20, 434
origin of, 3
pilocytic, 19
protoplasmic, 19
responses to injury of, 19–24, 31
Astrocytic gliosis, 19–23
in aging, 23
anisomorphic, 22
glial fibrillary acidic protein (GFAP) in, 20
granular cytoid bodies in, 22
isomorphic, 22
Rosenthal fibers with, 22
Astrocytomas, 297, 302–323, 368
anaplastic, 299, 301, 310–311
brainstem, 313–314, 319
cerebellar, 307, 309–310
cystic, 307, 308
dedifferentiation, 310, 311
differential diagnosis, 299
gemistocytic, 310
glioblastoma multiforme, 299, 300–301
clinical features, 311
grading of, 302
gross appearance, 311–313, 314
heterogeneity, 302
histopathology, 313, 315–319
low grade, 299, 300–310

[Astrocytomas]
clinical, 302
gross appearance, 302–304
histopathology, 302, 304–306
optic nerve, 314, 320, 321
pilocytic, 300, 305, 307, 308, 368
pleomorphic xanthroastrocytoma, 320, 322
protoplasmic (*see* Astrocytomas, cystic)
spinal cord, 368
subependymal giant cell, 300, 320, 322
association with tuberous sclerosis, 320
Ataxia
in galactosemia, 551
in Leigh disease, 538
in NARP, 537
Ataxia telangiectasia, 430–431
Atheroemboli, 62, 65, 83, 85, 101
Atherosclerosis
carotid artery, 63
clinical features, 62
complicated, 66
extracranial arteries, 64
and homocystinuria, 552
intracranial arteries, 64, 68, 69
neuropathology of, 62
ATPase, 605
copper transporting protein, 558
ATP-binding transporter protein, 513
Atrophy, hippocampal, 57
Atrophy, perifascicular skeletal muscle, in dermatomyositis, 576
Autofluorescence, in ceroid lipfuscinoses, 552
Autoregulation, 51
Axonal injury, 151, 159–162
Axonal regeneration, in diffuse axonal injury, 160
Axonal spheroids (neuro-axonal spheroids)
in adrenoleukodystrophy, 512
in adrenomyeloneuropathy, 512
[Axonal spheroids (neuro-axonal spheroids)]
in diffuse axonal injury, 160
in galactosemia, 551
in spinal cord injury, 168

Betz cells, 619
Bilirubin encephalopathy (kernicterus), 448
Binswanger's subcortical leukoencephalopathy (BSL), 78, 81
Bioenergetic deficit, 529, 542
Biopsy, 296–297
examination of, 298
Biopterin, 551
Biotinidase, deficiency, 538
Blood–brain barrier, 35–36
Blood–nerve barrier, 36, 631
Bone, tumors of, 374–377
Borrelia burgdorferi, 254
Boxing, 163–164
cavum septum pellucidum in, 164
neuropathologic findings, 164
Brain edema/swelling, 157
Brain herniation
cerebellar, 37, 38, 42
subfalcine, 37, 38, 42, 43, 94, 162
transtentorial (mesial uncal), 37–42, 162
Brain injury (*see also* Craniocerebral trauma)
hypoxic-ischemic, 51–52, 162–163
acute, 52
chronic, 52
clinical features, 52
Brain weights, 395
Branched chain amino acid disorders (BCAA), 549–551
glutaric aciduria type II (GA II), 550
maple syrup urine disease (MSUD), 550
Branched chain ketoacid (BCKA), 550
Bundle of Probst, 400 (*see also* Agenesis of the corpus callosum)

CADASIL (cerebral autosomal dominant arteriopathy with subcortical infarcts and leukoencephalopathy), 78, 82, 83
Calpain, 597
Campylobacter jejuni, in dysimmune neuropathy, 640–641
Canavan disease, 556–557
Capillaries
loss, in dermatomyositis, 573
in mitochondrial disease, 534, 537
in propionic acidemia, 546
Carbamyl phosphate synthase (CPS) deficiency, 548
Carbon monoxide (CO) poisoning, 53, 56
Carcinoma, metastatic to brain, 143
Carnitine, 586
deficiency, 544
Carnitine-acylcarnitine translocase, 586
Carnitine palmitoyltransferase I (CPT I), 542, 544, 586
Carnitine palmitoyltransferase II (CPT II), 542, 544, 586
Carotid artery, traumatic dissection of, 165
Catalase, 509
Caudate nucleus in Wilson's disease, 559
Central core disease, 590
Central pontine myelinolysis, 560–562
Centronuclear myopathy, 577, 609
Ceramide, 513, 517
Cerebellar aplasia (hypoplasia), 418–422
Joubert syndrome, 419
Pontoneocerebellar aplasia, 419
Cerebellar atrophy/degeneration
in alcohol abuse, 562
in Menkes kinky hair disease, 559
paraneoplastic, 504
Cerebellum, development, 415
Cerebral aqeduct, malformations of, 422–424
Cerebral atrophy
age-related, 156
in alcohol-induced disorders, 560
[Cerebral atrophy]
in argininosuccinate synthase (ASS) deficiency, 548
in boxers, 164
in ceroid lipofuscinoses, 555
in galactosemia, 551
in glutaric acidemia, 546
in homocystinuria, 552
Cerebral autosomal dominant arteriopathy with subcortical infarcts and leukoencephalopathy (CADASIL), peripheral nerve findings in, 631
Cerebral blood flow (CBF), 51
Cerebral cortex, formation of, 394
Cerebral edema
in argininosuccinate synthase (ASS) deficiency, 548
brain herniations with, 37–43
with cerebral infarct, 94
in fatty acid defects, 543
in maple syrup urine disease (MSUD), 550
mechanisms of, 36–37
in Reye's syndrome, 544
with spinal cord injury, 168
Cerebral palsy, 449
Cerebral perfusion pressure, 162
Cerebritis, 174, 175
Cerebroside sulphate, 518
Cerebrospinal fluid (CSF), 175
in Leigh disease, 538
in meningitis, 177
post-traumatic leakage of, 151
production of, 32
Cerebrovascular disease
in AIDS, 235
risk factors for, 61, 62
Ceroid, 552–556
Ceruloplasmin, 558
Charcot-Marie-Tooth neuropathy (*see* Neuropathy, peripheral)
Cherry red spots, 517, 521
Cholesterol, 510
Cholesterol lowering agents, 615

Cholesterol sulphate, 519
Chordoma, 299, 376–377
Choroid plexus, 30–31
  carcinoma, 299, 332
  papilloma, 299, 300–301, 331–332
  xanthomatous change in, 31
Chromatolysis
  central, 5–6
  peripheral, 5
Chronic progressive external ophthalmoplegia (CPEO), 538–540
Churg-Strauss syndrome, 631
Circle of Willis, 114
Cirrhosis
  in Alpers-Huttenlocher syndrome, 559–560
  in peroxisomal disorders, 510
Citrulline, 546
Cognitive impairment
  in boxing, 164
  in diffuse axonal injury, 162
Coma
  in argininosuccinate synthase (ASS) deficiency, 548
  with diffuse axonal injury, 162
  in fatty acid defects, 544
  in Reye's syndrome, 544
Complement, 572, 606
Complexes, respiratory chain, 529 (*see also* Mitochondrial diseases, 528–542)
Conduction defects, 536, 538
Congophilic angiopathy, cerebral, 121, 125, 128, 129, 472 (*see also* Amyloid angiopathy, cerebral (CAA))
Conjunctiva, in ceroid lipofuscinoses, 552
Connexin-32, 638
Contusions, 149, 156–159
  and behavioral disturbances, 157
  brain edema and, 157
  contrecoup, 149, 156
  coup, 149, 156
  distribution, 156
  fracture, 156–157
[Contusions]
  gliding, 157
  laceration-contusion, 156
  old, 157
  and post-traumatic epilepsy, 159
Copper, 558–559
Core diseases, 607–608
Corpora amylacea, 24
Corpus callosum
  agenesis, in fetal alcohol syndrome, 564
  hemorrhage, 159
Cortical dysplasia, 411–413 (*see also* Neuronal migration disorders)
  in glutaric aciduria, type II, 550
Corticospinal tracts, in motor neuron disease, 619
Craniocerebral trauma, 147–172
  blunt force injury, 149
  classification, types, 148, 151
  clinical features, 148
  contusions, 149, 156–159
  diffuse axonal injury, 151
  etiology, 148
  incidence, 148
  nonaccidental brain injury (NAI) in childhood, 164–165
  pontomedullary transection, 165
  primary brain injury, 149
  repetitive non-coma-producing, 163
  secondary brain injury, 149
  vascular ischemia, regional, 163
Craniopharyngioma, 299, 300, 351–353
Creatine kinase (CK), 604, 614
Creutzfeldt-Jakob disease (CJD; spongiform encephalopathy), 246–247
Critical care myopathy, 617
Crystallin, alpha β-, 558
Cuproenzymes, 559
Curvilinear bodies, 555
Cycas circinalis, 622
Cyclosporine, toxicity, 290
Cystathionine β-synthase (CBS), 552
Cystatin C protein (γ trace), 125
Cysteine, 552

Cysticercosis, 252, 254
Cysts, 380, 384–388
arachnoid, in glutaric acidemia, 546
colloid, 300, 386–387
dermoid, 301, 384–386
enterogenous, 387, 388
ependymal, 387
epidermoid, 301, 384, 385
leptomeningeal, 387
pineal, 387
Rathke cleft, 386–387
Cytochrome oxidase (COX), 530, 540
Cytochrome oxidase-succinic dehydrogenase (COX-SDH), 584–585, 591, 611
Cytomegalovirus (CMV) infection
congenital, 447
opportunistic (in AIDS)
of brain, 220–222, 224
of peripheral nerve and spinal nerve roots, 225
of retina, 218

D-methylmalonyl-CoA, 546
D-penicillamine, 616
Dandy-Walker syndrome, 415–418
Deafness
in Leigh disease, 538
in mitochondrial disease, 531
in peroxisomal disorders, 510
in Wolfram syndrome, 540
Debrancher enzyme deficiency (Cori-Forbes disease) GSD-III, 527
Degeneration, of nervous system, paraneoplastic, 503–505
Degeneration, Wallerian, 10, 122, 630 (*see also* Wallerian degeneration of axons)
Delayed neuronal death, 57
Dementia (*see also* Alzheimer's disease)
in NARP, 537
pugilistica (in boxers), 163
Dementias, non-Alzheimer
corticobasal degeneration, 481–482
diffuse Lewy body disease (DLBD), 482–484
[Dementias, non-Alzheimer]
clinicopathologic features of, 482–483
relationship to Alzheimer's disease, 483
ubiquitin and, 483
fronto-temporal (FTD), 475–477, 481
associated with motor neuron disease (MND), 477
genetics, 482
Pick disease, 476–479
miscellaneous, 484–485
vascular/multi-infarct/ischemic vascular, 75, 474–475
Demyelination, CNS (*see also* Multiple sclerosis)
in adrenoleukodystrophy, 511
Demyelination, in peripheral nerve, 628
Demyelination, post-infectious/parainfectious/inflammatory (non-MS)
acute disseminated perivenous encephalomyelitis (ADPVE), 287
acute/hyperacute hemorrhagic leukoencephalitis (AHL), 286–287
Denervation
in infancy, 576–577, 589, 591
in spinal muscular atrophy, 618
Dentate nucleus
in Leigh disease, 537
in MERRF, 535
Dentatorubropallidoluysian atrophy (DRPLA), 501
Dermatan sulphate, 519
Dermatomyositis (DM), 572, 593, 605–606
Descemet's membrane, 559
Desmin, 593
and myopathy, 610
Developmental malformations of nervous system, 392–431
associated with chromosomal disorders, 427–429
associated with genetic syndromes, 429–431
disorders of brainstem development,

[Developmental malformations of nervous system]
422–424
disorders of cerebellar development, 415–422
disorders of cerebral hemisphere formation, 402–404
disorders of midline formation, 399–402
disorders of posterior fossa formation, 413–415
neural tube defects, 395–399
neuronal migration disorders, 404–413
non-neural tube disorders of spinal cord development, 423–427
primary or secondary, 392
Diabetes insipidus, in Wolfram syndrome, 540
Diabetes mellitus
in Leigh disease, 538
in Wolfram syndrome, 540
Diffuse axonal injury, 151, 159–162
Diffuse Lewy body disease (DLBD) (*see* Dementias, non-Alzheimer)
Dihydrolipoyl dehydrogenase, 550
Dihydrolipoyl transacyclase, 550
Dissection, arterial, 67, 69, 74, 75
Down's syndrome (*see* Trisomy 21)
Duret hemorrhages, 38, 40 (*see also* Hemorrhage, brainstem, secondary)
Dystonia
in central pontine myelinolysis, 561
in glutaric acidemia, 546
in Leigh disease, 537
in maple syrup urine disease (MSUD), 550
Dystroglycan, 595
Dystrophin, 594–597
Dystrophy, muscular
Becker type, 595–598
Duchenne type, 595–598
Emery-Dreifuss type, 599–600
facioscapulohumeral, 600
limb-girdle, 597–598, 611
[Dystrophy, muscular]
myotonic, 600–601
regional, 601
scapuloperoneal, 601
Dystrophy, neuroaxonal (NAD); Hallervorden-Spatz disease, 502–503

Elastin, 559
Emboli
atheromatous, 65
cardiogenic, 83, 86–88
fat, 87
iatrogenic, 130, 134–135
miscellaneous, 87, 89
platelet-fibrin, 65, 86
tumor, 87, 88
Embryological development of the nervous system, 1–3, 392–395
Emerin, 597, 600
Empyema, subdural, 187
Encephalitis, 174, 175
arbovirus, 202–204
equine, 204
Herpes simplex, 194–195
chronic, 198
neuropathologic features, 196–197, 199–200
in newborns, 198, 447
mumps, 242
Rasmussen type, associated with epilepsy, 255–257
Encephalocele (Meningoencephalocele), 399
Encephalomyelitis, paraneoplastic, 504
Encephalopathy
in alcohol-related liver disease, 564–565
in glutaric acidemia, 546
Endarterectomy, 63
Endocarditis
infective/infectious, 86
non-bacterial thrombotic (marantic) (NBTE), 69, 85
Endoneurium, 44, 631 (*see also* Peripheral nerves)
Eosinophilia myalgia syndrome, 616

Ependymal cells
  origin of, 3
  response to injury, 27, 31
  tanycytic, 26
Ependymoma, 300–301
  anaplastic, 299, 328
  clinical, 326
  differential diagnosis, 299
  gross, 326, 328
  histopathology, 327–330
  myxopapillary, 369–370
  spinal cord, 369
  subependymoma, 299, 300, 328, 330, 331
Epilepsy
  in mitochondrial disease, 531
  myoclonic with ragged-red fibers, 534–535
  post-traumatic, 159
Epineurium, 44 (*see also* Peripheral nerves)
Epstein-Barr virus, CNS infection, 201
Excitatory amino acids (EAAs)/excitotoxicity, 60, 61, 457, 622
Excitotoxic (brain) injury (*see also* Excitatory amino acids)
  in mitochondrial disease, 542
Extradural hematoma/hemorrhage (*see* Intracranial hematoma)
Extrapontine myelinolysis, 561

Fabry disease, 520
Facial bones, 151
Facial dysmorphism, 563
Fahr's disease, 82
Familial fatal insomnia (FFI), 248
Fasciitis
  eosinophilic, 617
  necrotizing, 615
Fatty acids, 542 (*see also* Lipid disorders)
Fatty acyl-CoA, 542
Ferruginization, neuronal/axonal, 101, 104
Fetal alcohol syndrome, 448–449, 563–564
Fetal myosin, 579
Fiber type disproportion, 610
Fibrinoid necrosis, microvascular, 73, 121
Fibromuscular dysplasia (FMD), 65, 67, 70, 71
Fingerprint bodies/inclusions, 555, 607
Fistula, arterio-venous, 131, 133
Flavine adenine dinucleotide, 543
Focal axonal swelling, 14)
Fractures
  facial bones, 151
  skull, 151–153
Friedreich ataxia (FA), 501
Frozen sections, 296–297
  special processing, 296
  squash preparations, 296, 319, 325, 330, 345, 350, 360, 383
  touch imprints, 296, 337, 338

GM1-ganglioside, in dysimmune neuropathy, 640
GM2-ganglioside, 521
GM2 gangliosidosis, 602
Galactocerebrosidase, 518
Galactokinase (GALK), 551
Galactose, 513, 520, 551
UDP-galactose-4-epimerase, 551
Galactose-1–phosphate-uridyltransferase (GALT), 551
Galactosemia, 551–552
alpha-Galactosidase A, 520
beta-Galactosidase, 521
Gamma-aminobutyric acid (GABA), 565
Ganglion cell tumors, 332–334 (*see also* Neurocytoma, central)
  gangliocytoma, 333
  ganglioglioma, 299, 333–334
    anaplastic, 334
    desmoplastic infantile, 334
  ganglioneuroblastoma, 334
Gangliosidoses, 521–522
  GM1-gangliosidosis, 522
  Morquio B disease, 521
  Sandhoff disease, 521
  Tay-Sachs disease, 521

Gaucher disease, 517
Gelsolin, 634
Germ cell tumors, 299, 301, 353–354
  choriocarcinoma, 299, 354
  embryonal, 299, 354
  endodermal sinus (yolk sac), 299, 354
  germinoma, 299, 354
  mixed germ cell tumor, 354
  teratoma, immature, 354
  teratoma, mature, 354
Gerstmann-Straussler-Scheinker disease (GSSD), 247–249
Gitter cells (foamy macrophages/histiocytes), 100
Glioblastoma multiforme (*see* Astrocytomas)
Gliomas, 297, 302–331 (*see also* Astrocytomas; Ependymomas; Oligodendrogliomas)
  definition, 297
  mixed, 299, 326
  nasal, 314, 320
Gliomatosis cerebri, 558
Gliosarcoma, 299, 336
Globus pallidus
  in hepatic encephalopathy, 565
  in MERRF, 535
  in methyl malonic acidemia, 546
  in Wilson's disease, 559
Glucose, 513
α-Glucosidase, 527
Glutamate, 61
Glutaric acid, 546
Glutaric aciduria
  type I (GA I), 546
  type II (GA II), 550
Glutaryl-CoA dehydrogenase (GCDH), 546
Glycogen, 525
  accumulation in myophosphorylase deficiency, 590
  assessment in skeletal muscle, 586
Glycogen storage diseases, 525–528
  acid maltase deficiency, 525–527
[Glycogen storage diseases]
  debrancher enzyme deficiency (Cori-Forbes disease) GSD–III, 527
  myophosphorylase deficiency (McArdle disease), GSD–V, 527
  phosphofructokinase deficiency (Tarui disease), GSD–VII, 528
Glycosaminoglycans (GAGs), 523
Glycosphingolipids, 520
Gomori trichrome stain, 584–585, 615
Granular ependymitis, 27
Granular osmiophilic inclusions, 552
Granulovacuolar degeneration (of Simchowicz), 17
Growth factors, in devlopment, 393
Guam, 619
Guillain-Barré syndrome (*see* Neuropathy, peripheral, immune-mediated)
Gyri/gyration, 394–395, 406–411
  disorders of, 406–411
  formation of, 394–395

Head injury (*see* Craniocerebral trauma)
Heat shock protein, 558
Hemangioblastoma, 299, 301, 335–336, 366
  association with von Hippel-Lindau syndrome, 335
  differential diagnosis, 336, 382
Hemangioma, 128, 299
  cavernous, 130, 136
Hemangiopericytoma, 366–367, 368
Hematoma (*see* Intracranial hematoma; Subdural hematoma/hemorrhage)
Hemimegalencephaly, 406–407 (*see also* Neuronal migration disorders)
Hemorrhage
  brainstem, secondary (Duret), 94
  cerebral/encephalic, 61–62, 91, 126, 128
    with cerebral amyloid angiopathy (CAA), 127
    etiology, 116

[Hemorrhage]
hypertensive, 116, 120–121
chronic, 122
with leukemia, 140, 141
lobar, 125
miscellaneous causes, 133, 134, 142
with neoplasms, 134, 143
pathologic features, 123
epi/extradural, 101
intracranial, 101
intraparenchymal, 101, 112–113, 115
intraventricular, secondary, 115, 142
perinatal (*see also* Acquired lesions in developing brain, 435–439)
in propionic acidemia, 546
subarachnoid, 102–103, 105–106, 115, 128
complications of, 104, 106
miscellaneous causes, 111
subdural, 101
traumatic, 152–156, 159, 164, 165
Heparan sulphate, 519
Hepatic encephalopathy, 564–565
Hepatomegaly
in fatty acid defects, 544
in peroxisomal disorders, 501
Hereditary motor-sensory neuropathy (HMSN), 637–639
Herniations, brain (*see* Brain herniation)
Herpesvirus infections, opportunistic, 216–222
Heteroplasmy, 529
Hexosaminidase-A, 521
Hippocampal sclerosis, 58, 444
Holoprosencephaly, 402–404
alobar, 402–403
lobar, 403–404
semilobar, 403
Homocystinuria, 552
Homoplasmy, 529
Human herpesvirus-6, 201
Human immunodeficiency virus type 1 (HIV-1), 173, 205–207
immunolocalization in brain/CNS, 213
[Human immunodeficiency virus type 1 (HIV-1)]
infection of CNS, 207–208
polioencephalopathy, 214
progressive encephalopathy in children, association with, 208
Human T-cell leukemia virus type 1 (HTLV–1), 238
HTLV–1-associated myelopathy (HAM), 238
Huntington's disease/chorea (HD/HC)
clinicopathologic features, 489–491
molecular pathogenesis and genetics, 490–491
huntingtin, 490–491
Hurler disease, 523
Hyaline bodies, 601
Hydranencephaly, 444
Hydrocephalus, 32, 423
congenital, 423
ex vacuo, 32, 56
mechanisms of, 32, 423
obstructive, 153
post-subarachnoid hemorrhage, 104
3-Hydroxy-3-methylglutaryl coenzyme A (HMG-coA), 615
Hydroxylysine, 546
Hyperammonemia, 548
Hypoglycemia
in branched chain amino acid disorders, 550
in fatty acid defects, 544
Hypokalemia, 618
Hypokalemic periodic paralysis, 600
Hyponatremia, 561
Hypoxia, 162
Hypoxic-ischemic encephalopathy (*see* Brain injury, hypoxic-ischemic)

Immunofluorescence, in peripheral nerve disease, 628, 630
Immunohistochemical stains, 299
AFP, 299
CD-31, 299, 338
CD-34, 299, 338

[Immunohistochemical stains]
- CEA, 358
- chromagranin, 299
- cytokeratin, 299, 332, 358
- desmin, 345
- EMA, 299, 354, 356, 358, 367, 370
- factor VIII, 299, 335
- GFAP, 297, 299, 317, 320, 324, 328, 332, 333, 335, 336, 344, 347, 358, 369
- HMB-45, 299
- kappa light chains, 299
- Ki-67, 802
- L-26, 299, 340
- lambda light chains, 299
- LCA, 299
- Leu–7, 299
- muscle specific actin, 345
- myelin basic protein, 372
- neurofilament, 299, 320, 333, 335, 344, 346
- PCNA, 302
- PLAP, 299
- S-100 protein, 299, 348, 354, 356, 370, 372
- of skeletal muscle, 593–594
- synaptophysin, 299, 333, 335, 344, 346, 347
- UCHL–1, 299
- vimentin, 299, 354

Immunosuppression, 174

Inborn errors of metabolism, 545–552
- branched chain amino acid (BCAA) disorders, 549–551
- organic acidemias (OAs), 545–546
- single amino acid disorders, 551–552
- urea cycle defects (UCDs), 546–549

Inclusions
- Cowdry type A, intranuclear, 200
- curvilinear bodies, 555
- fingerprint, in ceroid lipofuscinoses, 555
- in mitochondrial disease, 530
- neuronal, in dementias, 476

Inclusion bodies
- fingerprint body, 607

[Inclusion bodies]
- in inclusion body myositis, 573
- reducing body, 607
- tubulomembranous, 607

Infarcts, brainstem, 106

Infarcts, cerebral, 52, 62
- acute, 92
- after subarachnoid hemorrhage, 104
- chronic, 98
- cystic (old), 95–97, 99, 102–103
- embolic, 82
- hemorrhagic, 85, 90
- lacunar, 78, 101, 108, 109
- liquefactive necrosis, 95
- microscopic changes, 99
- middle cerebral artery (MCA) territory, 94, 101
- in mitochondrial disease, 531
- neuropathologic features, 92
- posterior cerebral artery (PCA) territory, 98, 101, 107
- subacute, 92, 93
  - "cracking" artifact in, 97
- subcortical, 78
- vertebro-basilar territory, 101
- watershed, 53, 93

Infarcts, perinatal, 439–446 (*see also* Acquired lesions in developing brain)

Infection, central nervous system
- fungal, 174
  - cryptococcosis, 216–217
  - opportunistic, in AIDS, 215–216
- granulomatous, 180
  - etiology, 181
- opportunistic
  - bacterial, in AIDS, 234
  - miscellaneous (non-AIDS-related), 238–239
  - parasitic, 223, 226
- parasitic
  - helminthic, 251
  - protozoal, 250–251, 253
- prion (slow/atypical virus), 239, 244, 246–250
- purulent/suppurative, 177

[Infection, central nervous system]
rickettsial, 252
risk factors for, 177
viral, 173, 189, 191, 195
diagnosis of, 189
enterovirus, 203
neuropathologic features of, 193–194
opportunistic, in AIDS, 215–225
Infection, opportunistic, 173, 174
in AIDS, 208, 215–234
Inflammation
in adrenoleukodystrophy, 512
in astrocytomas, 310, 311
versus lymphoma, 299, 339, 341
Intracranial hematoma (*see also* Hemorrhage)
extradural, 153–154
subdural, 154–156
traumatic, 152
subarachnoid, 152–153
Intracranial pressure, raised, 60, 162 (*see also* Cerebral edema)
Intraoperative consultation (*see* Frozen sections)
Intraventricular hemorrhage, 153 (*see also* Hemorrhage, intraventricular)
Ion channels, 600
in Lambert-Eaton syndrome, 624
Ischemia, 162
Isobutyric acid, 550
Isoleucine, 545, 549, 551
Isovaleric acid, 550

JC virus, 219
in situ hybridization for, 231

Kaposi sarcoma, 235
Kayser-Fleischer rings, 559
Kearns Sayre syndrome (KSS) (chronic progressive external oph thalmoplegia [CPEO]), 538–540
Kennedy's syndrome, 619
Kernohan's notch, 38, 41
α-Ketoacid decarboxylase, 550
α-Ketoglutarate, 547, 560
Korsakoff psychosis, 560–561
Krabbe disease, 518
Kreb's cycle, 529
Kuru, 244

L-aspartic acid, 557
L-pipecolic acid, 509
Lacerations, brain, 156
Lactic acidosis, 531
Lambert-Eaton syndrome, 624
Laminar necrosis, cortical, 52–55, 57
Laminin-associated protein (LAMA 2), 600
Leader proteins, 541, 548
Leber's hereditary optic neuropathy (LHON), 535–537
Leigh disease, 537–538, 560
Leprosy, 631
Leucine, 549, 551
Leukemia, 341
Leukodystrophy, 518–520
in comparison to other white matter diseases, 288
Leukoencephalopathy, anoxic-ischemic, 285
Leukoencephalopathy, toxic, 287, 290–291
radiation- or chemotherapy-induced, 289
Leukomalacia, 139
Leukotomy, prefrontal, 290
Lewy bodies, 17, 482–484, 486–488
Lignoceroyl co-enzyme A, 512
Lipid disorders, 542–545
Lipofuscin, 15
Lipofuscinoses, 552–556
Lipohyalinosis, microvascular, 116, 121
Lipoma, 366
Lissencephaly, 406–409
"Locked-in" syndrome, 561
Locus ceruleus, neuromelanin in, 15
Long-chain acyl-coA dehydrogenase (LCAD), 544
Lyme disease, 254

Lymphoma, central nervous system
  in AIDS, 235–237
  clinical features, 337
  differential diagnosis, 299
  gross features, 337, 338
  histopathology, 337–340
  primary versus secondary, 337
  special processing of specimens, 296, 337, 339
Lymphomatoid granulomatosis (LG), 75, 80
Lysine, 546
Lysosomal storage disorders (LSDs), 513–524
Lysosomes, 513
Lysyl oxidase, 559

Magnetic resonance imaging (MRI)
  and boxing, 163
  in Canavan's disease, 556
  in chronic ethanol abuse, 562
  in diffuse axonal injury, 162
  in galactosemia, 551
  in glutaric acidemia, 546
  in hepatic encephalopathy, 565
  in Hurler disease, 523
  in spinal cord injury, 166, 169
Major histocompatibility complexes (MHC I and II), in inflammatory myopathy, 572, 603
Malaria, 251
Malformations, vascular, CNS
  classification, 131
  neuropathologic features of, 131
Malignant hyperthermia susceptibility (MHS), 608
Mallory body, 607
Mammillary bodies, in Wernicke-Korsakoff syndrome, 560
Maple syrup urine disease (MSUD), 550
Marchiafava-Bignami disease, 284–286, 562
  relationship to CPM, MNL, 285, 286
Marinesco bodies, 16
McArdle disease, 527, 586
Medium-chain acyl CoA dehydrogenase deficiency (MCAD), 543
Medulloblastoma (*see* Primitive neuroectodermal tumors (PNET))
Megalencephaly, 405–406
  in Alexander disease, 557–558
  in Canavan's disease, 556
Melanoma, primary, 367–368 (*see also* Neoplasms, metastatic)
Melanosis, diffuse meningeal, 367
Membranous cytoplasmic bodies (MCBs)
  in Hurler disease, 524
  in Tay–Sachs disease, 521
  in Zellweger's syndrome, 511
Meningeal sarcoma, 362, 365, 366
Meninges (leptomeninges), 32–35
  arachnoid plaques in, 35
  microscopic anatomy of, 32–35
Meningioma, 299, 300–301, 355–364, 370
  clinical aspects, 355–356
  gross appearances, 355–357
  histopathology, 356–364
    angiomatous, 359, 363, 364
    atypical, 362
    en plaque, 358
    fibroblastic, 358, 361
    malignant, 362, 364, 365
    meningothelial, 357, 358, 359
    papillary, 359
    psammomatous, 358
    secretory, 358, 363
    transitional, 358
  spinal cord, 370
Meningitis, 174
  granulomatous, 174–176
    fungal, 182, 185
    tuberculous, 181, 184
  lymphocytic, 174–176, 183, 186
  purulent/suppurative, 174–176, 178, 180, 182
    causal micro-organisms, 179
    complications of, 180
Meningocele, 387, 397–399 (*see also* Neural tube, defects of)

Meningoencephalitis, 174–175
Meningoencephalocele, 387
Meningomyelocele, 387, 397–399 (*see also* Neural tube, defects of)
Menkes kinky hair disease (MKHD), 559
Mental retardation, 449
Merosin, 593
Metabolism, cerebral, 51–52
Metastasis (*see* Neoplasms, metastatic)
Methionine, 545, 552
Methyl-malonyl-coA mutase, 546
2-Methylbutyric acid, 550
3-Methylglutaconic aciduria, 540
Methylmalonic acidemia, 546
Microaneurysms, cerebral, 87 (*see also* Aneurysms, Charcot-Bouchard type)
Microangiopathy, hypertensive, 101, 116, 121, 123
Microcephaly (microencephaly), 405
  in phenylketonuria, 551
Microglia, 27–31
  microscopic anatomy of, 27–29
  responses to injury, 29
Microglial scars (microglial nodules), 29, 160, 210–211
Miller-Dieker syndrome (lissencephaly), 406–409
Miller-Fisher syndrome (*see* Neuropathy, peripheral, immune-mediated)
Mitochondria, and COS-SDH mosaicism, 591, 603
Mitochondrial diseases, 528–542
  acquired mitochondrial dysfunction, 541
  and aging, 541
  classification, 529–530
  defects in nuclear DNA, 541
  histologic features, 530–531
  oxidative phosphorylation (OXPHOS), 529
Mitochondrial DNA (mtDNA), 528–531, 538–541
Mitochondrial encephalopathy, lactic acidosis and stroke-like episodes (MELAS), 81, 531–534
Mitochondrial neurogastrointestinal encephalomyopathy (MNGIE), 540
Mitochondrial proliferation (*see also* Ragged-red fibers)
  in Menkes kinky hair disease, 559
Mitochondrial trifunctional protein, 586
Mixed connective tissue disease (MCTD), 572, 604
Moebius syndrome, 442
Molecular diagnostics, in infectious diseases, 182–183, 201
Monoclonal gammopathy of unknown significance (MGUS), 635, 641
Mononeuritis multiplex, 626
Motor neuron disease (MND)/amyotrophic lateral sclerosis (ALS), 619–622
  clinicopathologic features, 493, 495–497
  molecular pathogenesis and genetics, 497–498
    superoxide dismutase mutations and, 498
Morquio B disease, 521
Moyamoya disease, 67, 72
Mosaicism, interfiber, in mitochondrial disease, 534
Mucopolysaccharidoses, 521, 523–524
Multicystic encephalopathy, 443
Multifocal motor neuropathy (*see* Neuropathy, peripheral, immune-mediated)
Multinucleated giant cells, associated with HIV-1 infection of CNS, AIDS encephalopathy/subacute encephalitis of AIDS, 212–213
Multiple sclerosis, 262–270
  clinical features, 264–265

[Multiple sclerosis]
and pregnancy, 265
diagnosis, clinical
evoked potentials, 265
neuroimaging modalities, 265
oligoclonal bands, in CSF, 265
epidemiology, 262–263
etiology
immunopathogenesis, 263–264
viral infection, 263
HTLV-1, HHV-6 as candidates, 263
pathologic features, 265–272, 274–278
in relation to other white matter diseases, 288
variants
acute, Marburg type, 268, 279
Balo's concentric sclerosis, 270
Charcot type, 268
diffuse sclerosis (Schilder's disease), 270
neuromyelitis optica (Devic's disease), 269–270, 280
Multiple sclerosis-like syndrome, in LHON, 536
Multiples system atrophy (MSA), 498–501
clinicopathologic features, 499
molecular pathogenesis, 500–501
tinucleotide repeats and, 501
olivopontocerebellar atrophy/degeneration (OPCA), 499–501
spinocerebellar degenerations, 498
Muscle biopsy, 570
interpretation of, 570–594
epimysium, 571
fiber size variation, 576–577
inflammation, 571–576
nuclei, 577–579
sarcoplasm, 579–583
special stains, 583–593
Muscle, inflammation, 571–576
eosinophilic, 576
granulomatous in sarcoidosis, 576
Muscle, skeletal
in glycogenoses, 525–528
histochemistry, 583–593
adenosine triphosphatase (ATPase), 588–589
cytochrome oxidase-succinic dehydrogenase (COX–SDH), 591
Gomori trichrome, 584–585
immunohistochemistry, 593–594
myophosphorylase, 586
nicotinamide adenine dinucleotide dehydrogenase (NADH), 590
oil red O, 586–588
periodic acid-Schiff (PAS), 585–586
ragged-red fibers, 531, 540
Muscle fiber
grouping, 589, 590
size variation, 576–577
splitting, 576
type, 588–589
Muscular dystrophy (*see* Dystrophy, muscular)
Myasthenia (myasthenia gravis)
acetylcholine receptors in, 623
autoimmune, 623
congenital, 624
drug-induced, 624
myasthenic syndrome, familial limb girdle, 611
neuromuscular junction in, 622
thymic hyperplasia in, 623
thymoma in, 623
Mycobacterium avium intracellulare (MAI), 229, 243
in skeletal muscle, 576
Myelin-associated glycoprotein (MAG), 641
Myelin
in development, 395
involvement in various diseases, 538, 556–558
Myelinolysis, central pontine (CPM), 272–273, 275, 278, 280–283, 560–562

Myelopathy
  HTLV-1-associated (HAM), 238
  paraneoplastic necrotizing, 505
Myeloschisis (*see also* Neural tube, defects of, 399
Myoclonic epilepsy with ragged-red fibers (MERRF), 534
Myoglobin, 614
Myoglobinemia, 614
Myoglobinuria, 614
  in ethanol abuse, 563
  in fatty acid defects, 544
  in glycogen storage diseases, 525
  in McArdle disease, 527
Myopathy
  centronuclear, 609
  congenital "structural," 606–611
  core diseases, 607–608
  critical care, 617
  cytoplasmic body, 593
  desmin, 610
  desmin-associated, 607
  distal, 595, 601
  drug-induced, 616
  fiber type disproportion, 610
  in glycogenoses, 525–528
  hypokalemic, 563
  with inclusions, 593, 610–611
  inflammatory, 602–606
  mitochondrial, 611–614
  myosin deficient, 617
  myotubular, 609
  nemaline rod, 608–609
  oculopharyngeal, 595
  spheroid body, 593, 607
  steroid, 616
  toxic, 614–618
  vacuolar, 527
  Myophosphorylase, 586, 590
Myophosphorylase deficiency (McArdle disease), GSD V, 527
Myosin, 593
Myositis (*see also* Myopathy, inflammatory)
  inclusion body, 572, 602–603
Myotonia, 600
[Myotonia]
  congenita, 600
  myotonic muscular dystrophy, 600–601
Myotonin protein kinase (MtPK), 597, 601

N-acetylaspartic acid (NAA), 556
N-acetylgalactosamine, 521
N-acetyl glutamate deficiency, 548
N-acylsphingosine, 513
N-methyl-D-aspartate (NMDA), 565
Neck, injury
  hyperextension, 165, 167
  hyperflexion, 165, 167
Necrosis
  of cerebral cortex in mitochondrial disease, 531
  of muscle fibers, 572, 579, 604, 614
  of muscle in McArdle disease, 527
  neuronal, 51
  in ornithine transcarbamylase (OTC) deficiency, 548
  of striatum in glutaric acidemia, 546
Necrotizing leukoencephalopathy, multifocal (MNL), 280–281, 283, 284
Negri body, 206
Nemaline rods, 585
  and myopathy, 608–609
Neonatal adrenoleukodystrophy (NALD), 510
Neoplasms, 295–390
  adult, 297, 300–301
  incidence, 295
  metastatic, 299, 376–384
    carcinoma, 300, 377–383
    melanoma, 384
  pediatric, 297, 300–301
Nerve, biopsy
  fiber density, 628
  immunofluorescence, 628
  interpretation, 631
  teased fiber preparation, 628
  technique, 626
Nerve conduction, 625

Neural folds, 1–2
Neural groove, 1–2
Neural plate, 1–2
Neural tube
  defects of, 395–399
  formation of, 1–2, 392–393
Neurilemoma (schwannoma), 299, 301, 370–371, 372
  acoustic neuroma, 354, 371
Neuroaxonal spheroids, 14
Neuroblastoma (*see* Primitive neuroectodermal tumors (PNET))
Neurocytoma, central, 299, 334–335
Neurodegenerative diseases
  classification of, incidence and genetics, 455
  clinicopathologic features, 454
  etiologic considerations, 453
  research approaches, 453
Neurofibrillary tangles, 17
Neurofibroma, 299, 301, 370, 371–372, 373
  neurofibromatosis type 1, 314, 372
  neurofibromatosis type 2, 354, 372
Neurofibromatosis, perineurial thickening in, 631
Neurofilaments, in motor neuron disease, 621
Neuroleptic malignant syndrome, and muscle fiber necrosis, 615
Neuromelanin, 15
Neuromuscular junction, 622
Neuronal apoptosis inhibitory protein (NAIP) gene, 619
Neuronal heterotopia, 411–412, 418
  cerebellar, 418
  laminar heterotopia, of cerebral hemisphere, 411–412
  subcortical band heterotopia of cerebral hemispheres, 411–412
Neuronal migration, in brain development, 393
Neuronal migration disorders, 404–413
  in fetal alcohol syndrome, 564
  in Zellweger's syndrome, 511
Neuronal proliferation, in brain development, 393
Neurons
  anoxic-ischemic (eosinophilic) change in, 5–6
  Golgi type I, II, 5
  microscopic anatomy of, 4–5
  origins of, 3
  pathologic inclusions of, 16–17
  responses to injury, 5–51, 31
  selective vulnerability in, 7, 34
Neuropathy, ataxia, and retinitis pigmentosa (NARP), 537
Neuropathy, peripheral, 625–642
  amyloid, 634–635, 637
  biopsy, 628
  demyelination, 628–629
  hereditary motor-sensory, 637–639
  immune-mediated, 637, 640–641
  and LHON, 536
  in metachromatic leukodystrophy, 518–520
  in mitochondrial disease, 540–541
  in peroxisomal disorders, 510
  tomaculous, 633
  in Wolfram syndrome, 540
Neurosyphilis, 174, 186–187, 234
Nicotinamide adenine dinucleotide, 543
Nicotinamide adenine dehydrogenase (NADH), 590
Niemann-Pick disease, 517
Nissl substance, 4
Nodes of Ranvier, 48 (*see also* Peripheral nerves)
Nodules of Nageotte, 43
Nonaccidental brain injury in childhood (NAI), 164–165
Nonperfused ("respirator") brain, 53, 57
Notochord, 1–2

Occipital cortex
  in Alpers-Huttenlocher syndrome, 559–560
  in mitochondrial disease, 534
Oligodendroglioma, 299, 300

[Oligodendroglioma]
anaplastic, 299, 326, 327
clinical, 324
gross, 324
histopathology, 324–326
Oligodendrocytes
inclusions of, 25–26
microscopic anatomy of, 25
origins of, 3
responses to injury, 25, 31
Olivary nucleus, inferior
in Leigh disease, 538
in MERRF, 535
Onion bulb formation, in peripheral nerve, 632
Ophthalmoplegia, chronic progressive external (CPEO), 538–540, 611
Opsoclonus-myoclonus, paraneoplastic, 504
Optic atrophy
in LHON, 535–537
in peroxisomal disorders, 510
in Wolfram syndrome, 540
Organic acidemias (OAs), 545–546
Ornithine, 546
Ornithine transcarbamylase (OTC) deficiency, 548
beta-Oxidation, 543
Oxidative phosphorylation (OXPHOS), 529, 542

Pachygyria, 409
in glutaric aciduria, type II, 550
in Zellweger's syndrome, 511
Paired helical filaments (PHF), in inclusion body myositis, 603
Pancytopenia, 540
Papovavirus, in PML, 219
Paramyotonia congenita, 600
Paraneoplastic disorders/degenerations of the CNS, 503–505
sensory neuronopathy, 641
Parkinsonism, post-encephalitic, 486
Parkinson's disease, 485–489
clinicopathologic features, 485–488
[Parkinson's disease]
and mitochondrial dysfunction, 541
molecular pathogenesis of, 488
Pearson marrow-pancreas syndrome (PMPS), 540
Perhexiline maleate, 616
Perineuritis, 631
Peripheral myelin protein (PM-22), 638–639
Peripheral nerves, 43–49
disease of, 625–646
microscopic anatomy of, 43–48
regeneration in, 48–49
responses to injury of, 48–49
Peripheral neuropathy (*see* Neuropathy, peripheral)
Periventricular leukomalacia 439–440 (*see also* Acquired lesions in developing brain)
Peroxisomes, 509–510
disorders of, 509–513
Persistent vegetative state (PVS), 52, 53, 60
Phenylalanine hydroxylase (PAH), 551
Phenylketonuria (PKU), 551
Phosphocholine, 513
Phosphofructokinase deficiency (Tarui disease), GSD VII, 528
Phytanic acid, 509
Pick (Pick's) disease, 7 (*see also* Dementias, non-Alzheimer)
Pick bodies, 18
Pigmentary retinopathy, 537
Pineal gland, 353–354 (*see also* Germ cell tumors)
pineoblastoma, 347
pineocytoma, 299, 354
Pituitary gland (*see also* Craniopharyngioma)
adenoma, 299, 300, 348–351
clinical, 348, 350
differential diagnosis, 350–351
gross appearances, 348
histopathology, 348–350
invasive, 351
carcinoma, 351

Plasma cell dyscrasia, 626
Plasmalogen, 510
Polyarteritis (periarteritis) nodosa, 75, 572
Polymerase chain reaction (PCR), 183, 201
Polymyositis (PM), 572, 593, 604–605
Polymicrogyria
  cerebellar cortical, 417–418
  cerebral cortical, 409–410
Pons
  in Leigh disease, 537
  in MERRF, 535
Pontomedullary transection, 165
Pontosubicular necrosis, 441
Porencephaly, 444
Presenilins, 473
Primitive neuroectodermal tumors (PNET), 341–343
  definition, 341–342
  ependymoblastomas, 346–347
  medulloblastoma, 299, 301, 342, 344–346
    clinical features, 342
    desmoplastic, 344, 346
    gross features, 344
    histopathology, 344–346
    medullomyoblastoma, 345
    pigmented papillary, 345
  medulloepithelioma, 346
  neuroblastoma, 299
    central, 345–346
    ganglioneuroblastoma, 334, 346
    olfactory, 347–348
  pineoblastoma, 347
  polar spongioblastoma, 347
  undifferentiated, 342
Procainamide, 624
Programmed cell death (PCD) (*see also* Apoptosis)
  in development, 394
Progressive multifocal leukoencephalopathy (PML), 25
  in AIDS, 218–219, 227–229, 230–231, 286
[Progressive multifocal leukoencephalopathy (PML)]
  in relation to other white matter diseases, 288
  ultrastructural features, 230
Progressive neuronal degeneration of childhood with liver disease (Alpers-Huttenlocher syndrome), 545–546
Progressive supranuclear palsy (PSP); Steele-Richardson-Olszewski syndrome, 491–493, 494
Propionic acidemia (PA), 545–546
Propionyl-coA carboxylase, 545
Purkinje cells
  in ethanol abuse, 563
  in galactosemia, 551–552
  in Leigh disease, 537–538, 560
  in Menkes kinky hair disease, 559
Putamen
  in hepatic encephalopathy, 565
  in Wilson's disease, 559
Pyruvate dehydrogenase complex (PDHC), in Wernicke-Korsakoff syndrome, 560

Quinidine, 624

Rabies virus infection, 173, 203–206
Ragged-red fibers, 530, 540, 584
  in aging, 541, 584
  in AZT (zidovudine) myopathy, 542
  in inclusion body myositis (IBM), 572, 603
  in mitochondrial myopathy, 611
Ramsay-Hunt syndrome, 535
Rectal mucosa, in ceroid lipfuscinoses, 552
Reducing body, 607, 611
Refsum's disease, infantile, 510
Regeneration, axonal, in diffuse axonal injury, 160
Renaut bodies, 46 (*see also* Peripheral nerves)

Repetitive, non-coma-producing head injury, 163
Repiratory insufficiency, in Leigh disease, 537
Respirator brain (*see* Nonperfused brain (NPB)
Retinitis pigmentosa, in NARP, 537
Retrograde degeneration of axons (*see also* Neurons, 7, 10, 14)
Reye's syndrome (RS), 544–545
  in fatty acid defects, 543
Rhabdomyolysis
  in ethanol abuse, 563
  myofiber necrosis in, 579
Rhizomelic chondrodysplasia punctata, 511
Rimmed vacuoles, 572, 581–593, 601–603
tRNA synthetase, 605
Rosenthal fibers, 307, 308, 309, 336, 353
  in Alexander disease, 557–558
Ryanodine receptor gene, 608

Sagittal sinus, thrombosis, 552
Sandhoff disease, 521
Sanfilippo disease, 523
SAP-1, 519
Sarcoglycans, 599
Sarcoidosis, 174
Sarcolemmal proteins, 593
Sarcoma, 299
  meningeal, 362, 365, 366
  neurogenic, 372
  osteogenic, 374–375
Sarcoplasmic vacuoles, 581–583, 615, 618
Sarcoplasmic reticulum, 601, 611
Satellitosis, 305
Scalp, avulsion injury, 151
Scherer, secondary structures of, 305
Schmidt-Lanterman incisures (*see also* Peripheral nerves, 46–47)
Schwann cells
  onion bulbs, 632
  response to injury, 632–633
Schwannoma (*see* Neurilemoma)
  spinal, post-traumatic, 169
Schwannosis, 169
Selective vulnerability, neuronal, 55, 57, 61
  in Parkinson's disease, 488
Senile dementia, Alzheimer-type (*see* Alzheimer's disease)
Septum pellucidum
  agenesis of, 401
  cavum, 401–402
Short-chain acyl CoA dehydrogenase deficiency (SCAD), 543
Shy-Drager syndrome, 488
Siderocalcinosis, vascular, 82, 84
Signal recognition particle (SRP), 605
Skin biopsy
  in fasciitis, 572
  in peripheral neuropathy, 625
Skull, fractures, 151–153
Spasm, arterial, 163, 168
Sphingolipidoses, 513–520
  Fabry disease, 520
  Gaucher disease, 517
  Krabbe disease, 518
  metachromatic leukodystrophy, 518–520
  Niemann-Pick disease, 517
Sphingolipids, 517 (*see also* Sphingolipidoses)
Sphingomyelin, 517
Sphingomyelinase, 517
Spina bifida (*see also* Neural tube, defects of, 397–399
Spinal cord
  malformations (*see also* Neural tube, defects of, 395–399, 423–427
    diastematomyelia, 425–426
    dimyelia, 425–426
    diplomyelia, 425–426
    hydromyelia, 424
    neural tube defects, 395–399
    syringomyelia, 424–427
  trauma, 165–169
  tumors of, 368–373
Spinal motor neuron (SMN) gene, 618

Spinal muscular atrophy (SMA), 576, 618–619
Spongioblastoma (*see* Astrocytomas, pilocytic)
Spongy change, in various disorders, 538, 548, 550, 551, 556, 559
Status epilepticus
  in Alpers-Huttenlocher syndrome, 559–560
  and myofiber necrosis, 615
"Status marmoratus," 441
Striatonigral degeneration, 501–503
Stroke (*see also* Cerebrovascular disease)
  clinical features, 73
  epidemiology, 61
  ischemic, 51
  in mitochondrial disease, 531
  in ornithine transcarbamylase (OTC) deficiency, 548
Strychnine, 616
Sturge-Weber-Dimitri syndrome, 431–432
Subacute sclerosing panencephalitis (SSPE), 242, 245
Subarachnoid hemorrhage, traumatic, 152–153, 165
  in arterial dissection, 165
  in NAI, 165
Subdural hematoma/hemorrhage, 154–156
Subependymoma (*see* Ependymoma)
Substantia nigra
  in Leigh disease, 537
  in MERRF, 535
  neuromelanin in, 15
Subventricular zone, in development, 393
Succinic dehydrogenase (SDH), 530, 584
Sudden death, in fatty acid defects, 543
Sudden infant death syndrome (SIDS), 450
Sulfatidase, 517
Sulfatide, 641
Superoxide dismutase (SOD), 621
Survival motor neuron (SMN) gene, 619
Syntrophin, 595
Syringomyelia (syrinx), 424–427
  post-traumatic, 168
Systemic lupus erythematosus (SLE), 81, 82, 572

Tay-Sachs disease, 8, 521
Teased fibers, in peripheral nerve biopsy, 628
Telangiectasia/telangiectases, capillary, 130, 138, 537
Tetrahydrobiopterin, 551
Thalamus
  in MERRF, 535
  in Wernicke-Korsakoff syndrome, 560
Thiamine, 560
Threonine, 545
Thrombosis
  arterial, 70
  and homocystinuria, 552
  venous, 70, 90–92
Thrombotic thrombocytopenic purpura (TTP), 82, 84
Thymic hyperplasia, 623
Thymoma, 623
Tobacco, and LHON, 536
Tomaculous neuropathy, 633, 639
Toxic shock syndrome, 616
Toxoplasmosis, 251
  in AIDS, 223, 226
  congenital, 447
  neuropathologic features, 231–234
Transgenic mice, in motor neuron disease research, 622
Transsynaptic degeneration, 8
Transthyretin, 634
Trauma, spinal, 165–169
Trichorrhexis nodosa, 549
Trinucleotide (triplet) repeats, 491, 500–501
  in myotonic dystrophy, 577, 601
Trisomy 13, 428–429
Trisomy 18, 428

Trisomy 21 (Down's syndrome), 427–428
Tropomyosin, 608
Trypanosomiasis, 251
Tryptophan, 546, 617
Tuberculosis (*Mycobacterium tuberculosis infection*), 181, 184, 234
Tuberous sclerosis complex, 429–430
Tubular aggregates, 585, 611
Tubulo-filamentous structures, 572
Tubulomembranous body, 607
Tumors (*see* Neoplasms)
Tyrosinase, 559
Tyrosine, 551

Ubiquitin, in inclusion body myositis, 603
Ulegyria, 56, 443
Urea cycle, defects (UCDs), 546–549
Uronic acid, 523
Uronidase, 523

Vacuoles, sarcoplasmic, 591
Vacuolar myelopathy of AIDS, 208–209
  similarity to subacute combined degeneration of spinal cord, 208
Vacuolation, of neuropil
  in Canavan's disease, 556
  in organic acidemia, 546
Valine, 545, 549, 551
Valproic acid, and Reye's syndrome, 544
Varicella zoster, CNS infection, 201
  opportunistic, in AIDS, 226
  "ventriculitis," 226
Vascular dilatation, in Menkes kinky hair disease, 559
Vascular injury, 153
Vascular malformations, of brain, 128
Vascular territories, 162
Vasculitis, 571, 606, 626, 631 (*see also* Angiitis; Arteritis)
  primary CNS, 71
[Vasculitis]
  systemic, CNS effects, 75
Vegetative state, persistent, after head injury, 160
Veins, bridging, 156
Ventricular zone, in development, 393
Ventriculitis, 178
Very long chain acyl-coA dehydrogenase, 586
Vertebral artery, dissection of, 165
Very long chain fatty acids, 510–513
Visual loss
  in Canavan's disease, 556
  in LHON, 535–537
Vitamin B12, in methylmalonic acidemia, 546

Walker-Warburg syndrome, 408 (*see also* Lissencephaly)
Wallerian degeneration of axons, 10, 630
  in diffuse axonal injury, 160
Watershed territories, arterial, 162
Wegener's granulomatosis, 75, 79
Wernicke's encephalopathy, comparison to Leigh disease, 537
White matter
  adrenoleukodystrophy, 512
  in Canavan's disease, 556
  contusional tears of, in NAI, 165
  rotational injury, 160
  vacuolation in Kearns-Sayre syndrome (CPEO), 540
Wilson's disease, 558–559
Wolfram syndrome, 540

X-chromosome, 595

Z-discs, 585, 605
Zebra body, 524
Zellweger's syndrome, 510
Zidovudine (AZT), 542
  and myopathy, 617